Management of Kidney Diseases

Your bonus with the purchase of this book

With the purchase of this book, you can use our "SN Flashcards" app to access questions free of charge in order to test your learning and check your understanding of the contents of the book. To use the app, please follow the instructions below:

1. Go to **https://flashcards.springernature.com/login**
2. Create an user account by entering your e-mail adress and assiging a password.
3. Use the link provided in one of the first chapters to access your SN Flashcards set.

MOREMEDIA

Your personal SN Flashcards link is provided in one of the first chapters.

If the link is missing or does not work, please send an e-mail with the subject "**SN Flashcards**" and the book title to **customerservice@springernature.com**.

Debasish Banerjee • Vivekanand Jha
Nicholas M. P. Annear
Editors

Management of Kidney Diseases

Springer

Editors
Debasish Banerjee
St George's University Hospitals NHS
Foundation Trust and St George's,
University of London
London, UK

Vivekanand Jha
The George Institute for Global Health
New Delhi, India

Nicholas M. P. Annear
St George's University Hospitals NHS
Foundation Trust and St George's,
University of London
London, UK

ISBN 978-3-031-09133-9 ISBN 978-3-031-09131-5 (eBook)
https://doi.org/10.1007/978-3-031-09131-5

This Springer imprint is published by the registered company Springer Nature Switzerland AG
The registered company address is: Gewerbestrasse 11, 6330 Cham, Switzerland

Foreword

There was a time, not that long ago, when nephrology was a speciality only practiced in a few high-income countries. There was a time when available nephrology experts were so few, and the cost of kidney replacement therapy so high, that it seemed nephrology would never expand beyond those countries. And there was little available evidence to guide the work of nephrologists, so the world hung on the expert advice of those few from high-income countries.

Happily those times are gone. Nephrology is now a worldwide speciality, recognising its unique clinical challenges in different parts of the world. True experts and authoritative teachers in nephrology come from almost every part of the world. There is a growing library of high-quality evidence to support the clinical work of nephrologists everywhere.

This book reflects those changes. It covers the whole gamut of nephrology in all parts of the world. Its editors and contributors come from many different heritages and practice in many different places.

The book presents all aspects of modern nephrology, with a clear focus on practical clinical management. And it is especially welcome that coverage includes topics which in recent years are gaining in importance as their contribution to the best nephrology care is being better understood. One such theme is transitional care for adolescents and young adults. Another is a more informed and balanced approach to the value of conservative care in the management of advanced kidney failure. Another is the increasing role of renal registries informing practice, assisting service planning, and providing a substrate for audit, research and clinical quality improvement.

The book provides the reader with a most approachable and clear knowledge base—case-based discussions and concise text; multi-coloured diagrams, flow charts, and tables which are easily assimilated; key practice points; the inclusion of current high-quality evidence; questions at the end of each chapter to help readers test their assimilation of knowledge.

The three lead editors and their many and diverse contributors have produced a first-rate text that will be much read and well used around the world. It will certainly be popular with specialist trainees equipping themselves for future practice and preparing for the examinations required of most before their training is completed. And it is a most handy reference for practice and teaching which will also be used by established specialist nephrologists.

Oakham, UK
October 2022

John Feehally

Preface

Worldwide, practicing nephrologists often need rapid and easily accessible information on evidence-based management for kidney patients, both in hospital and outpatient clinic settings. Kidney disease is a growing public health burden: patients with kidney disease have multiple associated health conditions and need care from a diverse group of healthcare professionals. The need for practical, evidence-based treatment recommendations for patients with kidney disease in all healthcare settings, that is mindful of available resources, has never been more evident than during the COVID-19 pandemic.

This book brings together the expertise of kidney health specialists from all over the world to provide practical management guidance for all regions, with variable healthcare resources and accessibility. The practice points integrated into each chapter are useful short practical reminders in the steps of management. Appropriate references, including recent guidelines, have been cited. The authors have incorporated recent KDIGO and other national guidelines, where available and appropriate. We are enormously grateful to KDIGO for endorsing the use of all available KDIGO guidelines and conference updates in the book.

The case-based approach is oriented towards illustrating the clinical picture, explaining the current understanding of the pathophysiology and management, which we hope will help outline the 'why' and 'how' aspects of routine patient care.

Updating knowledge in all aspects of kidney care can be daunting, not only for practicing nephrologists but also for trainees before examinations. The case-based, management focused, up-to-date approach to illustrating all kidney conditions, including kidney replacement therapies, will also aid contextualisation and revision for end-of-training examinations.

Another unique feature of this book is Springer's interactive flashcards, with 270 practice questions, authored by our international experts, which will help trainees—and fully trained nephrologists—consolidate their knowledge, monitor progress and learn from the available explanations.

We wish to thank all of our expert international authors for their fantastic work in putting together each chapter; to our publishing team, in particular Melissa Morton and Mahalakshmi Sathish Babu, for their tireless support throughout the development of this book; to our colleagues and trainees for continuing to inspire and motivate us; and of course most of all to our families for sacrificing the time, space and support to complete this important project.

London, UK Debasish Banerjee
London, UK Nicholas M. P. Annear
New Delhi, India Vivekanand Jha
July 2022

Contents

1 The Approach to the Patient with Kidney Disease

Debasish Banerjee, Nicholas M. P. Annear, and Vivekanand Jha

Clinical Scenario

A 40 year old female international traveller presents with a history of fever, dysuria and a serum creatinine of 208 μmol/L (2.35 mg/dL). She is assessed as confused in the emergency department, but has been found to be haemodynamically stable, with a temperature of 37 °C (98.6 °F), a blood pressure of 130/75 mmHg, and pulse of 70 beats per minute. She has indicated that she is due to fly back home in 2 days' time.

How would you proceed?

Introduction

Kidney disease is increasing in incidence worldwide, with increasing numbers of patients on kidney replacement therapy; more kidney patients are looked after by internists, general practitioners and other specialties than by nephrologists. Furthermore, kidney disease is now the 12th leading cause of death worldwide, and a staggering 14.5 million people are estimated to require kidney replacement therapy by 2030 [1, 2]. The initial approach to diagnosis of kidney disease, and management of patients on kidney replacement therapy requires a careful history, physical exam and initial laboratory tests, which are emphasised in this chapter.

D. Banerjee (✉) · N. M. P. Annear
St George's University of London, London, UK

St George's University Hospitals Foundation Trust, London, UK
e-mail: dbanerje@sgul.ac.uk; nannear@sgul.ac.uk

V. Jha
The George Institute for Global Health, New Delhi, India
e-mail: vjha@georgeinstitute.org.in

Common Kidney Patient Presentations

Kidney patients present may with symptoms, signs and abnormal investigations, with a hitherto unknown kidney disease. Careful history taking and a full physical examination can help the clinician to arrive at a provisional diagnosis for the kidney condition - these include common kidney syndromes, such as nephrotic syndrome, nephritic syndrome, chronic kidney disease and acute kidney injury (Fig. 1.1). A tailored investigation with urinalysis, blood tests and imaging can help to identify the cause of kidney disease, and formulate a management plan.

Patients with known kidney disease, on kidney replacement therapy may also present with complications of chronic kidney disease, or complications of their modality of kidney replacement therapy. For example, haemodialysis patients may present to the emergency department with shortness of breath—particularly following a prolonged interdialytic period, such as

D. Banerjee et al. (eds.), *Management of Kidney Diseases*,
https://doi.org/10.1007/978-3-031-09131-5_1

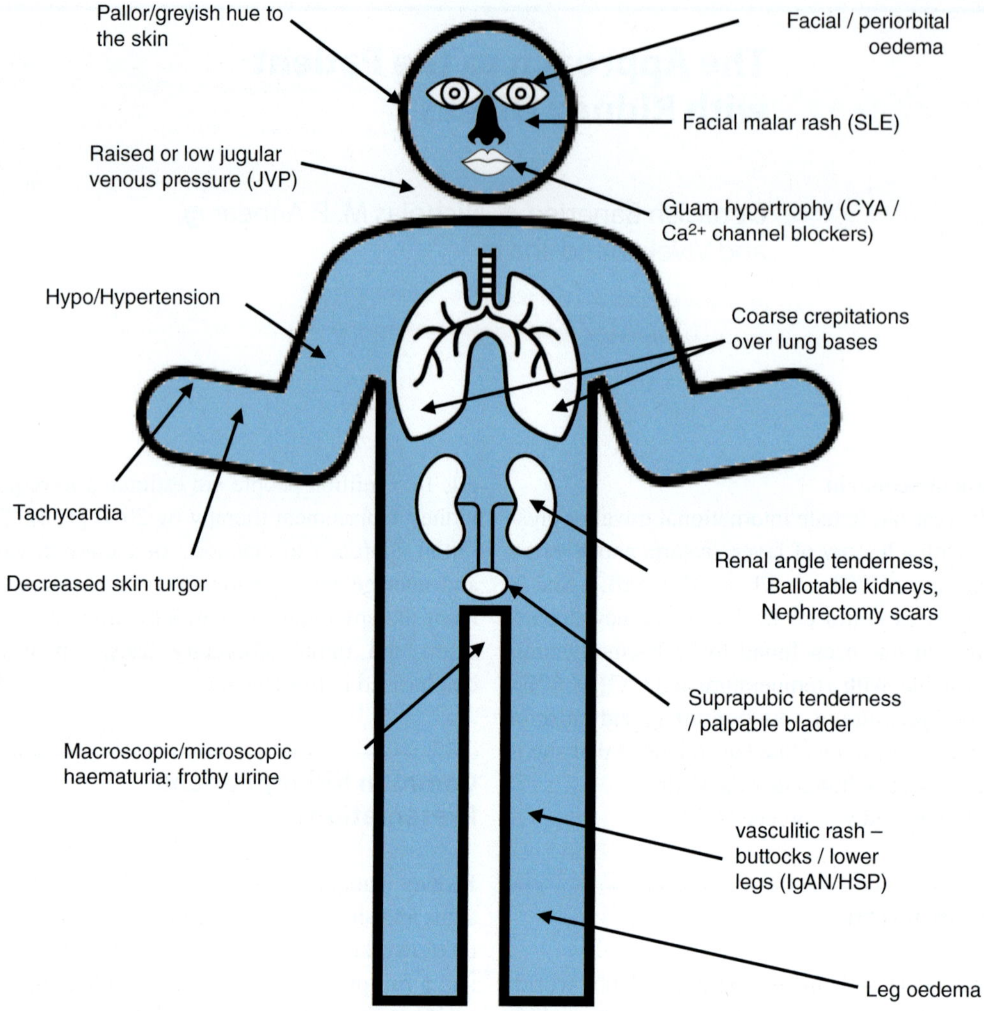

Also inspect groins, neck, precordium, and abdomen for scars/evidence suggestive of current or previous kidney replacement therapy (haemodialysis (arteriovenous fistula/dialysis catheter) /peritoneal dialysis (tenchkoff catheter) access and/or transplantation (J-shaped/Rutherford-Morrison scar)).

SLE – systemic lupus erythematosus; CYA – cyclosporin; Ca^{2+} channel blockers – Calcium channel blockers; IgAN – IgA nephropathy; HSP – Henoch Schonlein Purpura

Fig. 1.1 Physical signs that can be associated with kidney disease

after the weekend; peritoneal dialysis patients and kidney transplant patients may present with fever and abdominal pain, both requiring careful history and physical examination to arrive at a likely differential diagnosis, and start immediate treatment if necessary. Kidney replacement therapy is available in all countries; and patients are frequently managed by clinicians other than nephrologists, hence a good working knowledge about how to make a prompt diagnosis, and man-

Table 1.1 The approach to the kidney patient depends on the presence of a past history of kidney replacement therapy

Patients with no known kidney disease	Patients on dialysis, with kidney transplantation
Presents with symptoms or signs such as oedema, oliguria suggestive of kidney disease or urine abnormalities and rising creatinine	Presentation with general signs and symptoms such as breathlessness, fever or chest/abdominal pain in patients on kidney replacement therapy
Requires a careful history and physical examination to formulate a differential diagnosis from common kidney syndromes such as nephrotic syndrome, nephritic syndrome, chronic kidney disease or acute kidney injury	Requires a careful history and physical examination to formulate a differential diagnosis for causes of breathlessness, fever and chest/abdominal pain

age complications is important amongst nephrologists and non-nephrologists alike, in all regions of the world (Table 1.1).

Common Kidney Syndromes and Definitions

Haematuria: Abnormal number of red blood cells (RBCs) in the urine, either visible or detected on urine examination, >3 RBCs/high power field under the microscope.

Nephrotic syndrome: Significant proteinuria (>3 g/day), with oedema, hypoalbuminaemia, hypercholesterolaemia, and a hypercoagulable state.

Nephritic syndrome: Glomerular haematuria with proteinuria, dysmorphic RBCs, red cell casts, often a raised serum creatinine, and hypertension.

Acute kidney injury: A sudden rise in serum creatinine over hours or days (>50% from baseline).

Chronic kidney disease: Gradual, progressive and irreversible rise in serum creatinine over at least 3 months.

Kidney stones: Colicky loin pain, haematuria with graveluria.

Urinary tract obstruction: Inability to pass urine, with structural and functional abnormalities with urinary retention.

Kidney tubule defects: Abnormalities of electrolytes, acid-base in blood and urine.

Urinary tract infections: Infections of kidney, ureter, urinary bladder, prostate or urethra.

Anatomical Localisation of Kidney Diseases

The presenting signs, and symptoms, and presence of blood and urinary abnormalities are dependent on the anatomical structure of the urinary tract involved, as shown in the Table 1.2.

Table 1.2 Clinical features of kidney diseases, as determined by anatomical involvement of the urinary organs

Anatomical structure	Clinical features of presentation
Kidneys	Loin pain, hematuria, frothy urine, renal angle tenderness, oliguria, polyuria, nocturia, raised creatinine, electrolyte abnormalities
Ureters	Loin to groin pain, colicky in nature, haematuria, graveluria
Urinary bladder	Lower abdominal pain, dysuria, hematuria, suprapubic tenderness, leukocyturia
Urethra	Dysuria, hematuria at the initiation of micturition

Aetiology of Kidney Syndromes

Understanding the common causes of kidney syndromes can help to inform the approach to diagnosis and management. Some of the aetiologies may present with acute or chronic kidney diseases, the understanding of which helps with determining the reversibility of the pathological process and urgency of treatment (Table 1.3).

Table 1.3 Common causes of kidney syndromes

Kidney syndrome	Site affected	Causes
Haematuria	Kidney	Inflammation, infection, cancer, stone
	Kidney outflow tract	Stone, cancer, infection, inflammation
Nephrotic syndrome	Kidney limited (or idiopathic)	Minimal change, membranous, focal segmental glomerulosclerosis (FSGS)
	Systemic (or secondary)	Diabetes, mellitus lupus, Amyloidosis, Cancer: Lymphoma, Myeloma, Drugs: Gold, Antibiotics, NSAIDS, Heroin, Penicillamine, Infections: HIV, Hepatitis B, Hepatitis C, Malaria, Syphilis, Alport's syndrome, Nail-Patella syndrome
Nephritic syndrome	Kidney limited (or idiopathic)	IgA nephropathy, kidney limited vasculitis
	Systemic (or secondary)	Lupus, ANCA-associated vasculitis (AAV)
Kidney stones		Calcium oxalate, urate, struvite, cysteine
Urinary tract obstruction	Ureter	Stones, cancer
	Urethra/ bladder outflow	Stones, prostate cancer
Kidney tubular disorder	Acidosis	Renal tubular acidosis
Urinary tract infection (UTI)	Bacterial	*Escherichia coli, Klebsiella pneumoniae*
	Fungal	*Candida albicans*
	Viral	Cytomegalovirus (CMV), BK virus, adenovirus
Acute kidney injury	Pre-renal	Volume depletion, haemorrhage
	Renal	Acute interstitial nephritis (AIN), Acute Glomerulonephritis
	Post-renal	Urethral/bladder outflow obstruction
Chronic kidney disease		Diabetes mellitus, Hypertension, chronic glomerulonephritis, inherited kidney diseases

Approach to a Patient with Kidney Disease

A careful history and physical exam is necessary to identify the kidney syndrome and identify the cause. The duration of illness is important to determine the syndrome: for example, acute kidney injury (AKI) develops in hours to days, and chronic kidney disease (CKD) over months. The presence of fever, skin rash and joint pains indicates systemic disease. Visible haematuria indicates glomerular or renal tract bleeding. The presence of oedema may be associated with nephrotic syndrome, fluid retention or end stage kidney disease (ESKD). The physical is followed by tests of blood and urine (Tables 1.4 and 1.5).

Table 1.4 Approach to common kidney syndromes

Kidney syndrome	History	Physical examination	Investigations
Haematuria	Age of onset (malignancy if>50 years), gender (bladder cancer and prostate cancer is commoner in males, infection in females), associated symptoms: Fever, dysuria, flank pain, family history (Alport's), travel history (schistosomiasis), smoking, anticoagulation, pharyngitis (IgA nephropathy)	Hypertension, oedema, abdominal mass, palpable bladder	Urine microscopy for RBCs, dysmorphic RBCs, RBC casts, urinalysis for blood, leucocytes & nitrites (infection), proteinuria, test for myoglobin. Ultrasound, computerised tomography (CT), cystoscopy
Nephrotic syndrome (and non-nephrotic proteinuria)	Peripheral and facial oedema, frothy urine. History of diabetes mellitus, diabetic retinopathy. Fever, iv drug use, high risk sexual behaviour, malaria, filaria; drugs NSAIDS, gold, penicillamine	Dependent oedema, malar rash, scarring alopecia, telangiectasia, erythema nodosum, jaundice, spider naevi, leukonychia, yellow nails, dystrophic nails	Urine protein, albumin, cells, casts, lipids, urinary bence jones protein (BJP). Serum creatinine, liver function, full blood count. ANA, ANCA, anti-GBM, complement* (Table 1.5), ASOT, cryoglobulins, hepatitis B, C & HIV serology, ultrasound, kidney biopsy
Nephritic syndrome	Dark brown, tea-coloured or smoky urine, sore throat (IgA nephropathy) respiratory, skin infections (post-streptococcal), family history (Alport's syndrome), fever, skin rash, joint pain (lupus nephritis), haemoptysis (vasculitis)	Hypertension, oedema, hearing impairment (Alport's syndrome), skin lesion (Lupus, henoch-schonlein purpura (HSP), vasculitis, Fabry's disease)	Urine microscopy: dysmorphic RBC, casts, proteinuria >0.5 g/day, full blood count, serum creatinine, liver profile, ANA, ANCA, anti-GBM, complement*, ASOT, cryoglobulins, hepatitis B, C & HIV serology, ultrasound, kidney biopsy
Kidney stones	Haematuria, loin to groin pain, nausea, vomiting. High oxalate, high protein, high salt diet. Drugs triamterene, sulphonamides, indinavir. Hyperparathyroidism, sarcoidosis, bile salt depletion, short gut. Reduced fluid, excessive sweat	Fever, costo-vertebral 'renal angle' tenderness	Full blood count, serum calcium, phosphate, urate, pH Urinary RBC, WBC, pH, crystals. 24 h urine calcium, urate, citrate, oxalate, sodium Non-contrast helical CT of the kidneys, ureters and bladder (KUB), renal tract ultrasound
Urinary tract obstruction	Flank pain, suprapubic pain, suprapubic fullness. Urine frequency and urgency (partial obstruction). Anuria (urethral). Haematuria (stones, cancer) suprapubic fullness, frequency nocturia	Enlarged urinary bladder, enlarged prostate, uterine prolapse	Urine RBC, WBC, raised serum creatinine, hyperkalaemia, acidosis, renal tract ultrasound and CT scan

(continued)

Table 1.4 (continued)

Kidney syndrome	History	Physical examination	Investigations
Kidney tubular disorder	Renal stones, short stature, family history		Blood pH, electrolytes, urine electrolytes, pH
Urinary tract infection (UTI)	Urinary frequency and urgency, dysuria, cloudy urine, smelly urine, fever, flank pain	Suprapubic tenderness, flank pain/renal angle tenderness, signs of sepsis (fever, tachycardia, hypotension)	Urinalysis for blood, leucocytes & nitrites (infection), MSU culture to isolate causative organisms, FBC, blood urea, serum creatinine, electrolytes, CRP and blood culture if immune suppressed or signs of systemic sepsis. Ultrasound ± CT scan if obstruction or stones suspected, recurrent, or failure to resolve with first line therapy
Acute kidney injury	History of salt and water loss, drug history, fever, history of CKD, rash, hair loss, joint pain	Blood pressure & pulse, postural drop on assessing lying/standing blood pressure, dry mucus membranes, rash, alopecia, jaundice, ulcers, palpable bladder	Blood urea, serum creatinine, electrolytes. Urinary sodium, creatinine, osmolality, blood, protein, microscopy, RBC, casts, eosinophil Ultrasound of the renal tract, kidney biopsy
Chronic kidney disease	History of hypertension, diabetes, AKI, lupus, hepatitis, scleroderma, vasculitis, familial CKD. Polyuria, nocturia, haematuria, proteinuria. Anorexia, nausea vomiting	Blood pressure, pulse lying/standing, oedema, wasting, retinal exam, palpable kidney, urinary bladder	Full blood count, serum creatinine, electrolytes, calcium, phosphate, liver function, lipids. Urine protein, ultrasound of the renal tract

Table 1.5 Conditions causing abnormalities in complement levels

Complement levels	Condition
Low C3, Low C4	Lupus nephritis Cryoglobulinaemia Infective endocarditis Shunt nephritis Type 1 mesangio-proliferative glomerulonephritis (MPGN)
Low C3, Normal C4	Type 2 mesangio-proliferative glomerulonephritis (MPGN) Post-infective/post-streptococcal glomerulonephritis

Radiological Abnormalities

Radiological abnormalities of the urinary tract may be picked up incidentally, and should prompt further history taking, physical examination and tests to establish a diagnosis.

Haematuria

Haematuria is defined as an abnormal number of red cells in the urine i.e. more than 3 red blood cells seen under one high power field under the laboratory microscope. Haematuria may originate from the kidneys, or from the urinary tract. Table 1.6 can help with differentiating between the two:

Investigations for haematuria will be guided by the presentation, but may include urine microscopy, urinary protein quantification, ultrasound of the kidneys and urinary tract, and CT and cystoscopy if necessary (Tables 1.7 and 1.8).

Table 1.6 Clinical features of haematuria from kidney compared to that from urinary outflow tract

	Haematuria originating from the kidneys	Haematuria originating from the urinary outflow tract: ureters, urinary bladder & urethra
Age at presentation	Could be at any age	Usually >50 years
Urine colour	Dark red, brown, smoky	Bright red
Urinary clots	No	Yes
Mixed with urine	Yes	May be at beginning or end of micturition
Lower urinary tract symptoms	No	Yes
Proteinuria	Yes	No
Dysmorphic red blood cells (RBCs)	Yes	No
Oedema	Yes	No
Raised serum creatinine	Yes	No
Hypertension	Yes	No
Fever, rash, chest symptoms	Yes	No

Table 1.7 Common causes of haematuria

Category	Cause
Benign	Renal masses (angiomyolipoma (AML), oncocytoma Benign prostatic hypertrophy (BPH) Urethral strictures
Stones	Staghorn calculi Calcium stones Uric acid stones
Infective	Pyelonephritis Cystitis Urethritis
Trauma	Pelvic trauma Renal injuries Foreign bodies
Renal	IgA nephropathy Thin basement membrane disease Hereditary nephritis Medullary sponge kidney
Iatrogenic	Recent endoscopic procedure (e.g. transurethral resection of the prostate (TURP) Transrectal ultrasound (TRUS) guided prostate biopsy Traumatic catheterisation Radiation Indwelling ureteric stents Renal biopsy Extracorporeal shockwave lithotripsy (ECSWL)
Malignant	Renal cell carcinoma Transitional cell carcinoma Squamous cell carcinoma Urothelial cell carcinoma Prostate acinar adenocarcinoma

Table 1.8 Causes of red or brown urine

Endogenous substances	Foods	Drugs
Red blood cells Haemoglobin Myoglobin Bilirubin Porphyrins Melanin	Food colouring Beetroot Blackberries, Blueberries Fava beans Paprika Rhubarb	Rifampicin Adriamycin Chloroquine Deferoxamine Levodopa Methyldopa Metronidazole Nitrofurantoin Phenytoin Prochlorperazine Quinine Sulfonamides

Presentation of Kidney Failure Patients on Kidney Replacement Therapy

Common presenting features for kidney failure patients on kidney replacement therapy include, fever, breathlessness, chest pain, confusion, fatigue, falls and abnormal blood tests such as hyperkalaemia and rising serum creatinine in a kidney transplant patient. Infection and malfunction of dialysis vascular access are very common causes of acute admissions for patients on haemodialysis and peritoneal dialysis, followed by breathlessness due to fluid volume overload. Rapid ultrafiltration on haemodialysis and obligatory ultrafiltration with peritoneal dialysis can alternatively lead to volume depletion, hypotension and falls, particularly in elderly dialysis patients. Fatigue and tiredness due to anaemia and malnutrition are also common complaints in patients on renal replacement therapy.

A rising serum creatinine on routine blood test results is a common reason for hospital attendance in kidney transplant recipients, which could be due to acute transplant rejection, urinary infection, transplant urinary tract obstruction, transplant renal artery stenosis, or most commonly volume depletion (Table 1.9).

Table 1.9 Common causes to consider based on symptoms and blood results in patients on kidney replacement therapy

Common symptoms	Haemodialysis	Peritoneal dialysis	Kidney transplantation
Fever	Dialysis access related infection Infections of chest and urine	PD catheter exit site infection, peritonitis Infections of chest and urine	Urinary tract infection atypical infection of chest and blood stream e.g. CMV, EBV, TB
Breathlessness	Fluid overload Chest infection Anaemia, loss of native renal function	Fluid overload Chest infection Anaemia, loss of native renal function	Fluid overload Chest infection Anaemia
Fatigue	Anaemia Malnutrition	Anaemia Malnutrition	Anaemia
Falls	Hypotension due to excess ultrafiltration on dialysis Drug-induced hypotension Cardiac arrythmias, infection	Hypotension due to excess ultrafiltration on dialysis Drug-induced hypotension Cardiac arrythmias, infection	Volume depletion, infection
Hyperkalaemia	Missed dialysis High potassium diet	High potassium diet, underlying high cell turnover state	Tacrolimus High potassium diet Kidney transplant failure

Conclusions

Returning to the clinical scenario from the beginning of the chapter, the differential diagnosis with the available information is extremely broad, and includes an acute kidney injury, chronic kidney disease, a new presentation with glomerulonephritis, urinary tract infection, or an infective complication of known end stage kidney disease. Further clarification is only really possible through eliciting a careful medical history, and performing a thorough physical examination, which will in turn determine the most appropriate next investigations, and an appropriate, safe plan for management, including whether she is likely to be fit to fly home:

The patient had been assessed as confused because she was having difficulty communicating with staff in the emergency department: thankfully, one of the hospital nursing team was able to speak with her coherently in her native language. She shows the assessing clinician a letter from her nephrology team at home, which on translation, indicates that she has end stage kidney disease due to IgA nephropathy, and was transplanted with a deceased donor (donation after circulatory death (DCD)) kidney 5 years ago, and is chronically immune suppressed with tacrolimus and mycophenolate mofetil. Her most recent serum creatinine level was 200 μmol/L (2.26 mg/dL) 2 months ago, and she has a history of recurrent transplant urinary tract infections, most recently an *Escherichia Coli,* fully sensitive to standard antimicrobial agents.

A full physical examination reveals—in addition to the findings reported previously—a non-functioning right radiocephalic arteriovenous fistula from previous haemodialysis, a right-sided Rutherford-Morrison scar, overlying a non-tender mass. There is mild suprapubic tenderness. There was no peripheral oedema, but she had a mild resting tremor. Neither her white cell count nor CRP were raised; her tacrolimus trough level was 6 ng/mL, and her blood sugar was 5.6 mmol/L; Her urinalysis was positive for leukocytes and nitrites, but was otherwise clear. A transplant renal tract ultrasound revealed no evidence of obstruction, a small post-micturition bladder residual volume of 60 mL, and normal resistive indices (RIs) of 0.68.

A clinical diagnosis of kidney transplant urinary tract infection is made: given the absence of haemodynamic compromise, and a clear history of similar presentations, with a serum creatinine at her baseline, and on agreement with both the local nephrology, and her home nephrology teams, it was deemed appropriate to manage her in an ambulatory manner—avoiding admission—and encouraging oral fluid intake of 2–3 litres of fluid per day, and commencement of a course of oral antibiotics (amoxycillin + clavulanic acid 6750 mg orally tds for a 5 day course), with a view to being re-assessed by her local nephrology team in a week's time, on return to her native country.

Questions

1. A 22 year old black female presented with weakness, tiredness. On examination her pulse was 82/min, blood pressure was 165/80 mmHg and she had a red rash over her face. Urine examination showed blood and protein. Blood test showed low haemoglobin and creatinine was 187 μmol/L.

   What is most likely diagnosis
   A. Henoch Schulein purpura
   B. Systemic amyloidosis
   C. Systemic lupus erythematosus
   D. Essential cyroglobinimia
   E. Systemic vasculitis

Correct answer: young woman with low haemoglobin, haemo-proteinura and rash is most likely to be lupus.

2. A 45 year old black man presented with tiredness and frothy urine. On examination his pulse was 89/min, blood pressure was 130/82 mmHg. He had a white deposit over his tongue and inner side of his cheek. His urine protein:creatinine ratio was 300 mg/mol (Normal < 15). His kidney ultrasound showed bilateral normal size bright echogenic kidneys.

   What is the likely cause of his nephrotic syndrome?
   A. Amyloidosis
   B. Type 2 diabetes
   C. Hypertension
   D. HIV associated nephropathy
   E. Systemic lupus nephritis

3. A 23 year old female with lupus nephritis, end stage kidney failure on haemodialysis presented with fever and lethargy. She denied Joint pain, dysuria, cough, diarrhoea or rash. On examination pulse was 100/min, temperature 38 °C, blood pressure 110/60 mmHg. The exit site of her tunneled catheter was clean. Blood cultures were sent. Her white cell and CRP were raised.

   What is next best plan of management?
   A. Investigations for lupus nephritis.
   B. Investigations for lymphoma
   C. Start antibiotics for catheter related bacteremia
   D. Start oral steroids
   E. Start intravenous cyclophosphamide

Correct answer: C mostly cause of fever is catheter related bacteremia and lupus id less likely.

4. A 55 year old asymptomatic man was admitted to hospital from the transplant clinic with rising creatine 15 days post kidney transplant from 150 to 230 μmol/L. He was on mycophenolate 250 mg bd and tacrolimus 2 mg bd. His tacrolimus level was 5 ng/mL (target 10–15). His pulse was 78/min, blood pressure 130/60 mmHg. His urine had no blood pr protein. Ultrasound of the transplanted kidney was normal.

   What is the likely cause of his AKI
   A. Acute rejection
   B. Acute intestinal nephritis
   C. Tacrolimus toxicity
   D. Thrombotic microangiopathy related to tacrolimus
   E. Urinary tract infection

Test your learning and check your understanding of this book's contents: use the "Springer Nature Flashcards" app to access questions. To use the app, please follow the instructions below:

1. Go to https://flashcards.springernature.com/login.
2. Create a user account by entering your e-mail address and assigning a password.
3. Use the following link to access your SN Flashcards set: https://sn.pub/cz9Cok. If the link is missing or does not work, please send an e-mail with the subject "SN Flashcards" and the book title to customerservice@springernature.com.

References

1. Bikbov B, Purcell CA, Levey AS, Smith M, Abdoli A, Abebe M, et al. Global, regional, and national burden of chronic kidney disease, 1990–2017: a systematic analysis for the global burden of disease study 2017. Lancet. 2020;395(10225):709–33.
2. Liyanage T, Ninomiya T, Jha V, Neal B, Patrice HM, Okpechi I, et al. Worldwide access to treatment for end-stage kidney disease: a systematic review. Lancet. 2015;385(9981):1975–82.

Investigating Kidney Disease

2

Mukunthan Srikantharajah, Rukma Doshi, Debasish Banerjee, Vivekanand Jha, and Nicholas M. P. Annear

Clinical Scenario

A 50 year old male with a history of gout presents to the general nephrology clinic with a serum creatinine of 178 μmol/L (2.01 mg/dL). He is otherwise asymptomatic. His medications include allopurinol 200 mg po od, and ibuprofen 200 mg po prn. There is no significant family history of kidney disease or hypertension. His blood pressure is 170/90 mmHg, his pulse 70 beats per minute, but his physical examination is otherwise unremarkable.

How would you proceed?

M. Srikantharajah
Imperial College Kidney and Transplantation Institute, London, UK
e-mail: m.srikantharajah@nhs.net

R. Doshi
Epsom and St. Helier Hospitals NHS Trust, Epsom, UK
e-mail: r.doshi@nhs.net

D. Banerjee · N. M. P. Annear (✉)
St George's University of London, London, UK

St George's University Hospitals Foundation Trust, London, UK
e-mail: dbanerje@sgul.ac.uk; nannear@sgul.ac.uk

V. Jha
The George Institute for Global Health, New Delhi, India
e-mail: vjha@georgeinstitute.org.in

Introduction

The signs and symptoms of kidney disease are often non-specific, so pertinent further investigations can help either confirm or refute a diagnosis amongst differentials. For the kidney patient, key investigations include blood tests, urinalysis, imaging studies, histopathology and electrocardiography (ECG). DNA analysis may also be helpful in determining the diagnosis where certain clinical presentations are suggestive, or where there is a clear family history of kidney disease: we will discuss this in more detail in a later chapter. It is more often than not the combination of a careful history and physical examination, taken together with the results of key investigations that help clinicians to clinch the diagnosis, and define an appropriate management strategy [1–3].

Throughout the course of this textbook, you will encounter different kidney diseases and the investigative and management approach for each individually. In this chapter, we will look broadly at the investigations commonly used to investigate patients with possible kidney disease.

Blood Tests

Alongside blood pressure and urinalysis, a simple blood biochemical test assessing the serum creatinine stands as perhaps the single most widely used investigation for the practicing

D. Banerjee et al. (eds.), *Management of Kidney Diseases*,
https://doi.org/10.1007/978-3-031-09131-5_2

nephrologist: as a cheap, well-validated and easily available blood test, it is performed on most patients who attend hospital as an inpatient, and is frequently used to screen patients for kidney dysfunction in ambulatory, outpatient and community settings. Understanding the timeframe over which a serum creatinine result has become abnormal can help determine whether a kidney impairment is either acute or chronic; and using other widely available demographic data for the patient, including gender, age, ethnicity, alongside the serum creatinine, an estimate for the glomerular filtration rate (GFR) can be made. Alongside the serum creatinine, various other biochemical, haematological, immunological and virological blood tests that are used to further inform the clinician about the potential cause of kidney disease, and infer the chronicity and complications of kidney disease: we will set about describing them as follows (Tables 2.1, 2.2, and 2.3).

Serum Biochemistry

One of the key functions of the kidney is maintaining electrolyte homeostasis. Thus, measurement of blood urea, creatinine, electrolytes and pH can be used to assess the functions of the kidney in filtering and reabsorbing electrolytes, thus maintaining electrolyte concentrations and blood pH within a 'normal' range.

Table 2.1 Serum biochemistry tests in kidney disease

Test (Abbreviation) *Normal values–SI units (Conventional units)*	Raised levels associated with	Low levels associated with
Sodium (Na^+) *133–146 mmol/L (310–330 mg/dL)*	Fluid depletion	Drugs (loop/thiazide diuretics; proton pump inhibitors (PPIs); antipsychotic/antidepressant medications); Syndrome of inappropriate antidiuretic hormone secretion (SIADH)
Potassium (K^+) *3.5–5.3 mmol/L (14–20 mg/dL)*	1. Excess dietary intake; 2. Decreased excretion (AKI; decompensated CKD; drugs e.g. potassium sparing diuretics; liquorice); 3. High cell turnover states e.g. haematological malignancies	Drugs (loop/thiazide diuretics; renal tubular disorders (e.g. Barter's/Gitelman's syndromes)
Bicarbonate (HCO^{3-}) *22–26 mmol/L*	Renal tubular disorders	Insufficient renal production (decompensated AKI/CKD); drugs
Chloride (Cl^-) *98–106 mmol/L (340–370 mg/dL)*	Loss of body fluids from prolonged vomiting, diarrhoea, sweating or high fever (dehydration). High levels of blood sodium. Kidney failure, or kidney disorders. Diabetes insipidus or diabetic coma	Fluid loss/dehydration due to diarrhoea or vomiting
Urea *2.5–7.8 mmol/L (6–20 mg/dL)*	AKI; CKD; upper GI bleed	Nutrient insufficiency/low muscle mass
Serum creatinine *M 59–104 μmol/L (0.74–1.35 mg/dL) F 45–84 μmol/L (0.59–1.04 mg/dL)*	AKI; CKD; drugs (e.g. trimethoprim/co-trimoxazole)	Nutrient insufficiency/low muscle mass
Corrected calcium (cCa^{2+}) *2.2–2.6 mmol/L*	1. Excess dietary intake/drugs 2. Decreased excretion 3. High bone turnover (e.g. primary/secondary hyperparathyroidism; malignant myeloma; metastatic cancer)	Tertiary hyperparathyroidism Post parathyroidectomy 'hungry bone syndrome'

Table 2.1 (continued)

Test (Abbreviation) *Normal values–SI units (Conventional units)*	Raised levels associated with	Low levels associated with
Phosphate ($PO4^{3-}$) *0.87–1.45 mmol/L (3.0–4.5 mg/dL)*	Drugs (e.g. vitamin D enhances dietary phosphate absorption) Decompensated CKD	Hyperparathyroidism; vitamin D deficiency
Alkaline phosphatase (ALP) *30–130 U/L*	May be raised in liver dysfunction due to infection, alcohol, drugs or biliary obstruction. When isolated, may indicate increased bone turnover	n/a
Albumin *35–50 g/L (3.5–4.8 U/L)*	Fluid depletion	1. Insufficient production: Nutrient insufficiency/chronic inflammatory states; 2. Excess losses: nephrotic syndrome
Parathyroid hormone (PTH) *10–65 pg/L*	Primary & secondary hyperparathyroidism	Post parathyroidectomy/ectopic PTH production
Vitamin D *>50 nmol/L*	Dietary excess	Common in dietary insufficiency/seasonal variation
Glucose *4.0–6.0 mmol/L*	Diabetes mellitus	Insulinoma; exogenous insulin/oral antidiabetic drug administration
Ferritin *M & PMF 12–300 ng/mL (27–670 pmol/L) F 12–150 ng/mL (27–330 pmol/L)*	May be raised in acute inflammatory states	
Urate *M 200–430 μmol/L F 140–360 μmol/L*	1. Decreased excretion: Commoner in progressive CKD; certain forms of inherited renal disease e.g. UMOD; 2. Increased production: high cell turnover states e.g. haematological malignancy	Dilutional
Creatine kinase (CK) *M 40–320 U/L F 25–200 U/L*	Increased muscle breakdown e.g. marathon running/gym workouts; drugs e.g. statins, antipsychotic medication; exclude compartment syndrome	Dilutional
C-reactive protein (CRP) *<5 mg/L*	Acute and chronic infective or inflammatory states, including active autoimmune conditions	n/a

SI international system, *PMF* post-menopausal females

Urea and Electrolytes

Sodium, potassium, chloride and bicarbonate are all small ions, which are freely filtered and actively reabsorbed in the kidney.

Urea and Creatinine

Larger molecules like urea and creatinine are excreted and not resorbed by the kidney. Creatinine is a waste product of muscle metabolism and is excreted by the kidneys into the urine. Individuals with greater muscle bulk tend to have a higher serum creatinine level at baseline, as are individuals of black ethnicity, although the reason for this is uncertain. Serum creatinine is a sensitive marker of kidney function, and increases non-linearly as kidney function deteriorates. Most filtered creatinine is excreted by the renal tubule. It is important to note that this excretion can be blocked by certain medications such as the antibiotic trimethoprim/co-trimoxazole, which results in an increase in serum creatinine, that is not related to a change in glomerular filtration rate (GFR).

Table 2.2 Haematology tests in kidney disease

Test (Abbreviation) *Normal values–SI units (Conventional units)*	Causes of raised levels	Causes of low levels
Haemoglobin (Hb) *M 130–180 g/L* *F 115–165 g/L*	Polycythaemia may be primary, related to excessive EPO production in polycystic kidney disease, or upregulation of hypoxia inducible factor in tumour conditions such as VHL disease	Deficient EPO production by juxtaglomerular cells can lead to a normocytic renal anaemia
White cell count (WCC) Total WCC: *3.6–11.0 × 10⁹/L*	May be raised in infection or proliferative states	May be reduced in immune suppression, such as due to mycophenolate mofetil
Neutrophils: *1.8–7.5 × 10⁹/L*	Typically raised in bacterial infections	May be reduced in immune suppression, such as due to mycophenolate mofetil
Lymphocytes: *1.0–4.0 × 10⁹/L*	May be raised in viral infections	May be reduced acutely in viral infections
Eosinophils: *0.1–0.4 × 10⁹/L*	May be raised in interstitial nephritis	
Platelet count (Plt): *140–400 × 10⁹/L*	May be raised in acute inflammatory and infective conditions	May be reduced in haemolytic states
Mean cell volume (MCV): *80–100 fL*	May be raised in alcohol excess, thyrotoxicosis, B12 and folate deficiency—renal anaemia is typically normocytic	Reduced in microcytic anaemia and β-thalassaemia
Haemoglobin A1c (HbA1c) *<42 mmol/mol (6%)*	Raised in poorly controlled diabetes mellitus	n/a

Table 2.3 Immunolological and virological tests in kidney disease

Investigation	Description
Anti-neutrophil cytoplasmic antibody (ANCA)—marker of small vessel vasculitis	**c-ANCA** Diffuse **c**ytoplasmic staining, corresponding to antibodies against neutrophil proteinase-3 (PR3). Positive in 90% of patients with active granulomatosis with polyangiitis **p-ANCA** Perinuclear staining corresponding to antibodies against neutrophil myeloperoxidase (MPO). Positive in 60% of patients with microscopic polyangiitis and 30% of patients with Churg-Strauss syndrome
Anti-glomerular basement membrane (anti-GBM) antibody	Positive in anti-GBM disease (Goodpasture's disease). Patients can present "double positive" (ANCA vasculitis plus the presence of anti-GBM antibody)
Anti-nuclear antibody (ANA)	Many subtypes exist such as anti-Ro, anti-La and anti-Sm antibodies. Therefore, can be used in the diagnosis of many autoimmune disorders
Anti -dsDNA	Positive in 50% of patients with active SLE. Can be used to monitor disease activity in SLE
Complement concentrations C3 and C4	Low C3 + C4 (classical complement pathway activation). Used in SLE diagnosis and as a marker of activity. Isolated reduction in C3 (alternate complement pathway activation) is seen in C3GN and infection related GNs
Cryoglobulins	Present in various conditions associated with renal impairment (i.e. SLE, multiple myeloma, HIV). The most often quoted link is with Hepatitis-C related membranoproliferative GN
Viral serology: Hepatitis B, C and HIV	Hepatitis B and Hepatits C—associations with membranous nephropathy and mesangiocapillary GN HIV—associations with FSGS and HIV-associated nephropathy Virology is also key to perform when commencing patients on dialysis or immunosuppression

Table 2.3 (continued)

Investigation	Description
Serum (and urine) protein electrophoresis	Help detect production of single immunoglobulins (monoclonal antibodies). Relevant in Myeloma and Monoclonal gammopathy of renal significance
Serum free light chains (Kappa κ and Lambda λ)	Can help detect myeloma or light chain deposition disease. Mostly of significance when there is a significant difference between the ratios of kappa to lambda light chains. Kidney disease can cause elevation of both kappa and lamda light chains
Anti-phopholipase A2 receptor (anti- PLA2R) antibody	A relatively new component to the 'renal screen' (discovered in 2009) [4]. Associated with Primary membranous nephropathy (see Chap. 12)

The Glomerular Filtration Rate (GFR)

The Glomerular Filtration Rate (GFR), is the rate of blood flow through the kidney—and is commonly decreased in kidney disease. Gold standard tests for measuring the GFR (mGFR) include EDTA-GFR and iohexol. Each of these methods involve exogenous administration of a molecule that is filtered freely by the kidney, and not actively reabsorbed. This involves cost and complication, and low-level risk to the patient. Consequently, refinement of correcting equations for serum creatinine measurements to accurately estimate the GFR using patient demographics has allowed the widespread implementation of eGFR reporting, using the Cockroft-Gault (correction using weight and age), CKD-modified diet in renal disease (CKD-MDRD), and latterly CKD-Epidemiology Collaboration (CKD-EPI) formulae (Table 2.4) to correct for age, gender and ethnicity, and approximate the GFR. There are limitations in the accuracy of eGFR equations—with particularly large variation in children, adolescents, older adults, and different ethnicities, and with higher eGFR >60 mL/min/1.73 m^2, although this has improved with latter modifications to the formula. Other limitations include when creatinine excretion is directly blocked e.g. with trimethoprim/co-trimoxazole administration.

Importantly, most drug dosing recommendations are made based on Cockroft-Gault creatinine clearance, using age, weight and serum creatinine.

Alternative biomarkers to measure eGFR include measuring Cystatin C, which is an inert low molecular weight protein, produced by all nucleated cells in the body, and which is less influenced by muscle mass, gender and ethnicity. Levels of Cystatin C can still be influenced by medications, obesity and smoking, and the cost of measuring it remains significantly higher than that of measuring serum Creatinine. In global healthcare terms, its low cost and ready availability make serum Creatinine the most cost-effective marker of kidney function.

Table 2.4 Equations commonly used to calculate the estimated Glomerular Filtration Rate (eGFR)

Cockroft-Gault Equation:
$eGFR = \frac{(140 - age) \times weight \times 1.23\ [if\ Male]\ OR\ 1.04\ [if\ Female]}{SCr}$
MDRD eGFREquation:
$eGFR = 175 \times (SCr)^{-1.154} \times (age)^{-0.203} \times 0.742\ [if\ Female] \times 1.212\ [if\ Black]$
CKD-EPI Equation:
$eGFR = 141 \times \min(SCr/\kappa, 1)^{\alpha} \times \max(SCr/\kappa, 1)^{-1.209} \times 0.993^{(age)} \times 1.018\ [if\ Female] \times 1.159\ [if\ Black]$
κ = 0.7 (Female) or 0.9 (Male) α = -0.329 (Female) or -0.411 (Male) min = indicates the minimum of SCr/κ or 1 max = indicates the maximum of SCr/κ or 1
eGFR (estimated glomerular filtration rate) = mL/min/1.73 m^2 *SCr (standardized serum creatinine) = mg/dL or µmol/L* *Age = years*

Urine Tests

Urinalysis is a fundamental bedside test in helping investigate kidney disease. Fresh 'mid-stream' urine is most valuable to help reduce accidental contamination.

Appearance

Visible inspection of the urine can provide clues towards a diagnosis: changes in urine colour or consistency can be related to haemoglobin, myoglobin, proteins and crystals. For example, patients with nephrotic syndrome commonly observe 'frothy' urine—a sign of proteinuria. Table 2.5 highlights some of the commonly observed visual appearances of urine:

Urine should be dipped in a fresh mid-stream urine specimen, and then left to dry on the side for at least 1–2 min (depending on the manufacturer's recommendation), before being read against the manufacturer's colorimetric chart on the bottle (Fig. 2.1), or using an automated colorimeter where this is available (Tables 2.6 and 2.7).

Table 2.5 Common appearances of urine

Urine appearance		Significance
	Clear, Dilute	Well-hydrated /polyuric
	Clear, Pale yellow	Normal
	Concentrated	Fluid deplete / inadequate hydration
	Cloudy, turbid	May indicate infection
	Frothy	Protein – acts like a detergent and causes frothy or cloudy urine
	Orange	Medications such as rifampicin, sulfasalazine
	Blue or green	Dyes, food colouring, medication including Propofol and amitriptyline. Rarely by Pseudomonas aeruginosa
	Red	Blood, rifampicin, food colourings such as beetroot,
	Brown	Food such as fava beans. Medication such as nitrofurantoin and metronidazole

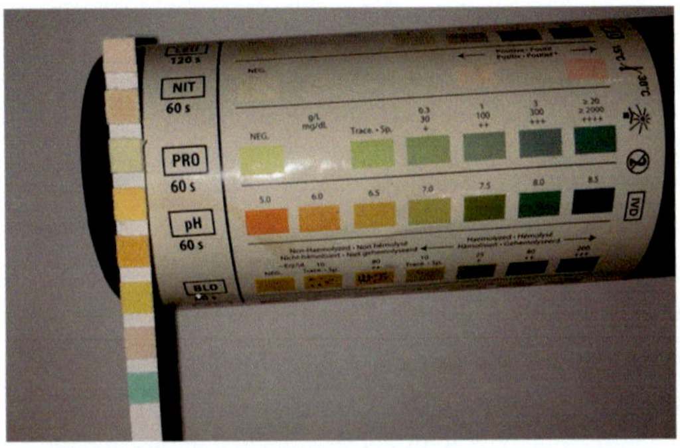

Fig. 2.1 Image of urine dipstick analysis

Table 2.6 The 'urine dipstick'/urinalysis

Urine dipstick component	Significance
Leukocytes	May indicate infection. Detected as leucocyte esterase activity
Nitrites	May indicate infection. Urinary nitrates are converted to nitrites in the presence of Gram-negative bacteria which produce nitrate reductase (e.g.*Escherichia coli*)
Protein	Standard dipsticks measure albumin only but may fail to pick up total protein as well as microalbuminuria (I.e. urine albumin 3-30mg/mmol creatinine). Proteinuria may equate to glomerular disease. Note – 70% of protein in the urine is albumin
pH	Normal urine pH is acidic. The pH can be used to investigate renal stone disease and suspected renal tubular acidosis.
Blood/Haemoglobin	May indicate haematuria (i.e. glomerular disease) however in the absence of haematuria can be due to intravascular haemolysis and rhabdomyolysis (myoglobinuria). Note – false negative results can occur in the presence of high vitamin C concentrations
Specific gravity	The measure of the amount of solute dissolved in urine. *Low specific gravity (<1.005)* – excess hydration / defect in ability of kidneys to concentrate urine *High specific gravity (>1.035)* – dehydration, glycosuria, proteinuria, contrast
Ketones	Ketonuria is associated with starvation, low carbohydrate diets, diabetic ketoacidosis, hyperthyroidism and alcoholism
Glucose	Positive when the serum glucose is high eg. Diabetes mellitus

Table 2.7 Summary of urine-based investigations when investigating kidney disease

Urine test	Significance
Visual inspection & urinalysis	See Tables 2.5 and 2.6
Microscopy	Urine is examined under a light microscope to demonstrate the presence of cells, bacteria, casts and crystals **Casts**—these are cylindrical structures formed in the distal renal tubules **Hyaline casts**—Most common type, typically innocuous (seen in concentrated urine i.e. dehydration) **Granular casts**—can result from degenerating cellular casts. Associated with inflammation and infection **Dysmorphic red cells and red blood cell casts**—indicate glomerular pathology **White cell casts**—can suggest infection such as pyelonephritis or tubulointerstitial nephritis **Crystals**—certain drugs such as anti-virals can cause this **Eosinophils**—suggests tubulointerstitial nephritis (TIN)
Urine culture	Useful in identifying infection. Pyuria (>8 × 10^6 white cells/L) without bacteriuria—think tuberculosis
Urine cytology	May identify urinary tract malignancy

Table 2.7 (continued)

Urine test	Significance
Urine protein quantification 24 h urine collections or single void specimens: Albumin: creatinine ratio (ACR) Or Protein: creatinine ratio (PCR)	**Urine ACR**: measures **only** albumin—to help detect glomerular disease **Urine PCR:** measures total protein. Therefore, will rise with any protein detected in the urine (i.e. low molecular weight proteins, light chains as well as albumin) *Urine PCR of 100 roughly equates to 1 g proteinuria per day*
Osmolality	Can help assess the ability of the kidneys to concentrate urine, free water clearance and cause of hypo/hypernatraemia. More accurate measure of urinary concentration than specific gravity. Raised in SIADH
Sodium	Fractional excretion of sodium (Fe_{Na}) can be used to determine the type of AKI. Low urinary sodium suggests normal reabsorptive function. High urinary sodium suggests renal salt wasting **Fe_{Na} <1%**—prerenal uraemia, hepatorenal syndrome **Fe_{Na} >2%**—ATN, CKD, osmotic diuresis A urine sodium >20 mmol/L may indicate diagnosis of ATN
Potassium	If <20 mmol/L or low TTKG—extra-renal potassium loss
Chloride	Can help distinguish between causes of metabolic alkalosis. A urinary chloride <20 mmol/L in a patient with metabolic alkalosis indicates volume contraction
Myoglobin	Can identify rhabdomyolysis
Urinary Bence Jones protein	This is an immunoglobulin light chain—its presence in urine is suggestive of a monoclonal gammopathy of renal significance (MGRS), or Multiple myeloma (MM)

TTKG transtubular potassium gradient = $\dfrac{\text{urine potassium / urine osmolality}}{\text{serum potassium / serum osmolality}}$

Radiological Imaging

The imaging modalities most often used in the initial assessment of the kidney patient are plain film radiography of the chest, and urinary tract ultrasound. Cross-sectional imaging using computed tomography (CT) or magnetic resonance imaging (MRI) is more frequently a second-line investigation.

Plain Radiography

Chest X-Ray

Breathlessness is a common presentation in kidney disease, thus a chest radiograph may be used to look for evidence of:

- Air space opacification:
  - Unilateral: when lobar and associated with lobar collapse, may be consistent with infection, and secondary AKI.
  - Bilateral: may be consistent with bilateral infection, pulmonary haemorrhage or—more commonly—fluid overload, particularly when associated with pleural effusions secondary to kidney failure or nephrotic syndrome (this may also be secondary to other transudative causes such as cardiac or liver failure).
- Hilar lymph node enlargement (associated with infection, autoimmune and inflammatory conditions such as sarcoidosis, and underlying

malignancy, particularly in the context of other spiculated lung lesions)

Abdominal X-Ray

Plain radiography of the abdomen (which can include imaging of the kidney, ureters and bladder) is not commonly used to investigate kidney disease. The renal outlines in plain films are often obscured by bowel gas shadows. Renal stones, namely calcium-containing, struvite and cystine stones (radiopaque) can be identified, however uric acid and xanthine stones (radiolucent) may not be effectively picked up (Fig. 2.2).

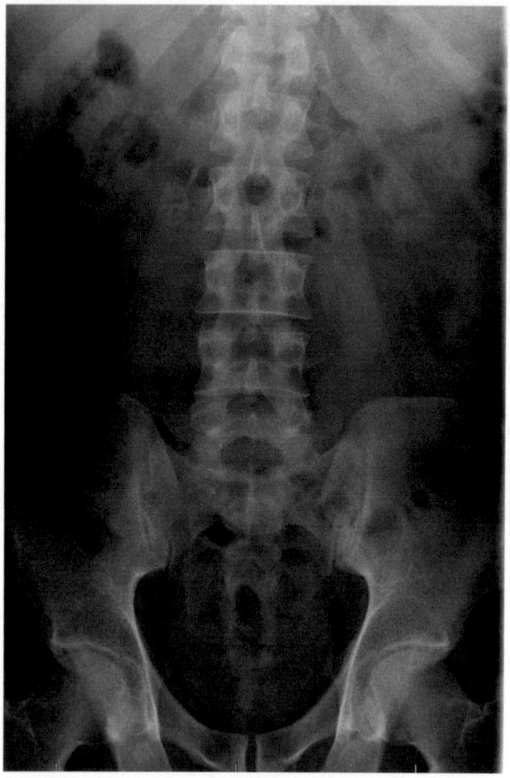

Fig. 2.2 Plain abdominal X ray. Normal Plain abdominal X ray—no radio-opaque kidney stones are demonstrated within the kidneys, ureters or bladder; the bowel gas pattern is normal

Intravascular Contrast Studies

Ultrasound has replaced most intravenous urogram/intravenous pyelogram examinations of the kidney.

Ultrasound

In the work up of a patient with a raised serum creatinine, an ultrasound scan of the renal tract is an invaluable non-invasive, first-line imaging modality. It can help determine kidney size, asymmetry, structural abnormalities (including differentiating between cystic or solid, and simple or complex renal parenchymal lesions), and identify and localise causes of urinary tract obstruction (Fig. 2.3).

Normal kidney size is approximately 10–12 cm and is normally proportional to height (Table 2.8). Ultrasound findings can also reveal

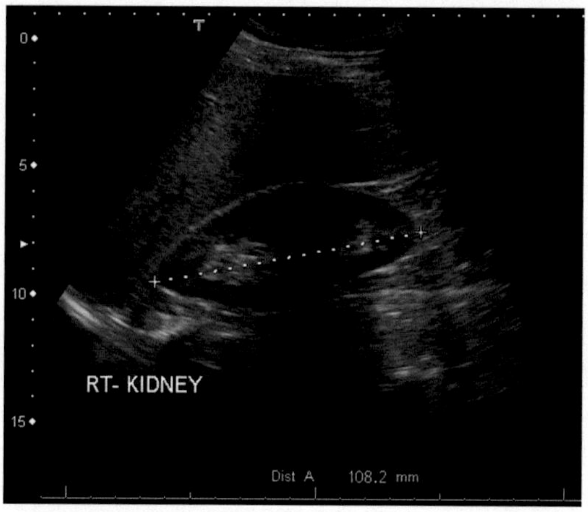

Fig. 2.3 Ultrasound imaging of the kidneys. A normal right kidney in the sagittal plane: the top of the ultrasound image is anterior; the bottom is posterior. Right on the image is towards the feet (caudal) and left is towards the head (cranial). The right liver lobe overlies the kidney; the right kidney cortex and medulla are well-differentiated; the interpolar length has been measured as 108.2 mm. Note areas of increased shadowing are produced by the ribs

Table 2.8 Causes of small and large kidneys on imaging

Small kidneys (<10 cm)	Large kidneys (>12 cm)
Chronic kidney disease	Diabetes mellitus
Renal artery stenosis	Acromegaly
Hypoplasia	Amyloidosis
	Lymphoma
	Polycystic kidneys

features related to chronic kidney disease, such as when the echo-consistency of the renal cortex is reduced compared to the medulla and the collecting system. The loss of this 'corticomedullary differentiation' is a sensitive but non-specific marker of chronic kidney disease.

Practice Point 1

Orienting the ultrasound image: the top of the ultrasound image is the location where the sound waves enter the patient first—so irrespective of position and tipping, the skin will always be at the top.

Renal Doppler Ultrasound Scans

Doppler ultrasound is a specialised ultrasound imaging that can evaluate the flow of blood in renal arteries and veins. They can help assess for renal vein thrombosis, renal artery stenosis, decreased renal perfusion and renal infarction.

Renal artery stenosis—may be identified if there is markedly peaked systolic velocity in the renal artery, particularly when compared to aortic peak systolic velocity.

Renal vein thrombosis—Since the kidneys are deep and retroperitoneal, doppler ultrasound of the native kidney is often insufficiently sensitive to make a diagnosis of renal vein thrombosis (e.g. related to nephrotic syndrome), so CT or MRI venography is preferred. However, transplant renal ultrasound is often the modality of choice in diagnosing renal vein thrombosis in a transplanted kidney, where the blood vessels are typically relatively superficial.

What Is the Resistive Index (RI)?

Resistive index (RI) = (Peak systolic velocity − End diastolic velocity)/Peak systolic velocity.

(Normal RI < 0.70)

The resistive index (RI) is a calculated flow parameter in ultrasound, derived from the maximum, minimum and mean doppler frequency shifts during the cardiac cycle. It works on the principle that as a vessel narrows and resistance to flow increases, the RI will increase. It can be used to monitor a kidney transplant blood vessel flow, particularly in the early post-transplant period. Causes for a raised RI in the transplanted kidney are multiple, and can be related to transplant renal vein and renal artery thrombosis, acute tubular necrosis, rejection, immunosuppressive toxicity, perinephric fluid collection, and transplant renal artery stenosis [5].

Computed Tomography (CT)

Cross-sectional urinary tract imaging using computed tomography (CT) can be used to provide additional or complementary information to the ultrasound, namely because a sharper resolution is obtained. It can be used to delineate the cause of obstruction and investigate masses in the kidney, including the staging of renal tumours. It is more effective at detecting ureteric calculi (non-contrast CT) and can help delineate the level of ureteric obstruction. However, it is less sensitive than ultrasound at differentiating between solid and cystic lesions in the kidney. CT angiography can help evaluate renal artery stenosis, in particular identifying the presence or absence of a post-stenotic dilatation in the affected renal artery (Fig. 2.4).

Iodinated radio-opaque contrast, used for CT imaging, poses the risk of nephrotoxicity, with the risk deemed greater for those with underlying kidney impairment. Pre-hydration with oral or intravenous fluid can be effective in reducing the risk of contrast induced nephropathy. N-acetylcysteine is no longer recommended to

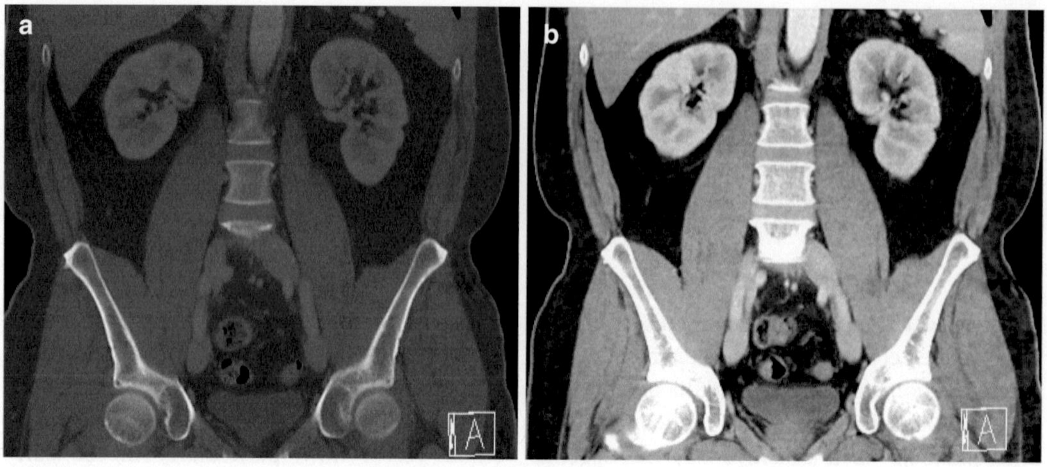

Fig. 2.4 Computed Tomography (CT) imaging of normal kidneys. Coronal CT scan of the normal kidneys and bladder—without contrast (**a**) and following administration of iodinated contrast (**b**)

prevent contrast nephrotoxicity (due to lack of any confirmed benefit).

Magnetic Resonance Imaging (MRI)

Magnetic resonance imaging (MRI) can be an effective method to study anatomical changes such as renal tumours, atherosclerotic vascular disease and renal vein thrombosis. Soft tissues are also visualised in greater detail than with CT or radiography; MRI has the additional benefit of no radiation exposure. MRI helps better delineate wall thickening and nodularity of renal lesions when compared to CT or ultrasound. This imaging modality also has a role in evaluating indeterminate renal lesions (i.e. diffusion weighted MRI may help in differentiating between inflammatory and malignant masses). Magnetic resonance angiography (MRA) with gadolinium can also be used to study renal artery stenosis, with greater accuracy than when compared to ultrasound [6] (Fig. 2.5).

Most MRI scanners comprise a very tight tunnel, and a loud 'banging' noise throughout the scanning process, which may make it difficult for patients who suffer with claustrophobia to tolerate. The advent of 'open MRI' scanners at certain centres may improve tolerability, but depending on availability, may also be in greater demand, leading to delays in the diagnostic process.

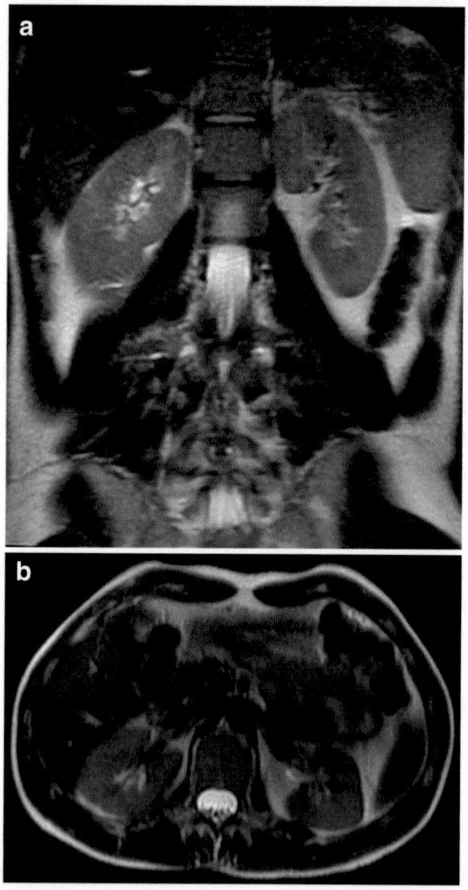

Fig. 2.5 Magnetic Resonance Imaging (MRI) of normal kidneys. Coronal (**a**) and Axial (**b**) T2-weighted MRI of the normal kidneys

Practice Point 2

- T1 MR images: 1 tissue type is bright—FAT
- T2 MR images: 2 tissue types are bright—FAT & WATER

Nephrogenic Systemic Fibrosis

The use of gadolinium has been linked to the development of nephrogenic systemic fibrosis (NSF). This is a rare syndrome that can involve fibrosis of skin, joints, eyes and internal organs. This is a particular risk to patients with end-stage kidney disease, and it remains recommended that gadolinium-containing contrast should be avoided in patients with an eGFR of <30 mL/min/1.73 m^2. As there is no definitive cure for this condition (although improvements in NSF symptoms have been seen following kidney transplant), ultimately treatment focuses on avoidance of the condition through minimising the use of gadolinium contrast where possible.

Nuclear Medicine Imaging: Renal Scintigraphy

Renal scintigraphy refers to several nuclear medicine examinations for the kidney using radiopharmaceuticals that evaluate the function and anatomy of the kidneys. Each of these techniques involve the injection of a radiopharmaceutical or radiotracer that emits a tiny amount of radioactivity into the patient. After injection, the radiotracer travels throughout the body to the kidneys, where it gives off energy in the form of gamma rays. This energy is detected by a device called a gamma camera. The camera works with a computer to produce special pictures offering details on both the structure and function of organs and tissues.

The different properties of each radiotracer allows for different information to be gleaned from each approach (Table 2.9). The three main radiopharmaceuticals used are: Technetium-99m diethylene triamine pentaacetic acid (^{99m}Tc-DTPA) and Technetium-99m mercaptoacetyltriglycine (^{99m}Tc-MAG3), Iodine-131-Hipuran (^{131}I-Hipuran), Technetium-99m glucoheptonate, and Technetium-99m dimercaptosuccinic acid

Table 2.9 Comparison of different renal nuclear medicine imaging modalities

^{99m}Tc-DTPA	^{99m}Tc-MAG3	^{131}I-Hipuran	^{99m}Tc-Glucoheptonate	^{99m}Tc-DMSA
• Filtered through the glomerulus	• Filtered through the glomerulus • Excreted by renal tubules	• Excreted by renal tubules	• Binds to renal cortex	• Binds to renal cortex
Perfusion • Vascular supply – Filtration • Measuring renal function (glomerular filtration rate) – Drainage • Detects obstruction	• Perfusion • Vascular supply – Filtration • Measuring renal function (glomerular filtration rate) • Drainage Detects obstruction • Diminished renal function • Kidney transplants	• Diminished renal function • Kidney transplants	– Renal scarring from chronic infection—Infarction – Renal mass – Differential renal mass (proportion of total renal mass contributed by each kidney)	• Renal scarring from chronic infection • Infarction • Renal mass • Differential renal mass (proportion of total renal mass contributed by each kidney)

(^{99m}Tc-DMSA). Local availability of radioisotopes is absolutely key to obtain simple radioisotope imaging.

Histopathology

A definitive diagnosis of kidney disease—particularly in diagnosing and grading severity of tubulointerstitial nephritis, glomerulonephritis and transplant rejection—often requires the direct examination of kidney tissue, which is obtained by percutaneous kidney biopsy. This is most often ultrasound or CT-guided, in order to minimise complications.

Kidney Biopsy

Despite medical advancements in recent years, the needle core kidney biopsy remains an invaluable tool for the nephrologist: It is an invasive investigation, in which samples of kidney tissue are obtained for histopathological study. Usually performed with local anaesthetic, with or without sedation, and under ultrasound or CT guidance, a specialised biopsy needle is guided retroperitoneally via the patient's back (native kidney biopsy—normally taken from the left lower pole when the anatomy is uncomplicated) or anteriorly over (transplant kidney biopsy) to obtain sample cores. Following the procedure, patients are required to have a period of bed rest (6–8 h), during which their vital signs are measured, and their urine monitored for visible haematuria (around 1:100). Bleeding is the major primary complication; in rare cases this may lead to significant retroperitoneal haemorrhage (around 1:1000) and the need for blood transfusions, and either radiological or surgical intervention to stop the bleeding. There is also a very small risk of death (<1:1000). The decision to undertake a kidney biopsy should therefore be made after careful evaluation of the risks and benefits of the procedure to the patient [7–8].

Indications

Kidney biopsies can help confirm a diagnosis (in particular for suspected glomerular pathologies), evaluate disease activity or establish disease stage/severity (e.g. lupus nephritis) and hence help determine disease prognosis (Table 2.10).

Although kidney biopsies have an invaluable role in providing a definitive diagnosis, there are certain situations where they are relatively or absolutely contraindicated, as the risk of the procedure potentially outweighs any conceivable benefit from a result (Table 2.11).

Table 2.10 Indications for renal biopsy

Indications forrenal biopsy
1.Acute kidney injury (after ruling out pre-renal and obstructive causes)
2.Unexplained chronic kidney disease
3.When suspecting glomerular pathology (acute glomerulonephritis andnephrotic syndrome)
4.Systemic diseases with kidney involvement
5.Kidney transplant dysfunction

Table 2.11 Contraindications to renal biopsy

Relative	Absolute
Single functioning kidney	Small kidneys
Limited patient cooperation	Uncorrectable bleeding diathesis / intravascular coagulopathy
Technical difficulties (for example due to large body habitus / unable to lie flat)	Uncontrolled hypertension

Light and Electron Microscopy

The kidney tissue samples are typically collected in formaldehyde for light microscopic evaluation, and, depending on centres—specialist fixation fluid for electron microscopic and RNA extraction where this is available and appropriate. An unfixed core is needed if immunofluorescence technique is used. Sometimes, a same-day preliminary result may be available and help guide immediate management of the kidney patient—but fixation of the sample can take up to 4 h of intense laboratory work, so a same-day result requires careful coordination, clear communication and swift transport between the clinician undertaking the biopsy, the histopathology laboratory team, and thence to the reporting histopathologist.

Light Microscopy (LM)

The light microscope uses visible light and a series of lenses to magnify cells from the biopsy sample up to a maximum magnification of around ×2000. Tissue samples are usually fixed in formalin, processed, cut into thin 2–3 micron thick serial sections and stained with Haematoxylin and Eosin (H&E) to enhance tissue contrast under the light microscope. This stain is helpful for general evaluation of the biopsy specimen (all 4 compartments; glomerular, tubular, interstitial and vascular). For kidney biopsies, there are additional specialised stains used to examine the pathology (Table 2.12 and Fig. 2.6):

Table 2.12 Different histochemical stains and their relation to renal histopathology

Stain	Significance
Haematoxylin & Eosin (H&E)	Evaluation of all four renal compartments and inflammation
Periodic acid-Schiff (PAS)	To examine the glomerular cell number, basement membrane, mesangium, tubular basement membrane, hyaline—red
Masson's trichrome	To assess fibrin, fibrosis and immune deposits. Extracellular glomerular matrix and tubular basement membranes—blue/green
Silver stain	To assess the basement membrane (i.e. to visualise spikes and double contours)—black and extracellular glomerular matrix
Congo Red	Amyloid
Von Kossa	Calcification
Acid Fuchsin-Orange G	Protein deposition (immune complex)
Sirius Red	Fibrosis

Immunohistochemistry

Immunohistochemical techniques are used to detect antigens by using 'tagged' antibodies, specific for that antigen. Antibodies can be conjugated to an enzyme that catalyses a reaction resulting in a colour change. Antibodies can also be tagged with a fluorescent compound that emits light on excitation by light. Specialised light microscopes can then be used to examine these samples. Certain antigens are routinely looked for, including:

- immunoglobulins (IgA, IgG, IgM) (Fig. 2.7)
- components of the classical and alternative complement pathways (C1q, C4)
- light chains (Kappa and Lambda)

Electron Microscopy

Electron microscopes use an electron beam (rather than a light beam) to create an image of a specimen. They are able to visualise samples using a much higher magnification—of around ×1,000,000, so the kidney tissue can be visualised to a resolution of around 0.2 nm. The kidney tissue is fixed in glutaraldehyde paraformaldehyde, and stained with toluidine blue to confirm the presence of glomeruli, after which the biopsy sample can be studied in greater detail (Fig. 2.8).

Tissue Examination and Interpretation of the Histopathological Report

When examining a kidney biopsy specimen, initially a low-power screening examination is useful to highlight any areas or defects. Furthermore,

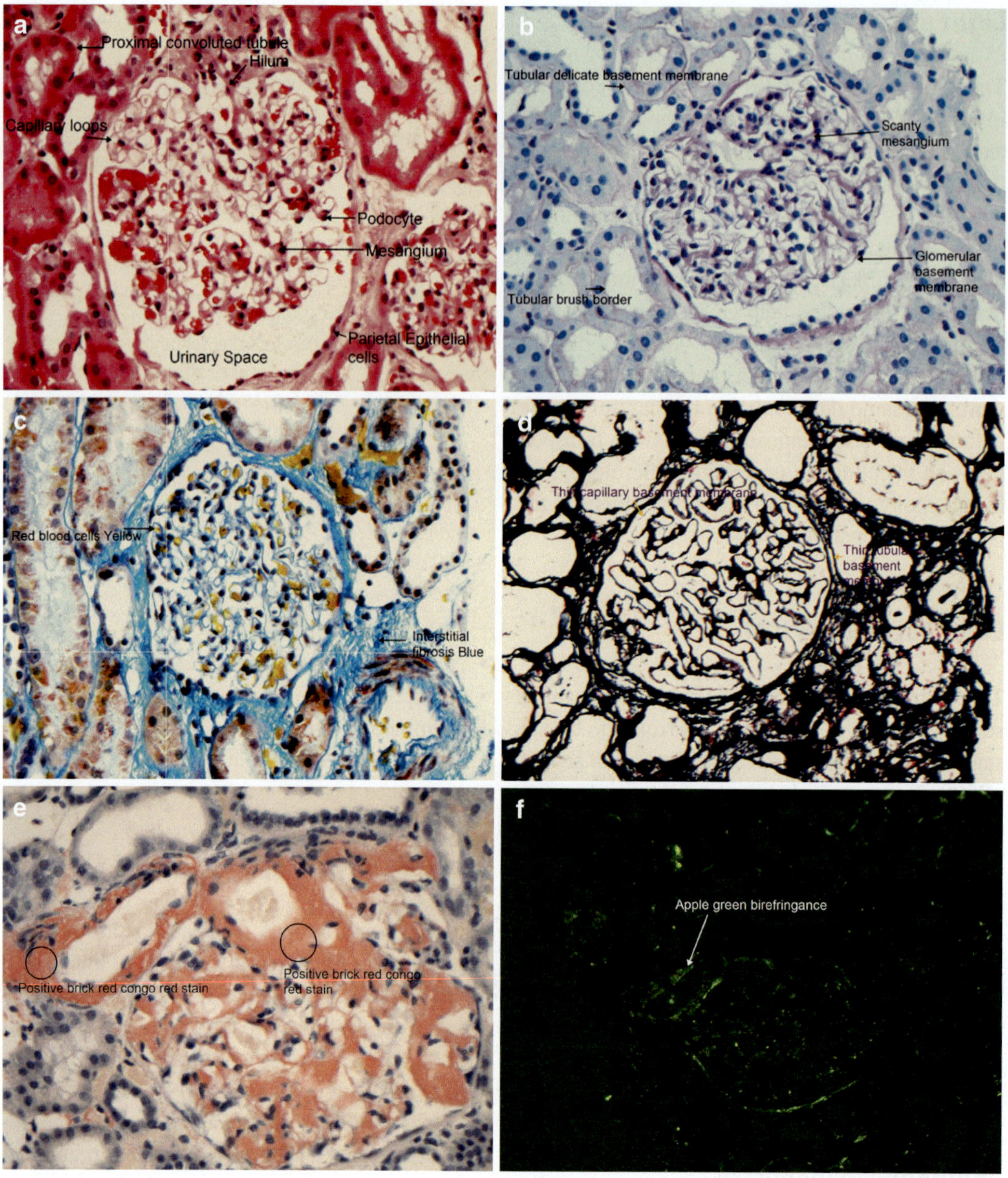

Fig. 2.6 Renal histopathological stains under light microscopy. Haematoxylin & Eosin (H&E) stain (**a**); Periodic Acid Schiff (PAS) stain (**b**); Masson's Trichrome stain (**c**) and Silver stain (**d**) of the normal glomerulus under light microscopy at ×40 magnification; Congo red stain illustrating amyloid deposition in the glomerulus (**e**); Apple green birefringence under polarised light reflecting amyloid deposition in the glomerulus (**f**); Sirius red stain of the normal kidney (**g**)

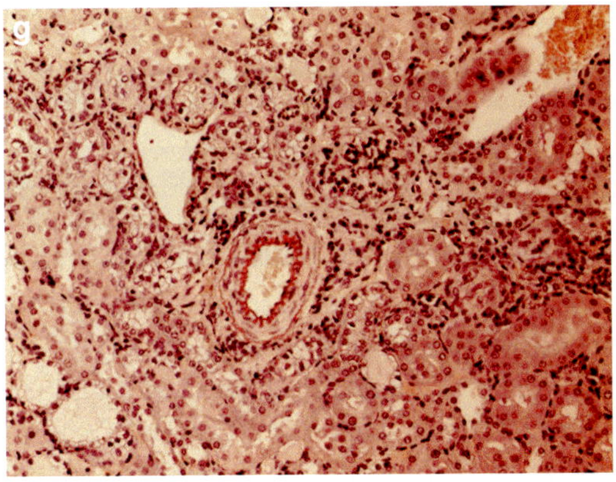

Fig. 2.6 (continued)

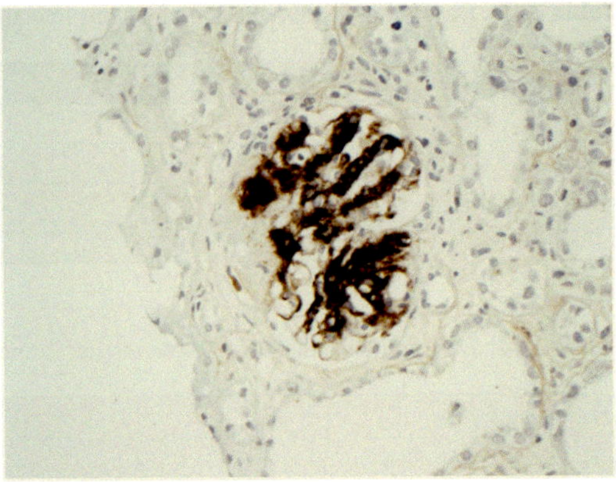

Fig. 2.7 Immunohistochemical staining. Immunoperoxidase staining for IgA deposition showing mesangial distribution of deposits in the glomerulus

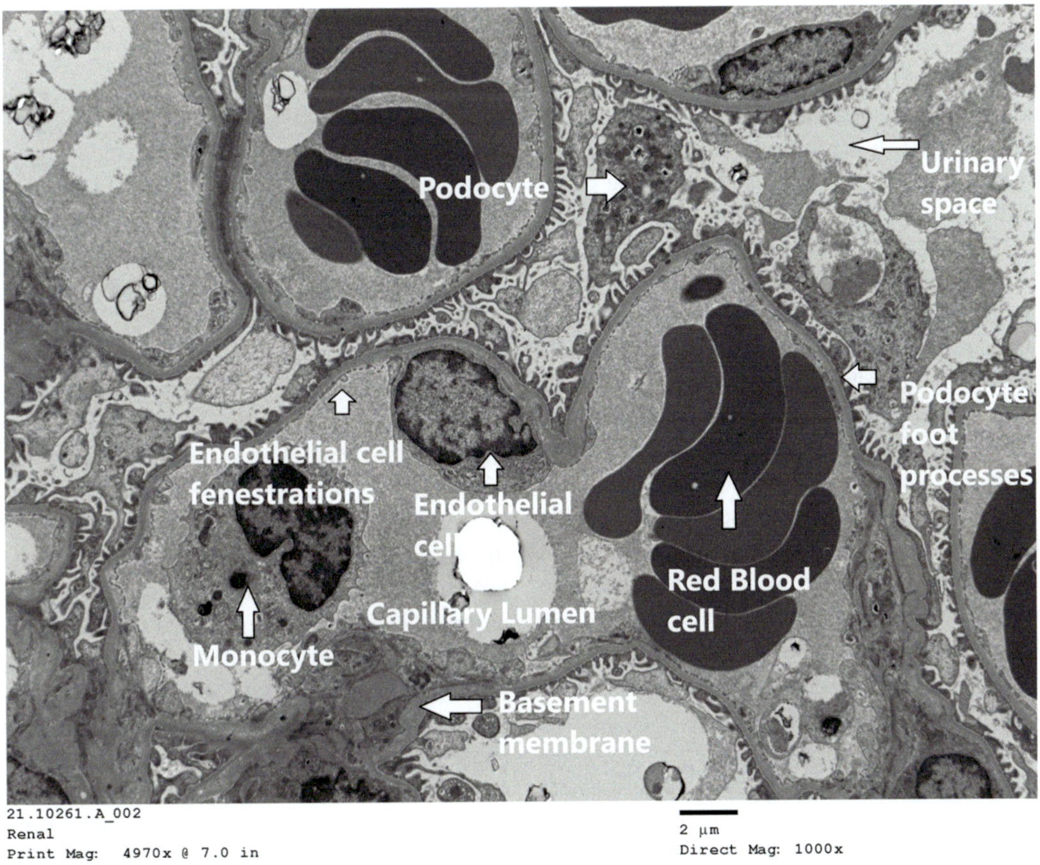

Fig. 2.8 Electron Microscopy Imaging. Annotated Electron Microscopy Image at ×1000 magnification of the normal glomerulus

Table 2.13 Describing the distribution of lesions affecting the glomerulus

Distribution	Definition
Focal	Changes affecting a few glomeruli only
Diffuse	Changes affecting all glomeruli
Segmental	Part of glomerulus is involved
Global	Whole glomerulus involved

Table 2.14 Descriptions indicating Active versus Chronic lesions in renal pathology

Active lesions	Chronic lesions
Proliferation of cells	Glomerulosclerosis
Necrosis/Apoptosis	Fibrous crescent
Cellular/Fibrocellularcrescent	Interstitial fibrosis
Oedema	Tubular atrophy
Active inflammation: Glomerulitis, interstitial nephritis, tubulitis, vasculitis	Vascular sclerosis

it will help with localizing whether there are defects in the glomerulus, tubule, interstitium or blood vessels. It is also important to be mindful of the distribution of lesions affecting the glomerulus (Table 2.13), and whether lesions seen in the biopsy appear active or chronic (Table 2.14):

Interstitial fibrosis and tubular atrophy can be summarised as a (visually estimated) percentage score, reflecting the level of background chronic damage in the kidney biopsy.

Where histopathological examination can give vast amounts of information, based on a single representative core of a patient's kidney tissue, the clinical nephrologist, with the help of the reporting histopathologist, are tasked with assimilating all of the available information, alongside the clinical history, examination, blood test and imaging data—to formulate the likely histopathological diagnosis.

Practice Point 3

- Appropriate investigations with blood tests, imaging—both structural and functional, and histopathological examination where appropriate—are all central to guiding the appropriate active management of kidney disease
- Certain clinical situations demand a more holistic approach—in particular to consider limiting the use of invasive investigations—for example amongst frail elderly multimorbid patients.

Conclusions

Returning to the clinical scenario from the beginning of the chapter, the differential diagnosis, based on the available information from the history and clinical examination is quite broad: Whilst the patient's history of gout and chronic NSAID use suggest two possible aetiologies, his poorly controlled hypertension may also be either contributory or secondary to his kidney disease. Further blood tests from his primary care practitioner demonstrate that his serum creatinine was 160 μmol/L (1.81 mg/dL) 2 years ago, and the presence of a raised serum, PTH, phosphate, urate and normocytic anaemia are all indicative of chronic kidney disease; his fasting serum glucose was 5 mmol/L, and the results of the rest of his acute nephritic screen were all within normal limits. His calculated

CKD-EPI eGFR is 43 mL/min/1.73 m^2, and his urinalysis demonstrated 1+ blood and 1+ proteinuria, with a measured urine PCR of 60 mg/mmol—(or around 60 mg of protein in 24 h) and ACR of 26.5 mg/mmol. In support of this, his kidney ultrasound demonstrated kidneys of 8 cm in bipolar length bilaterally. So, whilst the precise cause of his chronic kidney disease stage G3bA2 is uncertain (and may be related variously to chronic NSAID use, a chronic urate nephropathy, or hypertensive nephropathy), there are both relative (uncontrolled hypertension) and absolute (small kidneys) contraindications to a kidney biopsy in this gentleman's case. The most appropriate management plan is therefore likely to involve stopping all 'nephrotoxic' substances, in particular his NSAIDs, and rationalising other medications in light of his eGFR, (estimated using the Cockroft-Gault formula) (Table 2.4), and close control of his hypertension to a target average of <130/80 mmHg.

Questions

1. A 38-year old lady presented to the general nephrology clinic with a 2-day history of haematuria and left-sided flank pain. She had a background of primary membranous nephropathy, diagnosed 3 years previously. She was initially treated for this with the Ponticelli regimen, and had remained in complete remission for 2 years. On presentation today, she has noticed a 1-week history of frothy urine. On examination, she has oedema up to her ankles. She is normotensive, and she had bibasal crackles on auscultation of her chest. A urine dipstix test was positive for blood and protein. Her blood tests revealed hypoalbuminaemia and raised inflammatory markers, but her serum creatinine remains stable compared with her baseline, and her eGFR was over 60 mL/min/1.73 m^2. An ultrasound examination reported this morning demonstrated normal-sized kidneys.

   What is the next most appropriate investigation?

   A. Kidney biopsy
   B. Angiogram
   C. Flexible cystoscopy
   D. CT KUB with contrast
   E. Repeat ultrasound with doppler studies

Answer: D

A patient with oedema, hypoalbuminaemia and proteinuria has presenting features consistent with a 'nephrotic syndrome'. Her history of primary membranous nephropathy—previously treated with the Ponticelli regimen—mean that this presentation is consistent with a relapse of her condition. A nephrotic state in the setting of membranous nephropathy places her at enhanced risk of developing venous thromboembolism. In this case, her presentation with haematuria and loin pain, and clinical findings consistent with an underlying nephrotic state put renal vein thrombosis high on the list of differential diagnoses. Since the initial ultrasound scan of the kidneys was normal, and the clinical suspicion high, repeating this with doppler studies is less likely to be conclusive—particularly when scanning native kidneys, (although the more superficial transplant kidney may be much easier to image). Therefore, CT imaging with contrast enhancement is the modality of choice to diagnose renal vein thrombosis in this setting.

2. In which of the following scenarios is a kidney biopsy least warranted in the acute setting?

   A. 30-year-old lady with a background of SLE diagnosed 10 years previously, presents with 1-week history of lower limb oedema and worsening kidney function. No previous renal diagnosis.
   B. 45-year-old man with a background of IgA nephropathy presenting with macroscopic haematuria and acutely worsening kidney function for the last 2 weeks.
   C. 68-year-old lady with type 1 diabetes for the last 20 years presenting with progressive decline in kidney function. She is under active follow up with the local ophthalmology team, who have previously undertaken laser pan-retinal photocoagulation (PRP) for her diabetic retinopathy

D. 50-year-old lady with a 2-week history of rash, red eyes, haematuria and haemoptysis presenting with acute kidney injury
E. 28-year-old man with no past medical history presenting with a 1 week history of leg oedema and frothy urine. Urinalysis reveals 3.5 g/day of proteinuria

Answer: C

Option C is the least appropriate option for renal biopsy. Although it would be helpful to have a confirmatory diagnosis of diabetic nephropathy, the presence of diabetic retinopathy, particularly in type 1 diabetic patients, has a high sensitivity (>80%) for predicting diabetic nephropathy. The histological class of lupus nephritis is useful to help guide treatment and prognosis (scenario A). A native kidney biopsy in scenario B would help to identify or exclude a proliferative glomerulonephritis, that would determine prognosis. In scenario D, the clinical features are consistent with a rapidly progressing glomerulonephritis with systemic features, which requires a biopsy to help guide treatment and prognosis. A new diagnosis of nephrotic syndrome (scenario E) in an adult patient requires a kidney biopsy to provide information on the aetiology of the disease and thus guide treatment.

3. Which of the following diagnoses typically causes small kidneys?
   A. Diabetes
   B. Renal artery stenosis
   C. Polycystic kidney disease
   D. Amyloidosis
   E. Acromegaly

Answer: B

Renal artery stenosis is the only one of the options presented that typically leads to a 'small' kidney. The other listed causes typically result in enlarged kidneys—either due to enhanced growth, deposition or cysts.

4. A 35-year-old lady presents to the general nephrology clinic with fever and a rash. She has a past medical history of gastritis, for which she was on omeprazole (proton pump inhibitor) therapy. Her blood tests revealed a creatinine of 185 μmol/L (6 months ago it was 75 μmol/L). Microscopic examination of her urine reveals eosinophilic casts. What is the most likely cause of her kidney dysfunction?
   A. Acute tubular necrosis
   B. Acute interstitial nephritis
   C. Polycystic kidney disease
   D. IgA nephropathy
   E. FSGS

Answer: B

The presence of eosinophilc casts on urine microscopy, together with rash and fever point towards acute interstitial nephritis. The culprit in this case is most likely to be her proton pump inhibitor, omeprazole.

5. A 52-year-old man with a history of colorectal cancer presents to the renal clinic with frothy urine and swelling in his ankles. Blood pressure was 152/84 mmHg, and urinalysis was positive for protein. He had a serum albumin of 23 g/L, a serum creatinine of 89 μmol/L, and an ultrasound scan demonstrating normal-sized kidneys. A renal biopsy reported a thickened basement membrane, with subepithelial electron-dense deposits.

   Which antibody is this patient most likely to test positive for?
   A. Anti-phospholipase A2 receptor
   B. Anti-nuclear antibodies
   C. Anti-apolipoprotein L1
   D. Anti-Ro
   E. Anti-La

Answer: A

The patient in the question stem is most likely to have a diagnosis of membranous nephropathy, as confirmed by the histological findings on the kidney biopsy. Primary membranous nephropathy is recognised to be associated with antibodies against PLA2R. Approximately 70% of the patients with primary membranous nephropathy have anti-PLA2R autoantibodies in their serum [4].

6. A 65-year-old lady presented with nephrotic range proteinuria, progressive development of renal insufficiency, weakness, and weight loss. She had a past history of chronic inflammatory bowel disease for the last 10 years. A renal biopsy was performed which showed

acellular eosinophilic mesangial expansion. Which special stain will provide diagnostic information?

A. Silver stain
B. Martius Scarlet Blue
C. Congo Red
D. Sirius Red
E. Elastic Van Gieson stain

Answer: C

The mesangial expansion is due to deposit of amyloid which will stain brick red with Congo Red stain and will show apple green birefringence on polarized light. The type of amyloid deposited in the given history of chronic inflammatory bowel disease is likely type AA amyloid.

7. All of the following features seen on a renal biopsy suggest active disease except:

A. Fibrinoid necrosis
B. Fibrous crescent
C. Tubulointerstitial nephritis
D. Proliferation
E. Vasculitis

Answer: B

Cellular and fibro-cellular crescents suggest active disease. A fibrous crescent is indicative of a chronic disease process. Active and chronic lesions can coexist, suggesting an acute on chronic disease process.

8. A 75 year old man presented with 3 day history of profuse watery stools and vomiting. On presentation his BP was 100/70 mmHg, pulse 98/min. His creatinine was 257 μmol/L. Which of the following urine results suggest a 'pre-renal' cause for his presentation?

A. Urine sodium 9 mmol/L
B. Urine sodium 15 mmol/L
C. Urine sodium 40 mmol/L
D. Urine fractional excretion of sodium 2.5%
E. Urine fractional excretion of sodium 5%

Answer: A

Urine sodium 9 mmol/L. In the setting of volume depletion, urinary sodium should be low: typically less than 10 mmol/L, representing the normal renal physiological response, triggered to conserve sodium.

9. A 65 year old woman with a known colonic villous adenoma presents with a 10 day history of diarrhoea, volume depletion and acute kidney injury. Which set of biochemical blood and urine test results are most likely to reflect her illness?

	Serum creatinine μmol/L (60–100)	Serum potassium mmol/L (3.5–5.5 mmol/L)	Blood pH (7.35–7.45)	Urine potassium mmol/L
A	250	3.2	7.20	60
B	160	5.5	7.22	30
C	150	3.1	7.25	8
D	170	3.1	7.48	24
E	225	5.6	7.49	10

Answer: C

Colonic diarrhoea causes a hypokalaemic acidosis, due to loss of bicarbonate and potassium from the gastrointestinal tract, and with a low urinary potassium due to reduced renal potassium excretion in the setting of hypokalaemia.

10. A 35 year old woman is found to have a raised serum creatinine during her first pregnancy, of 180 μmol/L. On further questioning, she recalls suffering from several episodes of urine infections—between the ages of 15 and 25 years.

What is most likely result of her ultrasound scan?

A. Bilateral kidney cysts in medulla and cortex
B. Bilateral cortical kidney cysts
C. A horse-shoe kidney
D. Bilateral upper pole scarring
E. Unilateral duplex ureter

Answer: D

The scenario most likely reflects CKD, with the likely aetiology relating to the history of recurrent UTIs due to reflux nephropathy, leading to upper pole renal cortical scarring.

11. A 73-year-old man presented with a 3-day history of haemoptysis and 2-month history of lethargy and fever. He was also suffering from loss of smell, anorexia, reduced hearing and weight loss of 4 kg.

On examination, he appeared pale and had bilateral red eyes. Urinalysis showed blood 3+, protein 2+.

His blood results are as follows:

Creatinine 400 µmol/L (60–110) (baseline Creatinine 75 µmol/L one year ago)

Eosinophils 0.45 (0.04–0.40)

Lymphocytes 1.2 (1–4)

Neutrophils 7.8 (2–8)

CRP 310 (<10)

COVID PCR negative

CXR—bilateral patchy shadowing in lower zones. Consistent with COVID 19. Disease extent: Moderate.

What key investigation may help confirm a diagnosis?

A. Repeat COVID-PCR test
B. COVID antibody test
C. ANCA
D. MRI kidneys
E. Blood cultures

Answer: C

In the current era of clinical medicine, a patient presenting with respiratory symptoms and anosmia, COVID-19 is a key differential diagnosis to consider. However, this patient also has a constellation of other signs and symptoms together with an acute kidney injury which suggests a vasculitic process. Although the chest x-ray suggests a COVID diagnosis, it demonstrates relatively non-specific changes which could also be seen in patients presenting with pulmonary haemorrhage (Goodpastures syndrome). The initial COVID-PCR test is also negative. The presentation above is consistent with a pulmonary-renal syndrome (as evidenced by the systemic symptoms, haemoptysis and haemoproteinuria). Although initial blood tests have been performed, a renal or autoimmune screen is required to include blood testing for ANCA (Option C) and Anti-GBM. This patient will likely go onto have an ultrasound and kidney biopsy (an MRI is not indicated for this presentation). Blood cultures (Option E) are essential to rule out an infective process and may be a key initial investigation but it would not directly help to confirm the diagnosis here.

12. A 75-year-old lady presents with joint pain, leg swelling and nephrotic range proteinuria. An ultrasound reveals kidneys of 13 cm in size. She is referred for a kidney biopsy and the histopathologist makes a diagnosis of AL Amyloidosis. Which stain is useful in confirming the diagnosis of this condition (i.e. shows green birefringence with polarized light)?
    A. Congo Red
    B. Silver stain
    C. Sirus Red
    D. Trichrome
    E. Periodic acid-Schiff

Answer: A

The patient has a diagnosis of amyloidosis (evidenced by the presentation with nephrotic syndrome, kidneys being on the larger size on ultrasound and the confirmatory histological diagnosis). Congo red can be helpful in demonstrating the accumulation of amyloid. With light microscopy it stains a pink or light red colour and shows green birefringence with polarized light. Although this is the classical 'textbook' quoted description of amyloidosis, light microscopy in renal amyloidosis typically reveals diffuse glomerular deposition of amorphous hyaline material. These nodules stain weakly with PAS and methenamine silver stain. Silver stain may show spiking along glomerular capillary loops.

13. Which of the following statements are true in relation to performing a kidney biopsy?
    A. It can always be performed if the size of the kidneys are 7 cm
    B. It is necessary diagnostic tool in adult patients presenting with nephrotic syndrome
    C. Blood pressure does not influence the risk of bleeding post biopsy
    D. It can always be performed in patients with a single kidney

E. Patients should be told there is no risk in losing the kidney post biopsy

Answer: B

Adults with nephrotic syndrome should undergo a kidney biopsy in order to determine the underlying cause (unless there is a contraindication). In option A, the patient may have bilateral shrunken kidneys as a result of chronic kidney disease and a biopsy is contraindicated. Blood pressure needs to be controlled prior to a biopsy in order to minimise bleeding risk (option C) and a single functioning kidney is another contraindication to performing a biopsy. Patients should be counselled about the risks surrounding a kidney biopsy including pain, bleeding, the risk of losing the kidney and death (rare).

Test your learning and check your understanding of this book's contents: use the "Springer Nature Flashcards" app to access questions using https://sn.pub/cz9Cok. To use the app, please follow the instructions in Chap. 1.

References

1. Woodward S, Oliveira D. Renal medicine. 1st ed. London: Scion Publishing; 2016.
2. Goldsmith D, Jayawardene S, Ackland P. 2nd ed. Hoboken: Wiley-Blackwell; 2013.
3. Tarafdar S. Nephrology: a comprehensive guide to renal medicine. 1st ed. Hoboken: Wiley-Blackwell; 2020.
4. Beck LH, Bonegio RG, Lambeau G, et al. M-type phospholipase A2 receptor as target antigen in idiopathic membranous nephropathy. N Engl J Med. 2009;361(1):11–21.
5. Boote EJ. AAPM/RSNA physics tutorial for residents: topics in US: Doppler US techniques: concepts of blood flow detection and flow dynamics. Radiographics. 2003;23(5):1315–27.
6. Zhang J, Morrell G, Rusinek H, et al. New magnetic resonance imaging methods in nephrology. Kidney Int. 2014;85(4):768–78.
7. Visconti L, Cernaro V, Ricciardi C, et al. Renal biopsy: still a landmark for the nephrologist. World J Nephrol. 2016;5(4):321–7.
8. Agarwal S, Sethi S, Dinda A. Basics of kidney biopsy: a nephrologist's perspective. Indian J Nephrol. 2013;23(4):243–52.

Proteinuria and Haematuria

3

David Makanjuola and Dwomoa Adu

Clinical Scenario

A 24 year old white male is admitted to the Renal unit. He has a history of passing frothy urine for a few weeks. He has also noticed lower limb and peri-orbital swelling. His weight has increased by about 4 kg over the last couple of months. He has been short of breath and describes pleuritic left sided chest pain. His tests show the following:

- Urine dipsticks showed blood and proteinuria
- serum creatinine of 90 μmol/L (88–105 μmol/L)
- estimated GFR 78 mL/min/1.73 m^2
- serum albumin 22 mg/dL (35–50 mg/dL)
- serum cholesterol 7.2 mmol/L (2.5–5.0 mmol/L)
- urine total protein to creatinine ratio 530 mg/mmol (<15 mg/mmol)

Proteinuria

Introduction

Richard Bright, a physician at Guy's hospital in 1836, is credited with describing the association of proteinuria and kidney disease. He described 25 cases of dropsy (oedema) which he attributed to kidney disease. Many of these cases were found to have albumin in their urine. The triad of dropsy, albumin in the urine and kidney disease came to be called 'Bright's disease'.

This section will focus on proteinuria, in particular, how the kidneys handle protein excretion normally and in disease states, measurement of proteinuria, types of proteinuria and an approach to the management of the patient with proteinuria.

Pathophysiology

The kidneys receive about 25% of the cardiac output. In a 24 h period, about 70 g/L of protein passes through the kidneys. This equates to about 65 kg of protein, of which less than 100 mg appears in the urine. The glomerular capillary wall and the tubules play a major role in this.

Glomerular Barrier

The glomerular barrier is composed of the endothelial cell, an acellular basement membrane and the epithelial cell. The endothelial cells are fenestrated with 50–100 nm pores. The basement

D. Makanjuola (✉)
South West Thames Renal and Transplantation Unit, Epsom and St. Helier Hospitals NHS Trust, London, UK
e-mail: david.makanjuola@nhs.net

D. Adu
University of Ghana Medical School, Accra, Ghana

D. Banerjee et al. (eds.), *Management of Kidney Diseases*,
https://doi.org/10.1007/978-3-031-09131-5_3

membrane is about 300 nm thick, divided into the lamina rara interna, the lamina densa and the lamina rara externa. It is made up of different components including type IV collagen, laminin, and heparan sulphate proteoglycans. The foot processes (podocytes) of the epithelial cells interdigitate and form the outer layer of the basement membrane. The podocytes are separated by slit diaphragms, about 55 nm in width.

Low molecular weight proteins and water can freely pass through the glomerular capillary basement membrane, but larger molecular weight proteins have restricted passage due to their size and also their electrical charge, as most proteins are negatively charged and the basement membrane has a negative charge which repels most plasma proteins. In effect, the lamina rara interna is an impediment to charged molecules, the lamina densa further restricts passage of molecules based on their size and the slit diaphragm provides another barrier beyond this.

Despite this, there is still some passage of protein into the proximal tubule.

Tubular Reabsorption and Secretion

The protein that reaches the tubular lumen is endocytosed at the apical part of the cell membrane by megalin and cubulin. The endocytosed protein is then transferred to lysosomes and catabolised. The amino acids and other substances such as bound vitamins are returned to the circulation and the endocytosed receptors migrate back to the apical membrane.

Large molecular weight proteins can appear in the urine either by secretion from the tubules, or from desquamation of the tubular epithelial cells. Uromodulin (Tamm-Horsfall protein) is the major protein of renal origin, it is secreted from the cells in the thick ascending limb of the loop of Henle and tends to form casts by trapping substances such as albumin, red blood cells, white blood cells, or tubular debris. There is a suggestion that it might play a role in protecting against formation of kidney stones.

Normally therefore, only a small amount of protein reaches the urine, as the glomeruli limit the passage of large molecular weight proteins and the low molecular weight proteins are catabolised by the tubules. In healthy adults, 2–3 g of albumin is presented to the tubules each day, most of which is reabsorbed.

Definitions

Glomerular proteinuria—Glomerular proteinuria is due to increased filtration of protein across the glomerular capillary wall. The proteins are likely to be of large molecular weight and might be predominantly albumin (e.g. minimal change disease), or non-selective larger molecular weight proteins e.g. IgG in other glomerulopathies.

Tubular proteinuria—Interference with proximal tubular reabsorption, due for instance to tubulointerstitial diseases can lead to increased excretion of low-molecular-weight proteins. As described earlier, these proteins are normally freely filtered at the glomerulus, but almost completely reabsorbed and catabolised in the proximal tubule. They include beta 2-microglobulin and retinol-binding protein.

Overflow proteinuria—This is also sometimes called pre-renal proteinuria and is due to overproduction of a particular protein, leading to increased glomerular filtration and excretion. Conditions associated with this include myoglobinuria due to rhabdomyolysis and haemoglobinuria from intravascular haemolysis, but the most common cause is increased immunoglobulin light chains in multiple myeloma. In these conditions, the filtered load exceeds the tubular reabsorptive capacity.

Post-renal proteinuria—This can be seen in conditions such as urinary tract infections, although the mechanism is unclear. The excreted proteins are often non-albumin (often IgA or IgG), and leukocyturia is frequently present in such patients.

Orthostatic proteinuria—This is characterised by differences in protein excretion with changes in posture. Protein excretion is increased when the individual is upright and ambulant, but decreased in the recumbent position. Two to tenfold differences in urine albumin excretion have been reported and the mechanism is unclear. Total protein excretion is generally less than 1 g/

day in orthostatic proteinuria. It is more common in adolescents and is thought to be a benign condition that once confirmed, does not require extensive evaluation or specific therapy.

Measurement of Protein Excretion

Chemical methods used for measuring urine total protein, which are both accurate and precise, are generally adequate for patients with proteinuria >1 g/L. The problem arises when the protein excretion is in the much lower (mg/L) range. The differing urine proteins have variable chromogenicity for the different dyes used in measuring the urine total protein, resulting in different reference ranges. Also, at low total protein levels, the relative contribution of proteins secreted into the urine such as uromodulin, becomes more significant, thus masking within the total protein estimation small, but pathologically significant increases in other urine proteins, such as albumin. The US National Kidney Foundation Guidelines recommend β_2-microglobulin as a marker for tubulo-interstitial disease and albumin as the marker for chronic kidney disease due to diabetes, glomerular diseases and hypertension. Albumin performs well in this regard for determining microalbuminuria, but at higher concentrations of proteinuria, the requirement for repeated dilutions of the sample for accurate measurement of albumin adds considerably to the cost, so some guidelines now suggest that measurement of either urine albumin or total protein is acceptable for monitoring.

Urine Dipstick Test

The standard urine dipstick test for protein is a semi-quantitative chemical test based on the colour change of indicators such as bromophenol blue. The protein section of the dipstick strip contains an acid buffer to maintain the pH at a constant level. The test is more sensitive to albumin because albumin contains more amino groups to accept the hydrogen ions than other proteins.

At a pH level of 3.0, the indicator appears yellow in the absence of protein. However, as the protein concentration increases, the colour progresses through various shades of green and finally to blue. Readings are reported in terms of negative, trace, 1+, 2+, 3+ and 4+, or the semi-quantitative values of 30, 100, 300 or 2000 mg/dL corresponding to each colour change. Trace values are considered to be less than 30 mg/dL.

Interpretation of the reagent strips should be done with the understanding that false-positive readings are obtained when the reaction does not take place under acidic conditions. This would include situations in which:

- there is highly buffered alkaline urine (as seen in patients with urinary tract infections due to urea splitting organisms such as proteus) will override the acid buffer system, producing a rise in pH and a colour change unrelated to protein concentration.
- the reagent pad has remained in contact with the urine for a prolonged period, as this may remove the buffer.

Highly pigmented urine and contamination of the container with quaternary ammonium compounds, detergents, iodinated contrast agents and antiseptics also cause false-positive readings.

False negative readings for protein occur when the predominant protein being excreted is not albumin e.g. Bence-Jones proteins in myeloma, as the urine dipsticks predominantly detect albumin.

Timed Urine Collections

Measurement of urine protein or albumin as a concentration in milligrams or grams per litre does not take into account variations in urine flow rate. This can be corrected by collecting timed (usually 24 h) urine samples and expressing the results in protein mass per unit time (g/24 h).

Timed urine sample collections can be cumbersome and also inaccurate if the patient is not sure about when to start and finish the collection. Expression of the urine albumin or total protein as a ratio to creatinine concentration has been shown in numerous studies to be at least as reproducible as a timed urine collection and it is also more convenient, so most people have moved to using this, rather than timed urine collection to assess protein excretion.

Spot Urine Measurements (Albumin or Total Protein to Creatinine Ratio)

Due to the limitations of a 24-h urine collection described above, the urine albumin-to-creatinine ratio (UACR) or more commonly, the urine protein-to-creatinine ratio (UPCR) in a spot urine sample is measured. The urine protein concentration is measured in mg/dL and is divided by the urine creatinine concentration, measured in mg/dL, or mmol/L, yielding a number that estimates the 24-h protein excretion in grams per day.

There are two major limitations of using random spot urine samples to quantify proteinuria:

- The UPCR and UACR are heavily influenced by the urine creatinine concentration and therefore by the total daily creatinine production. The accuracy of the ratio is diminished if creatinine excretion is either markedly higher or lower than the average population value of 1000 mg/day. So, in individuals with large muscle mass, in whom creatinine excretion may be much higher than 1000 mg/day, the UPCR (or UACR) will underestimate proteinuria and conversely, in a patient with small muscle mass, in whom creatinine excretion may be much lower than 1000 mg/day, the UPCR (or UACR) will overestimate proteinuria.
- Urine protein excretion can vary throughout the day (especially resulting from exercise and posture) and from day to day.

It is well established that on a population level, the 24-h urine protein excretion and the spot UPCR are reasonably well correlated, but this may not necessarily hold true in the individual patient especially at lower levels of proteinuria as described above. It is important to remember this, as treatment decisions, such as the initiation or discontinuation of immunosuppressive agents and choice of anti-hypertensive therapy, are often based upon the degree of proteinuria in a given patient.

In order to address some of these limitations, some authors have devised another measure called the 'estimated albumin excretion rate' (eAER). It is calculated by multiplying the UACR by the expected 24 h creatinine generation, which can be calculated using a variety of equations. This may be particularly useful in patients who have very large or very small muscle mass. A similar calculation is also available for estimating the protein excretion rate (ePER) to creatinine ratio along the same principles.

Clinical Associations

Microalbuminuria

This term is used to describe an increase in urine albumin that is detectable by sensitive immunoassays but is below the limit of detection by chemical urine protein methods and dipstick tests. It is defined as an albumin excretion rate of 30–300 mg/24 h, or and albumin to creatinine ratio of 3–30 mg/mmol. Microalbuminuria is important, because studies have shown that it is a risk factor for micro- and macrovascular complications in patients with and without diabetes. Further studies have shown that microalbuminuria is associated with acute inflammatory conditions and is a reflection of systemic endothelial dysfunction. In some conditions, such as diabetes, microalbuminuria has been found to be reversible with interventions such as renin-angiotensin-aldosterone system (RAAS) inhibitors.

Isolated, Asymptomatic Proteinuria

This can be either transient or persistent. Transient proteinuria is essentially defined as happening when a subsequent qualitative test for proteinuria is negative. It can occur due to exercise, fever, or following a lower urinary tract infection.

If the proteinuria is persistent, orthostatic proteinuria should be considered. This can be ruled out by doing a 24 h urine collection, but split into two 12 h periods. The patient should collect urine during the waking hours, then collect a second sample overnight, including the first urine sample the following morning. Orthostatic proteinuria is confirmed if the urine protein excretion is normal in the recumbent sample, but high in the daytime sample.

Persistent isolated proteinuria needs full investigation for an underlying renal disorder by a nephrologist, as it might represent evolving glomerular or tubular disease.

Glomerular Proteinuria

A protein excretion rate of >3.0 g/24 h is unlikely to be solely due to tubular disease. This degree of loss of proteins is usually due to glomerular disease. The increased glomerular permeability may be associated with otherwise normal kidney function, acute kidney injury, or chronic kidney disease. Nephrotic syndrome is defined as proteinuria severe enough to cause hypoalbuminaemia, and the presence of oedema. The degree of proteinuria is usually in excess of 3 g/24 h.

The glomerular disease may be due to primary glomerular disorders such as minimal change disease or focal and segmental glomerulosclerosis, secondary to conditions such as diabetes, amyloidosis, or immunological conditions such as membranous glomerulopathy or lupus nephritis.

Some causes of the nephrotic syndrome are as follows:

Minimal change disease. On light microscopy, little if any abnormalities are seen, but on electron microscopy, there is effacement/fusion of the podocytes of the epithelial cells. The pathogenesis is not fully understood, but it is very common in children, less so in adults. It is usually very steroid responsive, but steroid resistant forms are also well recognised.

Membranous nephropathy. Primary (idiopathic) and secondary forms are recognised. Up to 70% of patients with the primary form have been found to have anti-phospholipase A2 receptor (PLA2R) antibodies. A smaller proportion have other antibodies such as anti-thombospondin type 1 domain containing 7A (THSD7A) antibodies. Secondary forms are due to class V lupus nephritis, Hepatitis B virus infection, drugs, and some cancers.

Focal and segmental glomerulosclerosis. The primary form is characterised by the nephrotic syndrome and the presence of focal sclerosis in a proportion of the glomeruli on light microscopy. Steroids are first line therapy, but the response is less good than is seen in patients with minimal change disease. It is also known to re-occur in the renal transplant.

Patients with the nephrotic syndrome also have abnormalities of other plasma proteins. There are changes in the concentration of circulating clotting factors. Anti-thrombin III, a natural anticoagulant, is lost in the urine and the serum levels of factors V, VII, VIII and IX are increased, leading to a prothrombotic state. Vitamin D and vitamin D binding globulin are also lost in the urine, which may lead to vitamin D deficiency. Hyperlipidaemia also occurs and this is believed to be due to reduced clearance and increased hepatic synthesis of very low density lipoprotein (VLDL) and low density lipoprotein (LDL), as well as increased urinary loss of high density lipoprotein (HDL). VLDL and LDL are potentially atherogenic and have been linked to the increased cardiovascular risk in these patients.

Tubular Proteinuria

In contrast to glomerular proteinuria, protein excretion in tubular proteinuria is usually less than 2 g/24 h. The dominant proteins are low molecular weight proteins <60,000 Da, rather than albumin. Under normal circumstances, the majority of filtered proteins are reabsorbed and catabolised by the tubules, but with tubular disease, the reabsorption of proteins, together with water, glucose, amino acids and other compounds such as bicarbonate, is impaired.

Glomerular proteinuria may also cause tubular disease, as absorption of the large amounts of plasma proteins being presented to the tubules causes inflammation and secondary tubular damage. In addition to the proteinuria, tubulo-interstitial disease can be associated with impaired handling of sodium, potassium, bicarbonate, amino acids, phosphate and uric acid.

The enzyme most commonly used to monitor tubular damage is N-acetyl β-D-glucosaminidase (NAG). It is a high molecular weight protein released by damaged tubular cells. Low molecular weight markers of tubular dysfunction include β_2-microglobulin and Retinol-binding protein.

Overflow Proteinuria

This can be defined as the occurrence of high amounts of proteins filtered through the glomeruli in the absence of any primary glomerular or tubular abnormality. Essentially, the increased amounts of protein delivered to the glomeruli exceed the tubular reabsorptive capacity causing the proteins to 'overflow' into the urine.

This includes conditions such as:

Myoglobinuria—myoglobin (Mb) has a molecular weight of 17,500 Da and is freely filtered at the glomerulus. It is released into the circulation when skeletal muscle damage (rhabdomyolysis) occurs. It is not just the presence of myoglobin in the tubules that causes the tubular injury, as infusion of pure myoglobin does not in general cause kidney damage. Acidosis as a result of the cause of the rhabdomyolysis may lead to the formation of metmyoglobin (Fe^{3+}Mb), which induces lipid peroxidation via reactive oxygen species.

Haemoglobinuria—Pure haemoglobin is not nephrotoxic, but a bit like myoglobin, acidosis and dehydration during severe haemolytic episodes may lead to formation of methaemoglobin and subsequent nephrotoxicity.

Bence Jones proteinuria—Bence Jones proteins characteristically precipitate between 45 and 60 °C (113 and 140 °F) and dissolve again between 90 and 95 °C (194 and 203 °F). In 1847, Henry Bence Jones, a Chemical Pathologist at St. George's hospital in London, surmised that these particular proteins, found in the urine, were a biomarker for patients with multiple myeloma. In the 1960s, other investigators, including Gerald Edelman showed that they were immunoglobulin light chains.

Free light chains (22–24,000 Da) are usually cleared from the circulation by glomerular filtration and then catabolised by the proximal tubules. The normal production rate is 500 mg/day and the tubular reabsorptive capacity is 10–30 g/day, so the production of the light chains must be substantially increased for overflow to occur. Multiple myeloma and other B-cell malignancies can lead to significantly increased amounts of light chains. With regards to causing tubular dysfunction, it is not just the amount, but also the type of light chains that seems to matter. Specific amino acid sequences in the variable (V_L) domain in particular produce a Fanconi syndrome. The light chains can also polymerise with Tamm-Horsfall protein, forming the typical myeloma casts.

Management

Once proteinuria is detected, it is important to determine whether it is transient or persistent. Patients with transient proteinuria can be reassured and do not need further investigation. Patients with persistent proteinuria however, need to have it looked into further to determine the cause and to institute appropriate management. An algorithm for management is shown in Fig. 3.1.

A full clinical and laboratory assessment should be carried out. This should include a renal

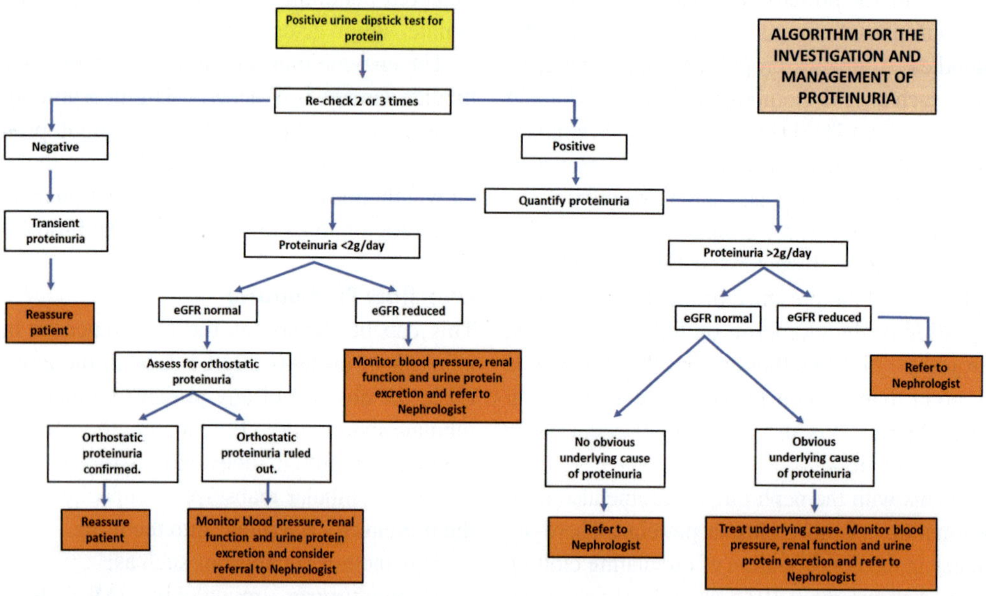

Fig. 3.1 Algorithm for the investigation and management of haematuria

biopsy in all patients with nephrotic range proteinuria unless it is not safe to do so, or if the biopsy is felt to be unlikely to change the management (e.g. in a patient with features very suggestive of diabetic nephropathy).

Other indications for performing a renal biopsy include:

- proteinuria persistently greater than 1 g/day
- co-existent glomerular haematuria
- reduction in estimated GFR

These measures will often identify underlying causes such as diabetes, hypertension, lupus nephritis, myeloma and amyloidosis. Specific treatment for these conditions should be instituted. It is important also to look for associated signs of cardiovascular disease and treat them.

Prognosis

Microalbuminuria has been found to be an independent risk factor for all-cause mortality, cardiovascular disease, and long-term end stage kidney failure. It is also a predictor of outcome in critically ill patients following insults such as major trauma, surgery and sepsis and this is even more marked in patients with underlying chronic kidney disease.

Isolated non-nephrotic proteinuria may have a much more benign course, although a fraction of such patients eventually develop renal dysfunction, especially those with higher amounts of proteinuria, though still in the non-nephrotic range.

Nephrotic-range proteinuria is however associated with poor renal outcomes in patients with primary and secondary glomerular diseases. Treatments to reduce proteinuria such as RAAS inhibitors have been found to be renoprotective.

Haematuria

Introduction

Haematuria can be microscopic (non-visible)—less than 3 red blood cells per microliter, or macroscopic (visible). The overarching anxiety about any observation of haematuria is the possibility of an underlying cancer and this dominates all the diagnostic guidelines. The anxiety is greater in individuals with asymptomatic microscopic haematuria who may be exposed to unnecessary and at times invasive procedures such as cystoscopy in an attempt to exclude a malignancy. The significance of haematuria varies significantly in different parts of the world. Thus, in Africa it is important to consider a diagnosis of schistosomiasis and also of sickle cell disease or trait. All patients with haematuria should have a careful history and clinical investigation.

Different countries have developed guidelines for the investigation of haematuria and indeed there is a guide to the guidelines [2]. We will not critique these guidelines but instead will provide a framework for the investigation of haematuria. Of the various guidelines, that of the UK Renal Association and British Association of Urological Surgeons combines clarity with simplicity [1] (Fig. 3.2).

It is unclear what proportion of patients with haematuria have nephrological as opposed to urological causes, because many patients with negative urological investigations do not have a renal biopsy. However, the most common causes of glomerular haematuria are IgA nephropathy and thin membrane nephropathy. There are several useful reviews of the causes of and investigations of haematuria [3, 4]. These also list the many causes of haematuria and so we will only discuss selected ones.

History

A careful history and examination may provide clues to the cause of the haematuria. Systemic symptoms and a family history may suggest the possibility of vasculitis or polycystic kidney disease and terminal haematuria suggests a bladder cause, for example. The causes of haematuria are summarized in Table 3.1.

Investigation of Haematuria

Dipstick Testing of Urine [5]

Microscopic haematuria is detected by dipstick testing of the urine. Cellulose strips impregnated with peroxidase, orthotolidine, and buffers detect

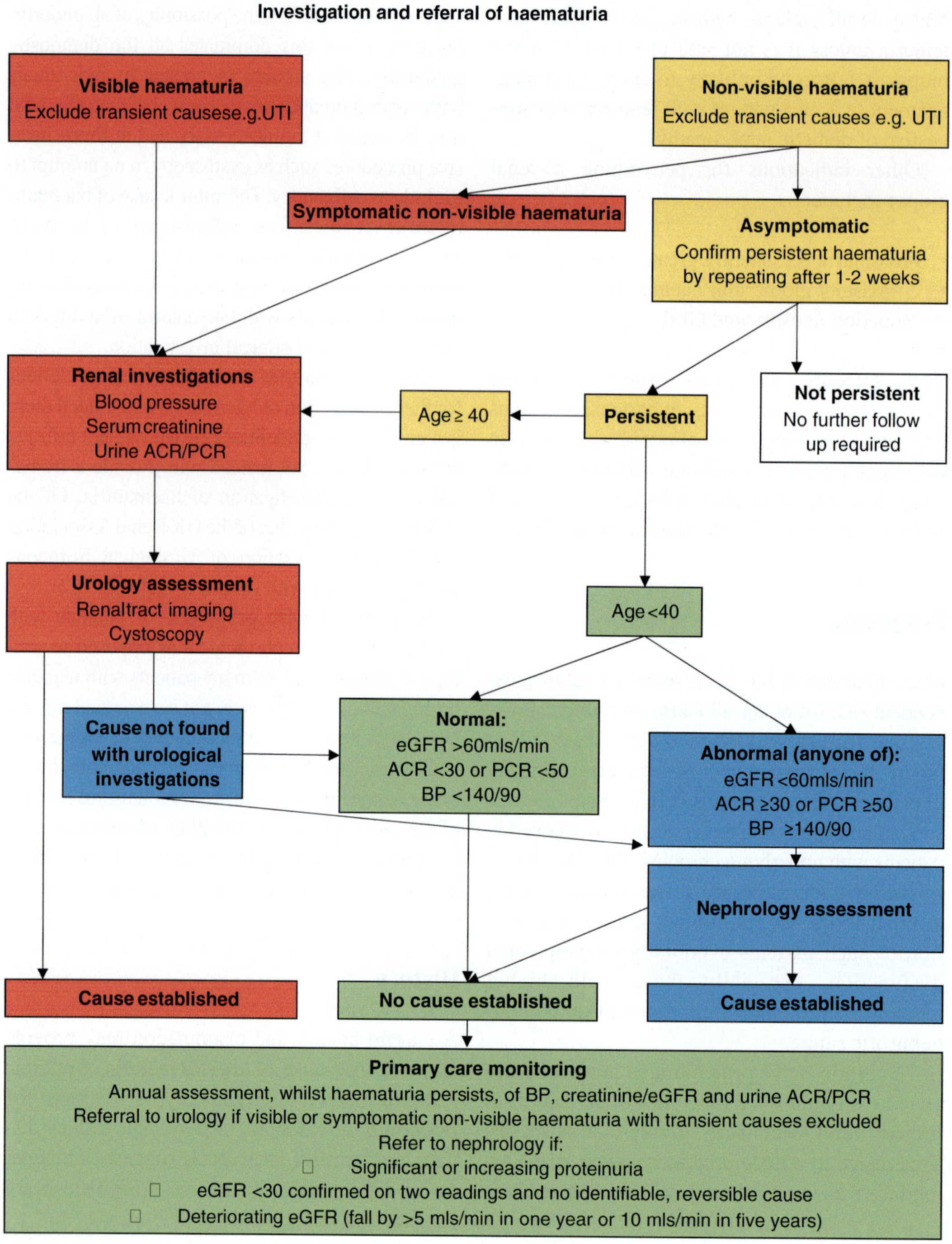

Fig. 3.2 Decision algorithm for the investigation and referral of haematuria (adapted from BUS/RA guidelines [1])

Table 3.1 Causes of haematuria

Causes of haematuria	
Extra-renal	Bladder and urothelial tumours Prostate tumour Ureter Benign prostatic hyperplasia Calculi Infection: Schistosoma haematobium
Renal parenchymal	Renal tumours-hypernephroma Sickle cell disease/trait Renal calculi Polycystic disease of the kidneys Medullary sponge kidney
Glomerular	IgA nephropathy Familial nephropathy/Thin glomerular basement disease Alport's syndrome
Other	Drugs: Heparin, warfarin, aspirin, cyclophosphamide Systemic bleeding disorders Trauma

the peroxidase activity of heme in urinary red blood cells (RBCs), haemoglobin, or myoglobin with a sensitivity of 91–100% and a specificity of 65–99%.

> **Practice Point**
>
> False negative haematuria dipstick tests will result if the urine contains a reducing agent (e.g. ascorbic acid), is acidic, or is diluted, voided after taking fluid. False positives will occur if the urine contains myoglobin, oxidising agents, contaminants, bacterial peroxidase, or if the urine is an early morning concentrated sample. Microscopic examination of the urine is mandatory if a dipstick test is positive. If, however, the result of a dipstick test is repeatedly negative, then further investigation is not necessary.

Microscopic Examination of the Urinary Sediment

Several factors can influence the microscopic detection of RBCs. RBCs are better preserved in acidic and concentrated urine and so the first morning urine sample should be used for urine microscopy. Strenuous exercise can lead to haematuria and should be avoided for 2–3 days before the collection of urine for microscopy. To reduce the likelihood of contamination, a midstream urine is used for the purpose of this examination. Birch and Fairly reported on a differentiation method of a group of diseases with haematuria, into glomerular and non-glomerular bleeding, based on morphological differences in urinary RBCs [6].

The presence of dysmorphic RBCs or cells with a low mean corpuscular volume is believed to indicate glomerular bleeding; isomorphic RBCs, or cells with a normal mean corpuscular volume are thought to originate from post-glomerular sources. The cause of the distortion which affects RBCs of glomerular origin is not known. The RBC morphology can be readily evaluated using light microscopy or phase-contrast microscopy [6].

Imaging Investigations

A wide variety of techniques for imaging the kidneys and urinary tract in patients with haematuria are now available. The optimal imaging technique is one which provides a definitive answer with the minimum of radiation and discomfort or danger for the patient. These choices are best made following consultation with radiological colleagues and many centres will have regular reviews of imaging involving radiologists, nephrologists and urologists.

In investigating a patient with renal disease, the ultrasound scan will establish the size of the kidneys, the nature of the renal parenchyma, the presence or absence of renal cysts, the presence or absence of obstruction to the urinary tract, and the integrity of the renal vasculature.

Cystoscopy

Many centers have established one-stop clinics for haematuria in which imaging of the kidneys and cystoscopy are performed [7–9]. These clinics have been reported to be cost effective. A study of the practice in Nordic countries recommended against cystoscopy in people with asymptomatic microscopic haematuria [10]. However microscopic haematuria at the time of bladder cancer diagnosis was associated with a lower disease stage than in patients with macroscopic haematuria [11]. We would recommend cystoscopy for patients aged over 40 years with persistent microscopic haematuria.

Microscopic Haematuria

The prevalence of microscopic haematuria varies widely. It is less common in children at between 0.6 and 4% and the prevalence increases with age affecting up to 20% of adults aged over 60 years as shown in a review [12]. The major causes of transient microscopic haematuria are urinary tract infection and repeated foot striking in exercise. Urine should be retested after the infection is treated and 3 days after exercise to confirm the haematuria. Persistent non-visible haematuria should be investigated.

Macroscopic Haematuria

Macroscopic haematuria is an alarm signal for cancer [10]. Of the patients with macroscopic haematuria, 18.9% had a malignancy and by contrast a malignancy was found in 4.8% of patients with microscopic haematuria. Cancer was more common in men (13.6%) than in women (9.1%) and was more commonly observed in people aged over 40 (12.8%) than in those aged <40 (3.4%) [13].

Causes of Haematuria

The causes of haematuria are many and varied and are summarized in Table 3.1.

Glomerular Disease

The commonest causes of glomerular haematuria are IgA nephropathy, thin basement membrane disease and diffuse proliferative glomerulonephritis. Patients with systemic symptoms may have a vasculitis or systemic lupus erythematosus. As a general rule, patients with potentially progressive glomerular disease will have albuminuria with a urine albumin:creatinine ratio in excess of 3.5 mg/mmol.

Cancer

Studies of the prevalence of cancers in patients with microscopic or macroscopic haematuria are subject to selection bias. However, 13.2–24.2% of subjects with macroscopic haematuria and 1.2–9.4% of those with microscopic haematuria had a cancer [8, 9, 13–15]. In adults an important cause of microscopic haematuria is urine infection [7].

The significance of haematuria is different in men and in women, in young and in older adults. The risk of cancer is higher with increasing age at 14.5% and 9.8% respectively in men and women aged over 40 years and 4.2 and 2% in men and women respectively aged <40 years [13]. Most of the cancers were picked up by cystoscopy and ultrasonography, making these the investigations of choice.

Urine cytology has poor sensitivity and is not recommended as a screening investigation for haematuria [16, 17]. In young people (<40 years), especially young females, cancer is an uncommon cause of asymptomatic non-visible haematuria, and a glomerular cause is more likely.

Schistosoma Haematobium Infection (Bilharzia): [18, 19]

Schistosoma haematobium infection is a neglected tropical disease that affects over 200 million people in Africa and is an important cause of haematuria. Humans acquire schistosomiasis following exposure to fresh water that contains cercariae. These cercariae are released by the intermediate host - freshwater snails, and cross the skin and settle in the peri-vesical plexus. Eggs laid by adult female worms pass into the bladder

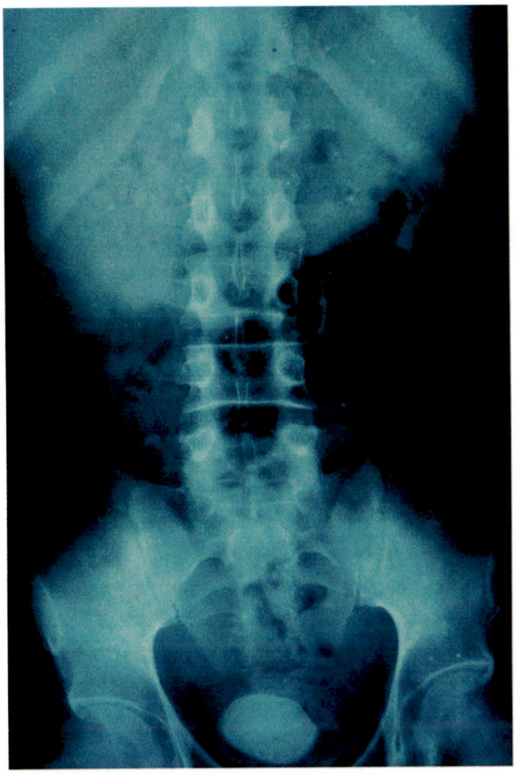

Fig. 3.3 Plain abdominal radiograph in a patient with Schistosoma haematobium infection showing a calcified bladder and a bladder stone

and genito-urinary tract where they cause inflammation, ulceration and haematuria.

With time, untreated schistosomiasis leads to bladder wall thickening and pseudo-polyps. Granulomata and inflammation at the ureteric orifice can lead to obstruction and hydronephrosis.

Cystoscopy shows sandy patches and pseudo-polyps and in late cases may show a cancer—usually squamous cell carcinoma of the bladder in 60% of cases and transitional cell carcinoma in 20% of cases. Diagnosis of schistosomiasis is with urine microscopy, which shows the typical eggs that have a terminal spine. Investigations include ultrasound scan and CT urography. A calcified bladder or ureters may be seen on abdominal radiographs and also calculi of infective aetiology (Fig. 3.3). Treatment with praziquantel results in high cure rates and when used community-wide in endemic areas, has been shown to reduce the prevalence of urinary tract abnormalities.

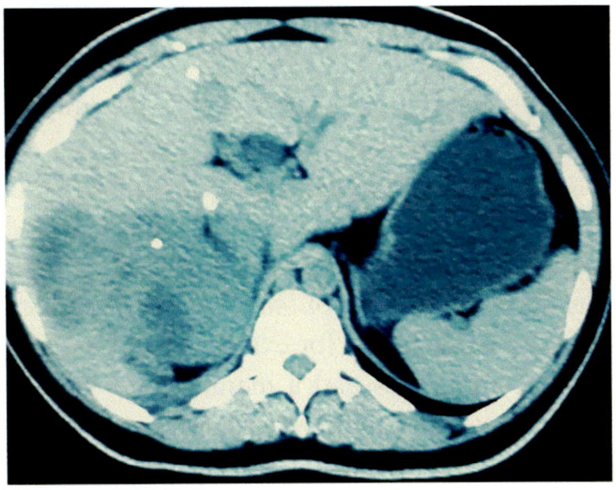

Fig. 3.4 CT scan of the abdomen in a patient with sickle cell trait (Haemoglobin AS) showing a heterogenous mass replacing the right kidney. Biopsy showed sheets of tumour cells with focal adenoid cystic-like pattern within desmoplastic stroma and admixed with neutrophils. Features were consistent with renal medullary cell carcinoma

Sickle Cell Disease and Trait

Sickle cell disease is a major public health burden in Sub-Saharan Africa and it is estimated that in 2010, 200,000–300,000 children were born with this disorder [20]. Microscopic haematuria is common in patients with both sickle cell disease and trait, and less commonly macroscopic haematuria, that may be persistent, is seen [21]. The usual management is with conservative measures only.

It is worthwhile screening for other causes of haematuria in these patients, e.g. schistosomiasis. Renal papillary necrosis is found in both sickle cell disease and sickle cell trait [21]. The clinical presentation is with haematuria that on occasion may be complicated by clot colic. Diagnosis is confirmed by CT urography, showing changes ranging from clubbing of calyces to a ring sign in which an often calcified, partly attached papilla is surrounded by a ring of contrast.

Renal medullary cell carcinoma is a rare malignant epithelial tumour that occurs in young individuals aged between 10 and 39 years with sickle cell trait [22]. The presentation is with macroscopic haematuria and abdominal pain and diagnosis is by ultrasound or CT scan (Fig. 3.4). The prognosis is poor.

Conclusions

The discussed case demonstrates the importance of the initial urine and blood tests in establishing the cause of proteinuria, this patient has nephrotic syndrome which required a kidney biopsy for establishing the diagnosis. The histopathology of the biopsied kidney guides the diagnosis; for example, positive anti PLA2R antibodies and a membranous pattern on biopsy may require immunosuppressive therapy guided by the antibody levels.

Questions

1. A 23-year-old woman presents with lower limb oedema and blood tests show a serum albumin of 22 mg/dL, cholesterol 8.7 mmol/L, creatinine 89 μmol/L. Her 24 h urine protein excretion is 7.5 g. Renal biopsy shows minimal change disease. Which one of the following statements is true?
   A. Minimal change disease accounts for about 50% of all adult nephrotic syndrome.
   B. The nephrotic syndrome may be associated with Indomethacin use.
   C. The nephrotic syndrome manifests with proteinuria, oedema and hyperalbuminaemia.
   D. The nephrotic syndrome is often accompanied by macroscopic haematuria.
   E. She is unlikely to have hypercholesterolaemia.
2. A 12-year-old boy is accompanied by his mother to the Emergency Dept. He developed a sore throat and joint pains. About 3 days later, he noticed macroscopic haematuria. His Hb was 14 g/dL, WBC 8.7 × 10^9/L, creatinine 66 μmol/L, clotting screen was normal. Urinalysis showed blood 3+ and protein 1+. Which one of the following is the most likely diagnosis?
   A. Reflux nephropathy.
   B. Diabetic glomerulosclerosis.
   C. Membranous glomerulonephritis.
   D. Light-chain nephropathy.
   E. Henoch-Schoenlein purpura.
3. A patient known to have type 1 diabetes for 15 years is found to have proteinuria. His blood tests show a creatinine of 155 μmol/L, urea 18 mmol/L, HbA1c 9.6%. 24 h urine protein excretion was 1.8 g. Which one of the following statements would be true of clinical diabetic nephropathy?
   A. It is unusual in patients with type 2 diabetes mellitus of <5 years duration from diagnosis.
   B. It is unlikely to occur in a patient free of proteinuria after 40 years of diabetes.
   C. It is usually associated with urinary albumin excretion of 50–100 mg/24 h.
   D. Renal functional decline can be halted by angiotensin II receptor blockers.
   E. It can be reversed by meticulous control of blood glucose.
4. A 45-year old lady presents with proteinuria, hypoalbuminaemia, normal renal function, oedema and hyperlipidaemia. A kidney biopsy shows membranous nephropathy. Which of the following is true?
   A. SLE is not a recognised cause of membranous nephropathy.
   B. Silver stain of the renal biopsy will show 'spikes' which represent new basement membrane growing between the immune deposits.
   C. Malignancy is a common cause of membranous nephropathy.
   D. Steroids are the treatment of choice in all cases, leading to complete remission in about 30% of patients.
   E. The M-type phospholipase A2 receptor (PLA2R) has been identified as a major antigen in ANCA positive glomerulonephritis.
5. A 35-year old male presents with repeated episodes of proteinuria and synpharyngitic haematuria. His renal function is normal. Which of the following statements is true?
   A. A biopsy should always be performed even in the absence of proteinuria, hypertension and renal impairment.
   B. IgA nephropathy never presents as a rapidly progressive glomerulonephritis.

C. In the presence of proteinuria (>1 g), a low protein diet and ACE inhibitors are indicated, aiming for a blood pressure of <140/80 mmHg.
D. Haematuria is not a marker of progressive disease.
E. Proteinuria is not a marker of progressive disease in IgA nephropathy.

6. A 78-year old man presents with proteinuria and oedema. His blood tests show a creatinine of 155 μmol/L, urea 18 mmol/L, 24 h urine protein excretion 6.8 g. The immunoglobulins were normal, but the serum free light chains showed elevated free kappa light chains and an abnormal kappa to lambda light chain ratio.

   Which one of the following statements is true?
   A. A renal biopsy would not be necessary for establishing the diagnosis.
   B. The proteinuria is most likely to be due to tubular damage from the free light chains.
   C. The Congo red stain is likely to be positive on the renal biopsy.
   D. Renal functional decline can be halted by angiotensin II receptor blockers.
   E. Further evaluation with a SAP scan is unlikely to be of benefit.

7. A 19-year old male is found to have proteinuria at a routine medical test. He is asymptomatic. His blood tests show a creatinine of 75 μmol/L, estimated GFR >90 mL/min, serum albumin 40 mg/dL. Which one of the following statements would be true with regards to orthostatic proteinuria?
   A. It is characterised by differences in protein excretion with changes in posture.
   B. The total protein excretion is usually more than 1 g/day.
   C. It is not thought to be a benign condition and if confirmed, requires evaluation and specific therapy.
   D. The diagnosis can be confirmed on the basis of two random urine samples done in the afternoon.
   E. It is more common in the elderly.

8. Which of the following statements about the renal handling of proteins is correct?
   A. Proteins, due to their positive charge, have free passage through the glomerulus.
   B. The slit diaphragm acts as a barrier to free movement of large molecular weight proteins on the endothelial side of the basement membrane.
   C. Megalin and Cubulin are situated on the baso-lateral aspect of the tubular cells.
   D. Proteins in the tubular fluid are endocytosed and catabolised into their constituent amino acids.
   E. The glomerular basement membrane has a net positive charge.

9. Which of the following statements is true?
   A. Tamm Horsfall proteins are secreted by the glomeruli.
   B. Bence Jones proteins precipitate at 4 °C, but dissolve on re-warming.
   C. Retinol binding protein is a marker of glomerular proteinuria.
   D. Tubular proteinuria is characterised by urine protein excretion greater than 3 g/day.
   E. Urine protein excretion can vary throughout the day.

10. A 24-year old white male is admitted to the Renal unit. He has a history of passing frothy urine for a few weeks. He has also noticed lower limb and peri-orbital swelling. His weight has increased by about 4 kg over the last couple of months. He has been short of breath and describes pleuritic left sided chest pain. His tests show the following:

    Serum creatinine 90 μmol/L (88–105 μmol/L).

    Estimated GFR 78 mL/min.

    Serum albumin 22 mg/dL (35–50 mg/dl).

    Serum cholesterol 7.2 mmol/L (2.5–5.0 mmol/L).

    Urine total protein to creatinine ratio 530 mg/mmol (<15 mg/mmol).

    Which of the following statements is correct?
    A. His chest pain is likely to be musculoskeletal and he should be given simple analgesia.
    B. The hypercholesterolaemia is an unusual finding in the nephrotic syndrome.

C. He is at an increased risk of venous thrombo-embolic disease.
D. Diuretic therapy will be sufficient treatment for his nephrotic syndrome.
E. The raised urine protein excretion is likely to be due to tubular proteinuria.

Answers

1. **B**

Minimal-change disease is the most common cause of the nephrotic syndrome in children. It accounts for 70–90% of cases in children who are younger than 10 years and 50% in older children. It is also an important cause in adults of all ages, accounting for 10–15% of cases. It manifests with oedema, hypoalbuminaemia and proteinuria. Macroscopic haematuria is not a feature of the syndrome. Hyperlipidaemia occurs due to reduced clearance and increased hepatic synthesis of very low density lipoprotein and low density lipoprotein, as well as increased urinary loss of high density lipoprotein. Non-steroidal anti-inflammatory drugs are recognised causes of the nephrotic syndrome.

2. **E**

Although proteinuria can be seen in all the other conditions listed, the macroscopic haematuria would be most likely to be seen in Henoch-Schoenlein purpura.

3. **B**

Diabetic nephropathy is unlikely to be the cause of *de novo* proteinuria after 40 years from diagnosis. It is not always clear for how long patients with type 2 diabetes mellitus have had the condition before they were diagnosed, so it is possible for diabetic nephropathy to be detected in some patients in whom the duration from the diagnosis of diabetes is less than 5 years. Diabetic nephropathy is by definition, present when there is overt proteinuria, rather than just microalbuminuria. The progression of renal disease in patients with diabetic nephropathy can be delayed by angiotensin converting enzyme inhibitors and also by angiotensin II receptor blockers, but they do not halt its progression. It cannot be reversed by meticulous control of blood glucose.

4. **B**

SLE is a recognised cause of membranous nephropathy (class 5 lupus nephritis). The 'spikes' on the silver stain on light microscopy of the renal biopsy represent basement membrane between the immune deposits. The M-type phospholipase A2 receptor (PLA2R) has been identified as a major antigen in patients with idiopathic membranous glomerulonephritis. Malignancy is a recognised association, but is not a common cause of membranous nephropathy. Steroids have been found to be useful as part of treatment regimens for membranous nephropathy, but they are not used in all cases.

5. **D**

IgA nephropathy is the most common glomerulopathy in the developed world. Synpharyngitic haematuria is the typical presentation for 50% of the cases, 40% are found on routine testing for renal abnormalities (any kind) and 10% have acute presentations (including RPGN and nephrotic syndrome).

Haematuria is not a marker of progressive disease. Proteinuria on the other hand reflects an abnormal permanent activation of mesangial cells causing permanent damage in the filter barrier and is a marker of disease progression. A biopsy is not usually performed in the absence of significant proteinuria, hypertension or renal impairment because the prognosis is excellent if these are absent. In proteinuric disease an ACE inhibitor (or angiotensin receptor blocker) is the initial drug of choice.

6. **C**

This patient is likely to have light chain induced renal disease and it would be important to do a renal biopsy to establish the diagnosis. Although the light chains can cause tubular toxicity, the degree of proteinuria suggests that there must also be glomerular disease. One manifestation of light chain induced renal disease is amyloidosis and the Congo red stain would be positive on light microscopy. A serum amyloid P (SAP) scan would be useful in determining the extent of organ involvement. Angiotensin receptor blockers will help attenuate the proteinuria but will not halt the disease process.

7. **A**

Orthostatic proteinuria is more common in adolescents and is characterised by differences in protein excretion with changes in posture. The total protein excretion is usually less than 1 g/day. Confirmation is by doing a 24 h urine collection, split into two 12 h periods. The patient should collect urine during the waking hours, then collect a second sample overnight, including the first urine sample the following morning. Orthostatic proteinuria is confirmed if the urine protein excretion is normal in the recumbent sample, but high in the daytime sample. It is thought to be a benign condition and if confirmed, does not require extensive evaluation or specific therapy.

8. **D**

The glomerular basement membrane has a net negative charge and proteins, due to their negative charge, have restricted passage through the glomerulus. The slit diaphragm is situated on foot processes (podocytes) of the glomerular epithelial cells. Megalin and Cubulin are situated on the apical aspect of the tubular cells and are believed to be responsible for the endocytosis on proteins in the tubular fluid. The proteins are then catabolised into their constituent amino acids.

9. **E**

Tamm Horsfall proteins are secreted from the cells in the thick ascending limb of the loop of Henle. Cryoglobulins precipitate at 4 °C, but dissolve on re-warming. Bence Jones proteins precipitate between 45 and 60 °C and dissolve again between 90 and 95 °C. Retinol binding protein is a low molecular weight protein and is a marker of tubular proteinuria. Tubular proteinuria is characterised by urine protein excretion less than 1 g/day. Urine protein excretion can vary throughout the day.

10. **C**

He is at an increased risk of venous thrombo-embolic disease. Changes in the concentration of circulating clotting factors, including anti-thrombin III, lead to a pro-thrombotic state. His chest pain is more likely to be due to pulmonary embolism and he will need further investigation e.g. CT pulmonary angiography for this. Hypercholesterolaemia is a common finding in the nephrotic syndrome. The cause of the nephrotic syndrome needs to be identified and appropriate treatment instigated. Diuretic therapy on its own is unlikely to be sufficient treatment for his nephrotic syndrome. The raised urine protein excretion is likely to be due to glomerular proteinuria.

Test your learning and check your understanding of this book's contents: use the "Springer Nature Flashcards" app to access questions using https://sn.pub/cz9Cok. To use the app, please follow the instructions in Chap. 1.

References

1. Anderson J, Fawcett D, Feehally J, Goldberg L, Kelly MJ, MacTier R, et al. Joint consensus statement on the initial assessment of haematuria. BAUS/RA Guidelines. 2008;2008:1–5.
2. Linder BJ, Bass EJ, Mostafid H, Boorjian SA. Guideline of guidelines: asymptomatic microscopic haematuria. BJU Int. 2018;121(2):176–83.
3. Kelly JD, Fawcett DP, Goldberg LC. Assessment and management of non-visible haematuria in primary care. BMJ. 2009;338:a3021.
4. Ingelfinger JR. Hematuria in adults. N Engl J Med. 2021;385(2):153–63.
5. Simerville JA, Maxted WC, Pahira JJ. Urinalysis: a comprehensive review. Am Fam Physician. 2005;71(6):1153–62.
6. Fairley KF, Birch DF. Hematuria: a simple method for identifying glomerular bleeding. Kidney Int. 1982;21(1):105–8.
7. Lynch T, Waymont B, Dunn J, Hughes M, Wallace D. Rapid diagnostic service for patients with haematuria. Br J Urol. 1994;73(2):147–51.
8. Ooi WL, Lee F, Wallace DMA, Hayne D. 'One stop' haematuria clinic in Fremantle Hospital, Western Australia: a report of the first 500 patients. BJU Int. 2011;108:62–6.
9. Madaan A, Kuusk T, Hamdoon M, Elliott A, Pearce D, Madaan S. Nurse-led one stop hematuria clinic:

outcomes from 2,714 patients. BJUI Compass. 2021;2(6):385–94.
10. Malmström P-U, Skaaheim Haug E, Boström PJ, Gudjónsson S, Bjerggaard Jensen J. Progress towards a Nordic standard for the investigation of hematuria: 2019. Scand J Urol. 2019;53(1):1–6.
11. Ramirez D, Gupta A, Canter D, Harrow B, Dobbs RW, Kucherov V, et al. Microscopic haematuria at time of diagnosis is associated with lower disease stage in patients with newly diagnosed bladder cancer. BJU Int. 2016;117(5):783–6.
12. Fogazzi GB, Edefonti A, Garigali G, Giani M, Zolin A, Raimondi S, et al. Urine erythrocyte morphology in patients with microscopic haematuria caused by a glomerulopathy. Pediatr Nephrol. 2008;23(7):1093–100.
13. Edwards TJ, Dickinson AJ, Natale S, Gosling J, McGrath JS. A prospective analysis of the diagnostic yield resulting from the attendance of 4020 patients at a protocol-driven haematuria clinic. BJU Int. 2006;97(2):301–5; discussion 5.
14. Khadra M, Pickard R, Charlton M, Powell P, Neal D. A prospective analysis of 1,930 patients with hematuria to evaluate current diagnostic practice. J Urol. 2000;163(2):524–7.
15. Tan WS, Feber A, Sarpong R, Khetrapal P, Rodney S, Jalil R, et al. Who should be investigated for haematuria? Results of a contemporary prospective observational study of 3556 patients. Eur Urol. 2018;74(1):10–4.
16. Chahal R, Gogoi NK, Sundaram SK. Is it necessary to perform urine cytology in screening patients with haematuria? Eur Urol. 2001;39(3):283–6.
17. Tan WS, Sarpong R, Khetrapal P, Rodney S, Mostafid H, Cresswell J, et al. Does urinary cytology have a role in haematuria investigations? BJU Int. 2019;123(1):74–81.
18. Barsoum RS. Urinary schistosomiasis: review. J Adv Res. 2013;4(5):453–9.
19. McManus DP, Dunne DW, Sacko M, Utzinger J, Vennervald BJ, Zhou X-N. Schistosomiasis. Nat Rev Dis Primers. 2018;4(1):13.
20. Piel FB, Hay SI, Gupta S, Weatherall DJ, Williams TN. Global burden of sickle cell anaemia in children under five, 2010-2050: modelling based on demographics, excess mortality, and interventions. PLoS Med. 2013;10(7):e1001484.
21. Akinkugbe OO. Renal papillary necrosis in sickle-cell haemoglobinopathy. Br Med J. 1967;3(5560):283–4.
22. Davis CJ Jr, Mostofi F, Sesterhenn IA. Renal medullary carcinoma. The seventh sickle cell nephropathy. Am J Surg Pathol. 1995;19(1):1–11.

Acute Kidney Injury

4

Indre K. Semogas, Jill Vanmassenhove,
Nishkantha Arulkumaran,
and Nicholas M. P. Annear

Clinical Scenario

A 75-year-old female presents to the emergency department with fever and rigors over the preceding 48 h. Her past medical history includes type 2 diabetes mellitus and chronic back pain. Her regular medications include metformin, gliclazide, ramipril, omeprazole, and ibuprofen. On arrival, she is hypotensive and tachycardic, with a temperature of 38 °C. Whilst being fluid resuscitated, and being given prompt broad spectrum antibiotics for presumed sepsis, her laboratory investigations are reported, showing a serum creatinine of 238 μmol/L (2.69 mg/dL); one week prior she had routine blood tests at which time her serum creatinine was 83 μmol/L (0.94 mg/dL).

Throughout this chapter, reflect on this case and consider the following:

- *Can you say with confidence that this represents an acute kidney injury (AKI)?*
- *From this limited information, what factors are likely to be contributing to AKI?*
- *What further information do you want to obtain in the immediate setting to clarify the cause, and identify life-threatening complications?*
- *What implications might concurrent AKI have on the management and prognosis of this patient's underlying diagnosis of sepsis?*

Introduction

Acute kidney injury (AKI) is a clinical syndrome characterized by a sudden decline in kidney function [1]. This is typically reflected through changes in serum creatinine and/or reduction in urine output. The 2012 KDIGO guidelines were published in order to standardize diagnosis, staging, risk stratification, prognostication, and care standards for AKI [1].

Despite the objective diagnostic criteria (Table 4.1), AKI presents heterogeneously, owing to the diversity of patient demographics, possible aetiologies, degrees of severity and resultant complications. The precise management of AKI is therefore reliant on a high degree of clinical acumen, taking into account each of

I. K. Semogas
Imperial College NHS Trust, London, UK

J. Vanmassenhove
Renal Division, Department of Internal Medicine, Ghent University Hospital, Ghent, Belgium
e-mail: jill.vanmassenhove@ugent.be

N. Arulkumaran
University College Hospitals NHS Foundation Trust, London, UK

University College London, London, UK
e-mail: nisharulkumaran@doctors.org.uk

N. M. P. Annear (✉)
St George's University Hospitals Foundation Trust, London, UK

St George's University of London, London, UK
e-mail: nannear@sgul.ac.uk

D. Banerjee et al. (eds.), *Management of Kidney Diseases*,
https://doi.org/10.1007/978-3-031-09131-5_4

Table 4.1 KDIGO diagnostic and staging criteria for acute kidney injury [1]

AKI Stage	Increase in serum creatinine:	Urine output:
Stage 1	≥ 1.5 x baseline creatinine * *or* ≥ 26.5 μmol/L (0.3 mg/dL) within 48 hours	<0.5 mL/kg/hour for 6-12 hours
Stage 2	2.0 – 2.9 x baseline creatinine*	<0.5 mL/kg/hour for ≥ 12 hours
Stage 3	3.0 x baseline creatinine* *or* Rise in creatinine to ≥ 353.6 μmol/L (4.0 mg/dL) *or* Initiation of kidney replacement therapy (KRT) *or* In patients aged 18 years or younger: reduction in eGFR to <35 mL /min per 1.73 m2	<0.3 mL/kg/hour for ≥ 24 hours *or* Anuria for ^{3} 12 hours
KDIGO = Kidney Disease Improving Global Outcomes. eGFR = estimated glomerular filtration rate. **Known or presumed to have occurred within 7 days*		

these variables, whilst incorporating evidence-based guidelines. This chapter highlights the fundamental considerations required in the assessment and management of AKI for the nephrology trainee, which is broadly applicable to most clinical contexts—from community to specialist outpatients, to higher-level inpatient care settings.

AKI, AKD, CKD and NKD

AKI and chronic kidney disease (CKD) represent common presentations for heterogeneous disorders. In practice, some clinical presentations of acute kidney diseases and disorders (AKD) do not meet the criteria for AKI or CKD. In principle, these presentations may be caused by the same diseases that cause AKI or CKD, which could be detected, evaluated, and treated before they evolve to AKI or CKD. By defining AKI as a subset of AKD, in harmony with the definitions of CKD, and further defining the absence of all of these presentations as no known kidney disease (NKD), KDIGO and the nephrology community has sought to develop management recommendations that could potentially improve care and outcomes for this wider group of patients with impaired kidney function not meeting the criteria for either AKI or CKD, but having adverse outcomes and requiring clinical care (Fig. 4.1).

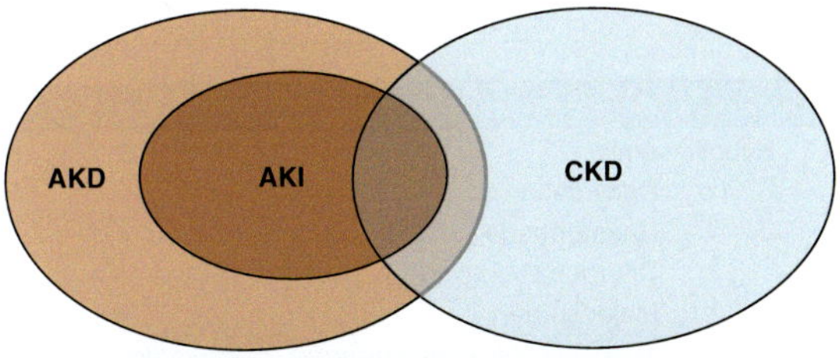

	AKI	AKD	CKD	NKD*
Duration	Within 7 days	≤ 3 months	> 3 months	
Functional Criteria	Increase in Scr by ≥50% within 7 days, OR Increase in SCr by ≥0.3mg/dL (26.5μmol/L) within 2 days, OR Oliguria for ≥4 hours	AKI OR GFR < 60 mL/min/1.73m^2 OR Decrease in GFR by ≥35% x baseline OR Increase in SCr by ≥50% x baseline	GFR < 60 ml/min/1.73m^2	GFR ≥60 ml/min/1.73m^2
Structural Criteria	Not defined	Marker of kidney damage (albuminuria/hematuria/pyuria most common)	Marker of kidney damage (albuminuria most common)	No marker of kidney damage

AKI, acute Kidney injury; AKD, acute kidney diseases and disorders; CKD, chronic kidney disease; NKD, no kidney disease.
•NKD implies no functional or structural criteria according to the definitions for AKI, AKD, or CKD.
Clinical judgment required for individual patient decision making.

Fig. 4.1 Conceptual model of the overlap of AKI, AKD, and CKD and diagnostic criteria [1–3]. Overlapping ovals show the relationships among AKI, AKD, and CKD. AKI is a subset of AKD. Both AKI and AKD without AKI can be superimposed upon CKD. Individuals without AKI, AKD, or CKD have no known kidney disease (NKD)

Epidemiology, Aetiology, and Risk Assessment

AKI carries around a five-fold increased risk of all-cause mortality, contributing to around 1.7 million deaths worldwide each year; the risk of death also increases with AKI stage [4, 5]. Around 1 in 5 adults, and 1 in 3 children admitted to hospital suffer from AKI, although the true incidence varies considerably according to geographic location, and the availability of healthcare resources to both identify and manage AKI [4]. Over 50% of AKI cases are thought to be community-acquired, highlighting the importance of detecting and managing AKI in the community [6, 7].

The majority of AKI cases are secondary to hypotension, or dehydration, with consequent kidney hypoperfusion [8]. Many other factors may be either independent causes or contributory factors, that may predispose to the development of AKI. Conceptually, it is still helpful to think of causes categorized as pre-renal, renal, and post-renal causes (Table 4.2).

Pre-renal causes result from kidney hypoperfusion. This can be due to true hypovolaemia, reduced effective circulation of blood volume, or impaired local autoregulation of kidney perfusion: Prolonged hypoperfusion may progress to ischaemic acute tubular necrosis. **Renal** causes can typically be categorized according to the location within the kidney which is primarily affected (Table 4.2). (certain conditions (e.g. multiple myeloma) can produce an acute kidney injury that is not limited to one anatomical segment. **Post-renal** causes relate to impaired or obstructed urine outflow, as a result of pathology that is either intrinsic, or extrinsic to the urinary tract.

Around a third of AKI cases are predictable, but the wide range of potential causes that may lead to AKI emphasizes the need for a targeted approach to screening: A risk assessment should therefore guide clinicians to screen for AKI amongst those with an exposure - including intercurrent or acute illness - or susceptibility/condition that may increase the risk of having AKI (Table 4.3).

Table 4.2 Causes of acute kidney injury

Location	Cause
Pre-Renal	• Hypovolaemia o Dehydration o Haemorrhage o Diarrhoea/vomiting o Major surgery o Third space losses e.g. *burns*, *pancreatitis* • Reduced effective circulating volume: o Reduced cardiac output: *e.g. cardiac failure* o Systemic vasodilation: *e.g. sepsis, anaphylaxis* • Medications affecting renal auto-regulation: o Angiotensin converting enzyme inhibitors/angiotensin receptor blockers o Non-steroidal anti-inflammatories
Renal**	• Glomerulonephritis • Acute tubular necrosis o Ischaemic *e.g. hypovolaemia, shock* o Toxins – endogenous (*e.g. rhabdoymolysis*) and exogenous (*e.g.iodine-based contrast*) • Acute interstitial nephritis o Infectious o Inflammatory or autoimmune o Drug/Toxin induced • Vascular o Malignant hypertension o Vasculitis o Thrombotic microangiopathy (*e.g. haemolytic uraemic syndrome*) o Pro-thrombotic or embolic conditions
Post-Renal	• Mechanical obstruction o Benign prostatic hypertrophy o Prostatic, pelvic or abdominal malignancy o Nephrolithiasis or urolithiasis o Retroperitoneal fibrosis • Neurogenic bladder

**List highlights common aetiologias and is not exhaustive*
***Note: Conditions causing intrinsic renal injury may not be limited to a single anatomical location, e.g. in the case of multiple myeloma*

Table 4.3 Causes of AKI: exposures and susceptibilities for non-specific AKI [1]

Exposures	Susceptibilities
Sepsis	Dehydration or volume depletion
Critical illness	Advanced age
Circulatory shock	Female gender
Burns	Black race
Trauma	CKD
Cardiac surgery (especially with CPB)	Chronic diseases (heart, lung, liver)
Major noncardiac surgery	Diabetes mellitus
Nephrotoxic drugs Radiocontrast agents	Cancer
Poisonous plants and animals	Anaemia

CKD **Chronic kidney disease,** *CPB* **cardio-pulmonary bypass**

This risk assessment should take into account variables such as inherent predispositions, co-morbidities, environmental and iatrogenic exposures, social conditions, and the patient's care setting.

Clinical Presentation

The absence of pathognomonic symptoms or signs in AKI means that patients' clinical presentations are highly dependent on both the cause, and complications. Patients may clearly show evidence of acute or intercurrent illness associated with AKI, or alternatively they may be asymptomatic, with AKI as an incidental finding.

The clinical presentation can provide significant insight into the aetiology of AKI, which is often multifactorial: a careful and thorough multi-system history and examination should be undertaken to identify all contributing factors. Key symptoms and clinical signs, that may indicate certain underlying pathologies are presented in Table 4.4.

The clinical presentation may also provide insight into the severity of AKI, by providing evidence of complications such as hypervolaemia or metabolic derangements (Table 4.5).

AKI is a complex physiological state, in which abnormalities in fluid balance can be key indicators of causal pathology, severity of AKI, or response to treatment. Frequent assessment of fluid status is therefore imperative in all cases of suspected or confirmed AKI. Haemodynamic parameters, jugular venous pressure, evidence of peripheral or pulmonary oedema, net fluid balance, and changes in weight can help guide efforts to achieve euvolaemia.

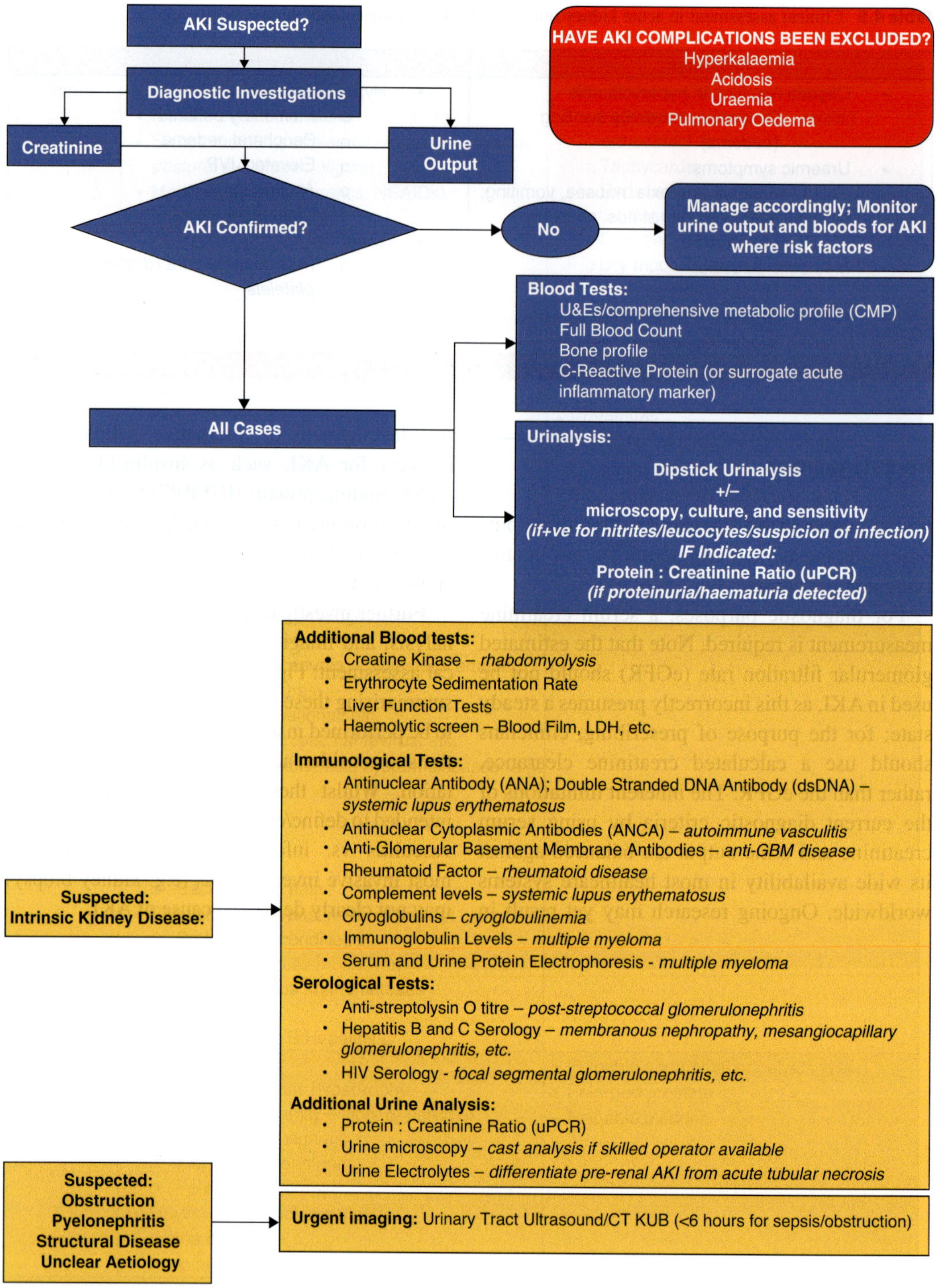

Fig. 4.2 Algorithm: Investigations to Consider in Patients with Suspected or Confirmed AKI

Differential Diagnosis

Due to its non-specific presentation, the differential diagnosis for patients presenting with AKI is broad when based on clinical features alone. Following biochemical confirmation of abnormal kidney function, the most frequent diagnostic dilemma occurs when differentiating AKI from CKD, or indeed AKD. If the baseline serum creatinine is not known, it is not possible to distinguish between these two conditions based on a single creatinine level. It is also important to recognize that these diagnoses are not mutually exclusive, as is illustrated in Fig. 4.1. Factors which might indicate underlying CKD include a history of predisposing conditions (e.g. diabetes, hypertension), presence of associated metabolic or haematologic abnormalities (e.g. hyperphosphataemia, anaemia), or reduced kidney size, thinning of the cortex, and loss of cortico-medullary differentiation on imaging. If diagnostic uncertainty remains, clinicians should evaluate and manage as AKI, ensuring appropriate monitoring is in place, with re-evaluation after the acute presentation has passed, so that the diagnosis of AKI, AKD or CKD may be established satisfactorily.

Management

Management strategies for AKI demonstrate a high level of heterogeneity, owing to diverse aetiologies alongside the wide variety of clinical contexts in which AKI presents. However, generally applicable principles can be utilized as a basic framework on which to build further management (Fig. 4.3). Ultimately, management will rely on treating the cause, minimizing further insults, and managing complications.

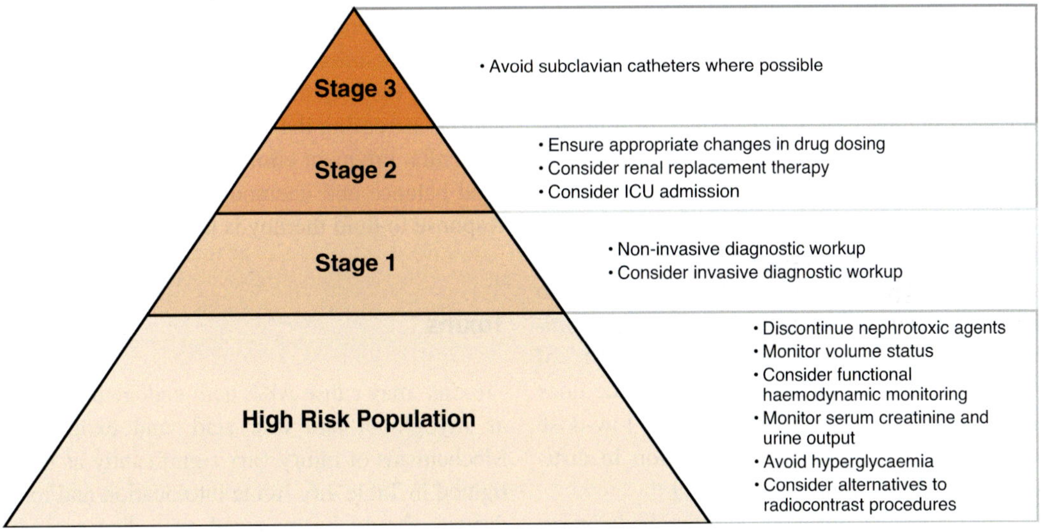

Fig. 4.3 KDIGO Guidance Regarding Stage-Based Management of AKI [1]. AKI requires management of underlying aetiology and resultant complications. Alongside this, consider generally applicable actions to be taken according to severity of AKI. Those listed under 'high risk population' should be taken in all cases, with additional actions building upon this—the extent of which is guided by stage

General Management Principles

As an 'aide-memoire', we have broadly divided the general management principles for AKI using the acronym 'SHTOP'—referring to Sepsis, Hypovolaemia, Toxins, Obstruction and Parenchymal causes:

Sepsis

Sepsis is a common cause of AKI. The precise mechanism for injury is debated: the simplest explanation cites kidney hypoperfusion due to factors including systemic vasodilation and endothelial dysfunction, although other contributing mechanisms may include renal parenchymal injury, due to the immune response to infection [10, 11].

No therapeutic agent specific for sepsis-associated AKI has been validated. Current management guidelines centre on standard practice for the treatment of sepsis and septic shock. This includes early targeted antibiotic therapy, source control of the infection (including careful consideration of the removal of infected lines, drainage of infected collections by an interventional radiological or surgical approach), and fluid resuscitation. Persistent hypotension despite adequate fluid resuscitation may prompt the initiation of vasopressors to maintain renal perfusion pressures: a target minimum mean arterial pressure (MAP) of 65 mmHg is recommended [1]. Evidence does not support the practice of initiating low-dose dopamine to increase renal perfusion in critically ill patients to prevent AKI [1].

The choice and dosing of antimicrobial therapy should be given careful consideration, given the risk of nephrotoxicity, or accumulation of the drug if renally cleared. Avoid aminoglycosides if possible; if necessary, ideally use once daily dosing ensuring appropriate monitoring of serum levels [1].

Hypovolaemia

Appropriate management of hypovolaemia should be guided by severity. In mild cases of AKI/AKD, oral fluid replacement may be appropriate. Otherwise, intravenous fluid replacement or resuscitation is appropriate. The choice of intravenous fluid should generally be crystalloid therapy, which is recommended over colloids [1], and should be administered alongside other intravenous therapies required specific to the clinical context, for example blood products or specific electrolyte replacement.

Management of hypovolaemia may be complicated due to numerous factors. Overzealous fluid administration may result in hypervolaemia: thus caution is advocated in managing patients with underlying cardiac or hepatic dysfunction, oliguric or anuric patients, the elderly, and those with known complex physiological states. Management strategies may also be less effective in states with increased extravasation of fluid (e.g. endothelial dysfunction, reduced oncotic pressures). Furthermore, progression of AKI may result in the development of oliguria or anuria, increasing the risk of transition to hypervolaemia. Frequent clinical review of a patient's fluid balance and haemodynamic parameters in response to fluid therapy is therefore essential.

Toxins

'Toxins' may cause AKI, both endogenous, such as myoglobin and uric acid, and exogenous. Mechanisms of injury vary significantly as highlighted in Table 4.6. Acute intoxication and toxidromes should be managed according to local and national toxicology guidelines. Specific management of toxin-induced AKI will depend on the mechanism of injury; note that pre-renal, renal, and post-renal pathologies may result. In all cases discontinue the offending agent unless

Table 4.6 Examples of exogenous toxins causing acute kidney injury* [9, 12]

Environmental/ Recreational Toxin Exposure	Therapeutic Exposures					
	Herbal Remedies	Medications				
		Mechanism of Injury				
		Altered Haemodynamics	Acute Tubular Necrosis	Acute Interstitial Nephritis	Crystalline Nephropathy
- Animal venoms e.g. snake bites - Heavy metal exposure - Herbicide exposure (e.g. glyphosate, paraquat) - Organophosphates - Illicit drug use - Hair dyes	- Traditional Herbal Remedies (e.g. Aristocholia sp., glycyrhetinic acid (licorice), colchicine, etc.)	- Non-steroidal Anti-inflammatories - Angiotensin Converting Enzyme Inhibitors - Angiotensin Receptor Blockers - Calcineurin Inhibitors	- Aminoglycoside Antibiotics - Glycopeptide Antibiotics - Radiographic - Contrast Agents - Cisplatin	- Proton Pump Inhibitors - Antiretrovirals - Beta-lactam Antibiotics - Sulphanomides - 5-Aminosalicylates - Allopurinol	- Aciclovir - Indinavir - Sulphonamides

**List is not exhaustive*

there is a critical indication for continuation; in these cases, consider dose-reduction where possible. Regardless of the cause of AKI, note that renally cleared toxins risk accumulation. Prevent this where possible by discontinuing or reducing dose of renally cleared medications according to creatinine clearance. Should accumulation and severe toxicity occur, extracorporeal removal through renal replacement therapy may be indicated; note that not all substances are amenable to removal through this method.

Incidence of AKI secondary to radiographic contrast use is still being established. At present, KDIGO guidance recommends assessing all those exposed to iodine-based contrast agents for risk of contrast-induced AKI (e.g. history of CKD, etc.). In those felt to be at risk, avoid exposure if possible. If necessary, use lowest dose of iso- or low-osmolar iodinated contrast media where possible [1]. Consider intravenous volume expansion using isotonic saline or sodium bicarbonate as a preventative measure [1].

Obstruction

Urinary tract obstruction causes acute kidney injury due to a cascade of effects resulting from reduced ability to excrete urine. Confirmation of obstruction is typically made using imaging such as ultrasound, showing distinct causal pathologies, bladder dilatation, or hydronephrosis.

If obstruction is causing AKI immediate relief is warranted. In simple cases of lower urinary tract obstruction such as bladder outlet obstruction (e.g. secondary to prostatic hypertrophy) or neurogenic bladder, attempt urinary catheterization. Definitive surgical management may ultimately be required; ensure referral to urology services is made promptly. AKI in the setting of upper urinary tract obstruction, including pyonephrosis, obstructed solitary kidneys, or bilateral upper urinary tract obstruction requires urgent referral to inpatient surgical services; interventions such as nephrostomy or ureteric stenting may be required.

It is important to note that following relief of obstruction patients may suffer post-obstructive diuresis, carrying a risk of dehydration and electrolyte imbalance.

Parenchymal

Causes of AKI primarily affecting the kidney parenchyma are diverse, including both local and multisystem pathologies: appropriate management is therefore specific to the clinical picture, and includes careful consideration of the risks and benefits of undertaking a kidney biopsy to confirm a histological diagnosis—which may serve to better define the management strategy, but may be considered unsafe, and hence delayed or avoided in certain clinical settings such as clinical frailty, or severe sepsis, complicated by coagulopathy. Management strategies for parenchymal causes include discontinuation of causal agents, such as in allergic interstitial nephritis, supportive measures where ATN is suspected, and immune suppressive treatment in glomerulonephritis. Sometimes concomitant antibiotic therapy is appropriate where concomitant bacterial infection is suspected. Indications and contraindications for kidney biopsy are outlined in Chap. 2, and the management of specific pathologies affecting the kidney parenchyma is dealt with in later chapters in this textbook.

Managing AKI Complications

Complications of AKI may occur, irrespective of the underlying aetiology: although the incidence and severity of complications typically correlate with increased AKI stage, numerous contributing factors may confound this relationship—such as the concurrent use of ACE inhibitors and potassium sparing diuretics in heart failure. Initial and continued assessments throughout the course of illness should therefore attempt to identify and manage complications appropriately, with consideration for the use of kidney replacement therapy (KRT).

Hyperkalaemia

Hyperkalaemia is a common complication of AKI—which can be life-threatening due to associated cardiac arrhythmias. Patients may be at a higher risk if the underlying illness includes a catabolic state (e.g. rhabdomyolysis, haemolysis). Figure 4.4 demonstrates a general approach to management. Basic principles should be implemented in all cases. Where serum levels are greater than 6.0 mmol/L, an active attempt to reduce serum concentration should be made through shifting potassium into cells (and enhancing excretion where appropriate). In cases with evidence of ECG changes ensure that therapy to stabilize the cardiac membrane is administered urgently and that cardiac monitoring is in place.

Acidosis

AKI disrupts acid-base homeostatic mechanisms, resulting in metabolic acidosis. Simple treatment measures for AKI itself may improve acidosis alongside renal function (for example, improving renal perfusion through intravenous fluid administration in hypovolaemia). If significant metabolic acidosis persists despite immediate resuscitative measures, intravenous bicarbonate may be indicated. If this is limited by the patient's volume status, renal replacement therapy may be required. Oral bicarbonate supplementation is only appropriate in mild cases (e.g. $NaHCO_3 > 18$ mmol/L).

Hypervolaemia

Oliguria or anuria as a result of AKI may lead to hypervolaemia and life-threatening consequences such as pulmonary oedema. Hypervolaemia can also quickly develop in AKI due to overzealous administration of fluid therapy for treatment of the primary aetiology (e.g. hypovolaemia or sepsis).

Management relies on frequent clinical assessment of fluid status to tailor therapy. Loop-diuretics

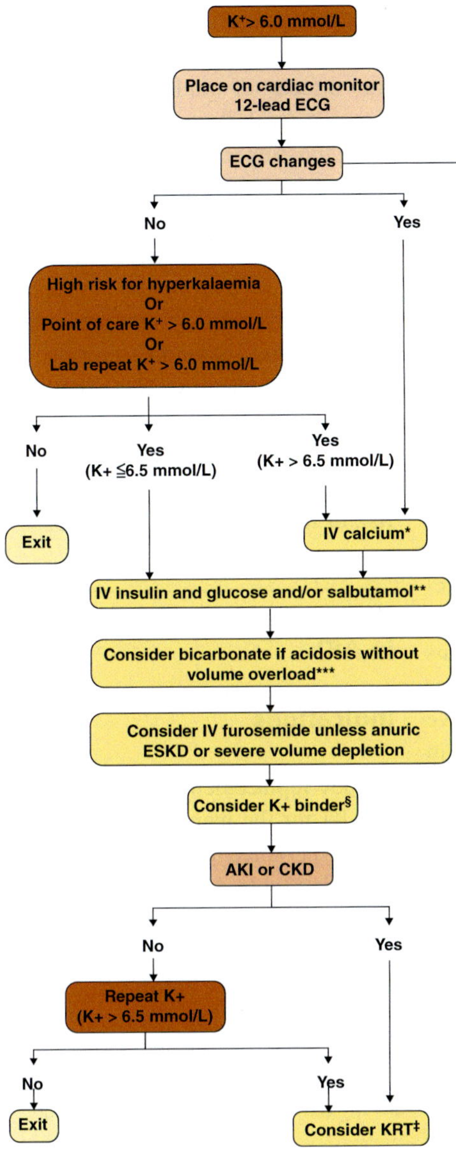

Serum K^+	Expected ECG Abnormality
5.5–6.5 mmol/L	Tall 'peaked' T waves with narrow base, best seen in precordial leads
6.5–8.0 mmol/L	Peaked T waves Prolonged PR interval Decreased amplitude of P waves Widening of QRS complex
>8.0 mmol/L	Absence of T wave Intraventricular blocks, fascicular blocks, bundle branch blocks, QRS axis shift, Progressive widening of QRS resulting in bizarre morphology 'Sine wave' patterns (Sinoventricular rhythm, VF, asystole

Fig. 4.4 Management Principles: Hyperkalaemia in AKI [13, 14]. Management of acute hyperkalemia in adults. The thresholds for actions are opinion based. Electrocardiogram (ECG) changes commonly reported with increasing potassium concentrations have been described in the literature. *IV 1 g calcium gluconate (3 × 10 mL of 10% solution, each containing 93 mg elemental calcium, 2.3 mmol) or calcium chloride (10 mL of 10% solution, 273 mg elemental calcium, 6.8 mmol). **IV regular insulin 5 units plus 25 g glucose (50 mL of 50%) is as effective as albuterol (salbutamol) 10 mg nebulized; insulin and albuterol may have an additive effect. Beware of hypoglycemia. ***IV bicarbonate (1 amp of 50 mL of 8.4% solution, Naþ 50 mmol, HCO_3–50 mmol) over 15 min. §Potassium binders: sodium polystyrene sulphonate 15–60 g p.o./p.r. (do not give with sorbitol) or zirconium cyclosilicate 10 g 3/day (patiromer not advisable as onset of action is 7 h). This guidance is suggestive as there are limited data on onset of action with no head-to- head studies between potassium binders. ‡Hemodialysis is the modality of preference. *AKI* acute kidney injury, *CKD* chronic kidney disease, *ESKD* end-stage kidney disease, *GFR* glomerular filtration rate, *IV* intravenous, *K*⁺ potassium, *VF* ventricular fibrillation

are the standard first-line therapy to promote diuresis. High doses may be required, particularly in patients with CKD or AKI, due to variable diuretic responsiveness. In the absence of hypervolemia, it is not recommended to use diuretic therapy in efforts to convert oliguric AKI to non-oliguric AKI [1]. If unable to restore adequate urine output with diuretic therapy, or in the context of clinical instability, renal replacement therapy may be indicated for fluid removal. As an interim measure respiratory support such as continuous positive airway pressure (CPAP) may be required in the management of pulmonary oedema.

Note that assessment of fluid status can rely heavily on non-invasive measures, such as blood pressure, jugular venous pressure, evidence of oedema, urine output, and changes in weight. Accurate clinical assessment of effective circulating volume may be difficult however; for example, in nephrotic conditions oedema is not solely attributable to intravascular hydrostatic pressure. Ultimately, invasive haemodynamic monitoring may be required in the context of critical illness and clinical instability.

Symptomatic Uraemia

Uraemia refers to high serum concentrations of uraemic toxins due to reduced renal excretion. It is worth noting that urea is used as a surrogate marker, and that the term uraemia encompasses the effects of multiple toxins. Symptomatic uraemia typically occurs at severe reductions in renal function (e.g. creatinine clearance <10 mL/min) [15], and may manifest as non-specific symptoms such as anorexia, malaise, nausea, vomiting, and pruritis. Further complications may occur such as uraemic encephalopathy, seizures, pericarditis, or pericardial effusion. Symptomatic uraemia warrants urgent renal replacement therapy. Note that altered mental status should not be attributed solely to uraemic encephalopathy without evaluation; uraemia may result in platelet dysfunction and increased risk of intracranial haemorrhage.

Kidney Replacement Therapy (KRT) in AKI

Indications

Kidney replacement therapy (KRT) is indicated in AKI for the management of severe or refractory hypervolaemia, hyperkalaemia, acidosis, or uraemia (Table 4.7). Timing is case and context dependent; no biochemical parameters (including creatinine levels) have been supported as broadly applicable cutoff values to dictate initiation of KRT [1, 13]. KRT can be initiated as an

Table 4.7 Indications for initiation of kidney replacement therapy (KRT) in AKI and relevant factors influencing the decision

Indications for KRT
• Refractory hyperkalaemia (K>6.5mM) • Refractory metabolic acidosis (pH<7.15) • Refractory fluid overload • End organ involvement (pericarditis, encephalopathy, neuropathy, myopathy, uraemic bleeding) • Certain poisonings (e.g. lithium, toxic alcohols)
Factors to consider in an assessment of the anticipated need/benefit of KRT
• Current levels and trajectories of biochemical parameters (K, pH, urea) • Uraemic solute burden (increased in tumour lysis syndrome, rhabdomyolysis, hypercatabolic states) • Requirement for intravascular space to allow administration of therapeutic interventions (e.g. blood products, nutrition) • Degree and duration of oliguria • Resolution/persistence of underlying renal insult • Presence of other organ dysfunction (affecting tolerance of uraemic complications) • Presence of other electrolyte disturbances (e.g. hypercalcaemia) that may be corrected by KRT

emergency measure to respond to the aforementioned complications, or alternatively may be started pre-emptively if development of such complications is felt likely based on the trajectory of illness. In addition, specific severe toxicities may require extracorporeal removal of the offending toxin through KRT if dialysable. It is of course important to recognize that KRT also carries a significant risk of complications – thus a careful consideration of and discussion with the patient and family members about the risks, benefits, and goals of care, prior to commencement of KRT, are vital to ensure a shared, patient-centred approach to decision making.

Modalities

Choice of modality for KRT in AKI may be influenced by clinical factors as well as the availability of resources and trained staff. Common modalities used include forms of continuous renal replacement therapy (CRRT), including continuous veno-venous haemofiltration (CVVHF), continuous veno-venous haemodialysis (CVVHD), and continuous veno-venous haemodiafiltration (CVVHDF); intermittent haemodialysis (IHD), and hybrid therapies such as extended duration dialysis (EDD), sustained low-efficiency dialysis (SLED) and the Genius system. Acute Peritoneal dialysis (PD) may also be used, although increasingly this has been restricted to paediatric and low-resource settings. Broadly, CRRT has the advantage of better haemodynamic tolerance due to more controlled fluid removal over a longer period, and gentler fluid shifts due to less intense solute clearance. Intermittent KRT results in faster fluid and solute removal which can lead to haemodynamic instability, metabolic fluctuations and shifts in fluid distribution. Intermittent KRT does offer the advantage of allowing the patient to mobilize and participate in active physiotherapy and rehabilitation. It also provides "down-time" for diagnostic and therapeutic procedures, and allows rapid solute clearance when this is necessary (e.g. in severe, refractory hyperkalaemia). No single modality is widely recommended as the optimal choice for KRT in AKI, given limited evidence regarding survival benefit [1]. A comparison of the considerations for different KRT modalities is illustrated in Table 4.8.

KDIGO provides general guidance regarding use of CRRT and IHD, summarized in Table 4.9. The International Society of Peritoneal Dialysis (IPSID) provides comprehensive guidance and management protocols for Acute PD in AKI, and we also deal with this topic in a later chapter [17].

Table 4.8 Comparison of KRT Modalities in AKI [1, 16]

Modality	Suitability in haemodynamically unstable patients	Solute clearance	Volume Control	Anti-coagulation
Peritoneal dialysis (PD)	Yes	Moderate high	Unpredictable	no
Intermittent haemodialysis (IHD)	Only with careful measures in place	High	Moderate	not essential
Hybrid techniques – e.g. Sustained Low Efficiency Dialysis (SLED)	Possibly	Moderate high	Good	not essential
Continuous Veno-Venous Haemofiltration (CVVH)	Yes	Moderate/high	Good	not essential
Continuous Veno-Venous Haemodialysis (CVVHD)	Yes	Moderate/high	Good	not essential
Continuous Veno-Venous Haemodiafiltration (CVVHDF)	Yes	High	Good	not essential

Table 4.9 KDIGO Recommendations for use of CRRT and IHD in AKI [1]

Choice of Modality	• Adapt choice of modality to changing patient needs • Use CRRT in preference to IHD for: o *Haemodynamically unstable patients* o *Patients ate increased risk of raised intracranial pressure or with generalized brain oedema*
Access	• Recommended site: o Avoid subclavian vein use: *risk of stenosis limiting use for permanent access* o Recommended order of preference: *right jugular vein, femoral veins, left jugular vein, left subclavian vein* • Procedural considerations: o Use an uncuffed non-tunneled dialysis catheter where possible o Use ultrasound guidance for placement o Confirm placement with chest x-ray after procedure and prior to first use o Do not use antibiotic locks for non-tunneled dialysis catheters – *risk of antimicrobial resistance, fungal infections, etc.*
Materials	• Use dialyzers with a biocompatible membrane – *attempt to avoid bioincompatabiliity phenomenon* • Use a bicarbonate buffer in dialysate and replacement fluid – *improved correction of acidosis and haemodynamic tolerance compared to lactate-based solutions*
Anticoagulation	• IHD o *Anticoagulation recommended in the absence of increased risk of bleeding or concurrent use of systemic anticoagulation* o *Use unfractionated heparin or low-molecular weight heparin* • CRRT o *Anticoagulation recommended unless concurrent use of systemic anticoagulation* o *Use regional citrate anticoagulation as first line method* o *If citrate is contraindicated, use unfractionated heparin or low-molecular weight heparin unless increased risk of bleeding*
Dosing	• Prescribe dose of KRT prior to each session, tailored to individual patient goals regarding solute and volume balance o IHD (*Recommended delivery of a Kt/V of 3.9 per week)* • CRRT o *Recommended delivery of an effluent volume of 20-25 ml/kg/h*

Discontinuation of KRT

Discontinuation of KRT may be appropriate for two reasons: the patient's kidney function has returned to an acceptable level for the individual patient, or continued KRT is not in line with goals of care [1]. Sudden discontinuation, or alternatively a gradual process of 'weaning' may be more appropriate: for example, gradual tapering of therapy through transfer from CRRT to IHD, or prolonged intervals in-between IHD sessions may provide an opportunity to more accurately assess recovery of kidney function until complete discontinuation is achieved: this may be facilitated through the judicious use of diuretic therapy to alleviate volume overload.

Palliative Care

Refer to the chapter on palliative care later in this book for guidance regarding principles of palliative care for patients with kidney disease. In all cases, ensure early discussion with the patient and caregivers regarding prognosis and care escalation giving consideration to patient wishes, current clinical condition, co-morbidities, and baseline functional status. This will facilitate decision-making in the patient's best-interests should clinical deterioration occur, particularly in the decision to initiate or continue KRT.

AKI and KRT Worldwide

Availability of KRT Worldwide for AKI may be limited. ISN 0 by 25 programme is trying to address that. In some low income countries PD may be used provided the PD solution is not very expensive.

Outcomes and Follow-up for AKI Patients

Outcomes in AKI depend on numerous factors such as aetiology, severity, duration, and co-morbidities. AKI is associated with increased short-term mortality, the risk of which escalates with increased severity of AKI [4]. AKI also carries long-term risks - irrespective of resolution of illness or return to premorbid kidney function. These include increased intermediate and long-term mortality, as well as risk of progression and faster progression to CKD [18, 19]. That said, not everyone with AKI has a poor outcome, and predictors of poor outcomes have been identified. Patients should therefore be followed up at 2–3 months following (or earlier if no recovery) resolution of acute illness to identify newly developed or worsening CKD (Fig. 4.5) [1, 3, 20]. Whilst an increased rate of adverse events amongst AKI patients makes careful follow-up of AKI patients—particularly after hospitalization and AKI stages 2–3 important, adherence to face-to-face follow up in specialist nephrology clinics may be limited by several barriers, including hospital fatigue, an excess of other hospital appointments, distance to travel, as has been demonstrated in one randomized controlled trial [21]. It is in this setting that the advent of remote AKI follow-up clinics may prove most effective, although

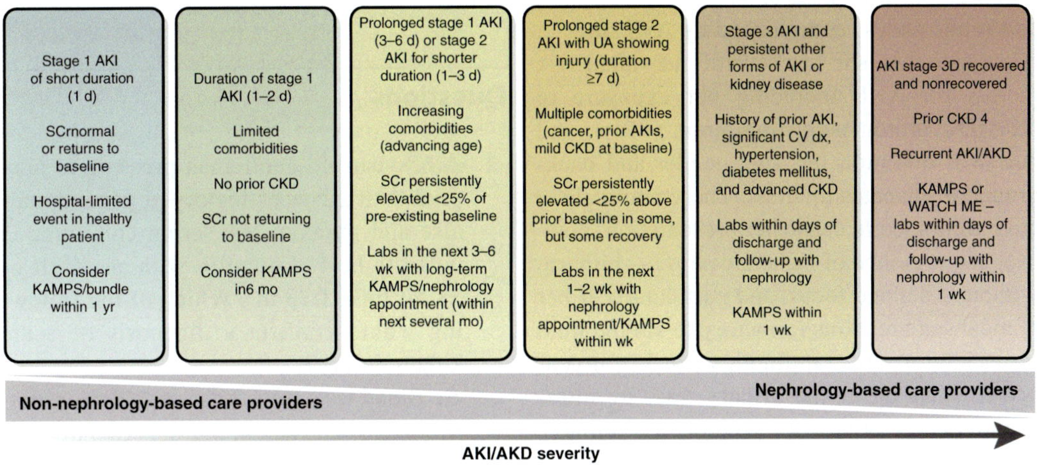

Fig. 4.5 Schematic for acute kidney injury/acute kidney diseases and disorders (AKI/AKD) follow-up [3]. The figure displays a potential paradigm for the care of patients who experience AKI/AKD. The degree of nephrology-based follow-up increases as the duration and severity of AKI/AKD increases. The timing and nature of follow-up are suggestions, as there are limited data to inform this process. Future research efforts should work to clarify the timing of AKI/AKD follow-up and which specific health-care providers should provide it. The items in each bucket follow the "OR" rule; therefore, each patient should follow the most-severe bucket even if they meet only 1 criterion in that bucket. For example, a patient with CKD G4, regardless of severity of AKI, should be followed by a nephrologist in 1 week. *AKI stage 3D* AKI stage 3 treated by dialysis, *CKD* chronic kidney disease, *CV* cardiovascular, *dx* diagnosis, *KAMPS* kidney function–advocacy–medications–pressure–sick day protocol, *SCr* serum creatinine, *UA* urine analysis, *WATCH-ME* weight assessment–access–teaching–clearance– hypotension–medications

there remains no consensus on the optimal strategy and duration of follow-up to improve short- and long-term outcomes.

Practice Points

- Common causes of AKI are sepsis, hypovolaemia, drug toxicity and obstruction
- The treatment includes SHTOP management of sepsis, correction of hypovolaemia, stopping toxins, relieving obstruction and treating parenchymal disease with consideration on role for a kidney biopsy

Conclusions

Returning to the clinical case from the beginning of the chapter, we can reflect that our 75-year-old female patient has a very common presentation in clinical practice: that of sepsis and septic shock, complicated by AKI stage 2. Alongside this, she has several individual risk factors for AKI, including her exposure to NSAIDs, proton pump inhibitors (PPIs), and her ACE inhibitor, her age, gender and background of diabetes mellitus. These could alone have combined to cause her presentation, however the presence of systemic sepsis—hitherto without a defined focus, and particularly if her clinical state remains refractory to simple fluid resuscitation and antibiotics—make urgent (<6 h) imaging of the urinary tract by ultrasound or CT vital—to exclude a drainable intra-renal collection, or another obstructive cause of AKI.

There are certain other elements that would help us in further evaluating her prognosis: the length of time she has been diagnosed with diabetes mellitus, her baseline blood sugar and blood pressure control, and whether she has significant microalbuminuria at baseline, as evidence of a potential underlying diabetic nephropathy. Further, for a lady of this age group, (her ethnic origin isn't stated)—and particularly if her renal function remains refractory to treatment, screening for other aetiologies—including vasculitis, multiple myeloma and HIV—that may make her more susceptible to infection—and to developing AKI. Furthermore, should her kidney function fail to recover, there should be a low threshold to screen for other underlying autoimmune causes of AKI.

Screening for AKI amongst such individuals presenting emergently to primary care, the emergency department, or acute medicine provides an important tool to help guide appropriate early interventions—including fluid resuscitation, antibiotics, drainage of infected collections, and relief of nephrotoxic medications (NSAIDs, possibly PPIs), and temporary withholding of ACE inhibitors and metformin until the patient recovers; thereafter, careful follow-up to chart recovery of kidney function, and ensure the timely reintroduction of appropriate medications (particularly ACE inhibitors and diabetic medications), and reinforce avoidance of nephrotoxic medications—particularly NSAIDs in this setting.

Questions

1. A 65-year-old gentleman presents to hospital with a 2-week history of general malaise and pyrexia. His serum creatinine is noted to be 184 mmol/L with an eGFR of 28 mL/min/1.73 m^2. Which of the following would confirm a diagnosis of acute kidney injury?
   A. Blood tests from 2 days ago demonstrating an eGFR of 40 mL/min/1.73 m^2
   B. Urine dipstick analysis positive for haematuria, leucocytes, and nitrites
   C. Bilateral hydronephrosis on urinary tract ultrasound
   D. Blood tests from 2 months ago demonstrating a creatinine level of 110 umol/L
   E. Blood tests from 2 days ago demonstrating a creatinine level of 160 umol/L

Answer: D

A. Incorrect: Diagnosis of AKI is dependent on serum creatinine levels rather than

eGFR (see KDIGO diagnostic and staging criteria).
B. Incorrect: These findings are suggestive of urinary tract infection, which is a known cause of acute kidney injury. However, this result alone cannot confirm that the patient's serum creatinine is indicative of AKI rather than chronic kidney disease.
C. Incorrect: This finding is suggestive of obstructive uropathy, which may cause AKI. As above, however, this result alone cannot confirm acute rather than chronic kidney disease.
D. **Correct:** This historic result would confirm that the serum creatinine value on presentation to hospital represents a rise greater than 1.5. × baseline. This would confirm that the patient is suffering a stage 1 AKI according to KDIGO criteria.
E. Incorrect: This result does not confirm that the patient is suffering an AKI as it does not strictly meet the KDIGO criteria of a 26.5 umol/L rise in creatinine over 48 h. However, this borderline result warrants attention as it may suggest that the patient is at risk of developing an AKI.

2. You confirm the above patient is suffering an acute kidney injury. Based on the provided information, which of the following medications must be held?
   A. Furosemide
   B. Sitagliptin
   C. Metformin
   D. Gentamicin
   E. Amlodipine

Answer: C

A. Incorrect: Further information is required to determine whether furosemide must be held. Furosemide may cause or worsen pre-renal kidney injury. Conversely, for certain aetiologies of AKI (e.g. cardiac failure), furosemide may be clinically indicated and aid recovery of renal function.
B. Incorrect: Sitagliptin does not need to be held based on available information, though it may require adjustment of dosing based on level of renal impairment.
C. **Correct:** Metformin should be held in all cases once eGFR is <30.
D. Incorrect: Aminoglycosides should ideally be avoided in AKI. However, where necessary they may be used to treat underlying infection with once daily dosing and monitoring of serum levels.
E. Incorrect: Amlodipine may be used in AKI. Refer to the renal drug handbook, or local pharmacy resources to confirm which medications are considered safe to use in different levels of renal function.

3. You are now able to access the patient's previous lab results. In comparison to his current serum creatinine of 184 mmol/L, over the past year and up to one-month prior his serum creatinine has been between 100 and 110 mmol/L. What is the correct diagnosis?
   A. Baseline renal function
   B. AKI Stage 1
   C. AKI Stage 2
   D. AKI Stage 3
   E. Chronic kidney disease

Answer: B

A. Incorrect: The degree in change of serum creatinine exceeds 1.5 times the baseline, therefore qualifying as acute kidney injury.
B. **Correct**: Acute elevation in creatinine is between 1.5 and 2 times the baseline level, therefore qualifying as AKI stage 1 according to KDIGO criteria.
C. Incorrect: These results indicate AKI stage 1.
D. Incorrect: These results indicate AKI stage 1.
E. Incorrect: There is not enough information available to diagnose chronic kidney disease, and irrespective of this an element of acute kidney injury is clearly present.

4. A previously fit and well 32-year-old gentleman is admitted to hospital with a stage 3 AKI. He reports a 2-week history of arthralgia, general malaise, and pyrexia. Which of the following is least suggestive of intrinsic renal pathology as the underlying cause of acute kidney injury?
   A. Microscopic haematuria
   B. Polyarthralgia
   C. Positive antinuclear antibody
   D. Increased renal parenchymal echogenicity on ultrasound
   E. Intermittent ibuprofen (NSAID) use

Answer: Question E

   A. Incorrect: Microscopic haematuria may indeed suggest an intrinsic renal pathology such as glomerulonephritis. It is imperative to note however that it may also represent other sinister pathology, such as urological malignancy.
   B. Incorrect: Polyarthralgia may be suggestive of systemic illnesses associated with intrinsic renal disease (e.g. rheumatoid arthritis association with amyloidosis, lupus nephritis, etc.)
   C. Incorrect: Positive ANA may indicate an underlying autoimmune disorder associated with intrinsic renal disease.
   D. Incorrect: Given the provided options, this is incorrect. Increased renal parenchymal echogenicity is a non-specific finding in acute kidney injury.
   E. **Correct**: In the above scenario, the patient is presenting with a short history of systemic symptoms, arthralgia, and AKI. This may alert the reader to an underlying pathology such as vasculitis or autoimmune disease which can be associated with intrinsic renal pathology. The patient may be using ibuprofen to manage these symptoms, however ibuprofen itself is known to cause AKI through pre-renal mechanisms. Therefore, intermittent ibuprofen use is the least suggestive of intrinsic renal pathology in this case vignette.

5. Which of the following is not a core aspect of management to improve prognosis of sepsis associated AKI?
   A. Antibiotic therapy
   B. Source control
   C. Fluid resuscitation
   D. Maintenance of mean arterial pressure of >65 mmHg
   E. Low-dose dopamine therapy

Answer: E

Correct answer: E. The core management strategy in all cases of acute kidney injury involves treating the underlying aetiology. Antibiotic therapy, source control measures, and fluid resuscitation are all pivotal in the management of sepsis itself, and in sepsis-associated AKI maintenance of a mean arterial pressure > 65 mmHg is advocated for to improve prognosis. Though historically low-dose dopamine therapy was used as a renoprotective agent in these cases, evidence of benefit is limited, and it is therefore not endorsed by KDIGO guidelines.

6. Which of the following is not a recognized complication of acute kidney injury (irrespective of aetiology)?
   A. Metabolic acidosis
   B. Metabolic encephalopathy
   C. Hypovolaemia
   D. Electrolyte abnormalities
   E. Toxin accumulation
   F. Pulmonary oedema

Answer: F

   A. Incorrect: Metabolic acidosis is a recognized complication of acute kidney injury.
   B. Incorrect: Uraemic encephalopathy is a recognized complication of acute kidney injury.
   C. **Correct:** Though hypovolaemia may indeed occur in specific contexts (e.g. sepsis, post-obstructive diuresis, overzealous diuresis), it is not a recognized complication of AKI in all cases. In severe AKI, renal dysfunction leads to inability to produce and excrete urine, resulting in hypervolaemia.

D. Incorrect: Electrolyte disturbances such as hyperkalaemia are recognized complications of AKI.
E. Incorrect: Toxin accumulation is a recognized complication of AKI due to reduced renal excretion.
F. Incorrect: Pulmonary oedema as a result of hypervolaemia is a recognized complication of AKI.

7. A 60-year-old female is admitted with acute-kidney injury secondary to glomerulonephritis. On clinical examination she has bi-basal crepitations on auscultation of her chest, a JVP of 4 cm, and peripheral oedema up to the level of her umbilicus. Her blood pressure is 160/100 mmHg and her pulse is 88 bpm. She has a measured urine output of 30 mL over the past 48 h despite receiving IV furosemide (Lasix) 80 mg twice daily. Morning blood tests are returned and reveal a potassium level of 6.7 mmol/L. Which of the following is the most appropriate therapy to urgently reduce whole body potassium levels?
   A. IV furosemide infusion
   B. Insulin and dextrose infusion
   C. Calcium gluconate infusion
   D. Renal replacement therapy
   E. Calcium resonium

Answer: Question D

A. Incorrect: Though furosemide may reduce serum potassium levels by increasing urinary excretion, it is not appropriate as the primary strategy in this case. This patient is borderline anuric despite receiving 160 mg IV furosemide over the past 24 h; further attempts at diuresis would likely be ineffective in urgently reducing potassium levels.
B. Incorrect: Though this strategy is useful to reduce serum levels by shifting potassium intracellularly, it will not reduce whole body potassium levels and will only have a temporary effect on serum levels. Though this may be a helpful interim strategy to reduce risk of cardiac arrhythmias associated with hyperkalaemia, as the patient is anuric further action is required.
C. Incorrect: Calcium gluconate does not reduce serum potassium levels. It is indicated in severe hyperkalaemia to stabilize cardiac cell membranes to protect against unwanted depolarization and resultant arrhythmia.
D. **Correct**: In this instance the patient has a critically high potassium level and is nearly anuric despite attempts at IV diuresis. The most effective way to effectively reduce whole body potassium levels would be through renal replacement therapy.
E. Incorrect: Calcium resonium is an ion exchange resin which promotes excretion of potassium through the gut. It has a limited role in acute hyperkalaemia due to relatively slow onset of action.

8. A 73-year-old female admitted with decompensated heart failure develops acute kidney injury while in hospital. Which of the following would be the greatest indication for consideration of urgent renal replacement therapy?
   A. Peripheral oedema resistant to diuresis
   B. Albumin level of 15
   C. Creatinine of 520 umol/L from a baseline of 140 umol/L
   D. Persistent anuria
   E. Urea level of 21 mmol/L

Answer: Question D

A. Incorrect: Peripheral oedema resistant to diuresis may further prompt consideration of whether renal replacement therapy might be appropriate dependent on the clinical context. However, it is alone not an indication for urgent renal replacement therapy.
B. Incorrect: Hypoalbuminemia can cause significant difficulties with fluid balance (e.g. resulting in significant peripheral oedema despite intravascular depletion). However, hypoalbuminemia itself is not an indication to start renal replacement therapy.
C. Incorrect: Elevated creatinine levels can indicate the severity of AKI. However, there is no cutoff in serum creatinine level at which renal replacement therapy

should be started. Rather, it is the complications of AKI (anticipated or already present) which should prompt consideration of urgent enal replacement therapy.

D. **Correct**: In this patient with decompensated heart failure and AKI, anuria is a concerning feature. Ongoing anuria may be a sign that certain complications are likely to develop such as pulmonary oedema or hyperkalaemia. If resistant to diuresis this should prompt urgent consideration of renal replacement therapy.

E. Incorrect: Though symptomatic uraemia is an indication for renal replacement therapy, this elevated urea level in itself is not.

9. Which of the following is not an advantage of continuous renal replacement therapy (CRRT) compared to intermittent haemodialysis (IHD) in patients with acute kidney injury?
   A. Greater control of fluid balance
   B. Reduced technical complexity
   C. Reduced risk of raised intracranial pressure
   D. Rapid removal of toxins

Answer: D

Correct Answer: D. In comparison to IHD, CRRT allows greater control of fluid balance and thus less risk of haemodynamic instability, and less risk of raised intracranial pressure. Though both require a significant amount of technical skill, CRRT is felt to be less technically complex than IHD. The correct answer is 4: speed of removal of toxins is relatively slower in CRRT than IHD.

10. Exogenous toxins cause acute kidney injury through various mechanisms. Which of the follow toxins is incorrectly matched with the mechanism through which it most commonly causes AKI?
   A. Acyclovir—crystalline nephropathy
   B. Aminoglycosides—acute interstitial nephritis
   C. Angiotensin-converting enzyme inhibitors—altered hemodynamics
   D. Proton pump inhibitors—acute interstitial nephritis
   E. Non-steroidal anti-inflammatories—altered hemodynamics

Answer: B

A. Incorrect: Crystalline nephropathy is a recognized complication of Acyclovir therapy.

B. **Correct**: Aminoglycoside antibiotics are known nephrotoxic agents. The mechanism of nephrotoxicity is complex but commonly attributed to acute tubular necrosis.

C. Incorrect: ACE Inhibitors cause nephrotoxicity through altered renal hemodynamics. ACE Inhibitors dilate efferent glomerular arterioles, reducing glomerular filtration pressure and thus glomerular filtration rate.

D. Incorrect: Proton pump inhibitors are known causes of acute interstitial nephritis.

E. Incorrect: Non-steroidal anti-inflammatories are known to cause altered renal hemodynamics, causing constriction of afferent glomerular arterioles and thus reducing glomerular filtration.

Test your learning and check your understanding of this book's contents: use the "Springer Nature Flashcards" app to access questions using https://sn.pub/cz9Cok. To use the app, please follow the instructions in Chap. 1.

References

1. Kidney Disease Improving Global Outcomes Group. KDIGO clinical practice guideline for acute kidney injury. Kidney Int Suppl. 2012;2(1). https://kdigo.org/wp-content/uploads/2016/10/KDIGO-20120AKI-Guideline-English.pdf.
2. Levey AS. Defining AKD: the spectrum of AKI, AKD, and CKD. Nephron. 2022;146(3):302–5. https://doi.org/10.1159/000516647.
3. Ostermann M, Bagshaw SM, et al. Controversies in acute kidney injury: conclusions from a kidney dis-

ease: improving global outcomes (KDIGO) conference. Kidney Int. 98(2):294–309.

4. Susantitaphong P, Cruz D, Cerda J, Abulfaraj M, Alqahtani F, Koulouridis I, Jaber B. World incidence of AKI: a meta-analysis. Clin J Am Soc Nephrol. 2013;8(9):1482–93.
5. Lewington A, Cerdá J, Mehta R. Raising awareness of acute kidney injury: a global perspective of a silent killer. Kidney Int. 2013;84(3):457–67.
6. Mehta R, Burdmann E, Cerdá J, Feehally J, Finkelstein F, García-García G, et al. Recognition and management of acute kidney injury in the International Society of Nephrology 0by25 global snapshot: a multinational cross-sectional study. Lancet. 2016;387(10032):2017–25.
7. Wonnacott A, Meran S, Amphlett B, Talabani B, Phillips A. Epidemiology and outcomes in community-acquired versus hospital-acquired AKI. Clin J Am Soc Nephrol. 2014;9(6):1007–14.
8. Mehta R, Cerdá J, Burdmann E, Tonelli M, García-García G, Jha V, et al. International Society of Nephrology's 0by25 initiative for acute kidney injury (zero preventable deaths by 2025): a human rights case for nephrology. Lancet. 2015;385(9987):2616–43.
9. Engelman DT, Ben Ali W, Williams JB, et al. Guidelines for perioperative care in cardiac surgery: enhanced recovery after surgery society recommendations. JAMA Surg. 2019;154(8):755–66. https://doi.org/10.1001/jamasurg.2019.1153.
10. Ronco C, Bellomo R, Kellum J. Acute kidney injury. Lancet. 2019;394(10212):1949–64.
11. Zarjou A, Agarwal A. Sepsis and acute kidney injury. J Am Soc Nephrol. 2011;22(6):999–1006.
12. Petejova N, Martinek A, Zadrazil J, Teplan V. Acute toxic kidney injury. Ren Fail. 2019;41(1):576–94.
13. Walker B, Colledge N, Penman I, Ralston S. Davidson's principles and practice of medicine. London: Elsevier Saunders; 2014.
14. Clase CM, Carrero J-J, Ellison DH, Grams ME, Hemmelgarn BR, Jardine MJ, Kovesdy CP, Kline GA, Lindner G, Obrador GT, Palmer BF, Cheung M, Wheeler DC, Winkelmayer WC, Pecoits-Filho R, Ashuntantang GE, Bakker SJL, Bakris GL, Bhandari S, Burdmann EA, Campbell KL, Charytan DM, Clegg DJ, Cuppari L, Goldsmith D, Hallan SI, He J, Herzog CA, Hoenig MP, Hoorn EJ, Leipziger JG, Leonberg-Yoo AK, Lerma EV, Lopez-Almaraz JE, Małyszko J, Mann JFE, Marklund M, McDonough AA, Nagahama M, Navaneethan SD, Pitt B, Pochynyuk OM, Proença de Moraes T, Rafique Z, Robinson BM, Roger S, Rossignol P, Singer A, Smyth A, Sood M, Walsh M, Weir MR, Wingo CS. Potassium homeostasis and management of dyskalemia in kidney diseases: conclusions from a kidney disease: improving global outcomes (KDIGO) controversies conference. Kidney Int. 2020;97(1):42–61.
15. Zemaitis MR, Foris LA, Chandra S, et al. Uremia. [Updated 2020 Feb 4]. In: StatPearls [Internet]. Treasure Island: StatPearls Publishing; 2020. https://www.ncbi.nlm.nih.gov/books/NBK441859/
16. Kanagasundaram S, Ashley C, Bhojani S, Caldwell A, Ellam T, Kaur A, Milford D, Mulgrew C, Ostermann M, Ivanov D transl., Kuchma I transl. The renal association clinical practice guideline acute kidney injury (AKI), August 2019. Kidneys. 2019;8(4):217–24. https://doi.org/10.22141/2307-1257.8.4.2019.185121.
17. Cullis B, Abdelraheem M, Abrahams G, Balbi A, Cruz D, Frishberg Y, et al. Peritoneal dialysis for acute kidney injury. Perit Dial Int. 2014;34(5):494–517.
18. Sawhney S, Marks A, Fluck N, Levin A, Prescott G, Black C. Intermediate and long-term outcomes of survivors of acute kidney injury episodes: a large population-based cohort study. Am J Kidney Dis. 2017;69(1):18–28.
19. Coca S, Singanamala S, Parikh C. Chronic kidney disease after acute kidney injury: a systematic review and meta-analysis. Kidney Int. 2012;81(5):442–8.
20. Fliser D, Laville M, Covic A, Fouque D, Vanholder R, Juillard L, et al. A European renal best practice (ERBP) position statement on the kidney disease improving global outcomes (KDIGO) clinical practice guidelines on acute kidney injury: part 1: definitions, conservative management and contrast-induced nephropathy. Nephrol Dial Transplant. 2012;27(12):4263–72.
21. Silver SA, Adhikari NK, Bell CM, Chan CT, Harel Z, Kitchlu A, Meraz-Muñoz A, Norman PA, Perez A, Zahirieh A, Wald R. Nephrologist follow-up versus usual care after an acute kidney injury hospitalization (FUSION): a randomized controlled trial. Clin J Am Soc Nephrol. 2021;16(7):1005–14. https://doi.org/10.2215/CJN.17331120. Epub 2021 May 21. PMID: 34021031; PMCID: PMC8425610.

5 Chronic Kidney Disease (CKD): Evaluation of the Cause and Prevention of Progression

Debasish Banerjee and Arpita Roychowdhury

Clinical Scenario

A 48 year old man presents with leg swelling and weakness. He is known to suffer from diabetes mellitus, with poor control of his blood sugar. His HbA1c is 113 mmol/mol (12.5%), and his blood pressure is 160/80 mmHg. His serum creatinine has been rising to now 180 µmol/L (2.04 mg/dL) with significant proteinuria 250 mg/mmol [protein:creatinine ratio]. He was prescribed Ramipril 10 mg OD, Atorvastatin 20 mg ON, and a basal-bolus insulin regimen. His adherence to therapy was poor.

Is this a common cause of chronic kidney disease (CKD)?

Is the rapid progression usual?

What can be done to slow or prevent progression of his CKD?

D. Banerjee (✉)
St George's University of London, London, UK

St George's University Hospitals Foundation Trust, London, UK
e-mail: dbanerje@sgul.ac.uk

A. Roychowdhury
Institute of Postgraduate Medical Education and Research, Kolkata, India

Introduction

Chronic kidney disease (CKD) is a condition diagnosed with an abnormal blood or urine test. CKD is defined as abnormal low kidney function with estimated glomerular filtration rate (eGFR) less than 60 mL/min/1.73 m^2, proteinuria, or abnormal structure, persistent for more than 3 months [1] (Table 5.1).

The global burden of CKD is increasing: and CKD results in high morbidity and mortality, particularly with its associated cardiovascular complications [1]—with significant impact on healthcare provision capabilities in many countries.

The major cause of CKD worldwide are diabetes mellitus and hypertension. With the rising prevalence of diabetes and hypertension, there has been an alarming increase in the prevalence of CKD particularly in India, China and sub-Saharan Africa. This rising prevalence of CKD is in turn associated with an increased prevalence of end stage kidney disease (ESKD). With limited resources, there is a huge gap between the number of patients at ESKD requiring kidney replacement therapy (KRT), and the number of patients actually receiving it.

Significant major advances have been made recently to prevent progression of CKD and its associated cardiovascular complications, particularly when associated with diabetes, how-

D. Banerjee et al. (eds.), *Management of Kidney Diseases*,
https://doi.org/10.1007/978-3-031-09131-5_5

Table 5.1 Criteria for diagnosis of CKD. Markers of kidney damage or deceased GFR, for more than 3 months: (adapted from KDIGO CKD guidelines 2012 [1])

Markers of kidney damage (one or more)	Albuminuria (AER 30 mg/24 hours; ACR 30 mg/g [3 mg/mmol]) Urine sediment abnormalities Electrolyte and other abnormalities due to tubular disorders Abnormalities detected by histology Structural abnormalities detected by imaging History of kidney transplantation
Decreased Glomerular Filtration Rate (GFR)	GFR < 60 ml/min/1.73 m^2 (GFR categories G3a-G5)

ever understanding the impact of increasing prevalence on healthcare resources and the health of individuals is extremely important particularly in healthcare resource-poor environments.

The Epidemiology of Chronic Kidney Disease

The prevalence of CKD varies worldwide: on average approximately 1 in 10 individuals worldwide is estimated to suffer from chronic kidney disease. The major causes of CKD worldwide are diabetes and hypertension. With increasing prevalence of diabetes particularly in the Southeast Asian, Chinese and sub–Saharan African population there will be further increase in number of patients with chronic kidney disease in this region. It is estimated about 700,000,000 patients suffer from chronic kidney disease. With increasing prevalence of chronic kidney disease number of patients reaching end stage kidney failure has been increased. It is estimated about 14.6 million people would require end stage kidney disease therapy by 2030. However such therapy will be available in five million people leaving a gap in therapy in more than nine million people worldwide.

The increasing prevalence of chronic in the disease is expected to be associated with rising morbidity and mortality putting further strain in already stretched healthcare resources in certain parts of the world. Hospital admissions due to acute coronary syndromes, heart failure and strokes in CKD patients is expected to rise worldwide.

In certain parts of the world particularly rural areas the cause of chronic kidney disease is uncertain, also known as CKD of unknown aetiology (CKDu). This etiology of chronic kidney disease due to unknown origin may be related to exposures to toxins, heavy metals and infections developing countries. CKDu affects often young hard-working people and progression of kidney disease can be rapid. The kidney biopsy may show varying degrees of chronic inflammation.

Almost one-third of the patients of chronic kidney disease are from India and China also the countries with two largest populations. In 2017 CKD ranked as the 12th leading cause of death worldwide as compared to being the 17th leading cause of death in 1990. Diabetes accounts for the possible singles largest contributed of CKD in about 31% our patience.

Another often unrecognised cause of chronic kidney disease is acute kidney injury which can be due to hypotension, sepsis, obstruction and drugs.

Pathophysiology of Chronic Kidney Disease

The most common causes of chronic kidney disease worldwide are diabetes and hypertension. Chronic kidney disease of unknown aetiology origin is an important cause in certain areas of India, Sri-Lanka, Nicaragua, Costa-Rica, Tunisia, El-Salvador. In the developed countries inherited kidney conditions such as polycystic kidney disease, chronic tubulo-interstitial fibrosis and chronic glomerulo-nephritis are also important cause of chronic kidney disease causing end stage kidney failure. The progression of chronic kidney disease depends on the rate of progression of fibrosis of the kidney parenchyma. The rate of progression of chronic kidney disease is variable and dependent on the causes of kidney disease.

Loss of functioning nephrons causes hyperfiltration in remaining nephrons. This hyperfiltration in individual nephrons leads to sclerosis of the glomeruli. Further nephron loss causes hyperfiltration in remaining functional glomeruli and thus the kidney disease progresses. Hence prevention of hyperfiltration using ACE inhibitors, angiotensin receptor blockers and more recently SGLT-2 inhibitors are important agents for prevention of progression of chronic kidney disease.

The Classification of Chronic Kidney Disease

Chronic kidney disease is divided into five GFR categories depending eGFR and three albuminuria categories depending on persistent albuminuria levels. This classification also emphasizes the increasing risk of adverse cardiac and renal outcomes, namely ESKD, acute coronary syndromes, heart failure and strokes heat map as shown in Fig. 5.1.

CKD can also be classified according to presence or absence of systemic diseases and which anatomical region in the kidney is affected kidney is affected by disease pathology as shown in Table 5.2.

Prognosis of CKD by GFR and Albuminuria Categories: KDIGO 2012				Persistent albuminuria categories Description and range		
				A1	A2	A3
				Normal to mildly increased	Moderately increased	Severely increased
				<30 mg/g <3 mg/mmol	30–300 mg/g 30–30 mg/mmol	<300 mg/g <30 mg/mmol
GFR categories (ml/min/1.73 m²) Description and range	G1	Normal or high	≥90			
	G2	Mildly decreased	60-89			
	G3a	Mildly to moderately decreased	45-59			
	G3b	Moderately to severely decreased	30-44			
	G4	Severely decreased	15-29			
	G5	Kidney failure	<15			

Green: low risk (if no other markers of kidney disease, no CKD); Yellow: moderately increased risk; Orange: high risk; Red, very high risk.

Fig. 5.1 Classification of Chronic Kidney Disease by stage (GFR and albuminuria) (reproduced with permission from KDIGO [1])

Table 5.2 Classification of kidney disease by histopathological diagnosis and systemic disease [1]

	Examples of systemic diseases affecting the kidney	Examples of primary kidney diseases (absence of systemic diseases affecting the kidney)
Glomerular diseases	Diabetes, systemic autoimmune diseases, systemic infections, drugs, neoplasia (including amyloidosis)	Diffuse, focal or crescentic proliferative GN; focal and segmental glomerulosclerosis, membranous nephropathy, minimal change disease
Tubulointerstitial diseases	Systemic infections, autoimmune disease e.g. sarcoidosis, drugs, urate, environmental toxins (lead, aristolochic acid), neoplasia (myeloma)	Urinary-tract infections, stones, obstruction
Vascular diseases	Atherosclerosis, hypertension, ischemia, cholesterol emboli, systemic vasculitis, thrombotic microangiopathy, systemic sclerosis	ANCA-associated renal limited vasculitis, fibromuscular dysplasia
Congenital and cystic diseases	Polycystic kidney disease, Alport syndrome, Fabry disease	Renal dysplasia, medullary cystic disease, podocytopathies

Genetic diseases are not considered separately because some diseases in each category are now recognized as having genetic determinants

ANCA antineutrophil cytoplasmic antibody, *CKD* chronic kidney disease, *GN* glomerulonephritis

*Note that there are many different ways in which to classify CKD. This method of separating systemic diseases and primary kidney diseases (modified from KDIGO CKD guidance 2012) [1]

Progression and Complications of Chronic Kidney Disease

Chronic kidney disease by nature is a progressive disease. The progression is estimated by serial estimation of GFR and albuminuria. With increasing creatinine and albuminuria the chronic kidney disease progresses towards kidney failure during which the patients experiences rising incidence of cardiovascular complications such as acute syndromes stroke and heart failure. A significant drop in eGFR is defined a drop in eGFR category with drop >25% in baseline. Rapid progression is defined as a loss of 5 mL/min/1.73 m^2 [or more] per year. The causes of progression include high blood pressure, high blood sugar control, older age, obesity, smoking, CV disease and use of nephrotoxins. The continuum of development, progression and complications are shown in the Fig. 5.2.

Several factors are associated with progression of CKD from early CKD to advanced CKD, including hypertension and diabetes mellitus (Table 5.3). Controlling such risk factors prevents progression.

With progression of chronic kidney disease, there are complications such as anaemia and chronic kidney disease-associated mineral bone disease (CKD-MBD). The anaemia is due to lack of production of erythropoietin (EPO) from peritubular interstitial cells. The erythropoietin producing cells sense hypoxia through stabilization

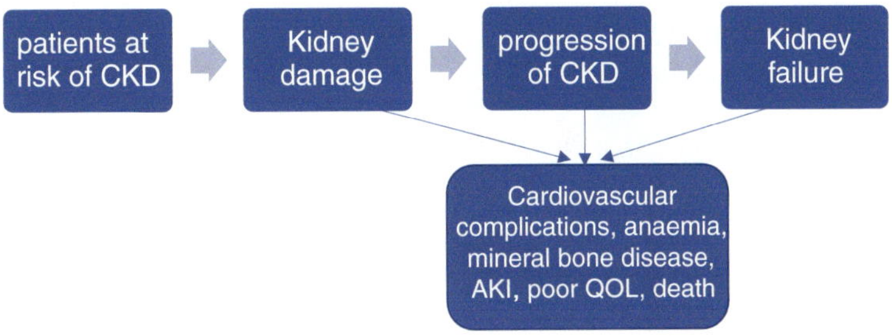

Fig. 5.2 The stages progression of CKD and emergence of complications [1]

Table 5.3 Risk factors for progression of CKD [1]

Non modifiable risk factors	Modifiable risk factors
Age	Elevated BP
Ethnicity	Hyperglycemia
Gender	Dyslipidemia
Cause of CKD	Smoking
Baseline eGFR	Obesity
Degree of albuminuria	Ongoing exposure to nephrotoxic substances

of hypoxia inducible factor-alpha (HIF-α), which in turn leads to activation of HIF target genes, including EPO.

CKD-MBD is due to phosphate retention by the failing kidneys, leading to hyperparathyroidism. The reduced activation of vitamin D causes poor calcium absorption from the gut, and low calcium levels leads to further hyperparathyroidism: hyperparathyroidism in this setting is a physiological homeostatic response to normalize calcium and phosphate. The stimulation of fibroblast growth factor 23 (FGF-23) is a further physiological response to normalize serum phosphate levels. Sustained kidney damage leads to persistent hyperparathyroidism, which leads to CKD-MBD (Fig. 5.3).

Progressive chronic kidney disease also causes hyperkalaemia, acidosis and fluid retention due to nephron malfunction.

The risk of complications are dependent on the level of eGFR and albuminuria. The relative risk rises with lower eGFR and high proteinuria. Estimates of risk may be useful in guiding patients about prognosis and planning management. With progression of CKD, the incidence of cardiovascular disease such as acute coronary syndromes and heart failure increases, together with the risk of dialysis requiring ESKD.

Online applications help with estimation of risk of progression e.g. https://kidneyfailurerisk.com/.

Figure 5.4 shows the relative risk of complications, dependent of different levels of GFR and albuminuria.

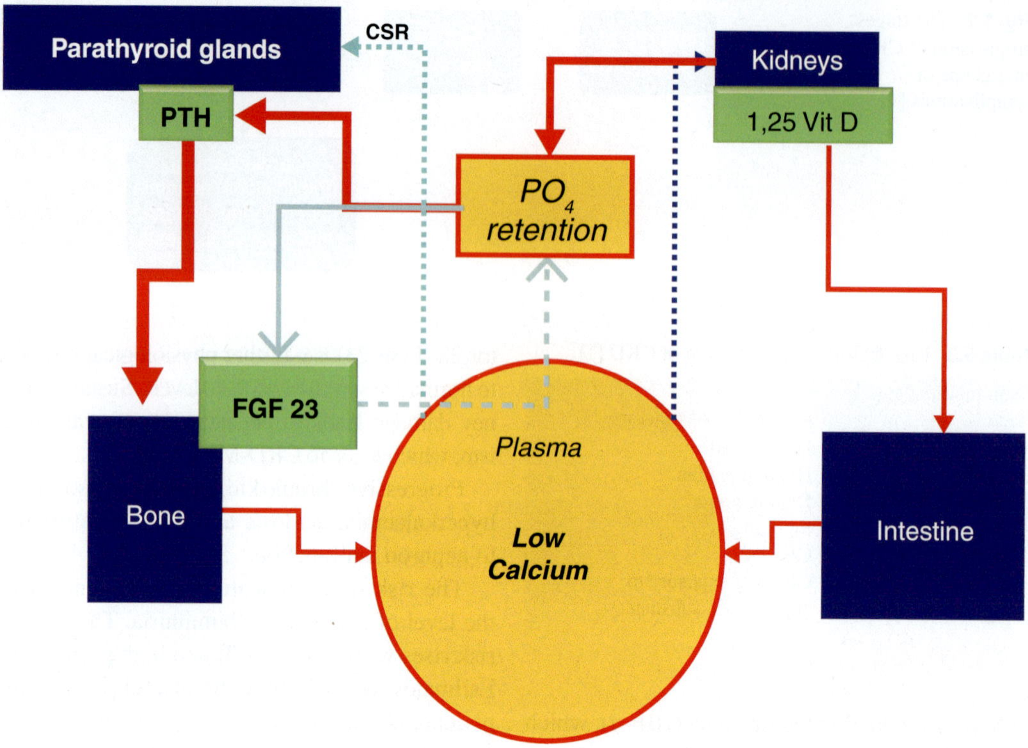

Fig. 5.3 Mechanism of chronic kidney disease mineral bone disease (CKD-MBD) [1]. Organs—Blue; Plasma—Yellow; Hormones—Green; Dotted lines: −ve feedback loop; solid lines: +ve feedback loop

Summary of relative risks from categorical meta-analysis (dipstick included) (–, ±, +, ≥++)

All-cause mortality

	ACR <10	ACR 10–29	ACR 30–299	ACR >300
eGFR >105	1.1	1.5	2.2	5.0
eGFR 90–106	Ref	1.4	1.5	3.1
eGFR 75–90	1.0	1.3	1.7	2.3
eGFR 60–75	1.0	1.4	1.8	2.7
eGFR 45–60	1.3	1.7	2.2	3.6
eGFR 30–45	1.9	2.3	3.3	4.9
eGFR 15–30	5.3	3.6	4.7	6.6

Cardiovascular mortality

	ACR <10	ACR 10–29	ACR 30–299	ACR >300
eGFR >105	0.9	1.3	2.3	2.1
eGFR 90–106	Ref	1.5	1.7	3.7
eGFR 75–90	1.0	1.3	1.6	3.7
eGFR 60–75	1.1	1.4	2.0	4.1
eGFR 45–60	1.5	2.2	2.8	4.3
eGFR 30–45	2.2	2.7	3.4	5.2
eGFR 15–30	1.4	7.9	4.8	8.1

Kidney failure (ESKD)

	ACR <10	ACR 10–29	ACR 30–299	ACR >300
eGFR >105	Ref	Ref	7.8	18
eGFR 90–106	Ref	Ref	11	20
eGFR 75–90	Ref	Ref	3.8	48
eGFR 60–75	Ref	Ref	7.4	67
eGFR 45–60	2.2	22	40	147
eGFR 30–45	56	74	294	763
eGFR 15–30	433	1044	1056	2286

Acute kidney injury (AKI)

	ACR <10	ACR 10–29	ACR 30–299	ACR >300
eGFR >105	Ref	Ref	2.7	8.4
eGFR 90–106	Ref	Ref	2.4	5.8
eGFR 75–90	Ref	Ref	2.5	4.1
eGFR 60–75	Ref	Ref	3.3	6.4
eGFR 45–60	2.2	4.9	6.4	5.9
eGFR 30–45	7.3	10	12	20
eGFR 15–30	17	17	21	29

Progressive CKD

	ACR <10	ACR 10–29	ACR 30–299	ACR >300
eGFR >105	Ref	Ref	0.4	3.0
eGFR 90–106	Ref	Ref	0.9	3.3
eGFR 75–90	Ref	Ref	1.9	5.0
eGFR 60–75	Ref	Ref	3.2	8.1
eGFR 45–60	3.1	4.0	9.4	57
eGFR 30–45	3.0	19	15	22
eGFR 15–30	4.0	12	2.1	7.7

Fig. 5.4 Risk of CKD complications with increasing albuminuria and decreasing GFR [2]. Summary of categorical meta-analysis (adjusted RRs) for general population cohorts with ACR. Mortality is reported for general population cohorts assessing albuminuria as urine ACR. Kidney outcomes are reported for general population cohorts assessing covariates and compared to the reference cell. Each cell represents a pooled RR from a meta-analysis; bold numbers indicated statistical significance at $P < 0.05$. Incidence rates per 1000 person years for the reference cells are 7.0 for all-cause mortality, 4.5 for CVD mortality, 0.04 for kidney failure, 0.98 for AKI, and 2.02 for CKD progression. Colours reflect the ranking of adjusted RR. The point estimates for each cell were ranked from 1 to 29 (the lowest RR having rank number 1, and the highest number 28). The categories with a rank number 1–8 are green, rank numbers 9–14 are yellow, the rank numbers 15–21 are orange, and the rank numbers 22–28 are coloured red. (For the outcome of CKD progression, two cells with RR < 1.0 are also green, leaving fewer cells as yellow, orange and red). *ACR* albumin to creatinine ratio, *AKI* acute kidney injury, *CKD* chronic kidney disease, *CVD* cardiovascular disease, *eGFR* estimated glomerular filtration rate, *ESKD* end stage kidney disease, *RR* relative risk. (Reprinted with permission from Macmillan publishers Ltd: Kidney International. Levey AS, de Jong PE, Coresh J, et al. The definition, classification, and prognosis of chronic kidney disease: a KDIGO controversies conference report. Kidney International 2011; 80: 17–28 [2])

Prevention of CKD

The at-risk group including patients with diabetes, hypertension and cardiovascular disease requires regular monitoring for detection of early CKD. In such patients, attention to risk factors for CKD such as blood sugar and blood pressure help delay the onset of albuminuria and declining kidney function.

Practice Points

- CKD is diagnosed with abnormal GFR, renal structure, proteinuria for more than 3 months.
- Important causes of CKD include diabetes, hypertension and CKDu.
- CKD is increasing in incidence world-wide.
- Complications of CKD include dialysis (or transplant), CV events, anaemia, MBD.
- The complications are dependent on stage of CKD and albuminuria.

Conclusions

The 48 year old patient with significant proteinuria suffered rapidly progressing CKD which is not uncommon in diabetic kidney disease; progressive chronic kidney disease is an independent risk factor for cardiovascular disease, end stage kidney disease (ESKD) and other complication. Identification of patients with rapid progression such as this allows them to be targeted for interventions to slow the progression of his chronic kidney disease with aggressive blood pressure and blood sugar control, and introduction of certain novel treatments, such as SGLT2 inhibitors.

Questions

1. A 65 year old man presents to his general practitioner. He has known hypertension and Type II diabetes which are treated with Ramipril and Metformin. His GP is concerned about how these conditions may affect his kidney function and investigates as follows:

   1st May: eGFR 57, ACR < 30 mg/g
   1st July: eGFR 54, ACR < 30 mg/g

   What can the general practitioner conclude from these results?

   A. No kidney disease
   B. Diagnose CKD G3aA1 with these results
   C. Repeat eGFR in August to confirm diagnosis
   D. Refer to nephrology
   E. Diagnose CKD G3bA1 with these results

   Answer: A. CKD is defined as an abnormal creatinine over 3 months

2. A 70 year old woman is diagnosed with CKD G3bA1. Which of these factors from her history is NOT a risk factor for development of CKD?

   A. Smoking
   B. Diabetes
   C. Hypertension
   D. Statin treatment
   E. Previous ITU admission for sepsis and AKI

   Answer: D. Statin treatment can rarely cause AKI due to rhabdomyolysis but does not cause CKD.

3. A 45 year old man presents to his general practitioner with increasingly swollen legs and notices he is short of breath on exertion. His past medical history is significant for poorly controlled Type I Diabetes.

   Which set of investigations is most appropriate to diagnose the likely cause of his symptoms?

A. Kidney biopsy
B. HbA1c, urine dip
C. CXR
D. eGFR, urinary ACR
E. Serum creatinine kinase

Answer: D. Measurement of eGFR and ACR will help with diagnosis of kidney failure or neprotic syndrome.

4. Which of these set of blood results would be typical in a diabetic patient with untreated CKD G4 A3?
   A. Hypoalbuminaemia, Hyperphosphataemia, Hyperparathyroidism, Hyperlipidaemia, Hyperkalaemia, Anaemia
   B. Hyperalbuminaemia, Hyperphosphataemia, Hyperparathyroidism, Hyperlipidaemia, Hypokalaemia, Anaemia
   C. Hypoalbuminaemia, Hypophosphataemia, Hyperparathyroidism, Hyperlipidaemia, Hyperkalaemia, Anaemia
   D. Hypoalbuminaemia, Hypophosphataemia, Hypoparathyroidism, Hyperlipidaemia, Normokalaemia, Anaemia
   E. Hypoalbuminaemia, Hypophosphataemia, Hypoparathyroidism, Hypolipidaemia, Normokalaemia, Anaemia

Answer: A. Stage 4 is associated with complications of high potassium, phosphate, parathyroid hormone, dyslipidaemia, erythropoietin deficiency

5. 60-year old female presented with worsening eGFR for 5 years from 54 to 45 mL/min/1.73 m^2. Her Blood pressure was 162/90, HBA1c 57 mmol/mol, haemoglobin 110 g/L, phosphate 1.9 mmol/L

   Which is the risk factor which requires most attention to prevent further progression?
   A. High blood sugars
   B. High blood pressure
   C. High phosphate
   D. Low haemoglobin
   E. Low vitamin D

Answer: B. Hypertension is the most important risk factor for prevention of CKD progression

6. 60 year old female presented with worsening eGFR for 5 years from 54 to 45 mL/min/1.73 m^2. Her Blood pressure was 162/90, HBA1c 57 mmol/mol, haemoglobin 110 g/L, phosphate 1.9 mmol/L

   What is the most likely adverse outcome
   A. Acute Kidney Injury
   B. Bleeding
   C. Cardiovascular event
   D. Dialysis
   E. Liver failure

Answer: C. Cardiovascular event

7. 60 year old female presented with worsening eGFR for 5 years from 54 to 45 mL/min/1.73 m^2. Her Blood pressure was 162/90, HBA1c 57 mmol/mol, haemoglobin 110 g/L, phosphate 1.9 mmol/L

   What is the most likely response from the body to manage high phosphate
   A. High erythropoietin
   B. High fibroblast growth factor 23
   C. High vitamin D
   D. Low calcitonin
   E. Low parathyroid

Answer: B. FGF23 is a phosphaturic hromone

8. 60-year-old diabetic female presented with worsening eGFR for 5 years from 54 to 45 mL/min/1.73 m^2. Her Blood pressure was 162/90, HBA1c 57 mmol/mol, haemoglobin 110 g/L, potassium 4.9 mmol/L, phosphate 1.9 mmol/L, ACR 2.1 mg/mol

   What is best initial agent to control his blood pressure?
   A. Amlodipine
   B. Bisoprolol
   C. Doxazocin
   D. Losartan
   E. Nifedipine

Answer: D. Losartan [ARB] reduces progression of CKD

9. 60-year-old diabetic female presented with worsening eGFR. Her Blood pressure was 162/90, HBA1c 57 mmol/mol, haemoglobin 110 g/L, potassium 4.9 mmol/L, phosphate 1.9 mmol/L, ACR 2.1 mg/mol, MCV 85

What is the most likely cause of anaemia

A. Iron deficiency
B. Folate deficiency
C. Erythropoietin deficiency
D. Vitamin B12 deficiency
E. Vitamin D deficiency

Answer: C. Low erythropoietin is possible cause for normocytic anaemia

10. 60-year-old diabetic female presented with worsening eGFR . Her Blood pressure was 162/90, HBA1c 57 mmol/mol, haemoglobin 110 g/L, potassium 4.9 mmol/L, phosphate 1.9 mmol/L, ACR 2.1 mg/mol, MCV 85, bilirubin 15

What is next best step in management

A. Coombs test
B. Hemoglobin electrophoresis
C. Measure ferritin and transferrin saturation
D. Measure serum iron and ferritin
E. Start erythropoietin

Answer: C. Ferritin and TSAT a good markers of iron stores

Test your learning and check your understanding of this book's contents: use the "Springer Nature Flashcards" app to access questions using https://sn.pub/cz9Cok. To use the app, please follow the instructions in Chap. 1.

References

1. KDIGO CKD guidelines 2012. https://kdigo.org/wp-content/uploads/2017/02/KDIGO_2012_CKD_GL.pdf.
2. Levey AS, de Jong PE, Coresh J, et al. The definition, classification, and prognosis of chronic kidney disease: a KDIGO controversies conference report. Kidney Int. 2011;80:17–28.

CKD: Management and Prognosis

6

Adeera Levin and Magdalena Madero

Clinical Scenario

You are caring for a 63 year old man with a history of diabetes mellitus, hypertension and gout, with one remote episode of Kidney stones. His eGFR 38 mL/min, urine albumin creatinine ratio (uACR) 48 mg/mmol; Hb 115 g/L; Transferrin saturation 0.20%; his electrolytes are normal apart from a slightly elevated potassium 5.1 mol/L. His HbA1C 7.9%, and his blood pressure is 138/85 mmHg. With a 24 h ambulatory BP monitor, you note that he does not have a nocturnal dip. He is currently on an ARB (Losartan), a diuretic (Chlorthalidone), lipid lowering agent (simvastatin), metformin and insulin.

Introduction

The prognosis of CKD is predicated on both underlying cause of the kidney disease, the GFR and the albuminuria levels, (CGA classification, KDIGO) [1]. This classification system helps to identify those at high risk of progression, and of other complications (cardiovascular events, hospitalization, infection, death, and AKI).

The management of CKD is then focused on addressing modifiable risk factors to improve patient outcomes, and reduce the incidence of events or delay progression of CKD and attendant CV and other system complications.

Epidemiology and Causes

The epidemiology of CKD is well described in multiple publications. The estimated prevalence around the world is approximately 10% in the adult population, with variability in estimates due to data capture, ability to obtain blood and urine samples, and regional differences in true prevalence. The causes of CKD may differ in different parts of the world, driven by local exposures and conditions. That being said, diabetes and hypertension remain the leading causes of CKD worldwide, as the incidence of these conditions rises, so will CKD. In addition, recurrent AKI episodes due to infections, malnutrition, diarrheal illness, heat stress or combinations thereof is well recognized in specific regions of the world. Kidney diseases may be classified according to cause, or into categories associated with anatomic locations (e.g. prerenal, intrinsic and post renal). Any sustained kidney injury, regardless off the etiology, could translate into CKD. As many conditions may coexist, or accrue over time within an individual, the

A. Levin (✉)
Division of Nephrology, University of British Columbia, Vancouver, BC, Canada
e-mail: ALevin@providencehealth.bc.ca

M. Madero
Division of Nephrology, Instituto Nacional de Cardiologia Ignacio Chavez, Ciudad de México, Mexico

D. Banerjee et al. (eds.), *Management of Kidney Diseases*,
https://doi.org/10.1007/978-3-031-09131-5_6

etiology of CKD is often multifactorial. Major categories of CKD include Congenital or Acquired conditions. Congenital conditions often include malformations of the genito-urinary system, which lead to a reduction in nephron mass or dysfunctional glomerular and tubular function, all of which culminate in progressive kidney decline. Inherited diseases contribute to approximately 4% of CKD worldwide, and include conditions such as APCKD, Alport's Syndrome, Fabry' disease amongst others. Acquired conditions include glomerulonephritidies, diabetes, stone disease, tubulointerstial diseases, due to drugs, toxins and environmental pollutants. It is beyond the scope of this chapter to delineate all the causes of CKD, but the reader is referred to Table 6.1.

Table 6.1 Causes of chronic kidney disease

Cause	Example
Tubulointerstitial nephritis	Acute or chronic due to analgesic medications (NSAIDS),antibiotics, toxins, heavy metals, herbal medications
Glomerulonephritis (primary)	IgA nephropathy, membranoproliferative glomerulopenprhitis, focal segmental glomerulosclerosis, membranous nephropathy
Glomerular disease (due to systemic illness)	Vasculitis, systemic lupus Erithematoso, amyloidosis, diabetes mellitis, trombotic microangiopathy
Hereditary diseases	Polycystic kidney disease, Alport syndrome, medullary cystic disease, Fabrys disease
Hypertension	Nephroangioesclerosis
Obstructive	Benign prostatic hyperplasia, posterior urethral valves, ureteral obstruction (litiasis, malignancy, congenital), vesicoureteral reflux
Large renal vascular disease	Renal artery stenosis (atherosclerosis or fibromuscular displasia)

Investigations

Chronic Kidney Disease is often under recognized and therefore not treated. Investigations that help to both prognosticate and manage CKD are listed in Fig. 6.1. The classification of CKD is based on eGFR and albuminuria determination. Staging patients with CKD according to cause, eGFR, and albuminuria enhances risk stratification for the major complications of CKD [1].

If available, imaging techniques (such as ultrasound) are important to assess size, symmetry and space occupying lesions intrinsic or extrinsic to the kidney.

Urinalysis in addition to urine albumin or protein determinations may add additional information. For example, red cells, white cells or casts may contribute to further diagnostic investigations (e.g., biopsy) or signal new or additional processes contributing to CKD progression.

CKD screening however is not recommended in the general population, screening should be done in high-risk populations such as age > 60 years, diabetes, hypertension, family history of kidney disease, history of kidney stones etc.

Note that regular monitoring of various parameters will help to determine responsiveness to therapy, and serve as excellent feedback for patients and the health care providers.

The regularity of monitoring depends on health care system resources as well as specifics of the patient. Recommendations in the table below presume access to resources for 'average' individuals, and would not apply to those whose other comorbidities (e.g. terminal cancers or advance heart failure), or advanced age, or both which would limit interventions or utility.

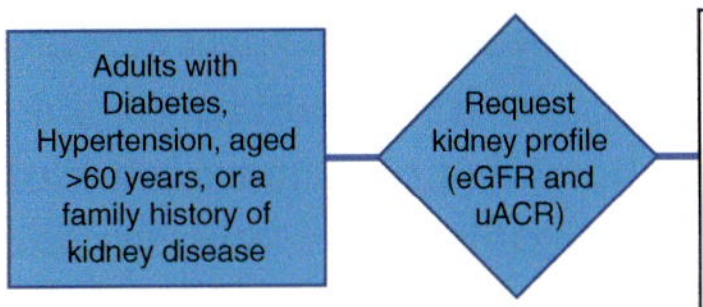

CKD is classified on the basis of: Cause (C) GFR (G) Albuminuria (A)			Albuminuria categories Description & range		
			A1	A2	A3
			Normal to mildly increased	Moderately increased	Severely increased
			<30 mg/g <3 mg/mmol	30-299 mg/g 3-30 mg/mmol	>300 mg/g >30 mg/mmol
GFR categories by eGFR (ml/min/1.73m²) Description & range: G1	Normal or high	>90	1	1	2
G2	Mildly decreased	60-89	1	1	2
G3A	Mildly to moderately decreased	45-59	1	2	3
G3B	Moderately to severely decreased	30-45	2	3	3
G4	Severely decreased	15-29	3	3	4+
G5	Kidney failure	<15	4+	4+	4+

Fig. 6.1 Risk of CKD Progression and Frequency of Assessment: Summary of recommendation statement (according to estimated glomerular filtration rate (eGFR) and albuminuria)

- The GFR and albuminuria grid depicts the risk of progression, morbidity and mortality by colour, from lowest to highest (green, yellow, orange, red, deep red)
- The numbers in the boxes are a guide to the frequency of assessment annually.
  - Green annual assessment for those at risk (Green can reflect CKD with normal eGFR and albumin-to-creatinine ratio (ACR) only in the presence of other markers of kidney damage, such as imaging showing Polycystic kidney disease or kidney biopsy abnormalities)
  - Yellow suggests assessment at least once per year
  - Orange suggests assessment twice per year
  - Red suggests assessment three times annually
  - Deep red suggests assessment four times annually
- These are general parameters only, based on expert opinion and must take into account underlying comorbid conditions and disease state, as well as the likelihood of impacting a change in management for any individual patient

(Kidney International 2013; 3 (Suppl):5 [1]. National Kidney Foundation. K/DOQI clinical practice guidelines for chronic kidney disease: evaluation, classification, and stratification. Am J Kidney Dis 2002; 39 (Suppl 1):S1 [2])

Management

The general management of the patient with CKD involves the following issues.

- Treatment of reversible causes of kidney dysfunction (e.g. obstruction, underperfusion).
- Preventing or slowing the progression of kidney disease.
- Treatment of the complications of kidney disease.
- Adjusting drug doses (or discontinuing) when appropriate for the level of estimated glomerular filtration rate (eGFR).
- Identification and adequate preparation of the patient in whom kidney replacement therapy will be required.

Treatment of Reversible Causes of Kidney Failure

hypovolemia, hypotension, nephrotoxic drugs (NSAIDS, Ace Inhibitors, antibiotics), Intravenous contrast material, obstruction, sepsis are common causes of reversible kidney injury and should always be assessed as an initial approach to kidney function deterioration.

Slowing the Progression of Kidney Disease

Treatment of the underlying cause of kidney disease should be targeted, i.e. APDKD, diabetes, glomerular disease, viral infections, liver disease, cardiac disease, malignancy etc. In those conditions there may be treatments or strategies that are suggested by the specificity of the diagnosis. Note that is some cases there may be more than one cause of CKD.

In addition, there are treatments that are universal for CKD patients: blood pressure control and proteinuria reduction. Blood pressure should be controlled to less than 120/80 mmHg using standardized office blood pressure measurement [2]. More intensive versus less intensive blood pressure control reduces the risk of end-stage renal disease (ESRD) in patients with proteinuric chronic kidney disease (CKD), but not in patients with nonproteinuric CKD. However, more intensive blood pressure lowering may reduce mortality in patients with CKD (whether they have proteinuria or not), even though there is no benefit on kidney endpoints among patients without proteinuria. The mortality benefit from aggressive blood pressure lowering noted in the Systolic Pressure Intervention Trial (SPRINT) [3].

The preferred antiypertensive agents in subjects with proteinuria are ACE inhibitors, ARB and mineralocorticoid receptor antagonists.

ACE inhibitors generally reduce protein excretion by approximately 30–35% in patients with nondiabetic or diabetic CKD. Similar results have been demonstrated with ARB [4]. The antiproteinuric effect is most prominent in patients who are on a low-sodium diet or who are treated with diuretics and it is dose dependent. Clinical trials have demonstrated a benefit of antihypertensive therapy with renin-angiotensin system (RAS) inhibitors, mostly angiotensin-converting enzyme (ACE) inhibitors, in patients with proteinuric nondiabetic chronic kidney disease (CKD). The renoprotective effect of angiotensin II receptor blockers (ARBs) has been best demonstrated in patients with diabetic nephropathy. It seems likely that they have a similar renoprotective effect as ACE inhibitors in nondiabetic CKD but supportive data are limited. ACE inhibitors or ARB should be given to proteinuric patients, with a recommendation of titrating either to maximal dose, however the combination of ACE and ARB has not been superior to individual treatment for CKD progression and has been associated with hyperkalemia and acute kidney injury [5].

Other Treatments

Patients who have proteinuric CKD (with or without diabetes) can benefit from treatment with SGLT2 inhibitors. Most of the trials including SGLT2 inhibitors have been performed in proteinuric patients although there is evidence to suggest that the benefit may be extended to non proteinuric CKD [6].

More recently newer non selective mineralocorticoid inhibitors such as finerenone reduced CKD progression in proteinuric diabetic kidney disease. More studies with these types if agents are required to confirm these findings [7].

Other targets for halting kidney disease progression should may protein restriction (0.8 g/kg/day), smoking cessation, weight management, glycemic control, healthy diet and physical activity.

Treatment of CKD Complications

The complications of kidney function include volume management, anemia, mineral bone disease, metabolic acidosis, hyperkalemia and malnutrition. These have been covered extensively in other chapters of this book, and are not dealt with here.

Drug Dosing and Adjustments in CKD

There are drugs which are nephrotoxic and should be avoided in CKD pts. (e.g. aminoglycosides, NSAIDs, some chemotherapeutic agents), or at least used with extreme caution.

There are other medications which require dose modification in CKD, and other which should be stopped at different GFR thresholds. A full list is beyond the remit of this chapter, but the reader is encouraged to review patient drug profiles, and before commencing new medications, to review the indications and potential side effects.

Drugs may impact kidney function through direct tubular or interstitial toxicity (e.g. Lithium, tenofovir, aminoglycosides); or promote progression fibrosis through multiple mechanisms (e.g. proton pump inhibitors, calceniurin inhibitors). Some drugs lead to a change in serum creatinine through interfering with creatinine secretion which is often confused with 'kidney damage': these changes are reversible with cessation of the drug (e.g. cotrimoxazole, cimetidine, fenofibrate).

Drugs that are excreted by the kidney require dose adjustments or cessation with advanced CKD (e.g. digoxin, novel anticoagulants e.g., apixiban).

Identification and Adequate Preparation of the Patient in Whom Kidney Replacement Therapy Will Be Required

Management of patients with CKD requires prognostication and anticipation of the need for Kidney replacement therapy in those who are eligible for it, or in whom it is appropriate. Use of the KFRE (kidney failure risk equation https://kidneyfailurerisk.com) [8] may help to identify those at highest risk for kidney failure within 2 years, and might help with planning of discussions.

The role of clinicians and clinical team members working with patients and families is to identify appropriate time points and educational materials which will help with decision making. There are data to suggest that decision making about complex choices (such type of dialysis, transplantation etc.) requires time, multiple interactions and appropriate tools to enhance understanding, Those who choose hemodialysis would ideally require placement of arterio-venous fistula at least 3–6 months prior to anticipated commencement of dialysis; those who choose peritoneal dialysis require catheter placement at least 2–4 weeks prior to commencement; and if living pre-emptive transplantation is required this process often takes between 6 and 9 months of preparation for donors and recipients. Thus, overall, best practices would suggest that discussions about kidney replacement therapy should commence at least 18 months in advance of anticipated need if possible, to optimize decision making and allow adequate time for discussion and procedures/processes to be put in place.

Conservative management options for those who either choose not to have KRT, or in whom it is not appropriate due to significant morbidity or futility should be offered. These include ongoing supportive care, symptom management and provision for palliative care services [9].

Health care system resources will vary around the world, and within jurisdictions. Not all countries or regions can offer KRT to individuals, and thus conservative care strategies should be clearly articulated and offered when KRT is not available [10].

Clinicians and their teams should have a good understanding of resources available in their jurisdiction, and how to access them to aid in appropriate timing for individuals patients.

Practice Points

Management of progressive CKD involves:

- Treatment of reversible causes of kidney dysfunction
- Prevention/slowing the progression ofCKD with BP control use of RAASi and SGLT2i
- Treatment of the complications of kidney disease, anaemia, CKD-MBD, hyperkalaemia
- Adjusting drug doses (or discontinuing) when appropriate for the level of eGFR
- Identification and adequate preparation of the patient for KRT

Conclusions

The 63 year old man has chronic kidney disease related to diabetes and may benefit from tighter blood pressure control. A calcium channel blocker may be started once the ARB and diuretic dose are maximised. Despite mild anemia treatment with iron or erythropoietin is perhaps not necessary at this stage. Tighter blood sugar control may not help but a SGLT2i may prevent progression of CKD and CV events.

Questions

1. What is the CKD stage on this patient?
   A. G3b A2
   B. G3A A1
   C. G1 A2
   D. G2 A2
   E. G4 A3

Answer: the correct answer is A, the patient has a GFR of 38 mL/min (stage G3B) and ACR of 48 g/g (stage A2).
EASY.

2. Based on his risk factors, how often does he need medical attention?
   A. Once a year
   B. Twice a year
   C. Three times/year
   D. Four times/year

EASY, Answer: based on the expert recommendations this patient risk is high for progression and cardiovascular events and should be monitored twice a year.

3. His target blood pressure should be:
   A. <120/80
   B. <130/80
   C. <140/90
   D. <110/70
   E. Between 130/80 and 140/90

Easy: The correct answer is A, based on data from SPRINT, CKD patients benefit from strict BP control. Current KDIGO guidelines recommend BP <120/80 in all CKD patients with and without albuminuria.

4. Based on his blood pressure, what would be the next step
   A. No change in management
   B. Increase losartan dose to a maximal dose
   C. Add an ACE inhibitor
   D. Start MRA
   E. Initiate SGLT2i

Easy; the correct answer is B, ARB dose should be maximized before adding another agent. The patient BP should be targeted to <130/80. Adding an ACE inhibitor to an ARB in DKD is no longer recommended. Mineralocorticoid receptor antagonists or SGLT2 inhibitors could be initiated once the patient is on maximal doses of ARB or ACE inhibitors.

5. Lowering blood pressure in this patient would:
   A. Delay the progression to ESKD
   B. Reduce cardiovascular complications
   C. Reduce all cause mortality
   D. No benefit
   E. B and C

Difficult; the correct answer is E, data from SPRInt showed BP reduction in CKD patients with small amounts of albuminuria benefit from cardiovascular and all cause mortality but does not halt CKD progression.

6. Adding SGLT2 inhibitor in this patient would result in:
   A. Delay in CKD progression
   B. Increase the risk of acute kidney injury
   C. Increase the risk for cardiovascular events
   D. Substantial glycemic control

The correct answer is A, SGLT2 inhibitors delay CKD progression even in normoalbuminuric (<30 mg/g), moderately increased albuminuria (30–299 mg/g) or large albuminuria (>300 mg/g), although the risk reduction is higher with higher ACR. SGLT2 inhibitors do not increase the risk of AKI (CREDENCE), are associated with a decrease in CV events. The glycemic control obtained from SGLT2 inhibitors is poor and the benefit is independent from glycemic control.

7. The estimated GFR calculations should not be used in the which of the following populations (Check all that apply)
   A. Amputees
   B. People at extremes of weight and height
   C. People of African descent
   D. People of Asian descent
   E. A and B

The correct answer is E, as the eGFR calculations are based on populations means, presuming height and weight distributions for age norms, and were never tested in those with severe cachexia or very high BMI, nor in those with amputations. Thus they should be used in caution with those individuals, or interpreted corrected for BSA.

8. Based on the new blood pressure guidelines, target BP should be established based on what type of blood pressure readings?
   A. Standardized Office Blood Pressure
   B. Manual Office Blood Pressure
   C. Home Blood Pressure readings
   D. Ambulatory Blood Pressure Measurements

The correct answer is A: standardized office BP measurement is recommended in preference to routine office BP measurement for the management of high BP in adults.

9. The recommended sodium intake in a patient with CKD and hypertension is:
   A. <1 g of sodium per day or <45 mmol per day or <2.5 g of sodium chloride per day
   B. <2 g of sodium per day (or <90 mmol of sodium per day), or <5 g of sodium chloride per day
   C. <4 g of sodium per day (or <180 mmol of sodium per day) or <8 g of sodium chloride per day
   D. Sodium restriction is not recommended if patients already of SGLT2 inhibitor

The correct answer is B. Targeting a sodium intake <2 g of sodium per day (or <90 mmol of sodium per day, or <5 g of sodium chloride per day) in patients with high BP and CKD is recommended.

10. Which of the following statements is correct:
    A. An AVF should be placed between 3 and 6 months before starting hemodialysis
    B. an AV graft could be placed within 2 weeks of hemodyalisis initiation and is the preferred choice
    C. a catheter can be placed for urgent hemodialysis initiation in those patients without mature AV fistula
    D. AV Fistulas are contraindicated in diabetic patients due to small vessel size
    E. A catheter should always be placed prior to starting RRT, regardless of other access planning

The correct answers are A and C. Although an AVgraft can be placed 2 weeks before hemodialysis initiation, it is not the preferred choice. Diabetic patients are suitable for AV fistulas although sometimes vessels are not ideal for fistula creation. If a patient already has an AVF or AVgraft, these can be used to start hemodialysis and catheters should be avoided.

Test your learning and check your understanding of this book's contents: use the "Springer Nature Flashcards" app to access questions using https://sn.pub/cz9Cok. To use the app, please follow the instructions in Chap. 1.

References

1. KDIGO. Summary of recommendation statements. Kidney Int. 2013;3 (Suppl):5.
2. Improving Global Outcomes (KDIGO) Blood Pressure Work Group. KDIGO 2021 clinical practice guideline for the management of blood pressure in chronic kidney disease. Kidney Int. 2021;99(3S):S1–S87.
3. SPRINT Research Group, Wright JT Jr, Williamson JD, Whelton PK, Snyder JK, Sink KM, Rocco MV, Reboussin DM, Rahman M, Oparil S, Lewis CE, Kimmel PL, Johnson KC, Goff DC Jr, Fine LJ, Cutler JA, Cushman WC, Cheung AK, Ambrosius WT. A randomized trial of intensive versus standard blood-pressure control. N Engl J Med. 2015;373(22):2103–16.

4. Kunz R, Friedrich C, Wolbers M, Mann JF. Meta-analysis: effect of monotherapy and combination therapy with inhibitors of the renin angiotensin system on proteinuria in renal disease. Ann Intern Med. 2008;148(1):30–48.
5. Fried LF, Emanuele N, Zhang JH, Brophy M, Conner TA, Duckworth W, Leehey DJ, McCullough PA, O'Connor T, Palevsky PM, Reilly RF, Seliger SL, Warren SR, Watnick S, Peduzzi P, Guarino P, VA NEPHRON-D Investigators. Combined angiotensin inhibition for the treatment of diabetic nephropathy. N Engl J Med. 2013;369(20):1892–903.
6. Heerspink HJL, Kosiborod M, Inzucchi SE, Cherney DZI. Renoprotective effects of sodium-glucose cotransporter-2 inhibitors. Kidney Int. 2018;94(1):26–39.
7. Bakris GL, Agarwal R, Anker SD, Pitt B, Ruilope LM, Rossing P, Kolkhof P, Nowack C, Schloemer P, Joseph A, Filippatos G, FIDELIO-DKD Investigators. Effect of Finerenone on chronic kidney disease outcomes in type 2 diabetes. N Engl J Med. 2020;383(23):2219–29.
8. Tangri N, Stevens LA, Griffith J, et al. A predictive model for progression of chronic kidney disease to kidney failure. JAMA. 2011;305(15):1553–9.
9. Davison SN, Levin A, Moss AH, Jha V, Brown EA, Brennan F, Murtagh FE, Naicker S, Germain MJ, O'Donoghue DJ, Morton RL, Obrador GT, Kidney Disease: Improving Global Outcomes. Executive summary of the KDIGO controversies conference on supportive care in chronic kidney disease: developing a roadmap to improving quality care. Kidney Int. 2015;88(3):447–59.
10. Harris DCH, Davies SJ, Finkelstein FO, Jha V, Bello AK, Brown M, Caskey FJ, Donner JA, Liew A, Muller E, Naicker S, O'Connell PJ, Filho RP, Vachharajani T, Strategic Plan Working Groups. Strategic plan for integrated care of patients with kidney failure. Kidney Int. 2020;98(5S):S117–34.

7 Management of Anaemia in Chronic Kidney Disease

Sunil Bhandari and Chuan-Ming Hao

Clinical Scenario

A 54 year-old man with Stage G4A3 CKD secondary to insulin-treated diabetes mellitus attended the renal outpatient clinic with increased lethargy and breathlessness. He had a previous history of a stroke, myocardial infarction, hypertension and had a fistula in situ. He was otherwise well.

On examination, his blood pressure was 156/72 mmHg and he was clinically pale. He was on Ramipril, Bisoprolol, Insulin, Furosemide, Atorvastatin and Aspirin.

Initial investigations found:

Haemoglobin	**106 g/L**	**(130–180)**
Platelet count	164×10^9/L	(150–400)
Serum ferritin	**130 μg/L**	**(15–300)**
Transferrin saturation	**18%**	**(20–50)**
Serum creatinine	383 μmol/L	(60–110)
eGFR (MDRD)	17 mL/min/1.73 m^2	(>60)

Does this gentleman have anaemia, and how common is it?

S. Bhandari (✉)
Hull University Teaching Hospitals NHS Trust, Hull, UK
e-mail: sunil.bhandari@nhs.net

C.-M. Hao
Division of Nephrology, Huashan Hospital, Fudan University, Shanghai, China
e-mail: chuanminghao@fudan.edu.cn

Introduction

Anaemia is common in chronic kidney disease (CKD). Iron deficiency and erythropoietin (EPO) deficiency are perhaps the most common causes of anaemia in patients with CKD, especially those requiring kidney replacement therapy (KRT/dialysis) [1–3]. The Renal National Service Framework and National Institute for Health and Clinical Excellence in the UK (NICE), and Kidney Disease Improving Global Outcomes (KDIGO), all advocate treatment of anaemia in patients with CKD [4–10]. Intravenous (IV) Iron therapy leads to a reduction in the use of erythropoietin stimulating agents (ESA). This reduction in ESA use may be potentially beneficial in certain cases such as reducing cardiovascular risk. The close relationship of anaemia, iron deficiency, CKD and cardiovascular disease make its therapy critical to improved clinical outcomes [11]. ESA therapy remains important after iron repletion to optimise haemoglobin concentrations to a KDIGO target range of 100–115 g/L. [5] Blood transfusions are infrequently required, and newer therapies such as Hypoxia-inducible factor (HIF) stabilisers are on the horizon [12–14].

Chronic kidney disease (CKD) is an increasing problem with over 850 million people suffering from kidney disease worldwide [7]. In the UK it affects approximately 4–6% of the adult population [3], 8–13% of the population in the

D. Banerjee et al. (eds.), *Management of Kidney Diseases*,
https://doi.org/10.1007/978-3-031-09131-5_7

USA [1] and 10.8% of the adult population of China [7]. The prevalence of cardiovascular morbidity and mortality is high in this patient population and the cost of caring for these patients presents a large economic burden to the health care systems. Indeed, kidney disease is the cause of almost 2.4 million deaths per year being the sixth fastest growing cause of death overall. It is the ninth leading cause of death in the USA, the 11th in Europe and 16th in China [1, 5, 7].

Definition of Anaemia in CKD

The World Health Organization (WHO) defines anaemia as an Hb concentration below a given threshold which is dependent on gender, age and menopausal/pregnancy status. However, this definition does not apply to CKD; an Hb between 100 g/L and 120 g/L is currently accepted as "normal" or at least adequate, based on National Institute of Health and Clinical Excellence, who define anaemia as an Hb < 110 g/L. [2, 8] Kidney Disease Improving Global Outcomes (KDIGO) 2012 guidelines recommend a target Hb of between 90 and <115 g/L. [7]

Prevalence

The prevalence of anaemia increases in the CKD population as renal function declines. The aetiology of anaemia in this group is multifactorial: relative erythropoietin (EPO) deficiency, iron depletion (absolute or functional), inflammation, higher levels of uraemic toxins and bleeding all contribute to the development of CKD-anaemia [7].

Anaemia of CKD is common in advanced CKD (Table 7.1). The median Hb in prevalent HD and peritoneal dialysis patients in the UK was 111 g/L, and 83.7% of them had a Hb of less than 120 g/L. [3]

Table 7.1 Prevalence of anaemia in USA, Europe and China in advanced CKD (stages 4 and 5)

	USA	Europe	China
	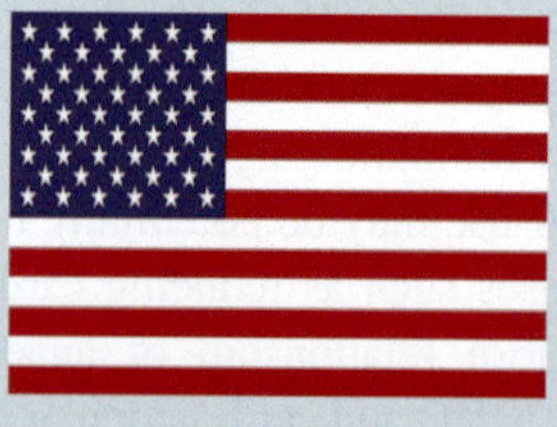	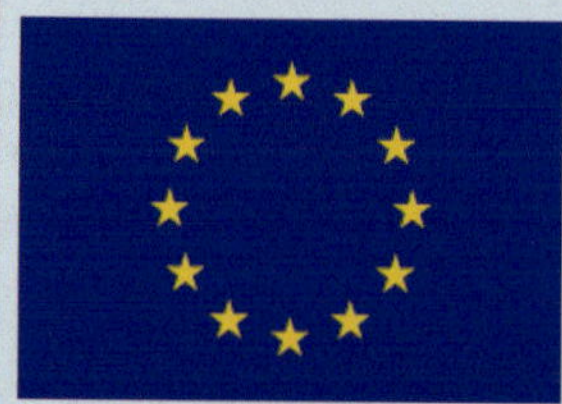	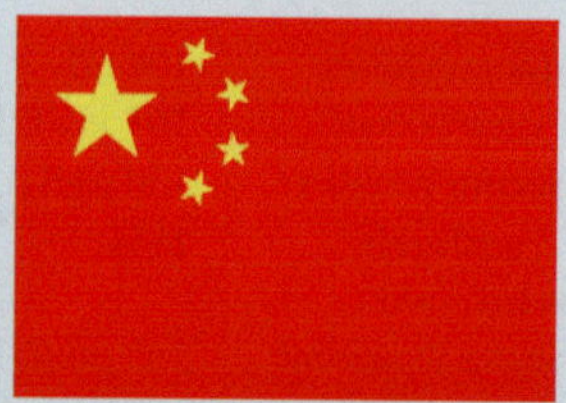
CKD Stage 4	64%	79.2%	76%
CKD Stage 5	72.8%	87%	90.2%

The Patient in the Clinical Scenario Has Diabetes, and Is Therefore more Likely to Have Anaemia

In patients with diabetes mellitus and CKD in comparison to those without diabetes mellitus, anaemia is more common even at modestly impaired eGFR values of <60 mL/min/1.73 m^2 (12% *vs.* 6%) and this increases dramatically as eGFR falls to a prevalence of over 50% in patients with and eGFR <30 mL/min/1.73 m^2 [15, 16].

What Factors Might Contribute to Anaemia

Most cases of anaemia in CKD are due to iron deficiency and anaemia of chronic disease, but other traditional and less common causes require consideration and exclusion (Fig. 7.1a and b). In a small cohort study of patients with CKD, 43% of the patients with identified anaemia and 15% of those without anaemia had iron and/or folate deficiency [17].

The hormone hepcidin, produced by the liver, is responsible for the control of iron absorption and macrophage iron recycling. In patients with CKD, levels of hepcidin are significantly elevated due to decreased renal clearance and inflammation induced production [18]. This leads to both true (absolute) and functional iron deficiency. CKD also leads to impaired production of erythropoietin, which reduces red cell production in the bone marrow. Inflammatory cytokines also contribute to suppression of erythropoiesis. Red cell lifespan is shortened due to inflammation and uraemia. Patients with CKD may have increased blood loss through haemodialysis circuits, frequent phlebotomy and in some cases chronic bleeding. The red bars demonstrate factors that contribute to anaemia; the green arrows indicate targets for treatment. ESA = erythropoiesis-stimulating agent.

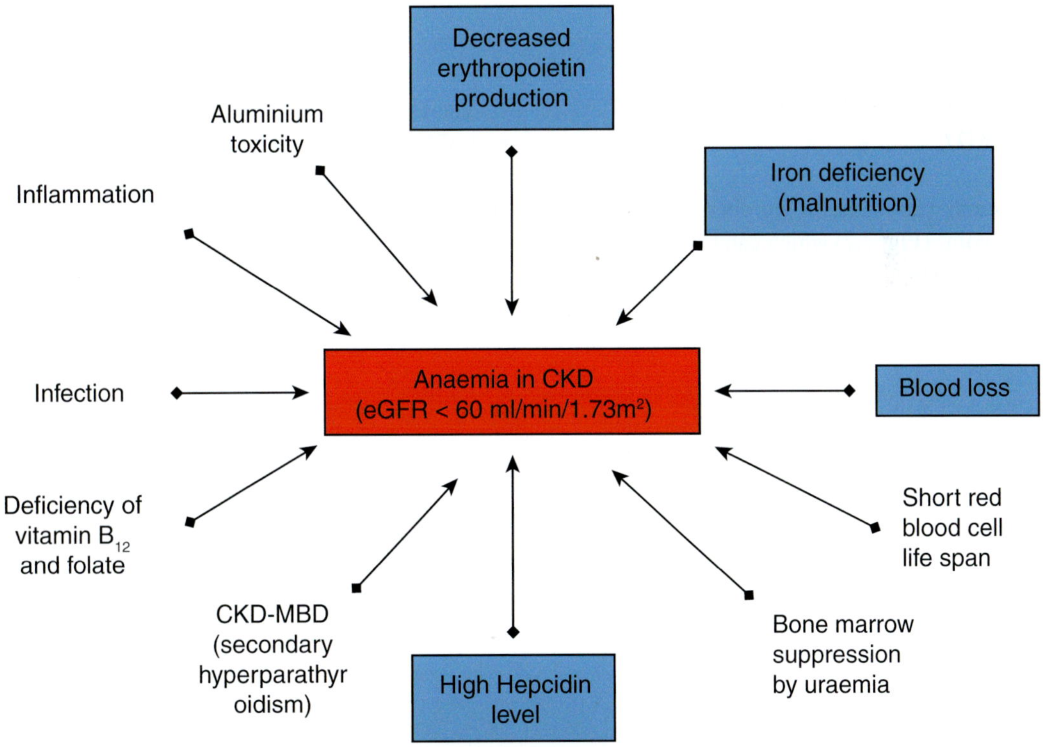

Fig. 7.1 (**a**) Causes of anaemia in CKD. *CKD-MBD* chronic kidney disease mineral bone disease. (**b**) Pathophysiology of anaemia in CKD

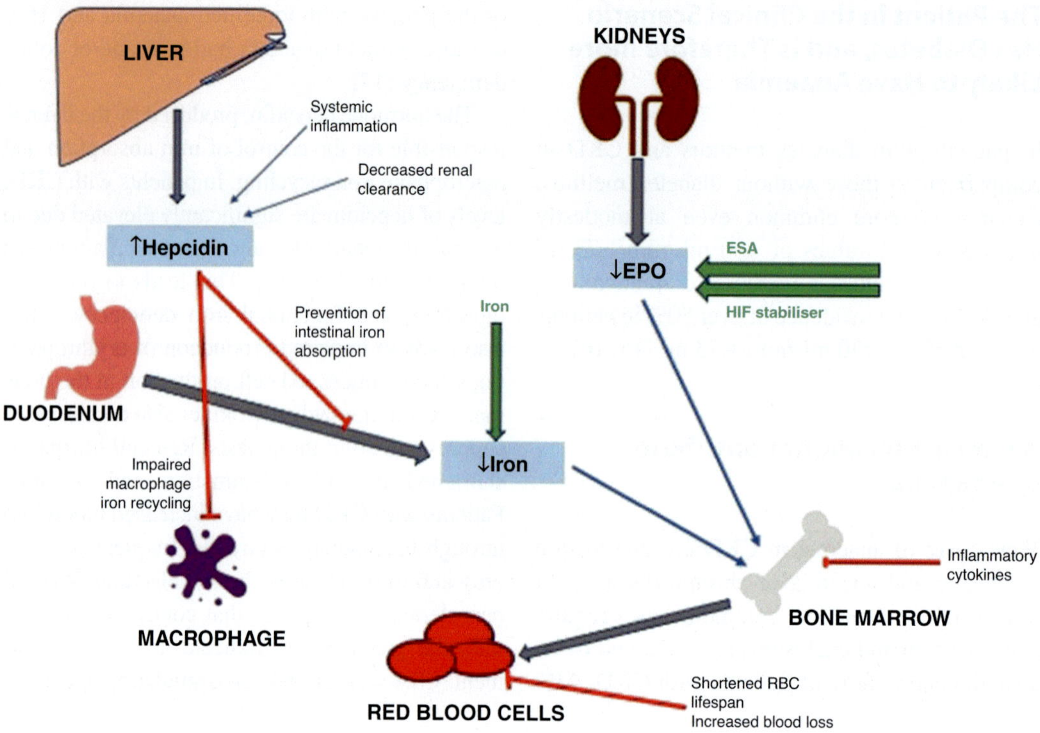

Fig. 7.1 (continued)

Why Treat this Patient's Anaemia of CKD?

Anaemia can cause a number of debilitating symptoms (Fig. 7.2) which can be improved with treatment (Fig. 7.3) [19]. Early management also improves prognosis, particularly cardiovascular risk (Table 7.2).

The FERWON-Nephro study of 1538 patients with CKD showed a 10-point increase in FACIT fatigue scores with IV iron, whilst the IRON-CKD study in 40 patients found improved physical component and mental state scores 1 month after IV iron and the Iron and Heart study a trend to improved quality of life scores [20–22].

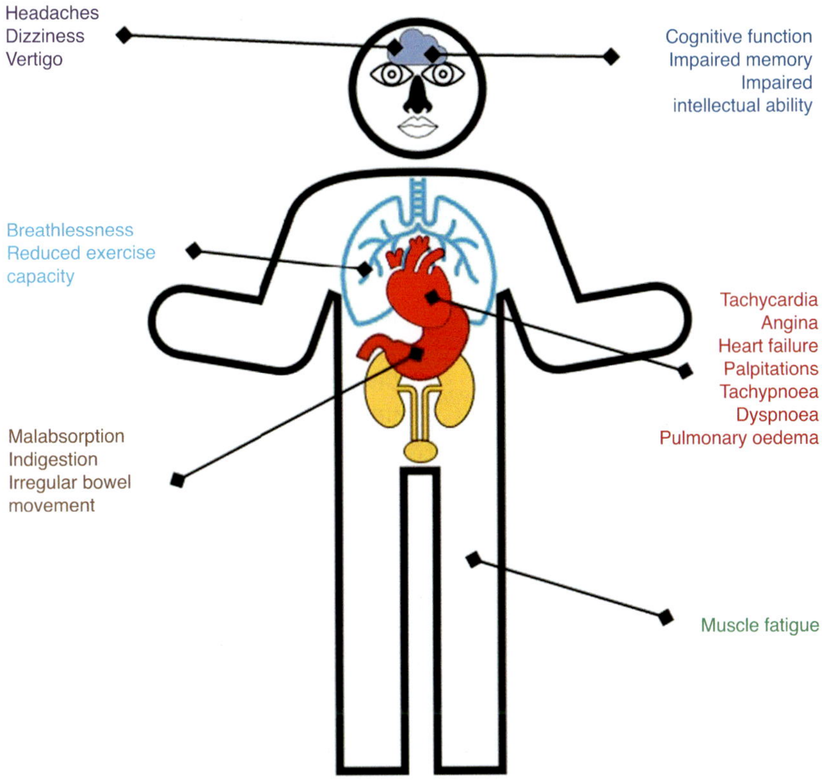

Fig. 7.2 Symptoms related to anaemia

Fig. 7.3 Effects of treating anaemia in CKD leads to a number of improvements

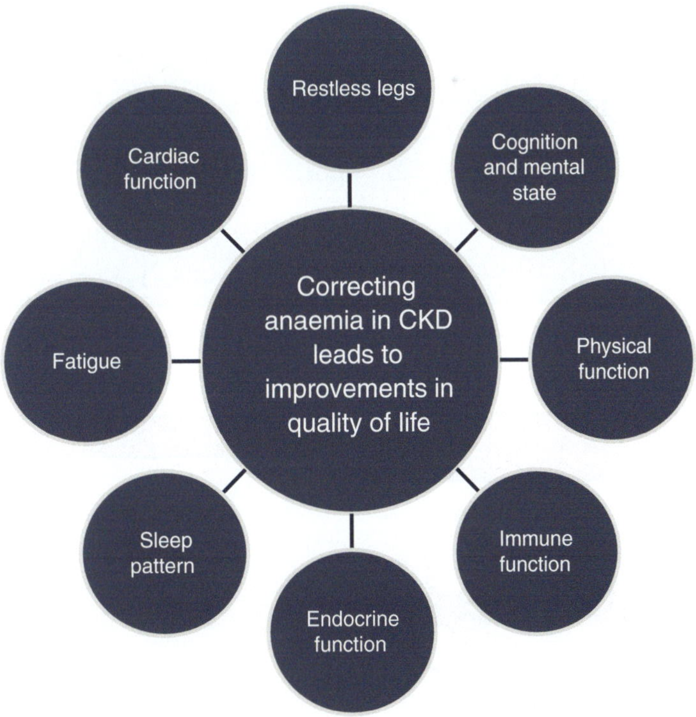

Table 7.2 Early management of anaemia of CKD may lead to improvements in prognosis

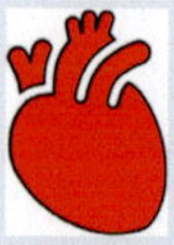

- There is a direct association with anaemia and iron deficiency and heart failure and CKD stage G5
- In the cycle of cardio-renal-anaemia syndrome, for every 10 g/L drop in mean Hb, there is a 25% increased risk of heart failure
- Anaemia increases CV events, heart failure admissions—a Hb <100 g/L in 9722 incident HD patients was associated with increased mortality at 6 months (HR 1.3 (1.14–1.49))
- Analysis of the DOPPS dataset among patients whose Hb was maintained above 110 g/L at 1 month following HD initiation at 1 year had half the mortality of those with a Hb < 80 g/L

Investigations for Iron Deficiency in CKD in our Patient

There are four main measurements to assess iron status available in most countries, but transferrin saturation (TSAT) and serum ferritin (SF) are the most commonly available and used (Table 7.3) [7].

Three treatment options are currently available (Fig. 7.4). All guidelines indicate that both absolute and functional iron deficiency require correction before subsequent effective use of ESA. Iron therapy should be considered when SF < 100 mg/mL or a TSAT <20%. The NICE guidelines suggest that correction of iron deficiency anaemia (IDA) is beneficial to CKD patients prior to commencing ESA (Fig. 7.5) [8].

Table 7.3 Tests of iron deficiency

Test strategy	Sensitivity	Specificity	Limitations
%HRC	82%	95%	• RBCs expand when blood is stored, so local analysis is required • % HRC >6% – indicates low iron availability
CHr	57%	93%	• Mean Hb content per reticulocyte <29 pg – indicates low iron availability and functional iron deficiency
TSAT	49%	64%	• Marked diurnal variation • May be influenced by inflammation, malnutrition and chronic disease
SF	39%	81%	• Acute-phase protein – Inflammatory conditions, infection, malignancy, hyperthyroidism, liver disease and heavy alcohol intake • Normal/high SF does not exclude FID

HRC hypochromic red cells, *RBCs* red bloods cells, *Chr* mean haemoglobin content or reticulocytes, *FID* functional iron deficiency

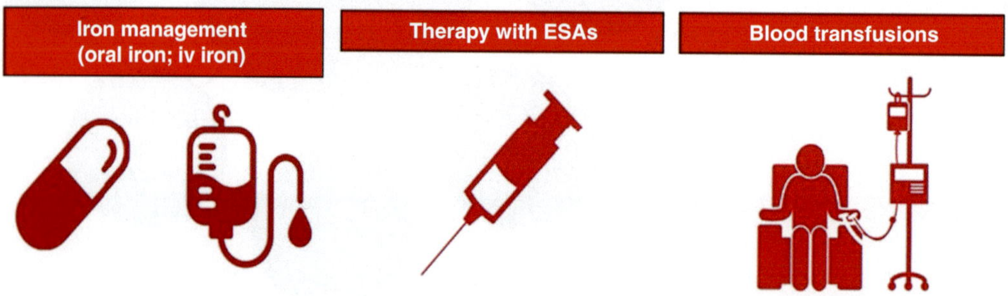

Fig. 7.4 What are the current management options for anaemia of CKD in our patient after correction of any folate or B12 deficiency?

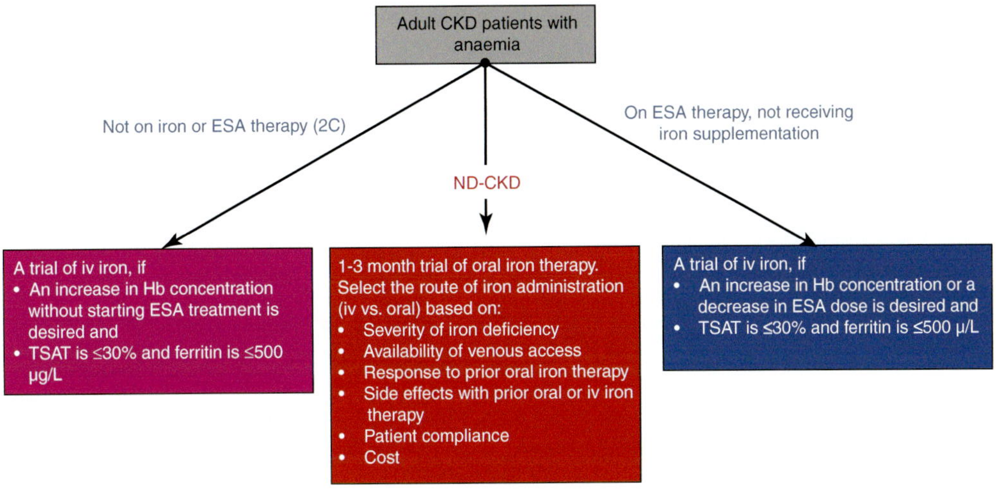

Fig. 7.5 Iron therapy in CKD—algorithm whether on or not on an ESA. *ND-CKD* non-dialysis dependent patients with CKD

Tables 7.4 and 7.5 Example protocols for third generation iron repletion regimes in CKD patients [7]. There are several regimes, the simplest being by body weight or a combination of body weight and Hb: protocols will vary depending on local practice for older preparations, which may require a longer administration period, and different dosing schedule

Body weight (kg)	<50	50 to <75	≥75
Dose of iron (mg)	500	1000	1500
Duration of infusion (min)	15	15	30-60

Body weight (kg)	50 to <75	≥75
Hb ≥100 g/L	1000 mg	15000 mg
Hb <100 g/L	1500 mg	2000 mg
Duration of infusion (min)	15-30	30-60

The FIND-CKD study of 626 patients showed that an IV iron strategy aiming for a higher ferritin range (400–600 ng/mL) led to a faster and greater Hb rise and was more likely to cause a greater than 10 g/L rise in Hb than a lower target driven repletion (100–200 ng/mL) or oral iron over 1 year follow-up ($p < 0.01$) [23].

The PIVOTAL study has reassured clinicians that in dialysis dependent CKD (CKD-HD), a proactive IV iron approach carries no increased risks of infection and cardiovascular events and indeed mortality and hospitalisations for heart failure were reduced. This was accompanied by a 19.4% reduction in ESA use and a 20% reduction in transfusion requirements [24]. In patients with CKD-HD, one would aim for a dosing regimen of 400 mg/month (if SF <400 or TSAT <30% while on ESA therapy) after a 600 mg loading dose in the first month, and withhold iron if the SF >700 µg/L or TSAT >40%. For non-dialysis dependent CKD (ND-CKD) patients, giving high doses infrequently would appear to be the best option, and a typical regime consists of either a weight-based single dose infusion or weight and haemoglobin-based regime (Tables 7.4 and 7.5) [7, 8].

Table 7.6 Available IV iron preparations, dosing and administration, monitoring and advice to patients [6, 7]

IV iron preparation	Brand name	Max dose at one sitting	Time taken to administer 1000 mg	Clinical implication	Monitoring	Advice to patient
Ferric carboxymaltose	Ferinject®/ Injectafer®	1000 mg	15 min in one sitting	Suitable when rapid infusion required (e.g. out-patient use)	Need to monitor phosphate levels Requires facilities for acute management of anaphylaxis	Oral iron therapy should be stopped at least 5 days before commencement of IV iron Contra-indicated if a history or previous anaphylaxis Not to give within 5 days of an active infection requiring antibiotics Potential side effects include urticaria, rashes, itching, nausea and shivering and myalgia and arthralgia
Ferric derisomaltose/ iron isomaltoside	Monofer®	20 mg/kg (total dose infusion), can be given at maximum rate of 250 mg/min	At a single session over 15–30 min	Suitable for out-patient use/ clinic visit use	All preparations require facilities for acute management of anaphylaxis	
Ferric derisomaltose/ iron isomaltoside	Diafer®	200 mg, as an IV bolus	Over 5 visits, dose must not exceed 1000 mg per week	As needs repeated infusions to achieve therapeutic effect, suitable for use in dialysis patients		
Ferumoxytol	Feraheme	510 mg given undiluted at rate of 30 mg/s	Over 2 visits between 3 and 8 days apart	Suitable for out-patient use but need two hospital visits		
Low molecular weight iron dextran	Cosmofer®	20 mg/kg (total dose infusion)	At a single session over 4–6 h	Useful in hospitalized patients		
Iron sucrose	Venofer®	200 mg, at 20 mg (1 mL of undiluted solution) per minute	Over 5 visits	Suitable for use in dialysis patients		
Ferric gluconate	Ferrlecit®	125 mg (can be given undiluted at rate of 12.5 mg/min or diluted in 100 mL Normal saline solution given over 1 h)	Over 8 visits (e.g. 8 sequential dialysis sessions)	Suitable for patients visiting hospitals for regular dialysis		

Prescribing Intravenous (IV) Iron

Used in isolation, IV iron leads to a 6–27 g/L rise in Hb concentration. Table 7.6 lists most of the commonly available iv iron preparations, dosing and administration, monitoring and advice to patients.

Potential Adverse Effects of Iron

The formulation of iron used is usually based on local recommendations and clinician preferences. Safety is critical, and has been demonstrated in several studies for the current available therapies. It is important to both

Risks of IV iron

Short-term issues

- Hypersensitivity reactions (anaphylactic reactions are rare)
- 'labile "Free" iron reactions' (all IV irons–too much too quickly)
- Transient Hypophosphataemia

Long-term issues

- Susceptibility to infections
- Increased inflammation
- Oxidative stree
- Cytotoxicity
- Endothelial dysfunction
- Iron overload
- Unknown long-term safety
- Cardiovascular events
- Mortality

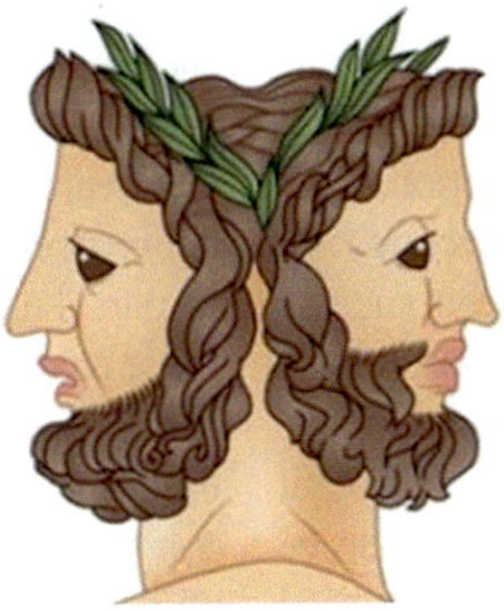

Benefits of IV iron

- Better bioavailability
- Rapid efficacy
- No compliance issues
- Greater Hb increase
- Reduced ESA needs
- Reduced transfusion needs

Fig. 7.6 The Risks and Benefits of IV iron

Table 7.7 Two clinical presentations of adverse effects of IV iron, and appropriate management strategies

Case 1	Case 2
35-year-oldlady with glomerulonephritis	62-year-old man; diabetic nephropathy
eGFR 32 ml/min/1.73m²; on ESA	eGFR 26 ml/min/1.73m²; no ESA
Hb 106 g/L SF 98 mg/l, TSAT 17%	Hb 96 g/L SF 66 mg/l, TSAT 19%
Developed dyspnoea, muscle aches; no change in BP 15 mins into IV Iron infusion. Patient and staff anxious	Developed urticaria & slight dyspnoea 10 mins into IV Iron infusion
Infusion stopped for 10 minutes • restarted without further problems	Infusion stopped • given prednisolone and chlorpheniramine
Probable labile iron (infusion) reaction	**Probable allergic reaction**
No further adverse effects with subsequent doses	Further treatment option to consider: • Give IV Iron with prophylactic steroid and chlorpheniramine – if mild • Try alternative Iron Preparation if mild • Avoid all IV Iron preparations if severe

understand and critically recognise the differences in adverse effects, such as the Fishbane Reaction to ensure the correct intervention (Fig. 7.6 and Table 7.7) [25].

Other Potential Risks of IV Iron

Infection Risk

It is advised to avoid administering IV iron to patients with an active systemic infection, as it remains unclear if IV iron increases infection risk. *In-vitro* studies have indicated that iron sucrose and iron gluconate cause significant inhibition of trans-endothelial migration of polymorphonuclear neutrophils, and may depress neutrophil intracellular killing capability. There may also be an increased bacterial proliferation and impaired phagocytosis. Comparative toxicological analysis in animals after injection of IV iron, have confirmed that iron sucrose appears to cause cell death perhaps via induction of MCP-1 generation in renal and extra-renal tissues leading to inflammation in addition to toxic effects on monocytes and macrophage. In the clinical setting, Hoen et al. in 985 dialysis patients demonstrated no increase in infection rates while a recent large epidemiological study of 776,203 exposures to IV iron has suggested that bolus dosing of less than 400 mg in HD was not associated with increased risk of infection [26]. An infection signal was not observed in the landmark PIVOTAL trial [24, 27]. Evidence in non-dialysis dependent CKD patients suggested no increased infection risk with IV iron compared to oral iron (FIND CKD) [23].

Oxidative Stress

The majority of IV iron when administrated is taken up by the reticuloendothelial system, where it combines to ferritin or transferrin for Hb production and storage. However up to 2% is released as free iron, a potential catalyst for the production of oxidant complexes and subsequent lipid peroxidation and cell damage.

Animal models have demonstrated that free iron causes glomerular dysfunction from oxidative stress and cell cytotoxicity (mesangial and endothelial cells). The effects seem to be iron preparation dependent. Ferric gluconate appears to reduce creatinine clearance and increase proteinuria while both ferric gluconate and iron dextran but not iron sucrose or ferric carboxymaltose increase tissue markers of oxidative stress. In clinical studies, Agarwal et al. has shown that the increase in oxidative stress markers from IV iron sucrose could, in part, be abrogated by N-acetyl cysteine [28]. More recent short-term data suggests the effects of IV iron on renal function are neutral [25]. Preliminary studies from Shah et al. in a small cohort of patients with either diabetes mellitus or no renal disease has shown that use of a chelator reduced the urinary catalytic iron with a subsequent improvement in kidney function. Further on the neutral effect of IV iron emanates from a post-hoc sub-analysis of the FAIR-HF (Ferinject assessment in patients with iron deficiency and chronic heart failure) study in a population of heart failure patients with iron deficiency anaemia and impaired renal function [29]. Additionally, newer IV iron products (ferric carboxymaltose, ferric derisomaltose) appear to be associated with a reduced generation of labile plasma iron [30].

The potential for long term harm from repeated total dose infusions of iron is unknown. There is a growing wealth of clinical data to reassure, but this remains the most critical element for the future use of newer iron preparations. Indeed, data in the dialysis population show there does not appear to be an increased risk of mortality with cumulative doses of IV iron but long-term data are lacking.

The Patient's Symptoms Improved with IV Iron, But His Haemoglobin Remains Low; Should He Start an ESA?

Based on the patient in our initial clinical scenario's history, and the data from the TREAT study [15] (Fig. 7.7 and Table 7.8), one should be cautious due to increased stroke and thrombotic risk, with recommendations summarised in Fig. 7.8.

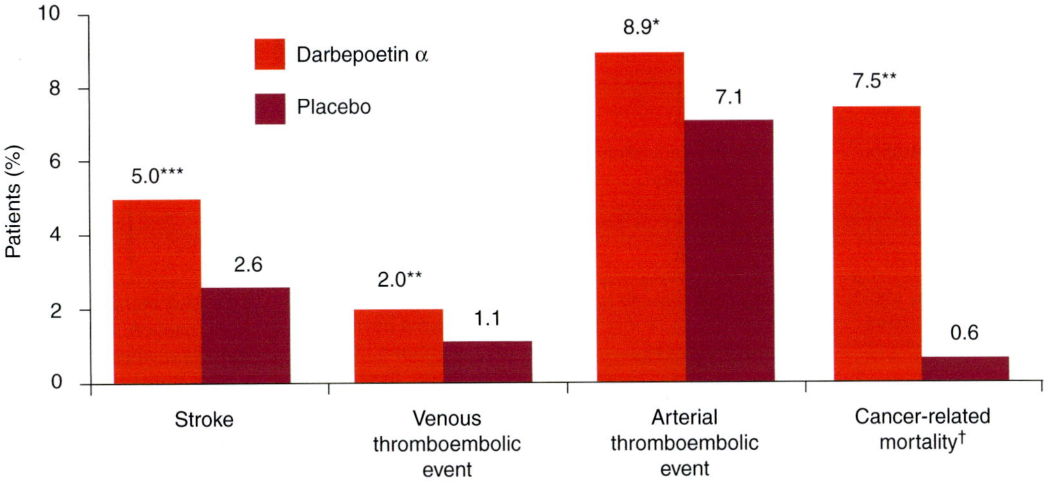

Fig. 7.7 Synopsis of findings from the TREAT study [15]

Table 7.8 Synopsis of the findings from the Normal haematocrit, CREAT, CHOIR and TREAT studies

Study	Hb (g/L) targets	Duration (months)	Results
NORMAL HEMATOCRIT TRIAL (N = 1233) [31]	100 140	29	• 30% increased risk of death or non-fatal MI (HR 1.3 (95% CI 0.9–1.9) in higher haematocrit group) • Terminated early
CREATE (N = 603) [32]	105–115 130–150	36	• No improvement in CV outcomes in higher Hb group • Terminated early
CHOIR (N = 1432) [33]	113 135	16	• 48% increased risk of death (P = 0.07) in higher Hb group • Terminated early
TREAT (N = 4038) [15]	130 90	29	• Increased risk of stroke (HR 1.92; 95% CI, 1.38–2.68; P < 0.001) in higher Hb arm

ESA therapy should be commenced when the Hb is less than 90 g/L for CKD-dialysis (CKD-HD) (evidence level D) patients and less than 100 g/L for non-dialysis CKD (ND-CKD) patients. Avoid initiating ESA therapy for ND-CKD patients with Hb ≥ 100 g/L unless symptomatic on an individualised basis in terms of quality of life and symptoms. In certain circumstances one should consider stopping ESA therapy (Table 7.9) [7].

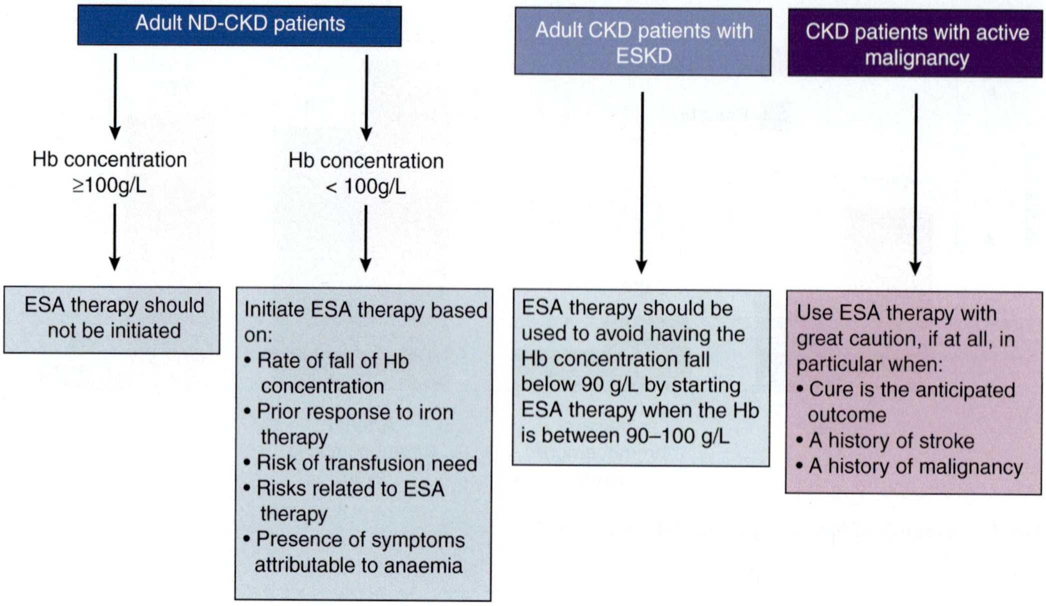

Fig. 7.8 Recommendations for management of CKD-related anaemia with necessary precautions [7]

Table 7.9 When to consider stopping ESA therapy or avoiding [7]

When to consider stopping ESA therapy or avoiding
Hb > 130 g/L
Development of cardiovascular disease
Thrombotic episode (arterial or venous)
Cancer—active malignancy
Uncontrolled BP (persistently >160/100 mmHg)
Development of pure red cell aplasia (PRCA)
Hyporesponsiveness—after exclusion or iron deficiency; hyperparathyroidism; Hb electrophoresis; blood loss; haemolysis; malignancy; ACEi effect; under-dialysis & inflammation such as periodontal disease or infection

Table 7.10 Practical administration of ESA [7]

Practical administration of ESA
• Determine the initial ESA dose using the patient's Hb concentration, body weight and clinical circumstances
• Adjust ESA dose based on the patient's Hb concentration, rate of change in Hb concentration, current ESA dose and clinical circumstance
• Reduce the ESA dose in preference to withholding ESA when a downward adjustment of Hb concentration is needed

Practical Administration of ESA

If anaemia remains despite repletion of iron, one should initiate an ESA, but also ensure that the BP is <150/90 mmHg, ideally to minimise the risk of stroke (Table 7.10). Several ESA agents are available and can be used either IV or subcutaneously (Table 7.11), and dosages should be adjusted according to Fig. 7.9 [7].

One should be aware of the two important concepts consisting of ESA hypo-responsiveness and loss of ESA response (resistance). Where no increase in Hb concentration from baseline is achieved after the first month of ESA treatment and repeated escalations of dose (>2× initial weight-based dose) this suggests ESA hypo-responsiveness. Loss of ESA response should be suspected where 2 increases in ESA dose >50% beyond the previously stable dose of ESA are not sufficient to maintain a previously stable Hb. In these patients avoid repeated escalations in ESA dose beyond double the dose at which they had been stable. Excluding reversible causes is important (Fig. 7.10) prior to concluding there is hypo-responsiveness [7].

Table 7.11 Prescribing ESA therapy and dose adjustments [7]

ESA product	Drug names	Recommendations	Dosing—initial dose IV or s/c	Maintenance dose	monitoring	Advice to patient
Darbepoetin Alpha	Aranesp	Maintain Hb in a range from 100–120 g/L based on NICE guidelines For KDIGO range is 100–115 g/L All products can be used in dialysis patients and patients with chronic kidney disease Caution with patients with cardiovascular history and history of stroke Avoid where possible in those with active cancer	450 ng/kg weekly Or 750 ng/kg fortnightly in non dialysis	According to response. Aim for 25% increased dose monthly	Titrate monthly Monitor BP Monitor serum potassium	May cause headache ESA should not be given if blood pressure is greater than 160/100 mmHg on two consecutive recordings
Erythropoietin alpha	Eprex Binocrit		50 units/kg ×3/week in all patients	25–100 mg/kg adjustments monthly		
Erythropoietin beta	Neorecormon		20 units/kg IV or s/c 40 units/kg	Titrate up to 80 units/kg		
Epoetin theta	Eporatio		20 units/kg	According to response—25% increased dose		
Epoetin zeta	Retacrit		50 units/kg	25% increased dose		
Methoxy polyethylene glycol epoiten beta	Mircera		600 ng/kg every 2 weeks-dialysis 1.2 mg/kg monthly—non dialysis patients	Double dose—titrate monthly		

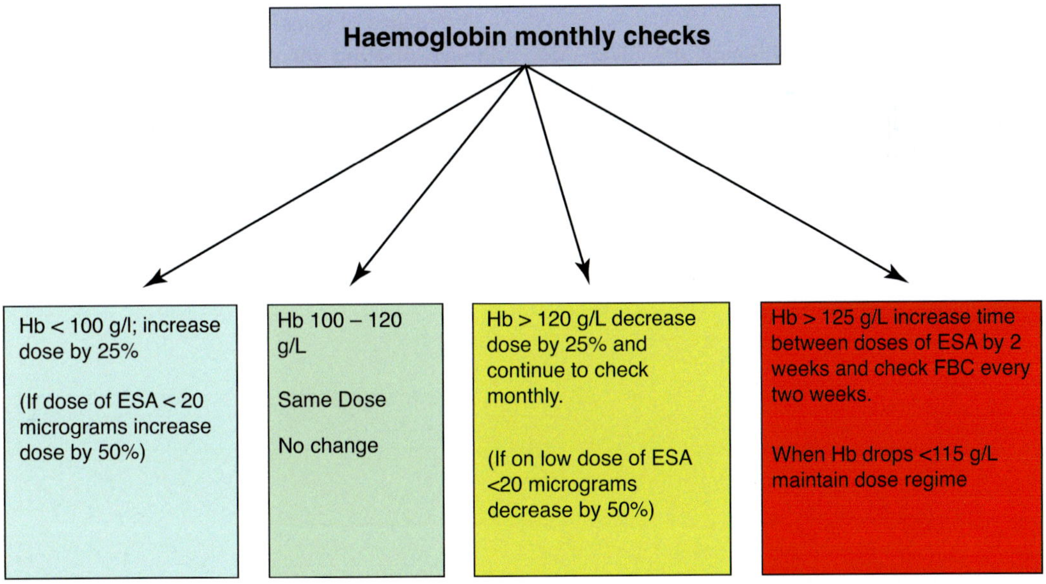

Fig. 7.9 Dose adjustments of ESA agents [7]

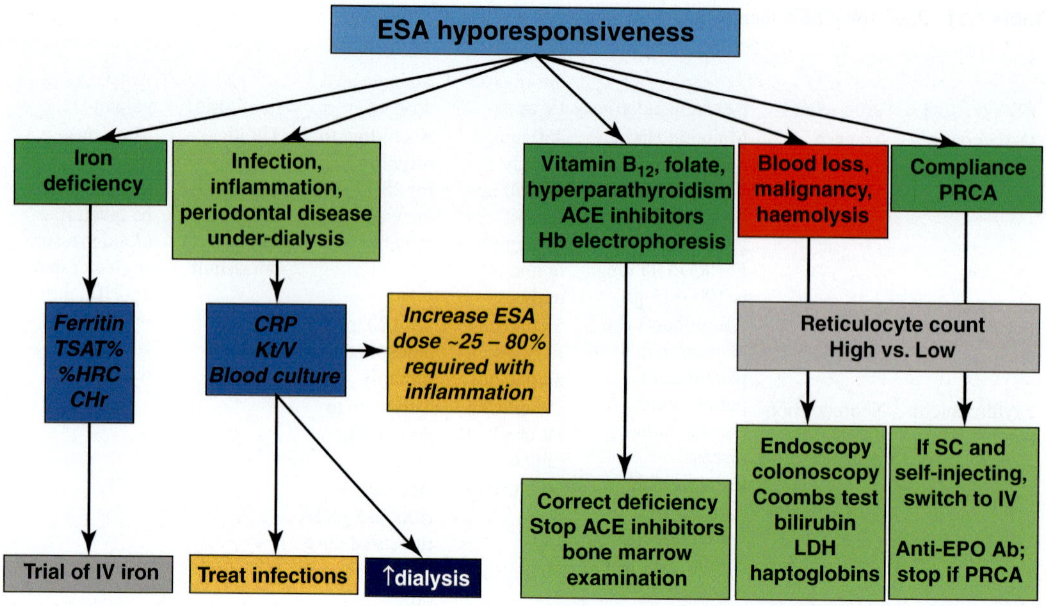

Fig. 7.10 Investigations to exclude ESA hyporesponsiveness or possible ESA resistance [7]. C-reactive protein (CRP); Kt/V (measure of dialysis adequacy); Angiotensin converting enzyme (ACE); pure red cell aplasia (PRCA); lactate dehydeogenacse (LDH); subcutaneous (sc), erythropoietin (EPO)

Despite Our Patient's History, He Is on the Transplant List: Why Should One Aim to Avoid Transfusions?

Red cell transfusions—although not ideal—do have a role in certain circumstances, where patients are unable to tolerate iron and/or ESA therapy, or have bone marrow failure. KDIGO recommends that transfusions should be avoided when feasible, to reduce the well-known potential risks associated with transfusions (Table 7.12) such as infection, blood transfusion resistance, and transfusion related lung disease [7].

Avoidance of transfusions is essential to limit allo-sensitisation for patients who may require future organ transplantation, as this reduces the risk of panel reactive antibody development, critical in future transplantation success. This can increase more than twofold with up to five blood transfusions administered (Fig. 7.11) [34].

Table 7.12 Recognised general risks associated with blood transfusions [7]

Estimated risk associated with blood transfusions per unit transfused (adapted from KDIGO 2012)	
Adverse event	**Estimated risk**
Graft versus host disease (GVHD)	Uncommon
Urticaria or other cutaneous reaction	1 in 50–100
Febrile reaction	1 in 300
Transfusion-related acute lung injury (TRALI)	1 in 5000
Haemolytic reaction	1 in 6000
Anaphylaxis	1 in 20,000–50,000
Fatal haemolysis	1 in 1,000,000
Transfusion-related infections	
Hepatitis B	1 in 137,000
West Nile Virus	1 in 350,000
Hepatitis C	<1 in 1,000,000
Death from bacterial sepsis	1 in 1,000,000
Human immunodeficiency virus (HIV)	<1 in 1,900,000

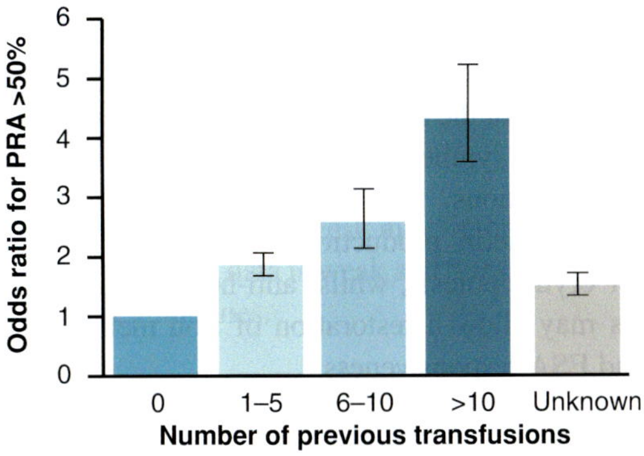

Fig. 7.11 Effects of transfusion on the odds of developing panel reactive antibodies (PRAs) [34]

Future Therapies

There are newer Iron Preparations, that appear to demonstrate improved absorption, tolerability and iron utilization:

- ferric maltol
- ferric citrate

Hypoxia-inducible factors (HIFs) are a family of oxygen-sensitive proteins that regulate the transcriptional response of cells to hypoxia. The

8. A 73-year-old Indian female was referred to the kidney clinic with a declining eGFR and increased tiredness. Her daughter suffered from chronic kidney disease and anaemia. On examination she was pale, blood pressure 137/90 mmHg, pulse 90/min.

Investigations:

Haemoglobin	98 g/L (115–165)
Platelet count	164 × 10^9/L (150–400)
Serum ferritin	120 μg/L (15–300)
Transferrin saturation	15% (20–50)
Mean corpuscular volume	72 fL (80–100)
Blood film	Microcytosis, hypochromic and target cells
Serum sodium	140 mmol/L (137–144)
Serum potassium	5.1 mmol/L (3.5–4.9)
Serum creatinine	323 μmol/L (60–110)

What is next best step in management?

A. Start IV hypoxia inducible factor stabilizer
B. Start subcutaneous erythropoietin
C. Start intravenous iron
D. Start intravenous erythropoietin
E. Start oral iron

Correct answer C

A. Incorrect—not part of clinical practice currently and no IV preparation available
B. Incorrect—need to correct iron deficiency first
C. Correct—a trial of intravenous iron as suggested by NICE probably the best option as the blood film consistent with Iron deficiency—haemoglobinopathy seems less likely given age but target cells present in both disorders.
D. Incorrect—see B
E. Incorrect

9. A 33-year-old Indian female was referred to the kidney clinic with declining eGFR and increasing tiredness. Her mother had suffered anaemia from an early age . On examination she was pale, blood pressure 137/90 mmHg, pulse 90/min. She was treated with 1000 mg of intravenous iron 2 months ago.

Investigations:

Haemoglobin	98 g/L (115–165)
Platelet count	164 × 10^9/L (150–400)
Serum ferritin	450 μg/L (15–300)
Transferrin saturation	40% (20–50)
Mean corpuscular volume	72 fL (80–100)
RDW (red cell distribution width)	14.1% (12.2–16.1)
Blood film	Microcytosis, hypochromic and target cells
Serum sodium	140 mmol/L (137–144)
Serum potassium	5.1 mmol/L (3.5–4.9)
Serum creatinine	323 μmol/L (60–110)

What is the likely main cause of her anaemia?

A. erythropoietin deficiency
B. haemolytic anaemia
C. iron deficiency
D. sideroblastic anaemia
E. vitamin B12 deficiency

Correct answer B

A. Incorrect—would benefit to measure levels as probably contributing but not main cause
B. Correct blood film and family history are suggestive of haemolytic anaemia; Haemoglobin electrophoresis demonstrated an alpha-thalassaemia. The RDW (red cell distribution width) tends to be higher in iron deficiency but not in the thalassaemias
C. Incorrect—the patient has received iron therapy and iron markers normal
D. Incorrect—no evidence of ringed sideroblasts on a peripheral smear which are pathognomic.
E. Incorrect no evidence from blood film

10. A 88-year-old female was seen in acute medicine unit with weakness, poor appetite, weight loss and a fall. She suffered from constipation. On examination she was pale and in atrial fibrillation. She suffered no bony fractures.

Her pulse was 110/min and irregular. Her BP was 120/68 mmHg. She was on bisoprolol, atorvastatin, bendroflumethiazide.

Haemoglobin	82 g/L (115–165)
Platelet count	220 × 10^9/L (150–400)
Serum ferritin	98 μg/L (15–300)
Mean corpuscular volume	78 fL (80–100)
Serum sodium	125 mmol/L (137–144)
Serum potassium	5.1 mmol/L (3.5–4.9)
Serum creatinine	458 μmol/L (60–110)

What is the most appropriate next step in establishing the cause of anaemia

A. measure blood vitamin B12 and folate levels
B. serum coombs' test
C. bone marrow biopsy
D. haemoglobin electrophoresis
E. request CT colonoscopy

Correct answer: E

A. Incorrect - MCV not raised
B. Incorrect - unlikely in this age group with low MCV iron deficicency
C. Incorrect
D. Incorrect - unlikely in this age group with low MCV
E. Correct a potential cause of iron deficiency anaemia is a colonic malignancy due to weight loss

Test your learning and check your understanding of this book's contents: use the "Springer Nature Flashcards" app to access questions using https://sn.pub/cz9Cok. To use the app, please follow the instructions in Chap. 1.

References

1. Centers for Disease Control and Prevention. Chronic kidney disease in the United States, 2019. https://www.cdc.gov/kidneydisease/publications-resources/2019-national-facts.html. Accessed September 2020.
2. The National Collaborating Centre for Chronic Kidney Disease: National Institute for Health and Clinical Excellence: Guidance. In: Chronic Kidney Disease: National Clinical Guideline for Early Identification and Management in Adults in Primary and Secondary Care, eds. Royal College of Physicians (UK) London: Royal College of Physicians of London; 2008.
3. UK Renal Registry. UK renal registry 22nd annual report—data to 31/12/2018, Bristol; 2020. renal.org/audit-research/annual-report.
4. Chronic kidney disease: assessment and management NICE guideline updated August 2021 [NG203]. https://www.nice.org.uk/guidance/ng203. Accessed 12 August 2022.
5. Locatelli F, Nissenson AR, Barrett BJ, et al. Clinical practice guidelines for anemia in chronic kidney disease: problems and solutions. A position statement from kidney disease: improving global outcomes (KDIGO). Kidney Int. 2008;74(10):1237–40.
6. Mikhail A, Brown C, Williams JA, Mathrani V, Shrivastava R, Evans J, Isaac H, Bhandari S. Renal association clinical practice guideline on anaemia of chronic kidney disease. BMC Nephrol. 2017;18(1):345.
7. Locatelli F, Barany P, Covic A, et al. Kidney disease: improving global outcomes guidelines on anaemia management in chronic kidney disease: a European renal best practice position statement. Nephrol Dial Transplant. 2013;28(6):1346–59.
8. National Clinical Guideline Centre: National Institute for Health and Care Excellence (NICE). Anaemia management in chronic kidney disease NG8. 2015. https://www.nice.org.uk/guidance/ng8/evidence/full-guideline-pdf-70545136. Accessed 26 June 2021.
9. Kidney Disease: Improving Global Outcomes (KDIGO) Anemia Work Group. KDIGO Clinical practice guideline for anemia in chronic kidney disease. Kidney Int Suppl. 2012;2(4):279–335.
10. Mikhail A, et al. Clinical practice guideline. Anaemia of chronic kidney disease. The Renal Association. 2020. https://ukkidney.org/sites/renal.org/files/Updated-130220-Anaemia-of-Chronic-Kidney-Disease-1-1.pdf. Accessed 14 September 2021.
11. De Silva R, Rigby AS, Witte KK, et al. Anemia, renal dysfunction, and their interaction in patients with chronic heart failure. Am J Cardiol. 2006;98(3):391–8.
12. Besarab A, Provenzano R, Hertel J, Zabaneh R, Klaus SJ, Lee T, Leong R, Hemmerich S, Yu KHP, Neff TB. Randomized placebo-controlled dose-ranging and pharmacodynamics study of roxadustat (FG-4592) to treat anemia in nondialysis-dependent chronic kidney disease (NDD-CKD) patients. Nephrol Dial Transplant. 2015;30(10):1665–73. https://doi.org/10.1093/ndt/gfv302.
13. Singh AK, Carroll K, McMurray JJV, Solomon S, Jha V, Johansen KL, Lopes RD, Macdougall IC, Obrador GT, Waikar SS, Wanner C, Wheeler DC, Więcek A, Blackorby A, Cizman B, Cobitz AR, Davies R, DiMino TL, Kler L, Meadowcroft AM, Taft L, Perkovic V. ASCEND-ND Study Group. Daprodustat for the treatment of anemia in patients not undergoing dialysis. N Engl J Med. 2021;385(25):2313–24. https://doi.org/10.1056/NEJMoa2113380. Epub 2021 Nov 5. PMID: 34739196.

14. Singh AK, Carroll K, Perkovic V, Solomon S, Jha V, Johansen KL, Lopes RD, Macdougall IC, Obrador GT, Waikar SS, Wanner C, Wheeler DC, Więcek A, Blackorby A, Cizman B, Cobitz AR, Davies R, Dole J, Kler L, Meadowcroft AM, Zhu X, McMurray JJV; ASCEND-D Study Group. Daprodustat for the treatment of anemia in patients undergoing dialysis. N Engl J Med. 2021;385(25):2325–35. https://doi.org/10.1056/NEJMoa2113379. Epub 2021 Nov 5.
15. Pfeffer M, Burdmann E, Chen C, Cooper M. A trial of darbepoetin in type 2 diabetes and chronic kidney disease. N Engl J Med. 2009;361:2019–32.
16. Solomon SD, Uno H, Lewis EF, et al. Erythropoietic response and outcomes in kidney disease and type 2 diabetes. N Engl J Med. 2010;363(12):1146–55.
17. Stancu S, Barsan L, Stanciu A, Mircescu G. Can the response to iron therapy be predicted in anemic non-dialysis patients with chronic kidney disease? Clin J Am Soc Nephrol. 2010;5(3):409–16.
18. Ganz T, Nemeth E. Hepcidin and disorders of iron metabolism. Annu Rev Med. 2011;62:347–60.
19. van Haalen H, Jackson J, Spinowitz B, et al. Impact of chronic kidney disease and anemia on health-related quality of life and work productivity: analysis of multinational real-world data. BMC Nephrol. 2020;21:88. https://doi.org/10.1186/s12882-020-01746-4.
20. Bhandari S, Kalra PA, Berkowitz M, Belo D, Thomsen LL, Wolf M. Safety and efficacy of iron isomaltoside 1000/ferric derisomaltose versus iron sucrose in patients with chronic kidney disease: the FERWON-NEPHRO randomized, open-label, comparative trial. Nephrol Dial Transplant. 2021;36(1):111–20. https://doi.org/10.1093/ndt/gfaa011. PMID: 32049331; PMCID: PMC7771981.
21. Kassianides X, Gordon A, Ziedan A, Sturmey R, Bhandari S. The comparative effect of intravenous iron on oxidative stress and inflammation in patients with chronic kidney disease (CKD). A randomized controlled-plot study. Kidney Res Clin Pract. 2021;40:89–98. https://doi.org/10.23876/j.krcp.20.120.
22. Bhandari S, Allgar V, Lamplugh A, Macdougall I, Kalra PA. A multicentre prospective double blinded randomised controlled trial of intravenous iron (ferric derisomaltose (FDI)) in iron deficient but not anaemic patients with chronic kidney disease on functional status. BMC Nephrol. 2021;22:115. https://doi.org/10.1186/s12882-021-02308-y.
23. Macdougall IC, Bock AH, Carrera F, Eckardt KU, Gaillard C, Van Wyck D, Roubert B, Nolen JG, Roger SD, FIND-CKD Study Investigators. FIND-CKD: a randomized trial of intravenous ferric carboxymaltose versus oral iron in patients with chronic kidney disease and iron deficiency anaemia. Nephrol Dial Transplant. 2014;29(11):2075–84. https://doi.org/10.1093/ndt/gfu201. Epub 2014 Jun 2. PMID: 24891437; PMCID: PMC4209879.
24. MacDougall IC, White C, Anker SD, Bhandari S, Farrington K, Kalra PA, McMurray JJV, Murray H, Tomson CRV, Wheeler DC, Winearls CG, Ford I, PIVOTAL Investigators and Committees. Intravenous iron in patients undergoing maintenance haemodialysis. N Engl J Med. 2019;380:447–58. https://doi.org/10.1056/NEJMoa1810742.
25. Kassianides X, Hazara A, Bhandari S. Improving the safety of intravenous iron treatments for patients with non-dialysis-dependent chronic kidney disease. Invited expert opinion. Expert Opin Drug Saf. 2020;20:23–35. https://doi.org/10.1080/14740338.2021.1853098.
26. Hoen B, Paul-Dauphin A, Kessler M. Intravenous iron administration does not significantly increase the risk of bacteremia in chronic hemodialysis patients. Clin Nephrol. 2002;57(6):457–61.
27. Macdougall IC, Bhandari S, White C, Anker SD, Farrington K, Kalra PA, Mark PB, McMurray JJV, Reid C, Robertson M, Tomson CRV, Wheeler DC, Winearls CG, Ford I, PIVOTAL Investigators and Committees. Intravenous iron dosing and infection risk in patients on hemodialysis: a prespecified secondary analysis of the PIVOTAL trial. JASN. 2020;31(5):1118–27. https://doi.org/10.1681/ASN.2019090972.
28. Agarwal R, Leehey DJ, Olsen SM, Dahl NV. Proteinuria induced by parenteral iron in chronic kidney disease—a comparative randomized controlled trial. Clin J Am Soc Nephrol. 2011;6(1):114–21.
29. Anker SD, Colet JC, Filippatos G, et al. FAIR-HF Trial: ferric carboxymaltose in patients with heart failure and iron deficiency. N Engl J Med. 2009;361:3426–2448.
30. Garbowski M W, et al. Haematologica. Intravenous iron preparations transiently generate non-transferrin-bound iron from two proposed pathways. 2021;106(11):2885–96.
31. Besarab A, Bolton WK, et al. The effects of normal as compared with low hematocrit values in patients with cardiac disease who are receiving hemodialysis and Epoetin. N Engl J Med. 1998;339:584–90.
32. Drueke TB, Locatelli F, Clyne N, et al. Normalization of hemoglobin level in patients with chronic kidney disease and anemia. N Engl J Med. 2006;355(20):2071–84.
33. Singh A, Szczech L, Tang KI, et al. Correction of anaemia with Epoetin Alfa in chronic kidney disease. N Engl J Med. 2006;355:2085–98.
34. Lawler EV, Bradbury BD, Fonda JR, Gaziano JM, Gagnon DR. Transfusion burden among patients with chronic kidney disease and anemia. Clin J Am Soc Nephrol. 2010;5(4):667–72.

Blood Pressure in CKD

8

Lisa Crowley and Indranil Dasgupta

Clinical Scenario

A 42-year old male is referred to the renal hypertension clinic with a 3-month history of persistent hypertension. Blood pressure readings were recorded in primary care of 171/92 mmHg. The patient has had 24-h ambulatory blood pressure monitoring, which demonstrated a daytime average BP of 172/89 mmHg and a night-time average of 151/87 mmHg. The patient has a strong family history of hypertension. His BMI is 32, and he smokes 15 cigarettes a day, although he is trying to cut down. He works long hours, and his diet consists of a great deal of convenience food because he is short on time. You are asked to see the patient to determine the cause of hypertension. Aside from his raised blood pressure, routine biochemical tests have shown a reduced eGFR of 52 mL/min/1.73 m^2. All secondary causes of hypertension have been excluded.

L. Crowley
Royal Derby Hospital, Derby, UK
e-mail: lisa.crowley5@nhs.net

I. Dasgupta (✉)
Heartlands Hospital Birmingham, Birmingham, UK

Warwick Medical School, University of Warwick, Coventry, UK
e-mail: indranil.dasgupta@uhb.nhs.uk

Introduction

Hypertension is an important risk factor for developing both cardiovascular and chronic kidney disease (CKD), and a major contributor to progression of CKD to end stage kidney disease (ESKD). Management of hypertension forms the cornerstone of managing CKD and reducing cardiovascular risk, and can be considered amongst the most important interventions in nephrology. There should therefore be a great emphasis on the accurate diagnosis of hypertension, and putting in place appropriate management strategies.

Clinic Blood Pressure and the 'White-Coat' Effect

The majority of major hypertension trials, and the guidelines that have resulted from them, are based on standardised office blood pressure (BP) measurements (Fig. 8.1). In contrast, when assessing blood pressure in the clinic, nephrologists often rely on routine office BP measurements. A standardised office BP generally means taking an average of 2 or 3 measurements following an appropriate period of relaxation in a quiet environment: a routine office BP measurement does not include any preparation before measurement. Measuring BP with the standardised technique inevitably requires more time and office space than may be available, but there is evidence that routine BP measurements are higher than those taken as routine in clinic. If treatment is

D. Banerjee et al. (eds.), *Management of Kidney Diseases*,
https://doi.org/10.1007/978-3-031-09131-5_8

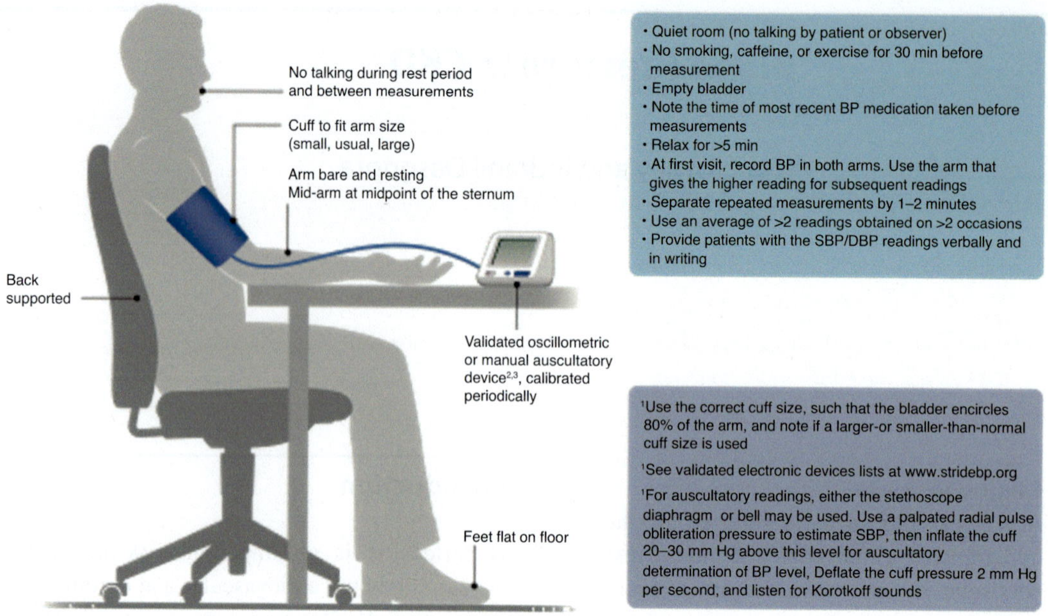

Fig. 8.1 How to measure blood pressure properly (standardised blood pressure measurement, adapted from KDIGO blood pressure guidelines 2021)[1]

to be instigated, it is important that we use the BP measurement technique that best accords with that adopted in the major clinical trials (Table 8.1).

There are some considerations for each individual patient in determining what the best method for measurement is:

- *Can the patient be seen face-to-face?*
- *Is the patient able to afford a home blood pressure monitor?*
- *Is the patient able to take their blood pressure and record the results?*

As far as possible we should be sure that each patient has access to accurate blood pressure measurements that allow physicians to optimise the management of their blood pressure.

Practice Point 1

- Accurate blood pressure measurement is crucial in ensuring correct treatment
- Most clinical trials are based on standardised blood pressure measurement
- Every effort should be made to give patients equitable access to accurate blood pressure measurements

Treating to a Target Blood Pressure

Measurement of standardised office blood pressure further confirms the findings of hypertension in this gentleman. He is given general lifestyle advice and referred to a dietitian to help him make changes to his diet that reduces his salt intake. However, his standardised office blood pressure is similar to his 24-h ambulatory measurement and the decision is made to institute anti-hypertensive treatment. As part of his work-up, he is also found to be proteinuric with a Protein Creatinine Ratio of 63 mg/mmol.

In the general population there is extensive evidence that lowering blood pressure reduces the risk of cardiovascular disease. This patient has proteinuric CKD, and so we are concerned with two related, but differing outcomes.

- What is the evidence for slowing progression of chronic kidney disease?
- What is the evidence for improving cardiovascular outcomes in patients with CKD?

Once we have reviewed this we can ask ourselves two further questions;

Table 8.1 Strengths and weaknesses of different techniques of BP measurement

	Standardised Office BP measurement	Home BP measurement	Ambulatory BP measurement
Description	• Measured in clinic setting • Patient should be relaxed in a quiet place with feet flat against the floor	• Self measure in quiet setting with back supported and feet flat on the floor • Taken in morning and evening usually	• Measure during routine daily activities • Obtained over 24 hours
Strengths	• Method used to guide treatment in clinical trials • Associated with outcomes	• Strong association with cardiovascular outcomes • Detects masked/'white - coat' hypertension	• Strong association with cardiovascular outcomes • Detects masked/'white-coat' hypertension • Measures BP throughout day including at night
Weaknesses	• Number of factors affecting results • Probably less accurate – only 1 or 2 measurements • Training and re-training of staff and space in clinic	• Patients may not correctly measure or report • Requires patient training • Home device may not be validated or calibrated	• Requires two hospital visits – to collect and bring back • Not tolerated by all • Limited equipment

- What target blood pressure should we be aiming for?
- What medications should we be using?

Practice Point 2

- Adults with high BP and CKD should be treated to a target systolic BP of <120 mmHg (as determined by standardised office BP measurement)

Slowing the Progression of CKD

The treatment of hypertension is one of the principal interventions available to a nephrologist for modifying progression of chronic kidney disease. The evidence for the lowering of blood pressure to slow progression to end stage kidney disease comes from landmark studies such as MDRD and AASK. For many years the results of these two trials in particular informed guidelines as to the management of BP in CKD patients (Figs. 8.2 and 8.3) [2, 3].

Meta-analysis of these two studies and another study (REIN-2) suggested that a lower blood pressure target was beneficial in slowing progression of CKD in patients with proteinuria of 300–1000 mg per day. The target blood pressure for patients with proteinuric kidney disease was therefore set by professional bodies at 130/80 mmHg which was, until recently, lower than the BP target for both non-proteinuric kidney disease and the general population [4].

LANDMARK TRIAL: THE MODIFICATION OF DIET IN RENAL DISEASE (MDRD)
• Investigated the effect of BP control and protein restriction on the progression of renal disease • Two randomised controlled trials, one with patients with a GFR of 25-55 ml/min/1.73 m^2 in 1,585 patients and one in patients with a GFR of 13-24 ml/min/1.73 m^2 • Protein restriction not found to have effect in slowing progression in more advanced CKD • In patients with proteinuria greater than 1g per day, more intensive blood pressure control (aiming for 125/75 mmHg) had a significantly slower rate of decline in kidney function

Fig. 8.2 Evidence of BP control (MDRD trial)

LANDMARK TRIAL: THE AFRICAN AMERICAN STUDY OF KIDNEY DISEASE (AASK)
• Randomised just over 1,000 non-diabetic hypertensive patients to a higher (140/90 mmHg) or lower blood pressure (125/75 mmHg) • The main study did not show a difference in death or progression of CKD, but a subgroup analysis showed a reduction in these primary endpoints in proteinuric patients

Fig. 8.3 Evidence for BP control AASK trial

Effect on Cardiovascular and All-Cause Mortality

Given the elevated rates of cardiovascular disease seen in CKD, blood pressuring lowering is key to improving cardiovascular outcomes and mortality. As seen above, the blood pressure target in proteinuric CKD patients was previously lower due to the observed effects on CKD progression. The most recent KDIGO guidelines however extend a lower BP target both to non-proteinuric CKD patients and to the general population [4].

There is evidence in the general population that the reduction in the risk of cardiovascular events is proportional to the reduction in blood pressure. Most of the larger general population trials do not include patients with chronic kidney disease. The recent SPRINT (Systolic Blood Pressure Intervention Trial) had a broader inclusion criteria and provided further evidence that a more intensive treatment target reduces cardiovascular events. SPRINT included a large subgroup with CKD in the trial. Based on this evidence the recent Kidney Disease Improving Global Outcomes (KDIGO) guideline recommend a target systolic BP in patients with CKD of <120 mmHg, when tolerated using standardised office BP measurement. However, this may not apply to all categories of CKD patients as discussed below (Fig. 8.4) [5–7].

The SPRINT trial examined cardiovascular outcomes in non-diabetic patients. It should be noted that the rate of decline in eGFR in the intensive treatment group was faster than in the less intensive treatment group. The effect was small and the limited number of events where serum creatinine doubled precluded firm conclusions from being drawn [8].

Studies in patients with diabetes with and without CKD have also examined the benefits of a more intensive treatment target. Some of these studies are summarised below:

- Hypertension Optimal Treatment (HOT)—suggested a lower diastolic blood pressure target in diabetic patients was associated with a reduction in CV events [9].
- UK-PDS (UK Prospective diabetes study) —suggested an intensive BP target reduced the risk of mortality and complications associated with diabetes [10].
- Appropriate Blood Pressure Control in Diabetes (ABCD) trial—Intensive blood pressure control associated with better mortality and reduced vascular complications [11].

None of these trials examined a blood pressure target of under 120 mmHg as the SPRINT trial did, therefore, given that the SPRINT trial excluded diabetics, we cannot say for certain that the target

LANDMARK TRIAL: SYSTOLIC BLOOD PRESSURE INTERVENTION TRIAL (SPRINT)

- **Compared the outcomes in two blood pressure groups, one treated to a target systolic BP of less than 140 mmHg and one to a target of less than 120 mmHg**
- 2500 patients with (non-diabetic) CKD with a mean eGFR of 48ml/min and minimal proteinuria (mean ACR 9 mg/mmol). Of note, SPRINT excluded patients with proteinuria >1 g/day, diabetes, polycystic kidney disease, and patients with eGFR <20 ml/min/1.73 m^2
- **Cardiovascular (CV) events and all-cause mortality both significantly lower in the intensive treatment group**
- **In CKD subgroup analysis the CV outcome difference was not significant but the mortality benefit was**
- **Significant reduction in dementia and cognitive impairment**
- **Benefits extended to older, frail patients**
- **The trail was terminated early due to significant benefits in intensive treatment group**

Fig. 8.4 Evidence for strict BP control SPRINT trial

of <120 mmHg is associated with mortality or cardiovascular benefits in diabetic patients. The ACCORD trial did examine the effect of an intensive blood pressure target in diabetics, it did show a difference in stroke but not in other cardiovascular events or mortality. Furthermore, ACCORD enrolled very few CKD patients [12].

Potential Exceptions to a Lower Target

The above trials leave some gaps in our knowledge in terms of groups that will benefit from an intensive treatment target [8]

- Patients with advanced CKD stages G4 and G5 who were not included in SPRINT (see below for treatment of blood pressure in dialysis patients)
- Patients with diabetic CKD
- Patients with significant proteinuria (>1 g/day)
- Patients with adult polycystic kidney disease
- Patients with glomerulonephritis treated or likely to be treated with immunosuppression
- Patients with a low diastolic BP—in theory an intensive target may be harmful and coronary perfusion depends on DBP
- Age > 90—balance of benefits and harms is unclear

In addition, in patients whose life expectancy is short or who have symptomatic postural hypotension due to autonomic neuropathy, then a pragmatic approach can be taken towards treatment of BP.

Practice Point 3

- In the general population, lowering BP is proportionally associated with improved cardiovascular outcomes
- A lower target for treating blood pressure has long been used to slow progression in proteinuric CKD and prevent cardiovascular events in diabetic patients
- The most recent evidence suggests an intensive BP target is beneficial in non-diabetic patients
- The most recent KDIGO recommendations are to treat adults with CKD to a systolic BP target of less than 120 mmHg

Management of Hypertension

Lifestyle and Blood Pressure

Lifestyle measures should not be overlooked as a means to improve blood pressure control. The patient in the case scenario is a smoker, overweight and likely has a diet high in salt. Aside from lowering blood pressure losing weight, stopping smoking and reducing salt intake has health benefits beyond simply lowering BP. Smoking cessation and regular exercise should be recommended to patients.

Dietary Salt Restriction

Practice Point 4

- Recommended sodium intake is <2 g (or <5 g sodium chloride) per day in patients with high BP and CKD.

Over the last few decades in Western countries, dietary habits have shifted from fresh to more processed foods. This has occurred in parallel to rising rates of hypertension and cardiovascular disease. The significance of this association was debated for many years. In 2010 a modelling study published in the New England Journal of Medicine based on data collected from surveys of sodium intake, estimated that 1.65 million deaths from cardiovascular disease could be attributed to a sodium consumption above 2.0 g per day. Most major health organisations recommend a sodium intake below this.

The relationship between salt and blood pressure has led to the design of dietary plans aimed at reducing salt intake and improving blood pressure. The most well-known and tested of these is the DASH diet (Dietary Approaches to Stop Hypertension) [13]. The diet has been written about and there are multiple books available although it only represents one potential method of improving dietary health (Table 8.2).

Does this dietary approach have an impact on both the general and chronic kidney disease populations? A meta-analysis of 17 randomised controlled trials suggested that in the general population, introduction of the DASH diet was associated with a significant reduction of both systolic and diastolic blood pressure. The effect in the CKD population is not as well tested. Small studies in diabetic and non-diabetics and populations with diabetes and significant albuminuria

Table 8.2 Example of recommendations from the DASH Diet

Food Group	Servings per day		Serving sizes	Notes	Significance of Food group to the eating plan
	2000 calories	2600 calories			
Grains	6-8	10-11	1 slice bread 1 oz dry cereal ½ cup cooked rice, pasta or cereal	Wholewheat bread, wholewheat pasta, brown rice, pitta bread, oatmeal, cereals	Major sources of energy and fibre
Vegetables	4-5	5-6	1 cup raw leafy vegetables ½ cup chopped raw or cooked vegetables ½ cup vegetable juice	Broccoli, carrots, spinach, green beans, potatoes, sweet potatoes, tomatoes, squash	Sources of potassium, magnesium and fibre

have suggested short-term reductions in blood pressure at least.

It is important to note that adoption of the DASH diet and use of sodium substitutes that are rich in potassium may not be appropriate for patients with advanced CKD or those with hyporeninemic hypoaldosteronism or other causes of impaired potassium excretion because of potential for hyperkalaemia.

While it is reasonable to assume that reductions in blood pressure will be associated with improvements in cardiovascular disease and mortality, there is insufficient trial data to confirm this. Considering that, as we shall see, high blood pressure is associated with progression of CKD, we can also reasonably assume that a diet that contributes to the lowering of blood pressure will be beneficial in protecting against advancement of CKD.

Barriers to a Healthy Diet

In supporting patients to follow a low salt diet it is important to be mindful of the barriers that exist for a patient. In surveys and academic work patients have identified a variety of barriers towards them cutting down on processed foods and following a healthier diet;

- Cost of fresh foods
- Time to prepare a fresh meal
- Acceptance of family in following the same diet/not being able to eat with family if following a different diet
- Not being able to eat out
- Preference for salt preserved foods
- Lack of taste
- Lack of awareness of sodium content in dishes

Patients do not exist apart from their social circumstances and any advice and intervention will be more effective if the health professional can tailor it towards the patient's individual experience.

Exercise

Practice Point 5

- Moderate physical activity for a cumulative duration of *at least 150 min** per week is recommended for patients with high BP and CKD
- **This recommendation should be tailored to a level compatible to each individual patient's cardiovascular and physical tolerance*

Regular exercise improves strength and physical fitness, lowers BP and reduces the risk of diabetes for those in the general population. While there is no specific evidence in CKD patients about the BP lowering effect of exercise it stands to reason that the benefits seen in the general population will carry over.

The CKD population encompasses a wide range of people including those for whom frailty and risk of falls precludes intensive exercise programmes. Therefore, given that physical activity is likely to improve health in the CKD population, an individualized exercise plan should ideally be offered, one that takes into account the patient's needs and capabilities.

Practice Point 6

- Public Health measures are part of the prevention and treatment of cardiovascular disease
- Smoking cessation, weight loss and exercise have proven benefits
- Dietary salt restriction such as in the DASH diet can be considered to help reduce blood pressure, though may not suitable for all patients
- Potential barriers to healthy eating and exercise in our patients should be recognised

Pharmacological Treatment of Hypertension in CKD

Practice Point 7

- There is limited evidence to guide the choice of antihypertensive agent in patients with CKD
- It is recognised that many people with CKD and high BP will need a combination of 2 or more antihypertensive drugs. (KDIGO) [4, 5]

Non-Diabetics

In non-diabetics with proteinuric CKD, treatment with drugs that block the renin-angiotensin system (ACE inhibitors and Angiotensin receptor blockers,RAASi)), is recommended. This class of drugs have been most extensively studied and this is where the best evidence exists on the effect on cardiovascular outcomes and progression of kidney disease [4, 5].

The largest study on the effect of ACE inhibitors (ACEi) is the Heart Outcomes Prevention (HOPE) Study. This trial of Ramipril versus placebo included a CKD subgroup. This subgroup analysis included 3394 patients. The results demonstrated a reduction in the risk of all-cause mortality by 20%, Myocardial Infarction by 26% and Stroke by 31%. This is the most well-known trial looking at the effect of a single agent [14].

A meta-analysis by Xie et al. examined renin-angiotensin system inhibition compared to placebo and looked at both kidney and cardiovascular outcomes. Both ACEI and angiotensin receptor blockers (ARBs) reduced the risk of kidney failure compared to placebo with high certainty, controls with moderate certainty. Both agents reduced major CV events compared to placebo but only ACEi reduced the odds of all-cause death compared to active controls [15].

Diabetics

In patients with CKD and diabetes with albuminuria RAAS inhibition is strongly recommended based on the evidence that this will slow progression of CKD and protect against adverse cardiovascular outcomes [16–19].

Studies have demonstrated that even aside from blood pressure control, ACEi or ARBS have a beneficial effect on the course of a patient's chronic kidney disease. This evidence is strongest in people with CKD stage 3 or 4 with severe proteinuria as seen in the IDNT and RENAAL studies.

The RENAAL study remaining on RASS inhibition treatment significantly delayed the onset of dialysis by a mean of 6 months. Analysis of the main studies also shows that RAAS inhibition delays the progression of moderate proteinuria to severe proteinuria. The studies are not as convincing in terms of demonstrating a reduction in cardiovascular events or all-cause mortality.

Combination of ACEi and ARB to treat hypertension in CKD is not recommended for it doesn't afford any additional benefit but on the other hand increases the risk of hyperkalaemia.

Monitoring a Patient on an ACEi or ARB

ACEi and ARB's counteract the vasoconstrictive effects of angiotensin II. By blocking the action of angiotensin II they cause vasodilatation of the of the efferent arterioles of the glomeruli and a decline in intraglomerular pressure. This leads to a decline in GFR and a rise in serum creatinine. Therefore, patients should be monitored after the initiation of one of these agents according to these principles;

- The rise in creatinine will occur in the first 2 weeks
- It should stabalise within 2–4 weeks assuming a normal salt and fluid intake
- Aside from an excessive rise in serum creatinine, patients should also be monitored for hyperkalaemia and hypotension

LANDMARK TRIAL: HEART OUTCOMES PROTECTION STUDY (HOPE)
• Assessed the role of Ramipril in preventing cardiovascular complications in patients not known to have heart failure with a low ejection fraction • Ramipril vs Placebo • Trial was a 2x2 factor design that included assessment of Vitamin E • 651 patients reached the primary endpoint (composite of MI, stroke, death from cardiovascular cause) vs 826 in the placebo group. • Treatment with Ramipril reduced the rates of death, stroke and myocardial infarction in patients not known to have left ventricular dysfunction • In CKD patients risk of stroke, MI and death reduced vs placebo (n=3394)

Fig. 8.5 Evidence of ACEi in CKD (HOPE study)

- Hyperkalaemia is a particular concern in patients with more advanced CKD and so monitoring should be adjusted appropriately
- Stopping the medications should be a last resort given their potential cardiovascular benefits but should be considered in patients with unacceptable creatinine rises of uncontrolled hyperkalaemia

The NICE CKD Guideline suggests checking serum potassium and eGFR before starting ACEi/ARB, and then repeating after 1–2 weeks of starting and after each dose increase (Fig. 8.5) [4, 5].

Other Agents

Mineralocorticoid Receptor Antagonist

There are small, short-term studies that demonstrate that Spironolactone and Eplerenone are effective in lowering blood pressure in people who are already on three anti-hypertensive agents. They also may lower albuminuria in patients with diabetic nephropathy. There are no long-term data and side-effects, particularly hyperkalaemia and decline in kidney function are a concern.

In patients without problems with high potassium and who have less advanced CKD, blocking aldosterone may be beneficial in controlling resistant hypertension.

A recent trial has demonstrated that in patients with CKD and type 2 diabetes, treatment with finerenone, a nonsteroidal, selective mineralocorticoid receptor antagonist, lowers the risk of CKD progression and cardiovascular events compared with placebo [20].

Calcium Channel Blockers, Beta-Blockers, Alpha Blockers and Diuretics

While all of the above medications are established treatments for hypertension and familiar to any nephrologist or primary care practitioner attempting to control a patient's blood pressure, there is little direct evidence of their benefit in terms of improving mortality and reducing cardiovascular events in patients with CKD. Instead, they should be thought of as the next line in drugs for a physician aiming for a blood pressure target in a CKD patient and their use will be determined by the patient's blood pressure, the potential side effects and their fluid status (Fig. 8.6).

Practice Point 8

- Drugs that block the renal-angiotensin system are the first-choice therapy for patients with chronic kidney disease and albuminuria
- In these patients RAAS inhibition has been shown to slow the progression on CKD towards end-stage kidney disease.
- Drugs blocking aldosterone might help in resistant hypertension but have important side effects that require monitoring
- Data on other drug classes is limited but all can be considered part of treating a patient to target

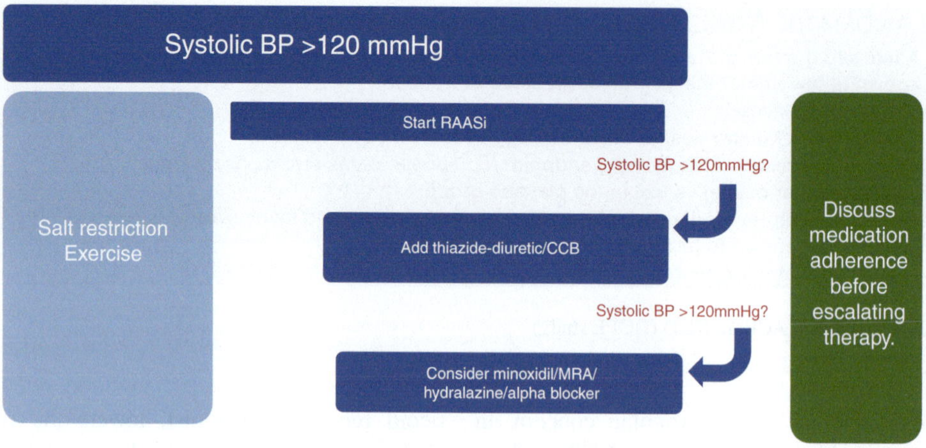

Fig. 8.6 Managing hypertension in non-dialysis dependent CKD patients

Blood Pressure Treatment in Dialysis Patients

Your patient confides to you that he is very worried about his blood pressure. His older brother had difficult to control blood pressure and ended up with kidney failure on dialysis. Since then his blood pressure has remained difficult to control and a couple of months ago he suffered a stroke which he has thankfully recovered from.

Hypertension is extremely common in patients on both Haemodialysis and Peritoneal dialysis. While the relationship between lowering blood pressure and improving cardiovascular outcomes is clear in the general population, it is not as clear cut in dialysis patients.

In Haemodialysis patients, there are a number of observational studies demonstrating a 'U' or 'J' shaped relationship between blood pressure and outcomes. In these studies, mortality is highest at both elevated systolic blood pressures and with low blood pressures. There are however, many factors which make true appreciation of the relationship between blood pressure and mortality difficult.

Firstly, pre-dialysis blood pressure is measured in sub-optimal conditions. Patients are rushing to start dialysis and may be frustrated at transportation delays and anxious about needling. Secondly, the fluid status and presence of uraemic toxins vary between dialysis sessions but would be at their peak in the pre-dialysis period. This may confound the measurements. Thirdly, a patient in end stage kidney failure may at this point have acquired a number of co-morbidities that confound blood pressure measurement including heart failure and malnutrition.

There are also considerations as to whether lowering BP is deleterious to HD patients. Intradialytic hypotension (IDH) complicates up to a third of HD sessions and is independently associated with increased morbidity and mortality. It is possible to lower BP by removing extracellular water to 'probe' the dry weight but this comes at the expense of increasing episodes of hypotension. There is evidence that IDH and increased ultrafiltration rates leads to myocardial stunning and LV fibrosis [21, 22]. Episodes of IDH contribute to fatigue and increased recovery time after dialysis, both outcomes that are important to dialysis patients. To read more about IDH, please refer to Chap. 18.

Ideally, we would have data from well conducted clinical trials that allowed us to develop a target blood pressure that was individualised to each patient depending on the patient's frailty, co-morbidities and how it affects a patient's

Management of Blood Pressure in the Haemodialysis Patient
• Attempt to collect as accurate blood pressure readings as possible through education of patients and dialysis staff. Choose the standardised office blood pressure method. • Fluid management is crucial. Consider extended sessions and extra ultrafiltration sessions if needed to improve fluid management and minimise ultrafiltration rate. • Counsel patients as to the importance of a low sodium diet • There is not sufficient evidence to make recommendations about which anti-hypertensive to use. Beta-blockers, calcium channel blockers and angiotensin receptor blockers (if potassium is controlled) are all reasonable choices. • In most patients, aim for a pre-dialysis BP of between 130/60 and 159/99 mmHg and a post HD BP of between 120/70 and 139/99 mmHg if tolerated. If there are issues with IDH then raise the BP goal or consider omitting antihypertensives immediately prior to dialysis. • If patients are motivated and able to measure home BP then aim for measurements of between 120 and 130 mmHg between sessions.

Fig. 8.7 Management of hypertension in dialysis patients [23]

overall well-being. Until such a time we should develop a practical approach to blood pressure management (Fig. 8.7).

Blood Pressure Management in Peritoneal Dialysis (PD) Patients

Hypertension is again, very common in PD patients. Hypertension generally improves after the initiation of PD and for the next 6–12 months after which BP control tends to decline. Observational studies have also suggested a similar 'J' shaped mortality curve as seen in the HD population although again this is confounded by co-morbidity. Fluid status is important again, subclinical hypervolaemia is more common in PD patients. Patients on PD also have differences in residual kidney function, peritoneal membrane characteristics and different capabilities in terms of salt handling that might have an impact.

The International Society of Peritoneal Dialysis (ISPD) guidelines recommend that BP should be recorded at home once weekly. They also recommend a target if less than 140/90 mmHg. Once again there is little data from randomized controlled trials and so this target has been extrapolated from previous targets set in the CKD and general populations. This is a reasonable target in the absence of further evidence.

The ISPD recommend optimising volume status in PD patients before initiating or increasing anti-hypertensive drugs.

Where pharmacotherapy is necessary, observational data does suggest some benefits in using RAAS inhibition in PD patients. There are small studies that benefits in terms of preserving residual kidney function with perhaps some effect on left ventricular function and mortality. These studies are limited and are not adequately powered randomised controlled trials but they provide a rationale for the use of RAASi in PD patients [22].

Practice Point 9

- In both HD and PD patients there is observation evidence of a 'j' shaped mortality curve with regards to blood pressure
- Studies are confounded by difficulties in accurate BP measurement, importance of fluid status and the frailty and co-morbidities in these populations
- A practical approach to blood pressure management is recommended in HD patients
- There is some, albeit limited, evidence that RAASi may be of benefit in PD patients

Blood Pressure Management in Transplant Patients

In a kidney transplant recipient the preservation of transplant function is added to the usual goals of blood pressure management. Patients gain a great deal from their improved quality of life compared to being off dialysis and, as a consequence, place considerable importance on preventing loss of the transplant. There are no trials testing specific blood pressure targets in this group and the current recommendation is to aim for a blood pressure of less than 130/80 mmHg. Transplant patients are still subject to higher rates of cardiovascular disease than the general population.

In terms of preserving kidney function, there is some evidence that treatment of blood pressure with dihydropyridine calcium channel blockers is associated with a reduction in graft loss. There is also perhaps some evidence that angiotensin receptor blockers are also associated with graft preservation. However, neither class of drug has been found to have an effect on all-cause or cardiovascular mortality. The recent KDIGO BP guideline suggest a dihydropyridine calcium channel blocker or an ARB be used as first line agent in adult kidney transplant recipients. There is no data supporting the use of other anti-hypertensives [5, 24].

Practice Point 10

- In treating transplant patients, preservation of graft function is as important a consideration to patients as the usual reasons to treat hypertension
- The recommendation is to treat to a blood pressure lower than 130/80 mmHg
- Calcium channel blockers are generally used as first line

Conclusions

The case of the 42 year old gentleman with CKD and hypertension from the beginning of this chapter illustrates the importance of measuring the blood pressure with an appropriate technique, providing guidance as to non-pharmacological interventions, for example dietary, exercise and smoking cessation advice, and design appropriate pharmacological therapy, an appropriate management plan and goals. The standardised BP is important in guiding management; whilst ACE inhibitors may be the first BP lowering agent of choice, most, including this patient—will likely need additional agents for adequate blood pressure control.

Questions

1. A 50-year-old man with chronic kidney disease was seen in the follow-up clinic. His blood pressure measured in sitting position after 15 min rest was 150/90 mmHg. His kidney function has deteriorated from 45 mL/min/1.73 m^2 to 41 mL/min/1.73 m^2 in 3 years and urine protein:creatinine ratio was 125 mg/mmol. His medications included amlodipine 5 mg once day and atorvastatin 20 mg once a day.

   What is the next best step in management of blood pressure?
   A. Increase amlodipine
   B. Start bisoprolol
   C. Start ramipril
   D. Start indapamide
   E. Wait for 3 months and remeasure blood pressure

Correct answer C: start ramipril and it is the agent most likely prevent progress of kidney disease.

2. A 50-year-old man with chronic kidney disease was seen in the follow-up clinic. His

blood pressure measured in sitting position after 15 min rest was 150/90 mmHg. His kidney function has deteriorated from 45 mL/min/1.73 m^2 to 41 mL/min/1.73 m^2 in 2 years and urine protein:creatinine ratio was 125 mg/mmol. His medications included amlodipine 5 mg once day and atorvastatin 20 mg once a day.

What is target BP (mmHg) for best results.

A. <120 systolic
B. 120/80
C. <130/80
D. <140/90
E. <125/75

Correct answer A: Less than 120 systolic as recommended by KDIGO BP guideline.

3. A 50-year-old man with chronic kidney disease was seen in the follow-up clinic. His blood pressure measured in sitting position after 15 min rest was 150/90 mmHg. His kidney function has deteriorated from 45 mL/min/1.73 m^2 to 41 mL/min/1.73 m^2 in 2 years and urine protein:creatinine ratio was 125 mg/mmol. His medications included amlodipine 5 mg once day and atorvastatin 20 mg once a day. He was started on losartan 50 mg daily and his eGFR declined to 35 mL/min/1.73 m^2.

What is the next best step in management?

A. Increase amlodipine
B. Increase losartan
C. Stop losartan
D. Start bisoprolol
E. Stop atorvastatin

Correct answer B: increase losartan.

4. A 45-year-old man with chronic kidney disease stage 4 was seen in the noisy kidney clinic. His blood pressure measured was 145/85 mmHg. He was on amlodipine 5 mg daily and ramipril 5 mg daily. His home blood pressure measured the night before was 115/75.

What is the best response to the blood pressure measurement?

A. Consider the clinic BP and increase amlodipine
B. Consider home blood pressure and decease amlodipine
C. Make no changes to his medications
D. Consider the clinic BP and increase ramipril
E. Consider home blood pressure and decease ramipril.

Correct answer C: make no changes in his treatment as home BP is well controlled.

5. A 55-year-old man with chronic kidney disease stage 3 was seen in the noisy kidney clinic. His blood pressure measured was 142/89 mmHg. He was on amlodipine 5 mg daily and ramipril 5 mg daily.

What is the best response to the blood pressure measurement?

A. Consider the clinic BP and increase amlodipine
B. Repeat the blood pressure under standard condition
C. Consider the clinic BP and increase ramipril
D. Start indapamide 1.5 mg daily
E. Start frusemide 40 mg daily

Correct answer is B: make no changes in his treatment.

6. A 65-year-old man with diabetic kidney disease stage 3 was seen in the diabetes clinic. His BP was 145/65 mmHg, eGFR 52 mL/min/1.73 m^2, HBA1c 66 mmol/mol, total cholesterol 6 mmol/L. He started in canagliflozin 100 mg daily and atrovatstain was increased to 40 mg.

Which is a mostly likely effect of the medication changes.

A. A drop in blood pressure
B. A drop in serum creatinine kinase
C. A rise in estimated GFR
D. A rise urine protein
E. A rise in haemoglobin A1c

Correct answer A: A drop in blood pressure.

7. A 65-year-old man with diabetic kidney disease stage 3 was seen in the diabetes clinic.

His BP was 145/65 mmHg, eGFR 52 mL/min/1.73 m^2, HBA1c 66 mmol/mol, total cholesterol 6 mmol/L. He started in canagliflozin 100 mg daily and atorvastatin was increased to 40 mg. His estimated GFR dropped to 48 mL/min/1.73 m^2

What is the most likely mechanism of the drop in eGFR?

A. Afferent arterial vaso-constriction
B. Afferent arterial vaso-dilatation
C. efferent arterial vaso-constriction
D. efferent arterial vaso-constriction
E. Decreased water delivery to distal tubule

Correct answer A: afferent arteriolar vasoconstriction due to increased salt and water delivery to distal tubule.

8. A 65-year-old man with diabetic kidney disease stage 3 was seen in the diabetes clinic. His BP was 150/65 mmHg, serum potassium 5.9 mmol/L, eGFR 52 mL/min/1.73 m^2, HBA1c 66 mmol/mol, total cholesterol 6 mmol/L. He was on ramipril 5 mg daily, aspirin 75 mg daily, atrovastatin 20, metformin. What is the nest best step in management of blood pressure?

A. Increase ramipril
B. Start spironolactone
C. Start indapamide
D. Start amlodipine
E. Start doxazocin

Correct answer C: start indapamide which will help reduce BP and hyperkalaemia.

9. A 46 year old man was found to have low eGFR of 52 mL/min/min and 50 mL/min/1.73 m^2 on two different occasion two different occasions 4 months apart. His BP was 146/70.

What is next best step in blood pressure control.

A. Exercise 150 min every week
B. Take <5 g of salt per day
C. Reduce alcohol intake to less than 2 standard drinks per day
D. All of the above
E. None of the above

Correct answer D: all of the above.

10. A 46 year Caucasian man was found to have low eGFR of 52 mL/min/min and 50 mL/min/1.73 m^2 on two different occasions 4 months apart. His BP was 146/70.

Which study provides the most relevant study guiding his BP target of <120 mmHg (systolic).

A. AASK
B. BENEDICT
C. SPRINT
D. SHARP
E. HOPE

Correct answer C: SPRINT trial.

Test your learning and check your understanding of this book's contents: use the "Springer Nature Flashcards" app to access questions using https://sn.pub/cz9Cok. To use the app, please follow the instructions in Chap. 1.

References

1. The KDIGO 2021 Blood Pressure in CKD Guideline https://kdigo.org/guidelines/blood-pressure-in-ckd/
2. Klahr S, Levey AS, Beck GJ, Caggiula AW, Hunsicker L, Kusek JW, Striker G. The effects of dietary protein restriction and blood-pressure control on the progression of chronic renal disease. Modification of Diet in Renal Disease Study Group. N Engl J Med. 1994 Mar 31;330(13):877–84.
3. Wright JT Jr, Bakris G, Greene T, Agodoa LY, Appel LJ, Charleston J, Cheek D, Douglas-Baltimore JG, Gassman J, Glassock R, Hebert L, Jamerson K, Lewis J, Phillips RA, Toto RD, Middleton JP, Rostand SG, African American Study of Kidney Disease and Hypertension Study Group. Effect of blood pressure lowering and antihypertensive drug class on progression of hypertensive kidney disease: results from the AASK trial. JAMA. 2002 Nov 20;288(19):2421–31.
4. Hypertension in adults: diagnosis and management: NICE guideline [NG136] https://www.nice.org.uk/guidance/ng136/chapter/recommendations#treating-and-monitoring-hypertension. Accessed 14 Jul 2021
5. Cheung AK, Chang TI, Cushman WC, Furth SL, Hou FF, Ix JH, Knoll GA, Muntner P, Pecoits-Filho R, Sarnak MJ, Tobe SW, Tomson CRV, Lytvyn L, Craig JC, Tunnicliffe DJ, Howell M, Tonelli M, Cheung M, Earley A, Mann JFE. Executive summary of the KDIGO 2021 clinical practice guideline for the management of blood pressure in chronic kidney disease. Kidney Int. 2021 Mar;99(3):559–69.
6. SPRINT Research Group, Wright JT Jr, Williamson JD, Whelton PK, Snyder JK, Sink KM, Rocco MV, Reboussin DM, Rahman M, Oparil S, Lewis CE, Kimmel PL, Johnson KC, Goff DC Jr, Fine LJ, Cutler

JA, Cushman WC, Cheung AK, Ambrosius WT. A randomized trial of intensive versus standard blood-pressure control. N Engl J Med. 2015;373(22):2103–16. https://doi.org/10.1056/NEJMoa1511939. Epub 2015 Nov 9. Erratum in: N Engl J Med. 2017 Dec 21;377(25):2506

7. Cheung AK, Rahman M, Reboussin DM, Craven TE, Greene T, Kimmel PL, Cushman WC, Hawfield AT, Johnson KC, Lewis CE, Oparil S, Rocco MV, Sink KM, Whelton PK, Wright JT Jr, Basile J, Beddhu S, Bhatt U, Chang TI, Chertow GM, Chonchol M, Freedman BI, Haley W, Ix JH, Katz LA, Killeen AA, Papademetriou V, Ricardo AC, Servilla K, Wall B, Wolfgram D, Yee J, SPRINT Research Group. Effects of intensive BP control in CKD. J Am Soc Nephrol. 2017 Sep;28(9):2812–23.
8. Dasgupta I, Zoccali C. Is the KDIGO systolic blood pressure target <120 mmHg for chronic kidney disease appropriate in routine clinical practice? Hypertension. 2022 Jan;79(1):4-11. doi: https://doi.org/10.1161/HYPERTENSIONAHA.121.18434. Epub 2021 Nov 17.
9. Hansson L, Zanchetti A, Carruthers SG, Dahlöf B, Elmfeldt D, Julius S, Ménard J, Rahn KH, Wedel H, Westerling S. Effects of intensive blood-pressure lowering and low-dose aspirin in patients with hypertension: principal results of the Hypertension Optimal Treatment (HOT) randomised trial. HOT Study Group. Lancet. 1998 Jun 13;351(9118):1755–62. https://doi.org/10.1016/s0140-6736(98)04311-6.
10. UK Prospective Diabetes Study Group. Tight blood pressure control and risk of macrovascular and microvascular complications in type 2 diabetes: UKPDS 38. UK Prospective Diabetes Study Group. BMJ. 1998;317(7160):703–13. Erratum in: BMJ 1999 Jan 2;318(7175):29
11. Schrier RW, Estacio RO, Jeffers B. Appropriate blood pressure control in NIDDM (ABCD) trial. Diabetologia. 1996 Dec;39(12):1646–54. https://doi.org/10.1007/s001250050629.
12. ACCORD Study Group, Cushman WC, Evans GW, Byington RP, Goff DC Jr, Grimm RH Jr, Cutler JA, Simons-Morton DG, Basile JN, Corson MA, Probstfield JL, Katz L, Peterson KA, Friedewald WT, Buse JB, Bigger JT, Gerstein HC, Ismail-Beigi F. Effects of intensive blood-pressure control in type 2 diabetes mellitus. N Engl J Med. 2010 Apr 29;362(17):1575–85. https://doi.org/10.1056/NEJMoa1001286.
13. Sacks FM, Svetkey LP, Vollmer WM, Appel LJ, Bray GA, Harsha D, Obarzanek E, Conlin PR, Miller ER 3rd, Simons-Morton DG, Karanja N, Lin PH, DASH-Sodium Collaborative Research Group. Effects on blood pressure of reduced dietary sodium and the Dietary Approaches to Stop Hypertension (DASH) diet. DASH-Sodium Collaborative Research Group. N Engl J Med. 2001;344(1):3–10.
14. Heart Outcomes Prevention Evaluation Study Investigators, Yusuf S, Sleight P, Pogue J, Bosch J, Davies R, Dagenais G. Effects of an angiotensin-converting-enzyme inhibitor, ramipril, on cardiovascular events in high-risk patients. N Engl J Med. 2000 Jan 20;342(3):145–53.
15. Xie X, Atkins E, Lv J, Bennett A, Neal B, Ninomiya T, Woodward M, MacMahon S, Turnbull F, Hillis GS, Chalmers J, Mant J, Salam A, Rahimi K, Perkovic V, Rodgers A. Effects of intensive blood pressure lowering on cardiovascular and renal outcomes: updated systematic review and meta-analysis. Lancet. 2016;387(10017):435–43. https://doi.org/10.1016/S0140-6736(15)00805-3. Epub 2015 Nov 7
16. The Heart Outcomes Prevention Evaluation (HOPE) Study Investigators. Effects of an angiotensin-converting-enzyme-inhibitor, Ramipril on cardiovascular events in high-risk patients. N Engl J Med. 2000;342:145–53. https://doi.org/10.1056/NEJM200001203420301.
17. Effects of Ramipril on cardiovascular and microvascular outcomes in people with diabetes mellitus: results of the HOPE and MICRO-HOPE substudy. Heart Outcomes Prevention Evaluation study investigators. Lancet 2000; Sep 2
18. Lewis EJ, Hunsicker LG, Clarke WR, Berl T, Pohl MA, Lewis JB, Ritz E, Atkins RC, Rohde R, Raz I, Collaborative Study Group. Renoprotective effect of the angiotensin-receptor antagonist irbesartan in patients with nephropathy due to type 2 diabetes. N Engl J Med. 2001 Sep 20;345(12):851–60. https://doi.org/10.1056/NEJMoa011303.
19. Brenner, et al. Effects of losartan on renal and cardiovascular outcomes in patients with type 2 diabetes and nephropathy. N Engl J Med. 2001 Sep 20;345(12):861–9. https://doi.org/10.1056/NEJMoa011161.
20. Bakris GL, Agarwal R, Anker SD, Pitt B, Ruilope LM, Rossing P, Kolkhof P, Nowack C, Schloemer P, Joseph A, Filippatos G, FIDELIO-DKD Investigators. Effect of finerenone on chronic kidney disease outcomes in type 2 diabetes. N Engl J Med. 2020 Dec 3;383(23):2219–29. https://doi.org/10.1056/NEJMoa2025845.
21. Hemodialysis-induced repetitive myocardial injury results in global and segmental reduction in systolic cardiac function
22. Burton JO, Jefferies HJ, Selby NM, CW MI. Clin J Am Soc Nephrol. 2009 Dec;4(12):1925–31. https://doi.org/10.2215/CJN.04470709.
23. Doulton TWR, Swift PA, Murtaza A, Dasgupta I. Uncertainties in BP management in dialysis patients. Semin Dial. 2020 May;33(3):223–35. https://doi.org/10.1111/sdi.12880.
24. van der Schaaf et al. Hypertension after renal transplantation: calcium channel or converting enzyme blockade. Jan 1995 Hypertension 25:77-81 doi: https://doi.org/10.1161/01.HYP.25.1.77.

Mineral and Bone Disorder in CKD 9

Miho Murashima and Takayuki Hamano

Clinical Scenario

An 80 year-old women with CKD stage G5D due to diabetic nephropathy was seen in the clinic. Her serum creatinine was 8.5 mg/dL [756 μmol/L], albumin was 3.6 g/dL [36 g/L], calcium was 9.4 mg/dL [2.35 mmol/L], phosphate was 3.5 mg/dL [1.1 mmol/L], and intact PTH was 753 pg/mL [80 pmol/L]. Calcitriol was started and her serum calcium increased to 11.0 mg/dL [2.7 mmol/L]. Intact PTH levels remain elevated above 500 pg/mL [53 pmol/L].

Introduction

CKD-MBD is a nearly universal complication of progressive loss of kidney function. Biochemical abnormalities in mineral metabolism lead to bone pain or increased incidence of fractures. Subsequently, abnormalities in mineral metabolism were shown to be associated with vascular calcification, and high cardiovascular morbidity and mortality. As a result, Kidney Disease Improving Global Outcomes (KDIGO) defined the CKD-MBD as follows [1]:

A systemic disorder of mineral and bone metabolism due to CKD manifested by either one or a combination of the following (Fig. 9.1):

- Abnormalities of calcium, phosphorus, parathyroid hormone (PTH) or vitamin D metabolism
- Abnormalities in bone turnover, mineralization, volume, linear growth, or strength
- Vascular or other soft tissue calcification

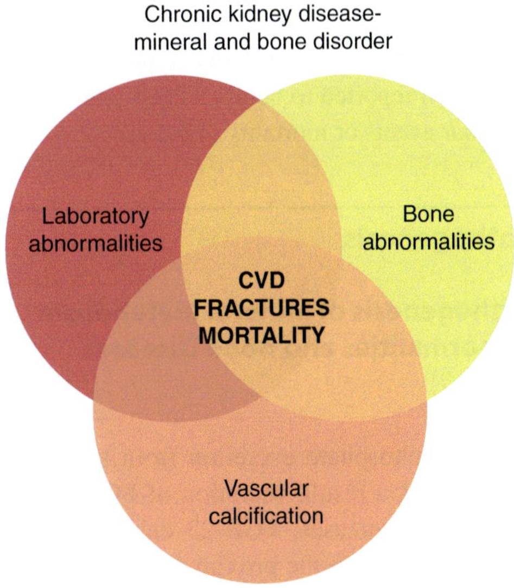

Fig. 9.1 The concept of chronic kidney-disease mineral and bone disorder

M. Murashima · T. Hamano (✉)
Department of Nephrology, Graduate School of Medical Sciences, Nagoya City University, Nagoya, Japan
e-mail: mmurashi@med.nagoya-cu.ac.jp; hamatea@kid.med.osaka-u.ac.jp

D. Banerjee et al. (eds.), *Management of Kidney Diseases*,
https://doi.org/10.1007/978-3-031-09131-5_9

Table 9.1 The association between traditional markers of CKD-MBD and mortality

Study	Design	Dialysis modality	Risk of mortality associated with markers of CKD-MBD					
			Calcium		Phosphate		PTH	
			Low	High	Low	High	Low	High
Block 2004 [2]	Retrospective	HD	↓	↑	NS	↑	NS	↑
Noordzij 2005 [3]	Prospective	HD, PD	NS	NS	NS	↑	NS	NS
Kalantar-Zadeh 2006 [4]	Prospective	HD	↑	↑	↑	↑	↑	↑
Melamed 2006 [5]	Prospective	HD, PD	NS	↑	NS	↑	NS	↑
Tentori 2008 [6]	Retrospective	HD	↑	↑	↑	↑	↑	↑
Block 2010 [7]	Prospective	HD	NS	↑	NS	↑	NS	↑
Floege 2011 [8]	Prospective	HD	↑	↑	↑	↑	↑	↑
Taniguchi 2013 [9]	Retrospective	HD	NS	↑	↑	↑	↑	↑
Soohoo 2016 [10]	Retrospective	HD	NS	↑	↑	↑	↑	↑
Waziri 2019 [11]	Prospective	HD, PD	NS	↑	NS	↑	NS	↑

CKD-MBD chronic kidney disease-mineral and bone disorder, *PTH* parathyroid hormone, *HD* hemodialysis, *PD* peritoneal dialysis, *NS* not significant

Epidemiology

Several observational studies have shown an association between deranged markers of CKD-MBD and poor clinical outcomes (Table 9.1). Hyperphosphatemia, hypophosphatemia, hypercalcemia, and high PTH levels were consistently associated with higher mortality and cardiovascular morbidity. Associations between hypocalcemia, low PTH levels and outcomes were somewhat controversial. In addition, high fibroblast growth factor 23 (FGF23) levels, high alkaline phosphatase (ALP) levels, hypomagnesemia have been reported to be associated with cardiovascular events or mortality [12–14].

Pathogenesis

Pathogenesis of Mineral Metabolism Abnormalities and Bone Diseases (Fig. 9.2)

In CKD, phosphate excretion from kidneys is reduced. As a result, secretion of FGF23 from osteocytes increases. FGF 23 enhances phosphate excretion in the proximal renal tubule by decreasing the luminal expression of sodium-dependent phosphate transporters. In addition, FGF23 reduces the synthesis of 1,25 dihydroxy vitamin D [$1{,}25(OH)_2D$] and enhances the

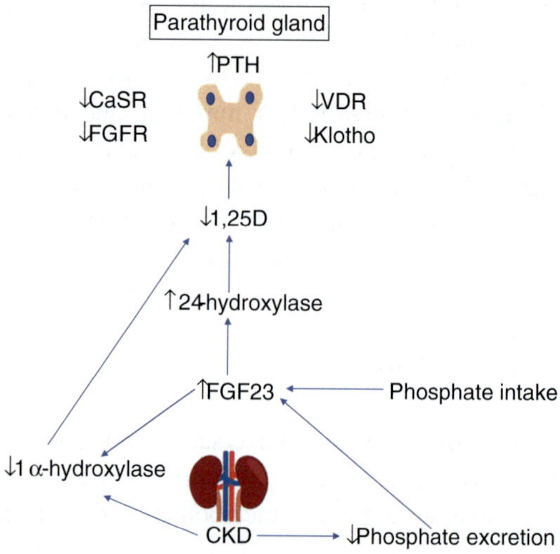

Fig. 9.2 Pathogenesis of secondary hyperparathyroidism in CKD. Impaired excretion of phosphate leads to increased levels of FGF23 which in turn reduces the synthesis, as well as enhancing the catabolism, of $1{,}25(OH)_2D$. Decreased levels of 1 α-hydroxylase also contribute to the deficiency of $1{,}25(OH)_2D$. The end result is a reduction in calcium absorption which leads to secondary hyperparathyroidism. As kidney function worsens, the responsiveness of the vitamin D and calcium receptors on the parathyroid decrease, further contributing to high levels of circulating PTH. In addition, expression of α-Klotho, the transmembrane protein required for the binding of FGF23 to its receptor, decreased with advancing CKD. This attenuates FGF23 mediated suppression of PTH and thus also contributes to secondary hyperparathyroidism. *PTH* parathyroid hormone, *CaSR* calcium-sensing receptor, *FGFR* fibroblast growth factor receptor, *VDR* vitamin D receptor, *1,25D* (1, 25) dihydroxy vitamin D, *FGF23* fibroblast growth factor 23, *CKD* chronic kidney disease

catabolism of 1,25(OH)$_2$D, thereby decreasing intestinal phosphate absorption. In the early stages of CKD, high levels of FGF23 attenuate hyperphosphatemia by increased excretion of phosphate from the kidneys at the expense of 1,25(OH)$_2$D suppression. As CKD progresses, 1α-hydroxylase synthesis in the kidneys decreases, which results in further decline in 1,25(OH)$_2$D levels. Suppression of 1,25(OH)$_2$D leads to secondary hyperparathyroidism and reduction in intestinal calcium absorption. With further worsening of kidney function, hyperphosphatemia ensues and further reduction of 1,25(OH)$_2$D leading to hypocalcemia and hyperparathyroidism. Other consequences of worsening kidney function include hyporesponsiveness of the vitamin D receptor and reduced expression of the calcium-sensing receptor on the parathyroid gland. FGF 23 requires α-klotho to enable it to bind to the FGF receptor. α-Klotho is a transmembrane protein expressed in the kidneys and parathyroid glands. With the progression of CKD, α-klotho expression decreases in the parathyroid glands, leading to attenuated suppression of PTH by FGF23. This also aggravates secondary hyperparathyroidism. Elevated PTH increases bone resorption and leads to osteitis fibrosa or high-turnover bone disease.

However, bone histology studies showed that bone diseases in dialysis patients are much more complex than expected [15, 16]. There were varieties of defects in bone mineralization, bone volume, and bone turnover. The abnormalities in bone were classified into severe osteitis fibrosa (high turnover from elevated PTH), mild osteitis fibrosa, osteomalacia (mineralization defect potentially from hypophosphatemia, hypocalcemia, or vitamin D deficiency), adynamic bone disease (low bone turnover from bone resistance to PTH or oversuppression of PTH by high-dose vitamin D or calcium load), and mixed renal osteodystrophy (increased turnover with abnormal mineralization) (Fig. 9.3). Those with osteitis fibrosa, adynamic bone disease, or osteomalacia tend to have high PTH, low PTH, or high ALP levels, respectively, but there are substantial overlaps in these bone markers for different bone histology. Currently, treatment decisions depend on these available bone markers, but we should note that these markers are not perfect predictors of bone histology and bone biopsy is indicated if there is a possibility that the result may change management.

Pathogenesis of Vascular Calcification (Fig. 9.4)

Recent evidence establishes that vascular calcification is a highly regulated cell-mediated process rather than passive deposition of calcium and phosphate to the vascular smooth muscle cells [17]. Features of vascular calcification in CKD is

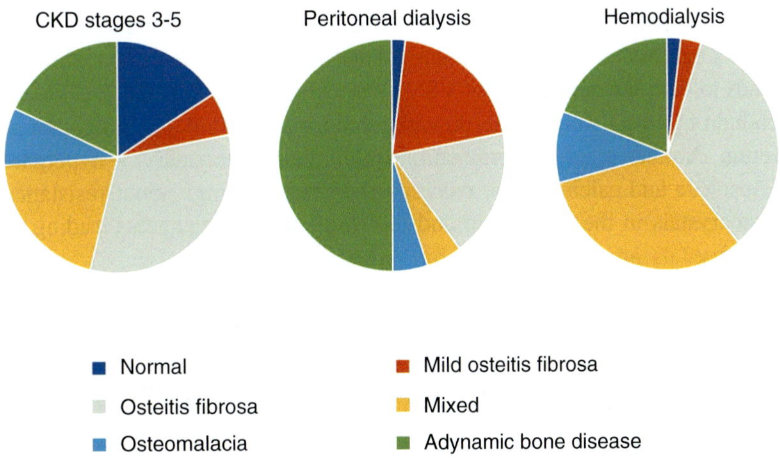

Fig. 9.3 Prevalence of types of bone disease as determined by bone biopsy in patients with chronic kidney disease-mineral and bone disorder. *CKD* chronic kidney disease (Modified from Kidney Int Suppl 2009; 113: S1–S130)

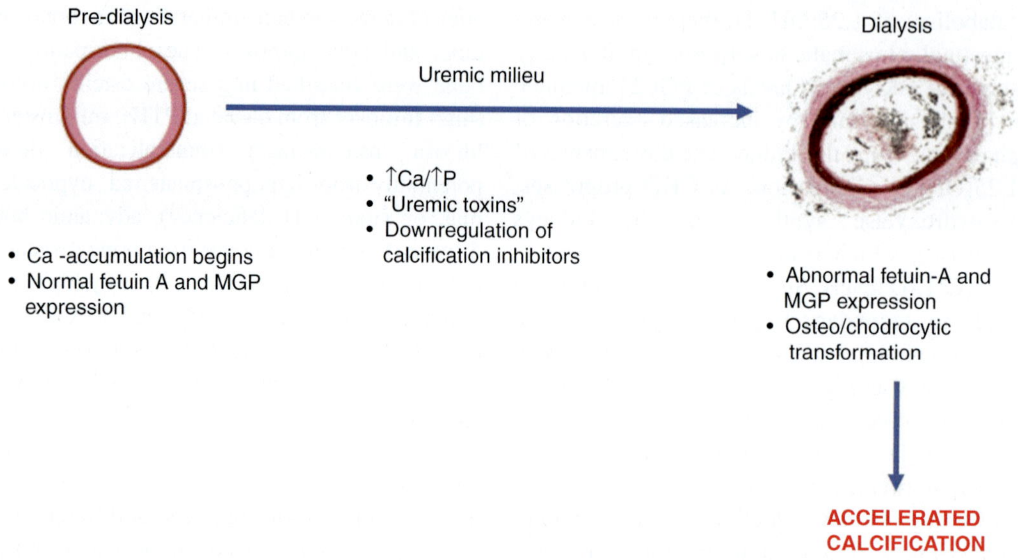

Fig. 9.4 Pathogenesis of vascular calcification in chronic kidney disease. *MGP* matrix G1a protein (Modified from J Am Soc Nephrol 2013; 24: 179–189)

medial calcification which involves sheet-like calcification in the tunica media with a concentric thickening of the vessel wall. Vascular smooth muscle cells (VSMCs) are of mesenchymal origin and under stress can differentiate to different mesenchymal-derived cell types such as osteoblasts or chondrocytes. In CKD, high circulating phosphate leads to phosphate uptake by VSMCs through sodium-dependent phosphate cotransporters. Under normal conditions, calcification of VSMCs does not occur, as mineralization inhibitors such as matrix G1a protein (MGP) and fetuin A work. However, when VSMCs are exposed to high phosphate levels in patients with CKD, Runx2 expression in VSMCs is upregulated. This leads to both the conversion of VSMCs to osteochondrocytes as well as the downregulation of fetuin A and other mineralization inhibitors. Phosphate and calcium form calcium-phosphate nanocrystals in the circulation and the resultant nanocrystals are phagocytosed by VSMCs and become the nidus of calcification. Nanocrystals also promote inflammation and osteochondrocytic differentiation of VSMCs, thus forming the vicious cycle of vascular calcification. Of note, vascular calcification is associated with lower PTH levels and adynamic bone disease [18]. This would suggest that adynamic bone cannot buffer calcium load either from dialysate or calcium-containing phosphate binders and it accelerates vascular calcification. Thus, there is a close relationship between bone diseases and vascular calcification in CKD patients.

Clinical Presentation

Severe hyperparathyroidism and osteomalacia may present with bone or joint pain. However, in most of cases, CKD-MBD was recognized in asymptomatic patients as biochemical abnormalities (elevated phosphate, PTH, and decreased calcium levels). Vascular calcification could be found on plain computed tomography. Severe secondary hyperparathyroidism sometimes brings about resistance to erythropoiesis stimulating agents leading to anaemia.

Investigations

The KDIGO guidelines recommend initiation of monitoring for biochemical abnormalities of CKD-MBD beginning in CKD G3a [1].

Table 9.2 Markers of chronic kidney disease-mineral and bone disorders

Marker	Frequency of measurements	Comments
Calcium Phosphate	Every 6–12 months in CKD G3a-G3b Every 3–6 months in CKD G4 Every 1–3 months in CKD G5	It is reasonable to increase the frequency of measurements for whom biochemical abnormalities are identified or monitor response to treatment
PTH	Every 6–12 months in CKD G4 Every 3–6 months in CKD G5	It is reasonable to increase the frequency of measurements for whom biochemical abnormalities are identified or monitor response to treatment
25(OH)D	Not stated	Vitamin D deficiency and insufficiency should be corrected using treatment strategies recommended for the general population.
Total alkaline phosphatase	Annually	A marker of osteoid formation and mineralization, inexpensive
Bone-specific alkaline phosphatase	No recommendation	More specific and a better surrogate marker of bone formation

CKD chronic kidney disease, *PTH* parathyroid hormone, *25(OH)D* 25-hydroxy vitamin D

Recommended laboratory tests and frequency of measurements are shown in Table 9.2. BMD testing is recommended to assess fracture risk where results will alter therapy.

Management

Overview

The essence of CKD-MBD management is largely to prevent the adverse consequences associated with secondary hyperparathyroidism and hyperphosphatemia. Treatment is dependent on well-established markers of disordered mineral bone metabolism. These markers are serum calcium, phosphate, and intact PTH. The current KDIGO guidelines recommend treatment based on the serial trends of these biochemical markers rather than single measurement [1].

Table 9.3 Guidelines on management of chronic kidney disease-mineral and bone disorder

		Recommended levels		
Group	Year	Corrected calcium (mg/dL)	Phosphate (mg/dL)	Intact PTH (pg/mL)
UKRA	2002	8.8–10.4	<5.6	<4 times upper normal range
K/DOQI	2003	8.4–9.5	2.5–5.5	150–300
CSN	2006	Within normal range	Within normal range	100–500
JSDT	2008	8.4–10.0	3.5–6.0	60–240
KDIGO	2009	Within normal range	Within normal range	2–9 times upper limit of normal
KDIGO	2017	Near normal range	Near normal range	2–9 times upper limit of normal

PTH parathyroid hormone, *UKRA* UK Renal Association, *K/DOQI* Kidney Disease Outcomes Quality Initiative, *CSN* Canadian Society of Nephrology, *JSDT* Japanese Society for Dialysis Therapy, *KDIGO* Kidney Disease Improving Global Outcomes

Several guidelines were published regarding management of CKD-MBD. There have been controversies on the target ranges of calcium, phosphate, and intact PTH levels (Table 9.3) and these guidelines have been largely opinion-based as the values derived mainly from observational studies. Recently, a randomized controlled trial (RCT) [19] examined the effect of strict vs. conventional phosphate lowering therapy in hemodialysis patients on vascular calcification and the trial showed the benefit of strict phosphate control, especially among elderly (65–79 years old). The result of the study might change the guideline in the near future.

Phosphate Restriction

Foods high in phosphate contents are shown in Table 9.4. In addition, phosphate is the main component of many preservatives and additive salts in processed foods. The intestinal absorptive rate of inorganic phosphate as in additives and beverages is between 80 and 100%, while that of plant-based phosphate such as nuts is between 20 and 40% [20].

The KDIGO guidelines recommend, "In patients with CKD G3a-G5D, we suggest limiting dietary phosphate intake in the treatment of hyperphosphatemia alone or in combination with other treatments". It is reasonable to consider phosphate source (e.g., animal, vegetable, additives) in making dietary recommendations.

Table 9.4 Dietary phosphate contents

P-to protein ratio	Foods	Serving	Phosphate contents (mg)
5–10 mg/g	Beef	3 oz	~160
	Chicken breast	1/2 breast	199
	Yellow fin tuna	3 oz	208
	Pork	3 oz	~185
10–15 mg/g	Soy protein isolate	1 oz	217
	Tofu, raw	1/2 cup	239
	Soy beans	1/2 cup	211
15–25 mg/g	Edamame	1/2 cup	284
	Mozzarella cheese	1 oz	149
	Cheddar cheese	1 oz	145
>25 mg/g	Biscuit	1 biscuit	562
	Milk (low fat)	1 cup	229

P phosphate
Modified from Clin J Am Soc Nephrol 2010; 5: 519–530

Phosphate Binders

Commonly used phosphate binders are shown in Table 9.5 [21]. Phosphate binders bind phosphate contained in food in the intestine and inhibit absorption of phosphate. They should be taken just before or after meals to be effective.

One RCT showed that prescription of phosphate binders to non-dialysis dependent CKD patients with normal serum phosphate levels resulted in modest decline in serum phosphate levels, prevented the increase in intact PTH, but promoted the progression of vascular calcification [22]. In this study, all phosphate binders were analyzed collectively, and the data suggested that the observed increase in coronary

Table 9.5 Commonly used phosphate binders

Agents	Estimated PO_4^- binding capacity	Advantage	Disadvantage
Calcium carbonate	~39 mg/g	Inexpensive	Hypercalcemia Concern for worsening vascular calcification
Calcium acetate	~45 mg/g	Less Ca absorption than Ca carbonate	Hypercalcemia Concern for worsening vascular calcification
Sevelamer HCl	~21 mg/g	Reduction in serum lipid level	Constipation Acidosis
Sevelamer carbonate	~21 mg/g	Reduction in serum lipid level No acidosis	Constipation
Bixalomer	Not known	Less GI side effects than sevelamer	Less lipid lowering effects than sevelamer
Lanthanum carbonate	90–135 mg/g	High binding capacity	GI side effects
Succroferric oxyhydroxide	260 mg/g	Improvement in iron parameters and anemia	GI side effects
Ferric citrate	46 mg/g	Improvement in iron parameters and anemia	GI side effects

GI gastrointestinal

artery calcification (CAC) was mainly driven by Ca-containing binders, and that those treated with Ca-free binders had no advantage over placebo in terms of progression of CAC. The implications of phosphate binders among non-dialysis dependent CKD with normal serum phosphate levels remain uncertain. As a result, the KDIGO guidelines recommend, "In patients with CKD G3a-G5D, we suggest lowering *elevated phosphate levels* toward the normal range". At present, phosphate binders are indicated for those with hyperphosphatemia.

There has been substantial debate on whether Ca-containing phosphate binders worsen vascular calcification compared with Ca-free phosphate binders. Multiple RCTs have been performed as summarized in Table 9.6. Several studies showed that progression of CAC might be worse with Ca-containing phosphate binders compared with sevelamer, though this could in part be attributed to the cholesterol-lowering effects of sevelamer. Comparison of the effect of Ca-containing binders and lanthanum carbonate on vascular calcification is inconsistent. At present, it is prudent to avoid use of high-dose Ca-containing phosphate binders and avoid oversuppression of PTH levels as adynamic bone is associated with vascular calcification.

There has been only one RCT comparing different Ca-free phosphate binders (Table 9.7). Although there was no significant difference in primary outcomes between sucrofferic oxyhydroxide and lanthanum carbonate groups, the study suggested a potential benefit of sucrofferic oxyhydroxide in younger patients.

Native Vitamin D

The KDIGO guidelines [33] recommend the measurement of 25-hydroxyvitamin D (25(OH) D) in patients with secondary hyperparathyroidism and renal transplant recipients. Moreover, it is reasonable to measure its level in patients with osteomalacia or rickets. If vitamin D is insufficient (less than 30 ng/mL or 50 nmol/L), it is recommended to administer cholecalciferol or ergocalciferol daily since intermittent pulsatile administration of native vitamin D is reported to increase bone fracture rate possibly by enhancing bone resorption independently of PTH suppression. Cholecalciferol is more useful than ergocalciferol in suppressing PTH since the biological availability of the former is higher than that of the latter. In the US, a modified-release (MR) oral formulation of calcifediol (calcidiol) was approved for the treatment of secondary hyperparathyroidism in patients with CKD G3 and G4. Since this agent does not increase endogenous FGF23 levels unlike calcifediol bolus therapy, endogenous $1,25(OH)_2D$ levels do not decrease but rather increase with this agent through the replenishment of vitamin D.

Active Vitamin D

Available formula for active vitamin D is shown in Table 9.8. It is intuitive to use active vitamin D for treatment of secondary hyperparathyroidism, as one of the inciting events in the development of secondary hyperparathyroidism is deficiency of $1,25(OH)_2D$. However, in patients with CKD G3a-G5 not on dialysis, the optimal PTH level is not known. Two RCTs examined the effects of active vitamin D on left ventricular hypertrophy (LVH) in non-dialysis dependent CKD G3a-G5 with elevated PTH levels and LVH [34, 35]. Both studies demonstrated that active vitamin D had no impact on change in LVH compared with placebo. As a result, the KDIGO guidelines state that the use of calcitriol and vitamin D analogs for patients with CKD G3a-G5 is not routinely recommended and should be reserved for those with CKD G4-G5 with severe and progressive hyperparathyroidism.

For those with CKD G5D, multiple observational studies demonstrated association between use of active vitamin D and lower mortality [36–38] or lower incidence of bone fracture [39, 40]. Although J-DAVID study failed to demonstrate cardiovascular benefit of active vitamin D for those with CKD G5D without secondary hyperparathyroidism, this does not preclude the use of vitamin D for treatment of secondary hyperparathyroidism for those with CKD G5D [41].

Table 9.6 Comparison of effects of Ca-containing and Ca-free phosphate binders on clinical outcomes

Study and country	Inclusion criteria	Exclusion criteria	Ca-containing binder	Ca-free binder	Results
Treat to Goal [23] (US, Germany, Austria)	Age > 19 Maintenance HD	PTH > 1000 pg/mL Ca > 11.5 mg/dL	Ca acetate or Ca carbonate (n = 101)	Sevelamer (n = 99)	Significantly less progression of CAC & aortic calcification in sevelamer Significant reduction in LDL-C in sevelamer group
Block 2005 [24] (US)	Incident HD Age > 18	CABG Af, AF Prior kidney transplantation	Any Ca-containing binders (n = 55)	Sevelamer (n = 54)	Significantly less progression of CAC in sevelamer group Significant reduction in LDL-C in sevelamer group
Asmus 2005 [25] (Austria)	Age > 18 Maintenance HD	Serious GI diseases Vasculitis Poorly controlled DM or HTN	Ca carbonate (n = 41)	Sevelamer (n = 31)	Significantly less progression of CAC or aortic calcification in sevelamer group
CARE-2 [26] (US)	Age > 18 HD > 3 months	PTH > 1000 pg/mL Ca > 11.5 mg/dL	Ca acetate + atorvastatin (n = 103)	Sevelamer ± atorvastatin (n = 100)	No significant difference in CAC progression No significant difference in LDL-C
Kakuta 2011 [27] (Japan)	Age > 20 Maintenance HD	Serious GI disorders, active malignancy, vasculitis	Ca carbonate (n = 92)	Sevelamer (n = 91)	Significantly less progression of CAC in sevelamer group Significant reduction in LDL-C in sevelamer group
INDEPENDENT-HD [28] (Italy)	Age > 18 Incident HD	Age > 75 Arrythmia	Any Ca containing binders (n = 234)	Sevelamer (n = 232)	Significantly lower all-cause and CV mortality in sevelamer group
Ohtake 2013 [29] (Japan)	Age > 20 Maintenance HD Hyper-phosphatemia	PTX	Ca carbonate (n = 26)	Lanthanum (n = 26)	Progression of CAC in Ca carbonate group Regression of CAC in lanthanum group No significant difference in LDL-C
LANDMARK [30] (Japan)	Maintenance HD PTH < 240 pg/mL Age > 65 Post-menopause DM		Ca carbonate (n = 1063)	Lanthanum carbonate (n = 1072)	No significant difference in CAC progression No significant difference in CV events or all-cause mortality
INDEPENDENT-CKD [31, 32] (Italy)	Age ≥ 18 CKD stage 3–4	CHF, CAD Nephrotic syndrome Liver diseases	Ca carbonate (n = 105)	Sevelamer (n = 107)	Significantly lower all-cause mortality in sevelamer group

Ca calcium, *HD* hemodialysis, *PTH* parathyroid hormone, *CAC* coronary artery calcification, *LDL-C* low density lipoprotein cholesterol, *CABG* coronary artery bypass grafting, *Af* atrial fibrillation, *AF* atrial flutter, *GI* gastrointestinal, *DM* diabetes mellitus, *HTN* hypertension, *CV* cardiovascular, *PTX* parathyroidectomy, *CKD* chronic kidney disease, *CHF* congestive heart failure, *CAD* coronary artery disease

Table 9.7 Comparison of effects of calcium-free phosphate binders

Study and country	Inclusion criteria	Exclusion criteria	Intervention	Control	Results
EPISODE [19] (Japan)	Maintenance HD Hyperphosphatemia CACS > 30 Age 20–80	PTH > 800 pg/mL Ferritin >300 ng/L TSAT>50% PTX	Sucrofferic oxyhydroxide (SO) (n = 53)	Lanthanum carbonate (n = 62)	No significant difference in CAC progression Significantly less CAC progression among young patients (age 20–64) in SO group

HD hemodialysis, *CACS* coronary artery calcification score, *PTH* parathyroid hormone, *TSAT* transferrin saturation, *PTX* parathyroidectomy, *CAC* coronary artery calcification

Table 9.8 Active vitamin D

	Oral or intravenous	Comments
Calcitriol	Oral and intravenous	
Paricalcitol	Intravenous	Less hypercalcemic than calcitriol or alfacalcidol
Alfacalcidol	Oral and intravenous	
Maxacalcitol	Intravenous	Less hypercalcemic than calcitriol or alfacalcidol
Falecalcitriol	Oral	Higher potency than calcitriol
Doxercalciferol	Oral and intravenous	Synthetic vitamin D2 analog that undergoes metabolic activation in vivo to form 1α,25-dihydroxyvitamin D_2 (1α,25-$(OH)_2D_2$)

Although there is a concern for worsening vascular calcification by the use of high-dose active vitamin D in animal studies, in clinical trials described in Table 9.6, the use of active vitamin D is more common and higher dose of vitamin D is used in Ca-free phosphate binders group. Despite more frequent use of active vitamin D in Ca-free phosphate binders group, the progression of vascular calcification was generally less in Ca-free phosphate binders group. There is no direct comparison of active vitamin D and calcimimetics. The choice of treatment for secondary hyperparathyroidism depends on biochemical abnormalities (e.g. Vitamin D for those with hypocalcemia and calcimimetics for those who develop hypercalcemia by active vitamin D treatment). The KDIGO guidelines state, "In patients with CKD G5D requiring PTH-lowering therapy, we suggest calcimimetics, calcitriol, or vitamin D analogs, or a combination of calcimimetics with calcitriol or vitamin D analogs" [1].

Calcimimetics

Calcimimetics are allosteric modulators of CaSR, activate CaSR, and thereby reduce the PTH levels. Calcimimetics also reduce serum calcium and phosphate levels partly through the suppression of bone turnover. Currently available calcimimetics are shown in Table 9.9.

Calcimimetics reduce the levels of serum calcium and phosphate, therefore, it raises the possibility that calcimimetics might prevent vascular calcification. In the ADVANCE study, cinacalcet with low-dose active vitamin D was compared with active vitamin D in terms of progression of vascular calcification. The study showed that progression of vascular calcification was less in the cinacalcet group [42].

The EVOLVE trial showed no significant difference in primary composite end point (all-cause mortality, hospitalization for angina, congestive heart failure, and peripheral vascular events) between cinacalcet and placebo group [43]. However, analyses adjusted for imbalances in baseline characteristics or sensitivity analyses accounting for patient nonadherence to the assigned drug demonstrated significant reduction in the primary composite endpoint and bone fracture in cinacalcet group [44]. It should be noted that cinacalcet reduced the incidence of congestive heart failure significantly even in the prespecified intention-to-treat analysis. Reduction of

Table 9.9 Calcimimetics

	Administration	Half-life	Comments
Cinacalcet	Oral	30–40 h	Metabolized by CYP3A4 and to lesser extent by CYP1A2, inhibits CYP2D6
Evocalcet	Oral	15–20 h	Less CYP2D6 inhibition and improved bioavailability compared with cinacalcet
Etelcalcetide	Intravenous at the end of dialysis	>7 days	Less gastrointestinal side effects No interaction with CYPs

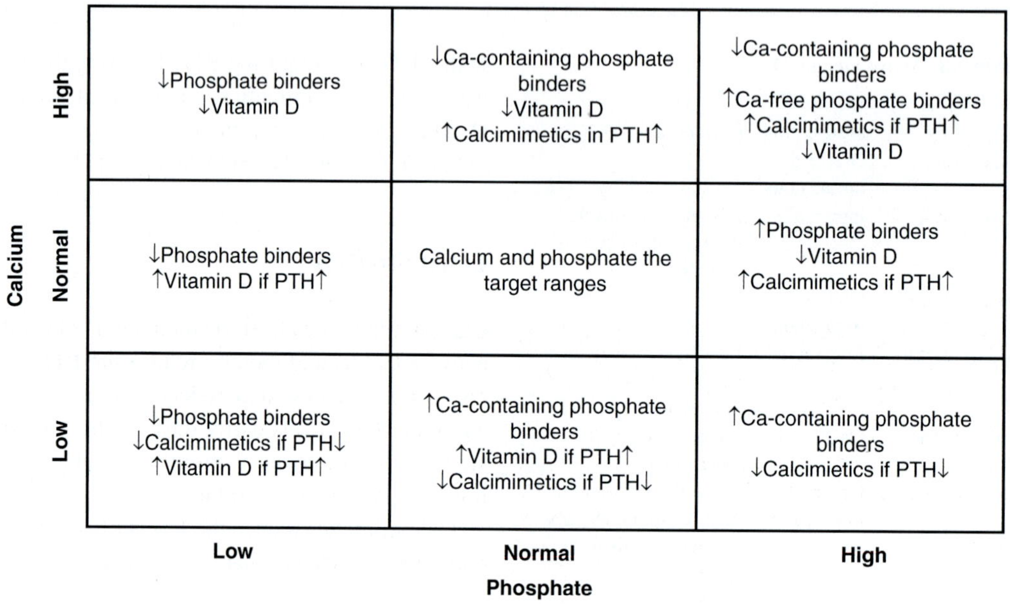

Fig. 9.5 Suggested management strategies for various combinations of biochemical abnormalities of chronic kidney disease-mineral and bone disorder. *PTH* parathyroid hormone

plasma FGF23 by cinacalcet might explain this phenomenon. Moreover, cinacalcet was shown to reduce the incidence of parathyroidectomy.

The difficulty in managing CKD-MBD is that when you treat one biochemical abnormality by a certain intervention, it can affect multiple other biochemical parameters of CKD-MBD. Suggested management for various combinations of biochemical abnormalities are shown in Fig. 9.5.

Parathyroidectomy

Parathyroidectomy remains a valid treatment option for those with severe secondary hyperparathyroidism and when other PTH-lowering therapies fail. An observational study demonstrated the association between parathyroidectomy (compared with medical therapy) and lower mortality [45], however it is extremely difficult to eliminate the indication bias inherent to observational studies. Hypocalcemia after parathyroidectomy should be treated appropriately, otherwise it might raise the early-term mortality post-parathyroidectomy.

Magnesium

Magnesium is an inhibitor of vascular calcification in vitro [46]. Among haemodialysis patients, hypomagnesemia was shown to be associated with higher all-cause and cardiovascular mortality [13]. Moreover, among hemodialysis patients with high serum magnesium levels, hyperphosphatemia was not associated with higher cardiovascular mortality [47], suggesting that magnesium is protective from detrimental effects of hyperphosphatemia on cardiovascular system. In an RCT, progression of vascular calcification was less among magnesium oxide group compared with usual care group among those with CKD stage 3–4 [48]. Despite the emerging evidence base for the use of magnesium, it is not yet in routine use nor featured in the KDIGO guidelines.

Calcium

KDIGO recommend maintaining calcium within the normal range and avoiding hypercalcemia. Mild, asymptomatic hypocalcaemia can be tolerated, particularly in the context of calcimimetic treatment, in order to avoid inappropriate calcium loading.

Future Perspectives

Tenapanor is an inhibitor of gastrointestinal sodium/hydrogen exchanger 3, and inhibits paracellular phosphate absorption from the intestine. The mechanisms of action of this drug is distinct from phosphate binders [49]. It was applied for Food and Drug Administration approval as a treatment of hyperphosphatemia in CKD.

Magnesium seems to be an important player in CKD-MBD and whether magnesium becomes a part of routine treatment for CKD-MBD remains to be seen. In Japan, dialysate with higher magnesium concentration has been approved. The benefits of this dialysate on clinically relevant outcomes are awaited.

Recently, hypoxia-inducible-factor prolyl hydroxylase (HIF-PH) inhibitors became available for treatments of anemia of chronic kidney disease. These medications upregulate HIF-1α, which is involved in the pathogenesis of vascular calcification. There is a concern that the use of HIF-PH inhibitors might aggravate vascular calcification. Further research is warranted to elucidate whether treatment for CKD-MBD should be changed due to the use of HIF-PH inhibitors.

Practice Points

CKD-MBD:

- is a nearly universal complication of progressive CKD, can lead to bone pain or increased incidence of fractures
- is associated with vascular calcification, and high cardiovascular morbidity and mortality
- management is targeted at preventing the adverse consequences of secondary hyperparathyroidism and hyperphosphatemia
- management with dietary phosphate restriction, phosphate binders before or after meals, active vitamin D supplementation, and calcimimetics—provides the mainstay of initial treatment

Conclusions

The clinical case demonstrates the typical biochemical abnormalities in patients advanced CKD-MBD. The hypercalcemia resulting from treatment highlights the difficulties in management and how treatment of one biochemical abnormality can lead to abnormalities in another. The treatment of hyperparathyroidism with active vitamin D resulted in significant hypercalcemia with only partial suppression of PTH. The clinical benefits of correcting the biochemical abnormalities are yet to be fully established. Hence, the treatment of the biochemical abnormalities should be guided by trends in all biochemical abnormalities evaluated together, avoiding abnormalities in one while correcting the other.

Questions

1. 80 years old women on hemodialysis is seen in the dialysis unit. Three months ago, her serum calcium was 8.8 mg/dL, albumin was 3.6 g/dL, phosphate was 3.4 mg/dL, and intact PTH level was 758 pg/mL on calcium carbonate. Calcitoriol was started and now her calcium is 11.0 mg/dL, albumin is 3.5 g/dL, phosphate is 6.5 mg/dL, and intact PTH is 565 pg/mL.

   Which of the following actions are inappropriate?

   A. Add cinacalcet
   B. Stop calcium carbonate
   C. Increase calcitriol
   D. Start lanthanum carbonate
   E. Start sevelamer

   Answer: C

   Although PTH is still elevated, increasing calcitriol would further aggravate hypercalcemia and hyperphosphatemia. Switching calcium-containing binders to calcium-free binders and adding calcimimetics are appropriate actions.

2. Which of the following is positively associated with vascular calcification?

   A. Fetuin-A
   B. Matrix G1a protein
   C. phosphate
   D. Magnesium
   E. Iron

   Answer C

   Fetuin-A, MGP, magnesium are inhibitors of calcification. Iron-containing phosphate binders decrease FGF23.

3. Which of the following is not associated with higher mortality?

   A. Hypercalcemia
   B. Hypophosphatemia
   C. Hypomagnesemia
   D. Hyperphosphatemia
   E. Low FGF23 levels

   Answer E

   Higher FGF23 levels are associated with higher mortality.

4. Which of the following statement is wrong about FGF 23?

   A. Suppress synthesis of 1,25 dihydroxy vitamin D3
   B. Increase phosphate excretion from the kidney
   C. Klotho is necessary for FGF 23 to bind to FGF receptors.
   D. FGF23 is secreted from kidneys.
   E. Higher FGF 23 levels are associated with left ventricular hypertrophy.

   Answer D

   FGF23 is secreted from osteocytes.

5. Which of the following is not high in phosphate content?

   A. Cheese
   B. Sausage
   C. Tofu
   D. Egg white
   E. Biscuit

   Answer D

   Although egg yolk is high in phosphate content, egg white is low in phosphate content.

6. Which of the following is not correct regarding phosphate binders?

   A. The use of phosphate binders in non-dialysis dependent CKD patients with normal serum phosphate levels results in less progression of vascular calcification.
   B. Several randomized controlled trials demonstrated that calcium-containing phosphate binders results in more rapid progression of vascular calcification compared with calcium-free phosphate binders.
   C. Sevelamer HCl causes metabolic acidosis.
   D. Lanthanum carbonate causes gastrointestinal side effects.
   E. Calcium acetate is less hypercalcemic than calcium carbonate.

   Answer A

   The use of phosphate binders for those with normophosphatemia is of unproven benefit.

7. Which of the following is correct regarding calcimimetics?

   A. Calcimimetics inhibit calcium-sensing receptors.
   B. Calcimimetics suppress PTH, causes adynamic bone, and vascular calcification.

C. Calcimimetics are allosteric modulator of calcium-sensing receptors.
D. Evocalcet inhibits CYP2D6 more than cinacalcet.
E. Etelcalcetide has shortest half-life among currently available calcimimetics.

Answer C

Calcimimetics activate calcium-sensing receptor. Calcium-sensing receptor are present on vascular smooth muscle cells and calcimimetics inhibits calcium uptake by vascular smooth muscle cells. Cinacalcet was shown to suppress the progression of vascular calcification in a clinical trial. Cinacalcet inhibits CYP2D6. Etelcalcetide has longest half-life among currently available calcimimetics.

8. Which of the following is correct regarding magnesium?
A. Hypermagnesemia is associated with higher mortality among hemodialysis patients.
B. Among those with hypomagnesemia, hyperphosphatemia was not associated with higher mortality.
C. Magnesium is an inhibitor of vascular calcification.
D. Magnesium oxide was shown to prevent vascular calcification among hemodialysis patients.
E. Hypomagnesemia was not associated with cardiovascular mortality.

Answer C

Hypomagnesemia was associated with higher all-cause and cardiovascular mortality. Among those with high serum magnesium levels, hyperphosphatemia was not associated with higher mortality, suggesting that magnesium is protective from detrimental effects of hyperphosphatemia. Magnesium oxide was shown to prevent vascular calcification among non-dialysis dependent CKD patients. The safety of magnesium oxide is unproven in hemodialysis patients.

9. Which of the following is correct?
A. The use of active vitamin D is not recommended in hemodialysis patients due to concern for vascular calcification.
B. Clacitriol is less hypercalcemic than paricalcitriol.
C. Several observations studies showed that the use of active vitamin D is associated with lower mortality among hemodialysis patients. However, J-DAVID trial demonstrated that alfacalcidol did not demonstrate beneficial cardiovascular effects among those with severe secondary hyperparathyroidism.
D. The use of active vitamin D among non-dialysis dependent CKD patients were shown to improve left ventricular hypertrophy.
E. In observational studies, the use of active vitamin D was associated with lower incidence of fracture among hemodialysis patients.

Answer E

J-DAVID showed that active vitamin D has no effect on cardiovascular outcomes among those with PTH < 180 pg/mL. Although there is a theoretical concern for vascular calcification by vitamin D use, in clinical trials, more use of vitamin D with calcium-free phosphate binders are associated with less progression of vascular calcification. In PRIMO and OPERA trials, active vitamin D has no benefit on LVH among non-dialysis dependent CKD patients.

10. Which of the following is correct?
A. Osteomalacia is the most common bone histology found among peritoneal dialysis patients.
B. ADVANCE trial demonstrated that cinacalcet causes progression of vascular calcification.
C. In EVOLVE trial, there was no significant difference in primary composite end point (all-cause mortality, hospitalization for angina, congestive heart failure, and peripheral vascular events) between cinacalcet and placebo group in main analyses, but there was substantial use of commercial cinacalcet in placebo group.
D. J-DAVID study included patients on hemodialysis with PTH > 180 pg/mL.

E. Hypoxia-inducible factor prolyl hydroxylase inhibitor may potentially inhibit vascular calcification.

Answer C

Adynamic bone disease is the most common bone histology found among peritoneal dialysis patients. In ADVANCE trial, cinacalcet was shown to ameliorate progression of vascular calcification. J-DAVID study included patients on hemodialysis with PTH < 180 pg/mL. HIF-PH inhibitor might promote vascular calcification.

Test your learning and check your understanding of this book's contents: use the "Springer Nature Flashcards" app to access questions using https://sn.pub/cz9Cok. To use the app, please follow the instructions in Chap. 1.

References

1. Kidney Disease Improving Global Outcomes (KDIGO) CKD-MBD Update Working Group. KDIGO 2017 Clinical practice guideline update for the diagnosis, evaluation, prevention, and treatment of chronic kidney disease-mineral and bone disorder (CKD-MBD). Kidney Int Suppl. 2017;7:1–59.
2. Block GA, Klassen PS, Lazarus JM, et al. Mineral metabolism, mortality, and morbidity in maintenance hemodialysis. J Am Soc Nephrol. 2004;15:2208–18.
3. Noordzij M, Korevarr JC, Boeschoten EW, et al. The Kidney Disease Outcomes Quality Initiative (K/DOQI) guideline for bone metabolism and disease in CKD: association with mortality in dialysis patients. Am J Kidney Dis. 2005;46:925–32.
4. Kalantar-Zadeh K, Kuwae N, Regidor DL, et al. Survival predictability of time-varying indicators of bone disease in maintenance hemodialysis patients. Kidney Int. 2006;70:771–80.
5. Melamed ML, Eustace JA, Plantinga L, et al. Changes in serum calcium, phosphate, and PTH and the risk of death in incident dialysis patients: a longitudinal study. Kidney Int. 2006;70:351–7.
6. Tentori F, Blayney MJ, Albert JM, et al. Mortality risk for dialysis patients with different levels of serum calcium, phosphorus, and PTH: the Dialysis Outcomes and Practice Patterns Study (DOPPS). Am J Kidney Dis. 2008;52:519–30.
7. Block GA, Zaun D, Smits G, et al. Cinacalcet hydrochloride treatment significantly improves all-cause and cardiovascular survival in a large cohort of hemodialysis patients. Kidney Int. 2010;78:578–89.
8. Floege J, Kim J, Ireland E, et al. Serum iPTH, calcium and phosphate, and the risk of mortality in a European haemodialysis population. Nephrol Dial Transplant. 2011;26:1948–55.
9. Taniguchi M, Fukagawa M, Fujii M, et al. Serum phosphate and calcium should be primarily and consistently controlled in prevalent hemodialysis patients. Ther Apher Dial. 2013;17:221–8.
10. Soohoo M, Feng M, Obi Y, et al. Changes in markers of mineral and bone disorders and mortality in incident hemodialysis patients. Am J Nephrol. 2016;43:85–96.
11. Waziri B, Musenge E, Duarte R, et al. Associations of plasma fibroblast growth factor 23 and other markers of chronic kidney disease-mineral and bone disorder with all-cause mortality in South African patients on maintenance dialysis: a 3-year prospective cohort study. PLoS One. 2019;14:e0216656.
12. Marthi A, Donovan K, Haynes R, et al. Fibroblast growth factor-23 and risks of cardiovascular and non-cardiovascular diseases: a meta-analysis. J Am Soc Nephrol. 2018;29:2015–27.
13. Sakaguchi Y, Fujii N, Shoji T, et al. Hypomagnesemia is a significant predictor of cardiovascular and non-cardiovascular mortality in patients undergoing hemodialysis. Kidney Int. 2014;85:174–81.
14. Blayney MJ, Pisoni RL, Bragg-Gresham JL, et al. High alkaline phosphatase levels in hemodialysis patients are associated with higher risk of hospitalization and death. Kidney Int. 2008;74:655–63.
15. Hutchison AJ, Whitehouse RW, Boulton HF, et al. Correlation of bone histology with parathyroid hormone, vitamin D3, and radiology in end-stage renal disease. Kidney Int. 1993;44:1071–7.
16. Sherrard DJ, Hercz G, Pei Y, et al. The spectrum of bone disease in end-stage renal failure-an evolving disorder. Kidney Int. 1993;43:436–42.
17. Shroff R, Long DA, Shanahan C. Mechanistic insights into vascular calcification in CKD. J Am Soc Nephrol. 2013;24:179–89.
18. London GM, Marty C, Marchais SJ, et al. Arterial calcifications and bone histomorphometry in end-stage renal disease. J Am Soc Nephrol. 2004;15:1943–51.
19. Isaka Y, Hamano T, Fujii H, et al. Optimal phosphate control related to coronary artery calcification in dialysis patients. J Am Soc Nephrol. 2021;32:723–35.
20. Hwang E, Choi BS, Oh KH, et al. Management of chronic kidney disease-mineral and bone disorder: Korean working group recommendations. Kidney Res Clin Pract. 2015;34:4–12.
21. Gutekunst L. An update on phosphate binders: a dietitian's perspective. J Ren Nutr. 2016;26:209–18.
22. Block GA, Wheeler DC, Persky MS, et al. Effects of phosphate binders in moderate CKD. J Am Soc Nephrol. 2012;23:1407–15.
23. Chertow GM, Burke SK, Raggi P, et al. Sevelamer attenuates the progression of coronary and aortic calcification in hemodialysis patients. Kidney Int. 2002;62:245–52.
24. Block GA, Spiegel DM, Ehrlich J, et al. Effects of sevelamer and calcium on coronary artery calcification in patients new to hemodialysis. Kidney Int. 2005;68:1815–24.

25. Asmus HG, Braun J, Krause R, et al. Two year comparison of sevelamer and calcium carbonate effects on cardiovascular calcification and bone density. Nephrol Dial Transplant. 2005;20:1653–61.
26. Qunibi W, Moustafa M, Muenz LR, et al. A 1-year randomized trial of calcium acetate versus sevelamer on progression of coronary artery calcification in hemodialysis patients with comparable lipid control: the Calcium Acetate Renagel Evaluation-2 (CARE-2) Study. Am J Kidney Dis. 2008;51:952–65.
27. Kakuta T, Tanaka R, Hyodo T, et al. Effect of sevelamer and calcium-based phosphate binders on coronary artery calcification and accumulation of circulating advanced glycation end products in hemodialysis patients. Am J Kidney Dis. 2011;57: 422–31.
28. Di Lorio B, Molony D, Bell C, et al. Sevelamer versus calcium carbonate in incident hemodialysis patients: results of an open-label 24-month randomized clinical trial. Am J Kidney Dis. 2013;62:771–8.
29. Ohtake T, Kobayashi S, Oka M, et al. Lanthanum carbonate delays progression of coronary artery calcification compared with calcium-based phosphate binders in patients on hemodialysis: a pilot study. J Cardiovasc Pharmacol Ther. 2013;18:439–46.
30. Ogata H et al. Presented at American Society of Nephrology, Kidney Week 2019.
31. Ogata H, Fukagawa M, Hirakata H, et al. Effect of treating hyperphosphatemia with lanthanum carbonate vs calcium carbonate on cardiovascular events in patients with chronic kidney disease undergoing hemodialysis: the LANDMARK randomized clinical trial. JAMA. 2021;325:1946–54.
32. Di Lorio B, Bellas A, Russo D, et al. Mortality in kidney disease patients treated with phosphate binders: a randomized study. Clin J Am Soc Nephrol. 2012;7:487–93.
33. National Kidney Foundation. K/DOQI clinical practice guidelines for bone metabolism and disease in chronic kidney disease. Am J Kidney Dis. 2004;42(suppl 3):S1–S202.
34. Thadani R, Appelbaum E, Pritchett Y, et al. Vitamin D therapy and cardiac structure and function in patients with chronic kidney disease: the PRIMO randomized controlled trial. JAMA. 2012;307:674–84.
35. Wang AY, Fang F, Chan J, et al. Effect of paricalcitol on left ventricular mass and function in CKD-the OPERA trial. J Am Soc Nephrol. 2014;25:175–86.
36. Naves-Diaz M, Alvarez-Hernandez D, Passlick-Deetjen J, et al. Oral active vitamin D is associated with improved survival in hemodialysis patients. Kidney Int. 2008;74:1070–8.
37. Teng M, Wolf M, Ofsthun MN, et al. Activated injectable vitamin D and hemodialysis survival: a historical cohort study. J Am Soc Nephrol. 2005;16:1115–25.
38. Shoji T, Shinohara K, Kimoto E, et al. Lower risk for cardiovascular mortality in oral 1 alpha-hydroxy vitamin D3 users in a haemodialysis population. Nephrol Dial Transplant. 2004;19:179–84.
39. Dey V, Farrah TE, Traynor JP, et al. Symptomatic fracture risk in the renal replacement therapy population. Nephrol Dial Transplant. 2017;32:1211–6.
40. Matias PJ, Laranjinha I, Azevedo A, et al. Bone fracture risk factors in prevalent hemodialysis patients. J Bone Miner Metab. 2020;38:205–12.
41. J-DAVID Investigators. Effect of oral alfacalcidol on clinical outcomes in patients without secondary hyperparathyroidism receiving maintenance hemodialysis. The J-DAVID randomized clinical trial. JAMA. 2018;320:2325–34.
42. Raggi P, Chertow GM, Torres PU, et al. The ADANCE study: a randomized study to evaluate the effects of cinacalcet plus low-dose vitamin D on vascular calcification in patients on hemodialysis. Nephrol Dial Transplant. 2011;26:1327–39.
43. Chertow GM, Block GA, Correa-Rotter R, et al. Effect of cinacalcet on cardiovascular disease in patients undergoing dialysis. N Engl J Med. 2012;367:2482–94.
44. Kubo Y, Sterling LR, Parfrey PS, et al. Assessing the treatment effect in a randomized controlled trial with extensive non-adherence: the EVOLVE trial. Pharm Stat. 2015;14:368.
45. Komaba H, Taniguchi M, Wada A, et al. Parathyroidectomy and survival among Japanese hemodialysis patients with secondary hyperparathyroidism. Kidney Int. 2015;88:350–9.
46. Diaz-Tocados JM, Peralta-Ramirez A, Rodriguez-Ortiz ME, et al. Dietary magnesium supplementation prevents and reverses vascular and soft tissue calcifications in uremic rats. Kidney Int. 2017;92:1084–99.
47. Sakaguchi Y, Fujii N, Shoji T, et al. Magnesium modifies the cardiovascular mortality risk associated with hyperphosphatemia in patients undergoing hemodialysis: a cohort study. PLoS One. 2014;9:e116273.
48. Sakaguchi Y, Hamano T, Obi Y, et al. A randomized trial of magnesium oxide and oral carbon adsorbent for coronary artery calcification in predialysis CKD. J Am Soc Nephrol. 2019;30:1073–85.
49. Block GA, Rosenbaum DP, Yam A, et al. Efficacy and safety of tenapanor in patients with hyperphosphatemia receiving maintenance hemodialysis: a randomized phase 3 trial. J Am Soc Nephrol. 2019;30:641–52.

10 Diabetes and CKD

Daniel Murphy, Vivekanand Jha, and Debasish Banerjee

Clinical Scenario

A 60 year old woman presents to your nephrology clinic. She has a history of hypertension and type 2 diabetes mellitus for 12 years, which are managed with amlodipine 5 mg OD and metformin 1 g OD. Her blood pressure was 146/80 mmHg, and her body mass index is 32 kg/m^2. She recently presented to her general practitioner with new-onset ankle oedema. Her albumin–creatinine ratio (ACR) was measured as 254.9 mg/g (25.5 mg/mmol) on an early-morning urine sample, her HbA1c was recently measured as 79 mmol/mol (9.4%), and creatinine 110 mmol/L (1.24 mg/dL). She was referred to you for clinical advice regarding (1) changes to her diabetic therapy and (2) initiation of renal-protective therapy.

D. Murphy
St. George's University Hospitals Foundation Trust, London, UK
e-mail: danajmurphy@doctors.org.uk

V. Jha
The George Institute for Global Health, New Delhi, India
e-mail: vjha@georgeinstitute.org.in

D. Banerjee (✉)
St. George's University Hospitals Foundation Trust, London, UK

St. George's University of London, London, UK
e-mail: dbanerje@sgul.ac.uk

Introduction

The global prevalence of diabetes mellitus is increasing. This is largely driven by an increase in prevalence of type 2 diabetes (T2DM) and its associated metabolic syndrome. However, there has also been a smaller but significant increase in prevalence of type 1 diabetes (T1DM).

T1DM is caused by autoimmune destruction of insulin-producing pancreatic β cells. T2DM is associated with peripheral insulin resistance and a decrease in insulin secretion. Solid-organ transplantation may result in post-transplant diabetes mellitus (PTDM). This is associated with immunosuppression, as well as risk factors for T2DM.

Hyperglycaemia caused by diabetes leads to microvascular changes within the kidney, which cause diabetic kidney disease (DKD/diabetic nephropathy). Combined DM and CKD (DM-CKD) increases cardiovascular morbidity and mortality, and is a leading cause of death in CKD patients.

The aim of the clinician in treating DKD should be primary prevention of progression to end-stage kidney disease (ESKD). This may be achieved via control of blood glucose, blood pressure, and body weight, and avoidance of nephrotoxic medications.

D. Banerjee et al. (eds.), *Management of Kidney Diseases*,
https://doi.org/10.1007/978-3-031-09131-5_10

Epidemiology and Causes

Prevalence of diabetes is closely linked to obesity and varies from <6% to >12% according to obesity rates. The prevalence of diabetes varies by country and by region (Table 10.1). Estimates are limited by diagnosis rates: more than half of individuals suffering from diabetes in Sub-Saharan Africa are thought to be undiagnosed. 537 million adults are living with diabetes and it is predicted that global rates of diabetes will increase to 734 million by 2045 [1].

T1DM accounts for <15% of the global diabetes burden and is more common amongst Northern European genetic groups. T2DM accounts for around 85% of cases, and its incidence is higher amongst South Asian, Afro-Caribbean, Polynesian, Middle Eastern, and Native American groups.

Studies in the USA have shown that 40% of individuals with CKD G1–5 have concurrent DM; there is little data available for other parts of the world. The incidence of PTDM following kidney transplantation has been estimated at 10–30%, with rates increasing with time after transplantation. It is important to note, however, that the prevalence of non-diabetic kidney disease (NDKD) in patients with diabetes ranges from 33 to 73% according to centres with high rates of kidney biopsy (although the predominance of atypical presentations amongst individuals who receive a kidney biopsy may lead to an over-estimation of this figure). Hence, a diabetic individual presenting with signs of kidney disease should not be assumed to have isolated DKD.

T1DM and T2DM cause DKD in the same way. Hyperglycaemia leads to a greater prevalence of glycated compounds in the blood and a greater oxidative stress load, leading to microvascular damage, increased glomerular capillary pressures, podocyte damage, and endothelial dysfunction. Other causes of kidney disease, such as hypertension or other primary kidney diseases, will accelerate the disease course.

Table 10.1 Prevalence of diabetes in adults aged 20–79 years according to IDF region (from IDF Diabetes Atlas 9th Edition)

IDF region	Prevalence of diabetes (age 20–79 years)
Africa	3.9%
Europe	8.9%
Middle East and North Africa	12.9%
North America and Caribbean	13.3%
South and Central America	9.4%
South-East Asia	8.8%
Western Pacific	9.6%

Table 10.2 Definitions of diabetes and associated conditions [2]

Condition	Definition
Diabetes mellitus	WHO criteria—any of: 1. Symptoms of hypoglycaemia **AND** raised venous glucose levels detected once (fasting glucose ≥ 7.0 mmol/L **OR** random glucose ≥ 11.1 mmol/L) 2. Raised plasma glucose (fasting ≥ 7.0 mmol/L **OR** random ≥ 11.1 mmol/L) on two occasions **OR** OGTT 2-hour glucose ≥ 11.1 mmol/L. 3. HbA1c ≥ 48.0 mmol/mol (i.e. ≥ 6.5%).
Impaired glucose tolerance	WHO criteria— • OGTT 2-hour plasma glucose 7.8–11.0 mmol/L • Fasting plasma glucose may be normal or elevated
Impaired fasting glucose	WHO criteria— • Fasting plasma glucose 6.1–6.9 mmol/L
Metabolic syndrome	International Diabetes Foundation (IDF) criteria— • Central obesity (BMI > 30 kg/m^2 or increased waist circumference according to ethnic groups • Plus two of: 1. Plasma triglyceride level > 1.7 mmol/L **OR** on treatment for hypertriglyceridaemia 2. Plasma HDL cholesterol < 1.0 mmol/L **OR** on treatment for cholesterol derangement 3. Systolic BP ≥ 130 mmHg or diastolic BP ≥ 85 mmHg, **OR** on treatment for hypertension 4. Fasting plasma glucose ≥ 5.6 mmol/L **OR** previously-diagnosed T2DM
Post-transplant diabetes mellitus	Diagnosis can be made by the above WHO criteria once a patient is stable on post-transplant immunosuppression.

BP blood pressure, *BMI* body mass index, *OGTT* oral glucose tolerance test, *T2DM* type 2 diabetes mellitus, *WHO* World Health Organization

Clinical Presentation

The vast majority of T1DM cases present during adolescence, but presentation may be at any age. Classic presenting features of T1DM are polyuria, polydipsia, and weight loss despite adequate nutritional intake, classically described as "starvation in the face of plenty". Patients may present for the first time in an acute setting with diabetic ketoacidosis.

Individuals with T2DM generally present >30 years of age, but it is increasingly being diagnosed in adolescents. It is associated with progression from a stage of impaired glucose tolerance and/or metabolic syndrome to frank diabetes (Table 10.2).

A patient may present completely asymptomatic or with severe complications of diabetes, depending on the length and severity of their disease. Complications to look for in the history and examination include diabetic retinopathy, neuropathy, signs or symptoms of macrovascular disease (e.g. stroke, myocardial infarction).

Diabetic nephropathy presents with a typically picture of proteinuric kidney disease. Oedema is a classical symptom and may be generalised, in gravity-dependent areas such as the ankles, or in areas of low tissue resistance such as the periorbital tissue. Patients may also present with frothy or bubbling urine, recurrent or resistant urinary tract infections, and other signs or symptoms of hypoalbuminaemia. The peak of presentation is in individuals who have had diabetes for 10–20 years.

Investigations

Standard investigations for diabetes include plasma glucose, capillary glucose, and HbA1c levels. These should be interpreted in the context of a patient's most recent glucose load (see Table 10.2). Blood glucose levels are particularly useful diagnostically following an oral glucose tolerance test, and acutely for diagnosing hypoglycaemia. Blood ketone levels should be taken to diagnose potential diabetic ketoacidosis when suspected.

The HbA1c is a useful marker of chronic hyperglycaemic load. HbA1c measurements are unreliable in certain patient groups: CKD G4–5; dialysis patients; those with any disease affecting lifespan of red blood cells (e.g. iron-deficiency anaemia, thalassaemia, recent acute blood loss, spherocytosis); those receiving HIV antiretroviral therapy; chronic liver disease; hypertriglyceridaemia. See annex Table 10.3 below for conversion of HbA1c units.

Renal biopsy is the only true way to confirm whether CKD in a diabetic patient is a direct result of the diabetes disease process. However in practice, a long history (>10 years) of diabetes, proteinuria, and signs of retinopathy are typically taken as sufficient criteria for a diagnosis of DKD. Any individual with a shorter history of diabetes should undergo a full CKD assessment looking for other causes. If a patient exhibits proteinuria with a diabetic history of <5 years, with no signs of microvascular complications, and the suspicion of systemic disease, a diagnostic kidney biopsy is recommended. Individuals with T2DM often have multiple renal pathologies, including primary glomerulopathies, age-related nephropathy, or damage from previous acute kidney injury. CKD in these individuals may therefore be a combination of DKD and NDKD.

Table 10.3 HbA1c values are variously reported worldwide as a measurement in mmol/mol or as a percentage; these units can be approximately compared using the table below

% HbA1c	HbA1c mmol/mol	% HbA1c	HbA1c mmol/mol	% HbA1c	HbA1c mmol/mol	% HbA1c	HbA1c mmol/mol
4	20	6.1	43	8.2	66	10.3	89
4.1	21	6.2	44	8.3	67	10.4	90
4.2	22	6.3	45	8.4	68	10.5	91
4.3	23	6.4	46	8.5	69	10.6	92
4.4	25	6.5	48	8.6	70	10.7	93
4.5	26	6.6	49	8.7	72	10.8	95
4.6	27	6.7	50	8.8	73	10.9	96
4.7	28	6.8	51	8.9	74	11	97
4.8	29	6.9	52	9	75	11.1	98
4.9	30	7	53	9.1	76	11.2	99
5	31	7.1	54	9.2	77	11.3	100
5.1	32	7.2	55	9.3	78	11.4	101
5.2	33	7.3	56	9.4	79	11.5	102
5.3	34	7.4	57	9.5	80	11.6	103
5.4	36	7.5	58	9.6	81	11.7	104
5.5	37	7.6	60	9.7	83	11.8	105
5.6	38	7.7	61	9.8	84	11.9	107
5.7	39	7.8	62	9.9	85	12	108
5.8	40	7.9	63	10	86		
5.9	41	8	64	10.1	87		
6	42	8.1	65	10.2	88		

Table 10.4 Differential diagnosis for diabetic nephropathy [2]

Primary nephropathy	Systemic conditions causing secondary nephropathy
Minimal change disease	Systemic lupus erythametosus
Membranous nephropathy	Rheumatoid disease
Focal segmental glomerusclerosis	Myeloma
Menbranoproliferative glomerulonephritis	Amyloidosis
	Infection (e.g. HIV, hepatitis B/C, malaria)

Differential Diagnosis

Differential diagnoses of diabetic kidney disease will include any proteinuric kidney disease. This may be primary renal disease (e.g. minimal change disease, membranous nephropathy) or renal disease secondary to a systemic condition (Table 10.4).

Diabetes Management

Glycaemic Control

Glycaemic control is the cornerstone of primary prevention in DM-CKD patients, and is monitored using HbA1c. Patients should be encouraged to meet an individual HbA1c "target" (see Table 10.5), which should be as close to normal as sustainably possible in order to reduce the risk of kidney disease progression. HbA1c targets <53 mmol/mol (7.0%) have been shown to reduce risk of progressive micro- and macroalbuminaemia compared with targets ≥53 mmol/mol (7.0%).

Routine monitoring of HbA1c should be twice-yearly. The frequency of monitoring can be increased in patients whose glycaemic targets are not met, or for patients undergoing changes in antihyperglycaemic therapy.

Self-monitoring of blood glucose levels is less useful as a marker of long-term glycaemic control. However, it is useful practise to prevent hypoglycaemic episodes. Patients taking anti-hyperglycaemic therapies that predispose to hypoglycaemia should be trained to self-monitor.

Due to the limitations of HbA1c, direct glucose monitoring is useful more accurate indicator of sugar control. The glucose can be monitored by repeated finger prick testing using a traditional glucometer or newer flash glucose monitoring system like "free style libra" device. Glycated albumin and serum fructosamine have been prosed as better indicators but further studies are needed for establishing the role of these two agents.

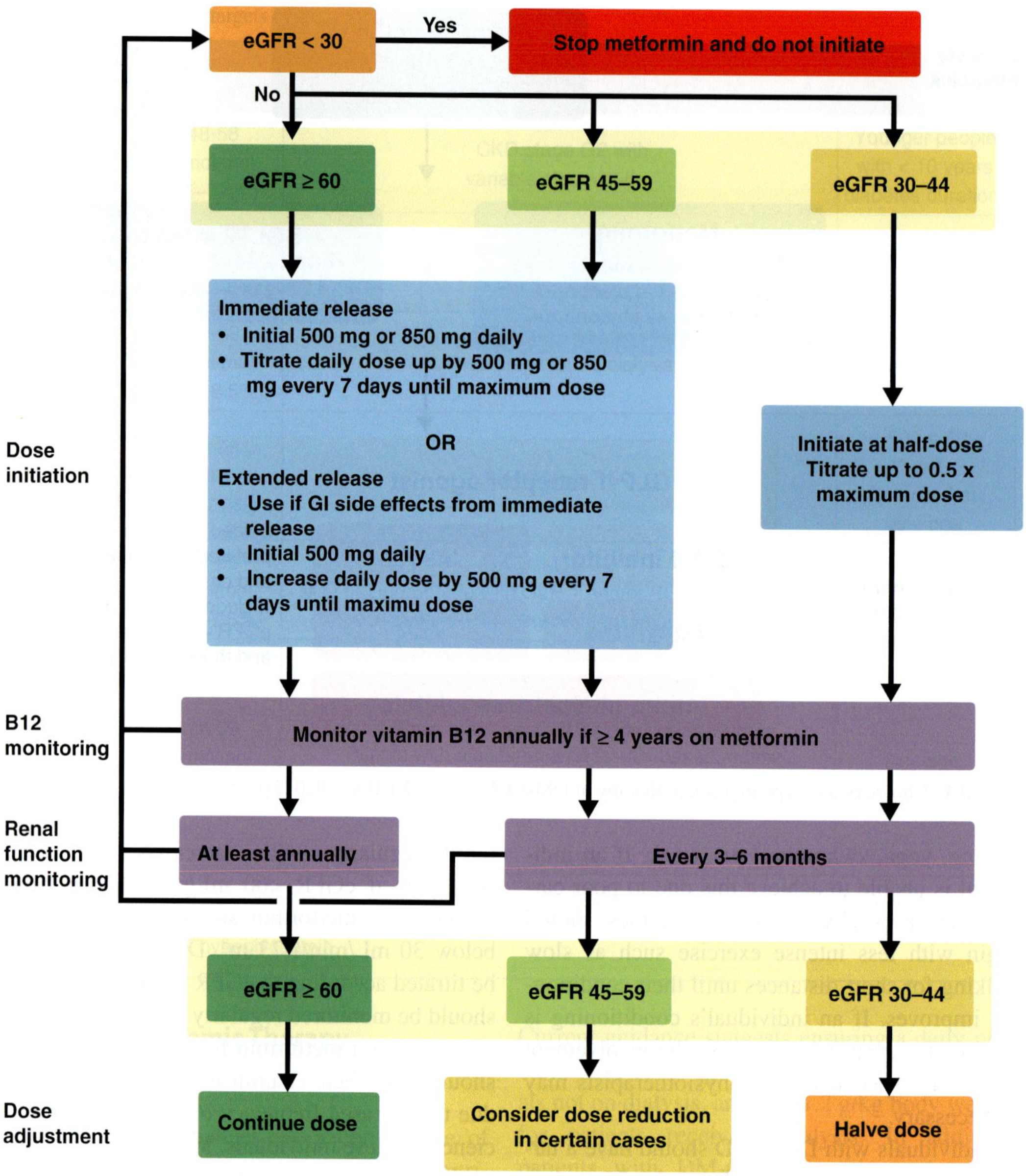

Fig. 10.2 Metformin dosing algorithm in CKD. (From KDIGO 2020 [2])

reabsorption. Inhibition of the co-transporter prevents glucose reabsorption and promotes urinary glucose excretion. There is strong evidence that SGLT-2 inhibitors prevent progression of DKD down to an eGFR of 30 mL/min/1.73 m^2. It is not recommended to initiate SGLT2 therapy in patients with eGFR <30 mL/min/1.73 m^2, however it may be continued if already begun.[2, 3]

There is strong evidence that SGLT-2 inhibitors reduce risk of (1) major adverse cardiac events, and (2) development and progression of heart failure in patients with T2DM with CVD risk factors.

Individuals taking SGLT2 inhibitors should be monitored for hypotension (especially if they also take diuretic medication) due to the drugs' diuretic effects, and for hypoglycaemia during at-risk peri-

Table 10.6 Choice of second-line antihyperglycaemic medication by clinical situation (adapted KDIGO 2020 [2])

Clinical situation	Suitable medications	Less-suitable medications
eGFR < 15 mL/min/1.73 m^2 or concurrent with dialysis	• DPP4 inhibitors • Thiazolidinedione • Insulin	• Thiazolidinedione
Co-morbid heart failure	• SGLT2i • GLP1 receptor agonists	• Thiazolidinedione
High-risk for atherosclerotic cardiovascular disease	• SGLT2i • GLP1 receptor agonists	
Higher-potency for glucose-lowering	• GLP1 receptor agonists • Insulin	• DPP4 inhibitors • Thiazolidinedione • -glucosidase inhibitors
To aid weight loss	• GLP1 receptor agonists	• Sulfonylureas • Insulin • Thiazolidinedione
To avoid hypoglycaemia	• GLP1 receptor agonists • DPP4 inhibitors • Thiazolidinedione • -glucosidase inhibitors	• Sulfonylureas • Insulin
To avoid injections	• DPP4 inhibitors • Thiazolidinedione • Sulfonylureas • -glucosidase inhibitors • Oral GLP1 receptor agonists	• GLP1 receptor agonists • Insulin
Low cost	• Sulfonylureas • Thiazolidinedione • -glucosidase inhibitors	• GLP1 receptor agonists • DPP4 inhibitors • Insulin

ods (e.g. illness, fasting, surgery) or if they take other medications which increase risk of hypoglycaemia (e.g. insulin, sulfonylureas). There has been evidence of increased risk of diabetic ketoacidosis associated with SGLT-2 inhibitor use.[2, 3]

Augmenting Therapy

There are several therapeutic options for individuals who do not meet their glycaemic targets on metformin and SGLT2 inhibitors (see Table 10.6). An overview of agents and doses to be utilised in different stages of CKD is provided in Table 10.7. Contraindications for glycaemic control medications are listed in Table 10.8.

GLP-1 Receptor Antagonists

GLP-1 receptor agonists (GLP-1 RAs) are often the first-choice second-line therapy. They are associated with gastrointestinal side-effects, so should be started at a low dose and titrated upwards as tolerated by the patient (see Table 10.9). Combination therapy using GLP-1 RAs with DPP4 inhibitors (DPP4i) is not recommended. These medications both act via the incretin pathway to stimulate insulin and inhibit glucagon release. Randomised controlled trials have not demonstrated benefits of combined therapy for glycaemic control [3].

GLP-1 RAs confer an increased risk of hypoglycaemia if used in conjunction with some other

Table 10.7 Antihyperglycaemic dosing in DKD. CrCl measured by Cockroft–Gault equation [2]

Class of drug	Drug	Stage 1 eGFR > 90	Stage 2 eGFR 60–90	Stage 3a eGFR 45–59	Stage 3b eGFR 30–44	Stage 4 eGFR 15–29	Stage 5 eGFR < 15
Biguanide	Metformin				Reduce dose to 500 mg BD	Potential role for 500 mg BD	
Sulphonylurea	Gliclazide	Monitor capillary blood glucose (CBG	CBG	CBG	Dose reduction advised, CBG	Off-licence. High risk of hypoglycaemia	
Meglitinide	Repaglinide	CBG	CBG	CBG	CBG	Dose reduction advised, CBG	
DPP-4 inhibitor	Sitagliptin			eGFR < 50 reduce dose to 50 mg	Reduce dose to 50 mg	Reduce dose to 25 mg	
	Saxagliptin			EGFR < 50 reduce dose to 2.5 mg	Reduce dose to 2.5 mg		
	Linagliptin						
Thiazolidinedione	Pioglitazone						
GLP-1 agonist	Lixisenatide			Caution if CrCl < 50 mL/min			
	Exenatide			Caution if CrCl < 50 mL/min	Conservative dosing advised		
	Exenatide MR			Stop if CrCl < 50 mL/min			
	Liraglutide					Dose reduction may be required	Off-licence
	Dulaglutide						
SGLT-2 inhibitor	Dapagliflozin			Reduce dose to 5 mg			
	Canagliflozin			Reduce dose to 100 mg			
	Empagliflozin			Reduce dose to 10 mg			
Insulin					Dose reduction may be required	Dose reduction required	

Table 10.8 Contraindications to antihyperglycaemic medications in diabetic complications [2]

Condition	Drug	Note
Biliary conditions	GLP-1 analogues	• Relative contraindication in active gallbladder disease
Bladder conditions	SGLT-2 inhibitors	• Relative contraindication of all medications in this class for individuals with (1) documented neuropathic bladder or (2) recurrent urinary tract infections • Relative contraindication / caution to initiation in individuals with (1) active bladder cancer or (2) unexplained and uninvestigated haematuria
	Pioglitazone	• Relative contraindication / caution to initiation in individuals with (1) active bladder cancer or (2) unexplained and uninvestigated haematuria.
Bone conditions	Pioglitazone	• Absolute contraindication in individuals with previous osteoporotic fractures • Relative contraindication in osteoporosis with neuropathy
	SGLT-2 inhibitors	• Relative contraindication in those with established osteoporotic fractures
Foot conditions	SGLT-2 inhibitors	• Absolute contraindication in diabetic foot disease with vascular complications or sepsis
Heart failure	Pioglitazone	• Absolute contraindication in established heart failure and when at-risk individuals have raised BNP
	Saxagliptin	• Absolute contraindication in established heart failure
Pancreatic conditions	GLP-1 analogues	• Absolute contraindication with previously-documented pancreatitis • Relative contraindication in those at risk of pancreatitis or with: (1) raised triglycerides; (2) on steroid therapy; (3) documented alcoholism; or (4) using other drugs associated with pancreatitis
Retinopathy	Pioglitazone	• Absolute contraindication in diabetic maculopathy
	Semaglutide	• Relative contraindication in marked hyperglycaemia (≥ 10.5%) who have diabetic retinopathy requiring ophthalmology input

Table 10.9 Dosing of GLP-1 RAs in CKD[2]

GLP-1 RA	Dose	CKD adjustment
Dulaglutide	0.75 mg and 1.5 mg once weekly	No dosage adjustment Use if eGFR >15 mL/min/1.73 m^2
Exenatide	10 μg twice daily	Use with CrCl >30 mL/min/1.73 m^2
Exenatide extended release	2 mg once weekly	Use with CrCl >30 mL/min/1.73 m^2
Liraglutide	0.6 mg, 1.2 mg, and 1.8 mg once daily	No dosage adjustments Limited data for severe CKD
Lixisenatide	10 μg and 20 μg once daily	No dosage adjustments Limited data for severe CKD
Semaglutide (injection)	0.5 mg and 1 mg once weekly	No dosage adjustments Limited data for severe CKD
Semaglutide (oral)	3 mg, 7 mg, or 14 mg once daily	No dosage adjustments Limited data for severe CKD

medications (e.g. sulfonylureas, insulin). If combined therapy using these agents is to be considered, patients should be started on low doses which should be titrated carefully and with close monitoring of blood glucose levels.

DPP-4 Inhibitors

Dipeptidyl peptidase-4 (DPP-4) inhibitors selectively bind to the DPP-4 enzyme and prevent breakdown of glucagon-like peptide 1 (GLP-1), leading to a moderate reduction in blood glucose levels. An advantage of their use lies in their favourable safety and tolerability profiles, as well as a low risk of hypoglycaemia. Because of this profile, DPP-4 inhibitors may be used in all CKD stages, including individuals on maintenance haemodialysis. Doses should be adjusted according to the stage of CKD.

Several trials have been conducted to understand the safety of DPP-4 inhibitor use in individuals with CVD. Large trials investigating sitagliptin (TECOS trial) and linagliptin (CARMELINA trial) have found no evidence of increased CVD risk in patients taking these medications compared with placebo. Retrospective analysis has also emphasised the safety of vildagliptin.

The EXAMINE trial found a mild increase in prevalence of heart failure in patients taking alogliptin, but no increase in hospital admissions due to heart failure. In contrast, the SAVOR-TIMI trial found that individuals taking saxagliptin with pre-existing risk factors for CVD were more likely to develop and be hospitalised for heart failure in the first 12 months after starting the medication. There was no increase in incidence of major adverse cardiac events.

Sulfonylureas

Sulfonylurea compounds act to decrease blood glucose levels in two principal ways. They act to close ATP-sensitive potassium channels in pancreatic β-cells, triggering insulin release via an intracellular cascade. Also, they stimulate activity of glucose receptors in muscle and adipose cells, increasing sensitivity to insulin. The sulfonylureas gliclazide and glipizide are metabolised by the liver into inactive metabolites, and are recommended as adjunct therapy for T2DM while eGFR >30 mL/min/1.73 m^2. Gliclazide has a more favourable cardiovascular safety profile. Dose reduction is advised with decreasing eGFR (see Table 10.6) and sulfonylureas are not licensed in individuals with eGFR <30 mL/min/1.73 m^2.

Other sulfonylureas such as glibenclamide, glimepiride, and tolbutamide are not recommended in CKD.

Key side effects of sulfonylureas are weight gain and hypoglycaemia. The risk of hypoglycaemia is greater in CKD than non-CKD individuals due to renal excretion of active and non-active metabolites. Due to this increased risk, co-prescribing with insulin is not recommended, and sulfonylureas should not be used in T1DM. Regular blood glucose monitoring should be considered.

Thiazolidinediones

Pioglitazone is licensed for use in T2DM. It acts to lower peripheral insulin resistance. Its advantages include a low risk of hypoglycaemia and its hepatic metabolism, due to which dose reduction is not required as renal function declines. Hence pioglitazone can be considered for individuals with any stage of CKD.

Disadvantages of pioglitazone include its association with increased fluid retention, and it should be avoided in heart failure and macular oedema and used with caution in known fluid-retainers. Pioglitazone is also associated with an increased risk of bladder cancer; it should be avoided in known cases and also in anyone with haematuria until cancer is excluded.

Meglitinides

Meglitinides (nateglinide, repaglinide) are compounds which act to increase insulin secretion in a similar manner to sulfonylureas. They act rapidly, and have the advantage of dosage flexibility with the concurrent drawback of multiple administrations. Repaglinide may be considered as monotherapy, while both compounds may be considered as adjuncts to metformin.

Both nateglinide and repaglinide have the potential to cause hypoglycaemia and doses should be reduced as eGFR declines. While repaglinide is secreted by the biliary system, nateglinide is excreted renally and hence carries increased risk of hypoglycaemia in CKD. For this reason, repaglinide is recommended at lower eGFRs. Both are partially metabolised by the cytochrome P450 system.

Post-transplant Diabetes Mellitus

In the immediate post-transplant period, patients should be actively monitored for hyperglycaemia while in hospital. Mild hyperglycaemia (<14 mmol/L) may be treated using oral therapy, while higher blood glucose levels should be managed via intravenous or subcutaneous insulin therapy. Following discharge and entering the maintenance phase of immunosuppressive therapy, post-transplant patients should be screened for PTDM yearly.

Recommended first-line therapy for patients with PTDM and eGFR ≥30 mL/min/1.73 m^2 is metformin (see Fig. 10.3). This may be augmented using sulfonylureas, DPP4 inhibitors, GLP1 RAs, and pioglitazone. SGLT2 inhibitors should be used with caution due to the risk of urinary tract infection in the immunocompromised patient. There is a low threshold for utilising insulin therapy in post-transplant patients if they display poor glucose management or symptomatic hyperglycaemia.

Management of Hypertension in DKD *[for details see* Chap. 8*]*

Type 1 Diabetes

Hypertension (HTN) is the greatest risk factor for the progression of CKD. Blood pressure targets for individuals with T1DM vary between 130/80 and 140/90 mmHg. Stricter targets are recom-

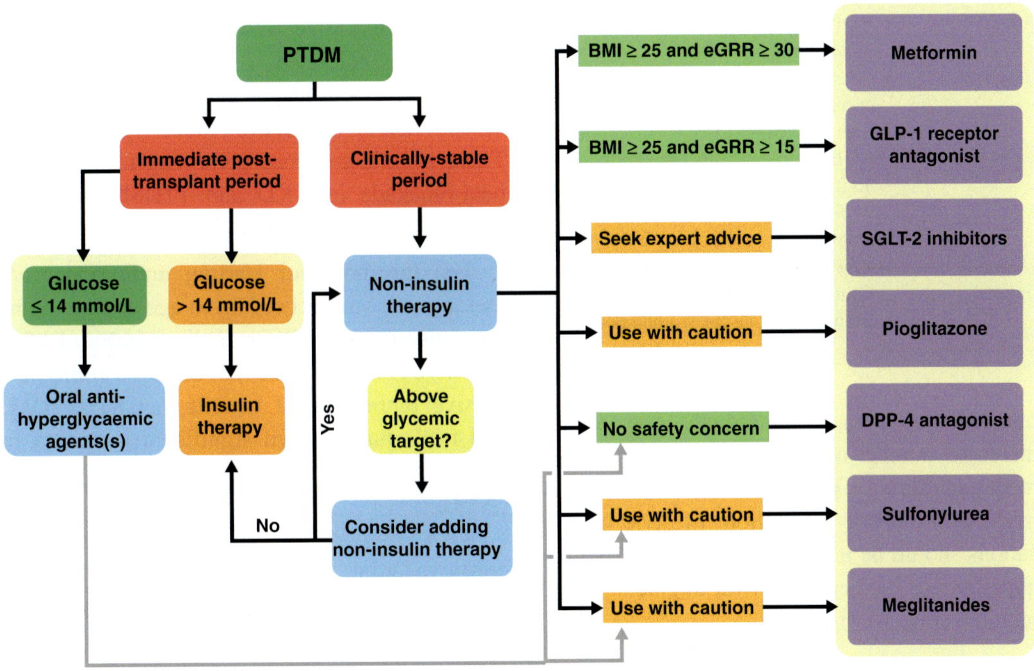

Fig. 10.3 Flow chart for glycaemic management of post-transplant diabetes mellitus (PTDM) [4]. On an individual basis, it should be considered whether immunosuppression represents a significant risk factor for the development of PTDM. It is currently recommended that the primary factor in deciding on immunosuppressive therapy should be to reduce the risk of allograft rejection, and there is no evidence to suggest that alterations to a patient's immunosuppressive regime will help to manage PTDM. However, in a patient starting immunosuppressive therapy for the first time who is at high risk of PTDM, a regime with lower risk of hyperglycaemia should be considered

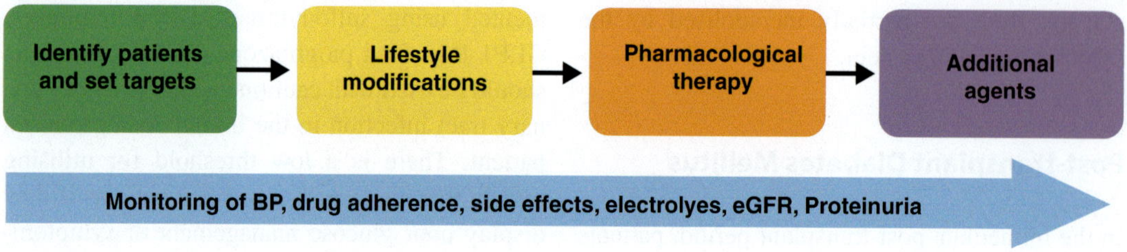

Fig. 10.4 Management principles of HTN in CKD. *BP* blood pressure, *eGFR* estimated glomerular filtration rate [from ABCD-RA guidelines on management of hypertension in diabetes 2021 [5])

Table 10.10 Lifestyle factors and hypertension in T1DM[2]

Lifestyle factor	Impact
Salt intake	• KDIGO guidance recommends a sodium intake of <90 mmol/day (equal to 2 g/day, or 5 g of sodium chloride) • Salt intake has greater impact on HTN risk in combined DM-CKD due to reduced renal excretion
Weight and Body Mass Index	• Abdominal obesity and high BMI are associated with HTN in T1DM • KDIGO guidance recommends maintaining a BMI of 20–25 kg/m^2
Exercise	• There is evidence that regular exercise reduces BP in individuals with T1DM • KGIDO guidance recommends 30 min of exercise five times per week, with intensity determined by tolerance
Alcohol intake	• KDIGO guidance recommends limiting intake to two standard drinks for men and one for women per day

mended in younger individuals due to the increased number of years at risk. The management paradigm for HTN in T1DM similar to that in the non-diabetic population: lifestyle modifications should be trialled first, followed by antihypertensive medications, with augmentation if required (Fig. 10.4).

Lifestyle factors and their impact on HTN in T1DM are outlined in Table 10.10.

Antihypertensive Medication in T1DM

ACE inhibitors are the recommended first-line antihypertensive therapy in individuals with CKD and T1DM. If ACEi medication cannot be tolerated, ARBs should be considered as a second-line alternative. Doses should be titrated upwards as tolerated. Spironolactone may be considered as a third-line agent, but carries a significant risk of severe, even fatal, hyperkalaemia. There is little evidence pertaining to the use of beta-blockade in CKD and T1DM, but some studies suggest a benefit to HTN.

The threshold for starting antihypertensive therapy will vary according to age and albumin-creatinine ratio (ACR), as outlined in Fig. 10.5.

There is no evidence that multiple antihypertensive therapy is of benefit in CKD-T1DM, and trials have shown significant increases in risk of hyperkalaemia and acute kidney injury (AKI).

RAASi medication is associated with fetal cardiovascular, neurological, and renal abnormalities in pregnancy, and so should be

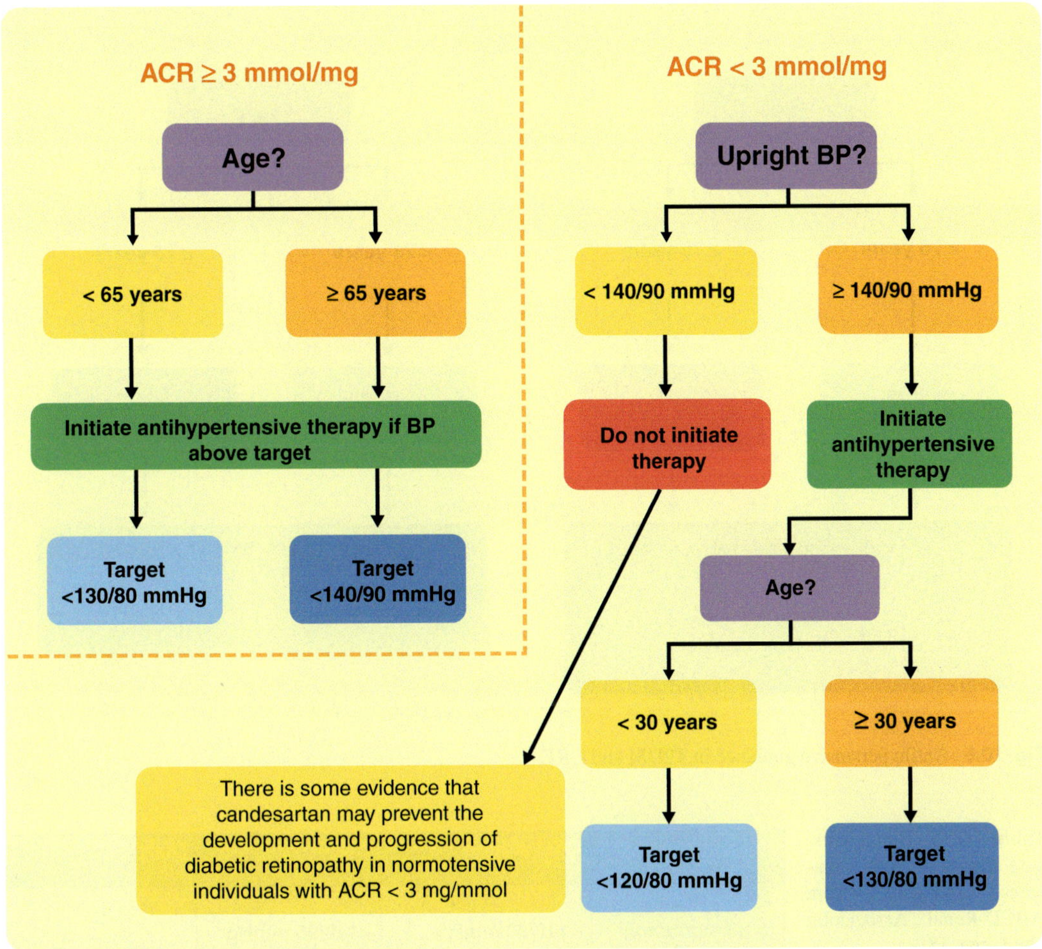

Fig. 10.5 Guidance on initiating antihypertensive therapy in patients with CKD and T1DM (adapted from ABCD-RA guidance [5])

stopped if an individual is pregnant or planning a pregnancy.

Type 2 Diabetes Mellitus

Lifestyle modifications recommended for HTN in T2DM are similar to those in T1DM (Table 10.8). Also similarly to T1DM, thresholds initiation of pharmacological therapy will depend on age and ACR (Fig. 10.6). In individuals with an ACR < 3 mg/mmol, there is no specific recommended first-line agent in DKD. If ACR ≥ 3 mg/mmol, ACEi medication—or ARB if ACEi is not tolerated—is recommended. The target blood pressures are summarised below (Table 10.11):

Practice Points

- Insulin resistance increases in early CKD, which worsens sugar control
- Insulin clearance decreases in advanced CKD, eGFR <20 mL/min/1.73 m^2, which makes patients prone to hypoglycaemia
- Blood sugars may fall during haemodialysis due to relatively low dialysate glucose and removal of glucagon
- Fluid assessment and therapy in DKA can be challenging in patients on dialysis
- Blood glucose rises during peritoneal dialysis and reduces ultrafiltration
- HbA1c may not be accurate due to altered red cell life span

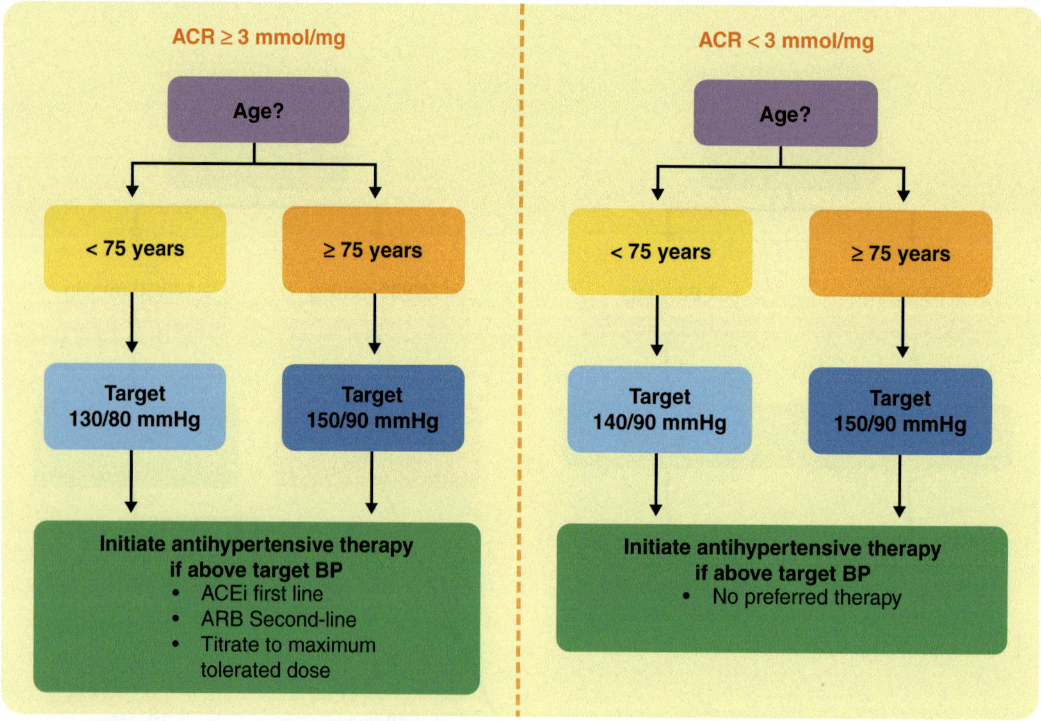

Fig. 10.6 Antihypertensive guidance in T2DM and CKD

Table 10.11 Blood pressure targets in Type 2 diabetes (adapted from ABCD-Renal Association Guidelines [5])

	CKD stages 1-3	CKD stages 4-5	Dialysis
ACR<3mg/g (> 30 mg/mmol)	<140/90 mmHg	<140/90 mmHg	<140/90 mmHg
ACR>3 mg/g (> 30 mg/mmol)	<130/80 mmHg	<130/80 mmHg	

Conclusions

Returning to our case from the beginning of the chapter—the patient has a long history of diabetes mellitus, with a likely clinical diagnosis of diabetic kidney disease. She has comorbidities, including clinical obesity, suboptimal blood sugar control, and suboptimal blood pressure control. The next steps in her management in clinic should include:

- Establishing her diagnosis from her long history of diabetes mellitus, and the presence of diabetic retinopathy
- Starting an ACE inhibitor (or angiotensin receptor blocker)
- Achieve more optimal blood pressure control <130/80 mmHg
- Achieve better blood sugar control (target HbA1c 52–58 mmol/mol for Type 2 DM associated CKD stage G3A3)
- Start dapagliflozin
- Monitor creatinine, potassium, Blood pressure and HBA1c

Questions

1. A 57 year-old woman presents to nephrology clinic for the first time following referral for new-onset significant proteinuria. She has a three-year history of type 2 diabetes which has so far been controlled with lifestyle modifications. Her BMI is 31.1 kg/m^2 and she has no other past medical history. Her eGFR is measured as 54 mL/min/1.73 m^2. Which of the following is the most appropriate initial action?
   A. As her diabetes has been controlled by lifestyle modifications, it would be appropriate to monitor her HbA1c and initiate pharmacological therapy when it is >48 mmol/mol (6.5%)
   B. Initiate metformin and an SGLT2 inhibitor as first-line therapy as eGFR ≥30 mL/min/1.73 m^2 and discharge to her general practitioner for follow-up.
   C. Refer to ophthalmology to examine for diabetic retinopathy before starting glucose lowering therapy.
   D. Perform a full CKD assessment looking for causes other than diabetes.
   E. Initiate GLP1 receptor agonist therapy as this is recommended to aid weight loss.

   Answer: D

   A. **Incorrect**: in all cases of diabetic kidney disease with an eGFR of ≥30 mL/min/1.73 m^2, dual therapy with metformin and an SGLT2 inhibitor is recommended.
   B. **Incorrect**: as this patient has a short (<10 years) history of diabetes and no known evidence of microvascular complications, she should undergo a full assessment for other potential causes of CKD.
   C. **Incorrect**: While she should have annual screening for retinopathy this would not necessarily need to precedent the commencement of glucose-lowering treatment.
   D. **Correct**: as mentioned, due to the short and relatively well-controlled history of diabetes, this patient requires a full workup to look for other causes.
   E. **Incorrect**: in all cases of diabetic kidney disease with an eGFR of ≥30 mL/min/1.73 m^2, recommended first-line therapy is with metformin and an SGLT2 inhibitor.

2. A 65 year-old man with G3aA2 CKD and T2DM presents to clinic for a follow-up appointment. He currently takes metformin with dapagliflozin and pioglitazone for diabetes management. He was recently had an echocardiogram demonstrating a left ventricular ejection fraction of 35–40% and blood tests returning a NT-proBNP level of 1200 pg/mL. Which of the below is the most appropriate immediate action?
   A. Stop metformin with dapaglifozin as dapaglifozin is contraindicated in G3a CKD.
   B. Stop pioglitazone and replace with another agent as thiazolidinedione medications are contraindicated in heart failure.
   C. Continue current antihyperglycaemic therapy and add an ACE inhibitor .
   D. Continue current antihyperglycaemic therapy and add a beta blocker.
   E. Continue current antihyperglycaemic therapy and add a GLP-1 agonist to control hyperglycaemia and reduce cardiovascular risk.

   Answer: B

   A. **Incorrect**: dapaglifozin is contraindicated in G3b CKD. In G3a CKD dose reduction is advised.
   B. **Correct**: thiazolidinediones can cause fluid retention and are contraindicated in heart failure.
   C. **Incorrect**: while an ACE inhibitor may be beneficial for patients with combined CKD-HF, current antihyperglycaemic therapy should not be continued as thiazolidinediones are contraindicated in heart failure.
   D. **Incorrect**: as above, thiazolidinediones are contraindicated in heart failure.

E. **Incorrect**: as above, thiazolidinediones are contraindicated in heart failure.

3. A 59 year-old woman with G2 CKD and recently-diagnosed T2DM is referred to the renal clinic by her GP for advice on medications. She has started metformin immediate-release 500 mg with dapagliflozin 10 mg daily for glycaemic control, and her latest HbA1c is 65 mmol/mol (8.1%). She has a history of hypertension and gastro-oesophageal reflux disease, and her blood pressure in clinic is 153/91 mmHg. She currently takes nifedipine 30 mg daily. Which of the below is the most appropriate option?
   A. Increase metformin to 1000 mg and send urine sample for ACR testing.
   B. Add a GLP-1 agonist and send urine sample for ACR testing.
   C. Increase metformin to 1000 mg and increase nifedipine to 60 mg daily.
   D. Add a GLP-1 agonist and increase nifedipine to 60 mg daily.
   E. Add a DPP-4 inhibitor and change nifedipine to ramipril.

   Answer: A

   A. **Correct**: since the patient is only taking a low dose of metformin, it is appropriate to titrate the dose upwards. In addition, it is important to know her ACR as if it is ≥3 mmol/mg, she should be taking an ACE inhibitor as first-line antihypertensive therapy.
   B. **Incorrect**: the patient is only taking a small dose of metformin; it would be more appropriate to up-titrate the dose before switching drug classes.
   C. **Incorrect**: while it is appropriate to up-titrate the dose of metformin, we must check the patient's ACR to determine what her ideal antihypertensive therapy should be.
   D. **Incorrect**: we should first up-titrate the metformin dose and also must send a urine sample for ACR to determine optimal antihypertensive therapy.
   E. **Incorrect**: We should first up-titrate the metformin dose and also must send a urine sample for ACR to determine optimal antihypertensive therapy. There is no one preferred therapy for those with an ACR < 3 mmol/mg.

4. A 52 year-old man is an inpatient on the renal ward having been admitted via the Emergency Department with abdominal pain, nausea and vomiting. He received a kidney transplant 6 months ago. Nursing staff are routinely monitoring his blood glucose levels and call you to report that the latest measurement is 16.4 mmol/L. His latest eGFR is 35 mL/min/1.73 m^2. What is the most appropriate management?
   A. Start metformin 500 mg and continue monitoring blood glucose.
   B. Start a variable-rate insulin infusion.
   C. On discharge, request his GP to begin antihyperglycaemic therapy.
   D. Start dapagliflozin 10 mg and continue monitoring blood glucose.
   E. Start subcutaneous long-acting insulin injections.

   Answer: B

   A. **Incorrect**: oral therapy is an option for inpatient management of post-transplant diabetes, but as this patient's blood glucose level is >14 mmol/L, insulin therapy is a more appropriate option.
   B. **Correct**: the patient is not "clinically stable" and his blood glucose is >14 mmol/L, therefore oral antihyperglycemic therapy would not be appropriate.
   C. **Incorrect**: the patient's blood glucose is high enough to warrant inpatient management and it would be inappropriate to ask the GP to begin therapy after this admission.

D. **Incorrect**: not only is insulin therapy is more appropriate in this situation, but SGLT-2 inhibitors should not be used in immunocompromised patients due to an increased risk of urinary infection.
E. **Incorrect**: long-acting insulin would not be appropriate as initial management alone in the context of acute illness and vomiting

5. Which of the following statements is false with regard to contraindications of antihyperglycemic medications in CKD?
   A. All SGLT-2 inhibitors are contraindicated in patients with unexplained haematuria.
   B. All pioglitazones are contraindicated in patients with heart failure.
   C. All DPP-4 inhibitors are contraindicated in patients with heart failure.
   D. Metformin is contraindicated in patients with eGFR <30 mL/min/1.73 m^2.
   E. All GLP-1 agonists are contraindicated in patients with a history of pancreatitis.

   Answer: C

   A. **Incorrect**: this statement is true.
   B. **Incorrect**: this statement is true.
   C. **Correct**: only saxagliptin is contraindicated in heart failure.
   D. **Incorrect**: this statement is true.
   E. **Incorrect**: this statement is true.

6. A 65 year old man with heart failure (EF 30%) was seen in diabetes clinic. His HBA1c was 54. He was on metformin 2000 mg and ramipril 10 mg daily. What is the next best medication to control his blood sugar?
   A. Acarbose
   B. Dapagliflozin
   C. Gliclazide
   D. Insulin
   E. Pioglitazone

   Correct answer is B dapagliflozin

7. His eGFR declines from 65 to 60 mL/min/1.73 m^2 after 2 weeks. His dapagliflozin should be stopped.
   A. True
   B. False

   Correct answer B False: this drop in eGFR is seen acutely and does not have any long-term side effects

8. What is the cause of the acute decline in eGFR?
   A. Efferent arteriolar vasodilatation
   B. Tubuloglomerular feedback

   Correct answer is B: tubuloglomerular feedback

9. The dapagliflozin will continue provide benefit even if the eGFR<30 mL/min/1.73 m^2
   A. True
   B. False

   Correct answer is True: it reduces the chance of ESKD (End Stage Kidney Disease)

10. The dapagliflozin is unlikely to reduce the chance of hospitalisation
    A. True
    B. False

    Correct answer is false: Dapagliflozin reduces heart failure hospitalisations

Test your learning and check your understanding of this book's contents: use the "Springer Nature Flashcards" app to access questions using https://sn.pub/cz9Cok. To use the app, please follow the instructions in Chap. 1.

References

1. IDF Diabetes Atlas | Tenth Edition https://diabetesatlas.org/
2. Navaneethan SD, Zoungas S, Caramori ML, Chan JCN, Heerspink HJL, Hurst C, Liew A, Michos ED, Olowu WA, Sadusky T, Tandon N, Tuttle KR, Wanner C, Wilkens KG, Lytvyn L, Craig JC, Tunnicliffe DJ, Howell M, Tonelli M, Cheung M, Earley A, Rossing P, de Boer IH, Khunti K. Diabetes management in chronic kidney disease: synopsis of the 2020 KDIGO clinical practice guideline. Ann Intern Med. 2021;174(3):385–94. https://doi.org/10.7326/M20-5938. Epub 2020 Nov 10. PMID: 33166222.
3. Heerspink HJL, Stefánsson BV, Correa-Rotter R, Chertow GM, Greene T, Hou FF, Mann JFE, McMurray JJV, Lindberg M, Rossing P, Sjöström CD, Toto RD, Langkilde AM, Wheeler DC, DAPA-CKD Trial Committees and Investigators. Dapagliflozin in patients with chronic kidney disease. N Engl J Med. 2020;383(15):1436–46. https://doi.org/10.1056/NEJMoa2024816. Epub 2020 Sep 24. PMID: 32970396.
4. Chowdhury TA, Wahba M, Mallik R, Peracha J, Patel D, De P, Fogarty D, Frankel A, Karalliedde J, Mark PB, Montero RM, Pokrajac A, Zac-Varghese S, Bain SC, Dasgupta I, Banerjee D, Winocour P, Sharif A. Association of British Clinical Diabetologists and Renal Association guidelines on the detection and management of diabetes post solid organ transplantation. Diabet Med. 2021;38(6):e14523. https://doi.org/10.1111/dme.14523. Epub 2021 Feb 11. PMID: 33434362.
5. Banerjee D, Winocour P, Chowdhury TA, De P, Wahba M, Montero R, Fogarty D, Frankel A, Goldet G, Karalliedde J, Mark PB, Patel D, Pokrajac A, Sharif A, Zac-Varghese S, Bain S, Dasgupta I. Association of British Clinical Diabetologists and The UK Kidney Association. Management of hypertension in patients with diabetic kidney disease: summary of the joint Association of British Clinical Diabetologists and UK Kidney Association (ABCD-UKKA) Guideline 2021. Kidney Int Rep. 2022;7(4):681–7. https://doi.org/10.1016/j.ekir.2022.01.004. PMID: 35497783; PMCID: PMC9039464.

Cardiovascular Complications of CKD

11

Rebecca Shone, Charles A. Herzog, and Debasish Banerjee

Clinical Scenario
A 55 year old gentleman of South East Asian background was seen in the cardiorenal clinic. He has stage 3 chronic kidney disease along with a past medical history of ischaemic heart disease with previous coronary artery bypass grafting. He reported chest pains and feeling tired. He is no longer able to walk to the bus stop. His has a left ventricular ejection fraction of 25%. He had previously been prescribed ramipril but this was held after his potassium reached 6.1 mmol/L. He has been referred to the clinical for advice regarding re-initiation of ramipril or consideration of Entresto (Sacubitril-Valsartan).

R. Shone
St George's University of London, London, UK
e-mail: rshone@sgul.ac.uk

C. A. Herzog
University of Minnesota, Minneapolis, MN, USA
e-mail: Charles.Herzog@cdrg.org

D. Banerjee (✉)
St George's University of London, London, UK

St George's University Hospitals Foundation Trust, London, UK
e-mail: dbanerje@sgul.ac.uk

Introduction

The interrelationship between chronic kidney disease (CKD) and cardiovascular disease is widely established; the presence of CKD increases the risk of cardiovascular events and vice versa. As the glomerular filtration rate worsens the rate of cardiovascular events rises dramatically, and, alongside it, the risk of death from these events. Research has shown that 40–50% of deaths in patients with advanced (stage 4 and 5) CKD are attributable to cardiovascular disease, compared with 26% of deaths in patients without CKD [1]. The cause of CVD in CKD patients is multifactorial (Fig. 11.1). Traditionally, patients with CKD, particularly stages 4 and 5, have been excluded from the plethora of research into cardiovascular diseases which has led to challenges in the management of this patient group. This chapter will aim to draw together the key elements of cardiovascular disease management in the CKD patient population with particular focus on the following:

- Coronary artery disease
- Arrhythmias
- Heart failure
- Valvular heart disease

Please refer to Chap. 8 for a thorough review of hypertension.

D. Banerjee et al. (eds.), *Management of Kidney Diseases*,
https://doi.org/10.1007/978-3-031-09131-5_11

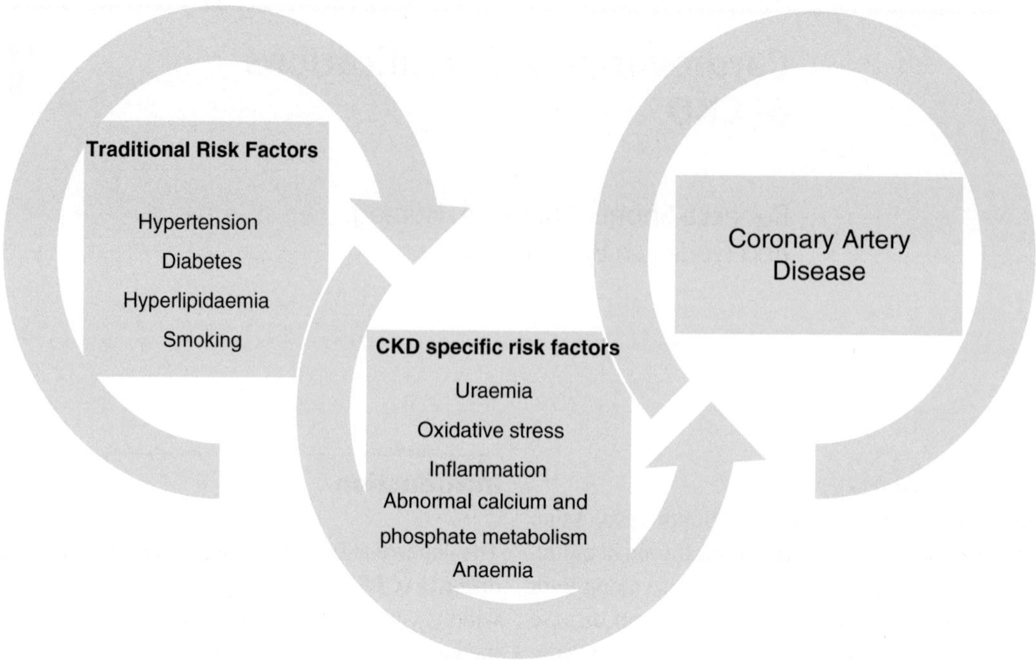

Fig. 11.1 Factors contributing to cardiovascular disease in patients with CKD

Coronary Artery Disease

Chronic kidney disease (CKD) is a major risk factor for the development of coronary artery disease (CAD). The probability of developing CAD increases in proportion to the deterioration in estimated glomerular filtration rate (eGFR) [2].

Even accounting for those patients with CKD who have the traditional cardiovascular risk factors such as hypertension and diabetes, there are additional risk factors to which these patients are exposed to such as uraemia and abnormal calcium and phosphate metabolism which further increase the risk of cardiovascular events. The pathophysiological milieu in which cardiovascular disease progresses in the patient with CKD is therefore different to the patient without underlying renal dysfunction.

Clinical Presentation

Classical angina symptoms are less common in patients with CKD, and ischaemia is often silent or atypical in presentation. In the setting of acute coronary syndrome, non-ST elevation myocardial infarction (NSTEMI) is a more common event than STEMI [2].

Investigations

The optimum means of investigating the presence of CAD in patients with chronic kidney disease is not well established. From biochemistry to radiology, the presence of co-existent CKD not only makes the results of commonplace investigations more challenging to interpret, but it also puts the patients at higher risk of serious consequences. For instance, acute kidney injury following coronary angiography. A further complicating factor is that the majority of risk stratification scores either do not take into account, or do not give sufficient weight to, the diagnosis of CKD, which complicates the selection of investigation [2].

No study to date has suggested that there is any benefit to be derived from pre-emptive revascularization in asymptomatic patients with CAD. It follows from this that only patients who report symptoms of angina warrant further investigation via the pathway suggested below.

On balance, pharmacologic stress testing is used with greater frequency in patients with CKD than in those without though it is not without its limitations as described in Table 11.1. Previously data surrounding the use of stress testing in CKD patients was derived from studies of transplant candidates and its generalizability to the dialysis/non-transplant population was therefore limited [2, 3]. More recent data on utility of stress testing shows that event rates continue to be high but coronary interventions may not be useful hence an individualised approach in symptomatic patients may be the most effective.

Practice Point 1

Given the uncertainties that exist, it is important to take an individualised approach to the selection of investigation in the CKD patient.

Table 11.1 Summary of cardiac investigations

	Description	Clinical use	Limitations
Biomarkers			
Cardiac troponins (cTn)	Biomarkers for the detection of myocardial damage	Diagnosis of acute coronary syndrome—serial assays A routine outpatient measurement of troponin helpful to establish "baseline" in stable CKD [2]	Frequently elevated in advanced CKD in the absence of ACS Specificity of troponin to detect acute ischaemia falls with GFR [3]
B type naturetic peptide (BNP)	Peptide hormone released in response to ventricular stretch	Diagnosis of heart failure Has a high negative predictive value	Indicator or volume overload which may be non-cardiac, particularly in the CKD population
Imaging			
Echocardiography	Cardiac ultrasonography Transthoracic most commonly used approach. Transoesophageal offers more detailed valvular assessment	First line investigation for patients with suspected CAD or heart failure	Operator dependent
Cardiac MRI	Cardiovascular magnetic resonance Provides information on both cardiac structure and function Use of gadolinium can aid assessment of the myocardium	Diagnosis of inflammatory diseases of the myocardium, cardiomyopathies, myocardial fibrosis and assessing presence of scar	Some patients may not be able to undergo MRI due to implanted devices Risk of **nephrogenic systemic fibrosis**, a rare but potentially fatal condition caused by gadolinium administration in those with eGFR <30. The American College of Radiologists divides gadolinium-based contrast agents (GBCAs) into three groups based on the level of risk associated with each agent. The risk is deemed low to non-existent with use of Group II agents. The lowest dose possible should be selected. In dialysis patients, it is recommended that GBCA enhanced MRI is undertaken as closely before haemodialysis as possible, to enable prompt post-procedural haemodialysis. Nonetheless, there is little evidence to support this approach [4, 5]

(continued)

Table 11.1 (continued)

	Description	Clinical use	Limitations
Dobutamine stress echocardiography	Stress echocardiography—compares regional wall motion and thickness of myocardium at rest and after stress	Presence of regional systolic dysfunction suggests presence of CAD **Screening investigation of choice for patients with symptomatic CAD or asymptomatic transplant patients**	Operator dependent Often difficult to obtain adequate acoustic windows Result interpreted as positive or negative by reporting individual Limited sensitivity and specificity Existing data has evaluated DSE in the context of asymptomatic transplant patients, the results may not extrapolate onto the non-transplant CKD population
Myocardial perfusion scintigraphy	Radionucleotide test—compares perfusion of myocardium at rest and then after "stress" (e.g. dipyridamole dobutamine)	In normal coronary arteries, applying "stress" results in vasodilation. However, diseased coronary arteries are already maximally dilated so there is no increase in blood flow after stress. These regions will be recognized as areas of decreased perfusion A reversible defect is sign of ischaemia A fixed defect (decreased perfusion regardless of stressor) represents infarction	Result interpreted as positive or negative by reporting individual Left ventricular hypertrophy can cause attenuation artefact leading to a false positive result. Significant but balanced ischaemia (i.e. triple vessel disease) can give false negative result Radiation dose administered Limited sensitivity and specificity Possible decreased responsiveness to the effects of dipyridamole as stress agent in CKD patients with arterial calcification or diabetics with autonomic neuropathy [6] Existing data has evaluated MPS in the context of asymptomatic transplant patients, the results may not extrapolate onto the non-transplant CKD population
Exercise ECG	Patient exercises on treadmill while attached to ECG. Symptoms and BP response checked continuously	Symptoms of angina or ischaemic changes on ECG suggest underlying CAD	High proportion of CKD patients have abnormal ECG at baseline which limits assessment of changes brought on by exercise (e.g. LVH) Many CKD patients may not be able to achieve an adequate peak workload Result interpreted as positive or negative by reporting individual
Coronary artery calcium score	CT used to detect the presence of calcium in plaque on walls of coronary arteries. A calcium score is then derived, calculated as a total of all calcified lesions in the coronary arteries. A high score is associated with a higher risk of cardiovascular disease	Investigation of symptomatic cardiac ischaemia/asymptomatic potential transplant recipient	Radiation exposure Modest specificity and sensitivity (67% and 77% respectively) [2]

Table 11.1 (continued)

	Description	Clinical use	Limitations
CT angiography	CT which also enables computerized reconstruction of coronary arteries and assessment of vessel wall and lumen	Investigation of symptomatic cardiac ischaemia/asymptomatic potential transplant recipient Lesions can be isolated to a specific vessel rather than a vascular territory Can demonstrate soft atheromatous plaques in vessel walls which may be missed in conventional angiography	Radiation exposure Risk of contrast associated nephropathy Cannot intervene on findings as in conventional angiography
Coronary angiography	Coronary artery catheterization—can be performed as both a diagnostic and interventional procedure	Gold standard investigation for detection of CAD	High cost Risk of complications Radiation exposure Risk of contrast associated AKI Operator dependent interpretation of results

Management

Medical management of traditional cardiovascular risk factors is the cornerstone of managing coronary artery disease, both in patients with and without CKD. However, the treatment of the CKD patient population is complicated by the underrepresentation of this group in the clinical trials which have provided the evidence base for many of these medical therapies (Fig. 11.2).

Some studies have attempted to assess whether pre-emptive intervention in the asymptomatic patient with stable coronary disease has a prognostic benefit. To date, no study has shown an interventional invasive approach to stable coronary disease to be of greater benefit than optimal medical therapy (OMT), even taking into account the difficulties in establishing what constitutes OMT amongst the CKD population. In fact, the recently published ISCHAEMIA-CKD trial has shown that for patients with CKD stage 4–5 who have moderate to severe ischaemia on stress testing, there is no benefit to be gained from revascularisation when compared to OMT in terms of the primary end points of death or acute MI. Furthermore, there was no improvement in angina-related health status in those who were managed with an invasive strategy. It is important to bear in mind that patients with an ejection fraction of <35%, those who had had a recent acute coronary syndrome or heart failure and those who were very symptomatic were excluded from the trial so caution is needed in interpreting the findings in those populations [7].

Lipid Modification

All patients with CKD should be evaluated with a lipid profile (total cholesterol, LDL cholesterol, HDL cholesterol, triglycerides). The purpose of this initial testing is to rule out severe hypercholesterolaemia and/or hypertriglyceridemia and to identify any potentially reversible underlying cause (see Table 11.2). Though there is no evidence-base for specific values which should trigger referral for a specialist opinion, KDIGO suggest that fasting triglyceride (TG) levels above 11.3 mmol/L (1000 mg/dL) or LDL-C levels above 4.9 mmol/L (190 mg/dL) should prompt consideration of specialist further evaluation. In many cases lipid lowering treatment is recommended based on cardiovascular risk and underlying co-morbidities, rather than absolute cholesterol levels. Once treatment has been commenced, there is no benefit to be gained from repeated lipid measurements, as no absolute cholesterol levels are targeted in this population [8].

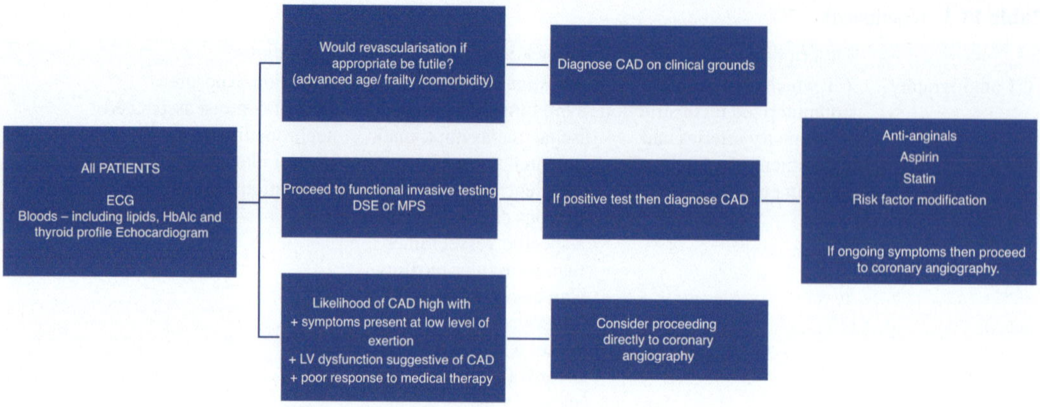

Fig. 11.2 Investigation and management of suspected CAD in patients with CKD

Table 11.2 Medical conditions and medications that can cause secondary dyslipidaemia (adapted from KDIGO Clinical Practice Guideline 2013)

Medical Conditions	Nephrotic syndrome Hypothyroidism Diabetes Alcohol Excess Cholestatic liver disease
Medications	Thiazide diuretics Beta blockers Oral oestrogens Atypical antipsychotics Antiretrovirals

The benefits of statins have been clearly established in the general population in terms of reduction in cardiovascular risk and this benefit appears to extend to patients with early CKD. As the eGFR declines, these benefits appear to diminish, and research to date has not demonstrated any benefit from initiating lipid lowering treatments for dialysis patients. if a patient is already taking a statin and / or ezetimibe at the time of dialysis initiation then this should be continued. Further research is required to establish if statins are beneficial in dialysis patients with prevalent CAD as this group was under-represented in the major statin trials. For patients with pre-dialysis diabetic nephropathy its advisable to use statins and target cholesterol levels of <4 mmol/L [LDL-C < 2 mmol/L; Non HDL < 2.5 mmol/L] (Fig. 11.3).

New and emerging lipid lowering therapies such as protein convertase subtilisin/kexin type 9 (PCSK9) inhibitors are being increasingly employed in the management of dyslipidaemia in cases where statin monotherapy fails to achieve sufficient cholesterol reduction. Though more research is required to evaluate these drugs in patients with advanced CKD, they appear to be safe and effective in patients with mild to moderate CKD [9].

Revascularisation

Patients with angina refractory to optimal medical therapy or those with significant multivessel disease will need multidisciplinary evaluation regarding the optimum means of revascularisation: **coronary artery bypass grafting (CABG) or percutaneous coronary intervention (PCI)**. For certain patients the decision is straightforward with only one of these options being feasible; for instance, left main stem disease requiring CABG, or PCI for a patient with an unfavourable surgical risk profile. Nonetheless, for the majority of patients where both options are clinically possible, careful patient centred discussions are required with input from cardiothoracic surgeons, cardiologists and nephrologists.

What is known is that the short-term procedural risks are higher in patients with CKD than those without CKD, with both CABG and PCI. Observational data has indicated that the short-term risks of CABG are greater than PCI in terms of death, stroke and incidence of AKI [10]. A meta-analysis has suggested that CABG decreases the risk of subsequent MI and need for repeat revascularisation without affecting sur-

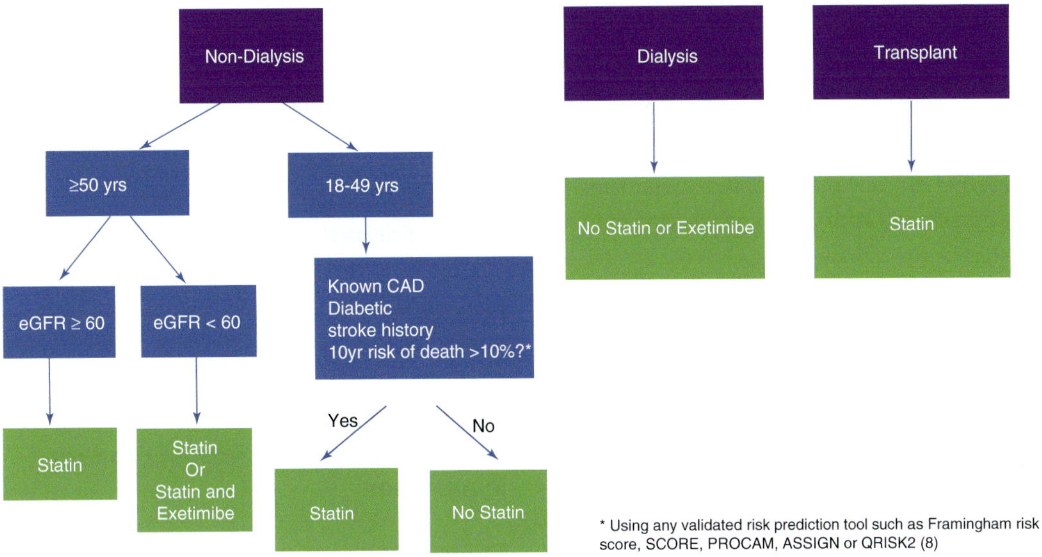

Fig. 11.3 Algorithm for Lipid Management

Fig. 11.4 Relative Benefits of Coronary Artery Bypass Grafting versus Percutaneous Coronary Intervention with regards to short- and long-term outcomes in patients with CKD

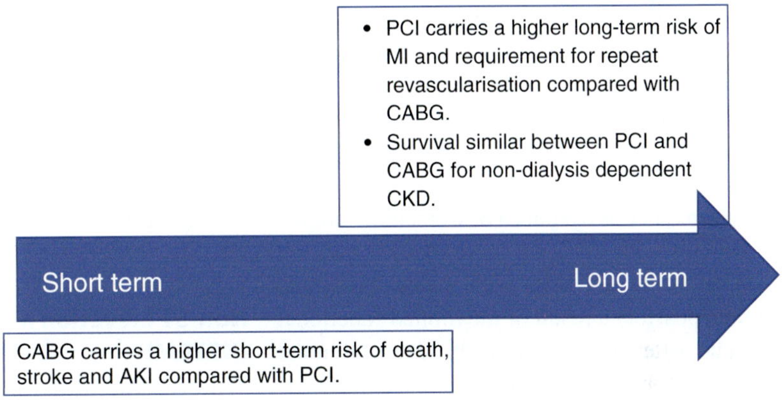

vival when compared to PCI in patients where both options are equally feasible. However, this meta-analysis included very few patients with advanced CKD and none with stage 5 or 5D CKD so these outcomes are largely confined to patients with stage 3 CKD (Fig. 11.4) [11].

There are several important additional considerations when considering revascularisation in a patient with CKD, these include:

- Risk of AKI and measures to mitigate this.
- Access site for cardiac catheterisation and potential implications on vascular access for dialysis.
- Duration of antiplatelet therapy.

Given the lack of robust data to guide decision making around optimum mode of revascularisation it is key that all decision making is **multidisciplinary and patient-centric** in nature.

Acute Coronary Syndromes

Acute coronary syndrome (ACS) encompasses a range of conditions resulting from acute myocardial ischaemia, including unstable angina, non-ST elevation myocardial infarction (NSTEMI) and ST elevation myocardial infarction (STEMI).

KDIGO recommends that the level of care for ischaemic heart disease offered to patients should not be prejudiced by their CKD. Nonetheless, many patients do not receive optimal care due to a lack of knowledge and concerns about the safety and efficacy of appropriate treatments [1]. Indeed, patients with CKD and an acute coronary syndrome are challenging to manage because they are at high risk of both ischaemic and bleeding complications.

Clinical Presentation

It is important to note that acute coronary syndrome presentations can be atypical, with less obvious chest pain and more prominent heart failure when compared with non-CKD populations [12]. One study found that only 44% of dialysis patients presenting with an acute MI reported chest pain [13]. Patients with diabetes who are often represented in CKD populations are also more likely to present with atypical symptoms. Therefore, physicians need to have a low index of suspicion to suspect an acute coronary syndrome in a patient with CKD, with particular attention to symptoms such as dyspnoea or worsening fatigue.

Patients with CKD are more likely to present with an acute MI than with stable exertional angina, possibly a result of the limited functional capacity often associated with advanced renal disease. Of the acute MI presentations, NSTEMI is more common than STEMI [1].

Investigation and Diagnosis

Any patient with CKD presenting with an ACS must be jointly managed by the cardiology and renal teams. Particular consideration should be given to the prevention and management of acute deterioration in kidney function, including discussion between the patient and responsible teams regarding a plan for renal replacement therapy should this become necessary (Figs. 11.5 and 11.6; Table 11.3).

- ECG within 10 minutes of presentation
- Clinical Assessment
- If evidence of ST elevation on ECG then primary PCI indicated
- High sensitivity troponin at 0 and 1 hours (+/- 3 hours)
- Echocardiogram

Fig. 11.5 Work up required for patients presenting with suspected acute coronary syndrome (adapted from European Society Cardiology Guideline)

Revascularisation in Acute Coronary Syndromes

ST Elevation Myocardial Infarction (STEMI)

International guidelines recommend primary percutaneous coronary intervention (PPCI) in patients presenting with STEMI, with a target time of 120 min to PPCI. In cases where the reperfusion time is anticipated to be longer than 120 min then fibrinolysis in indicated [14]. Given the time critical nature of these decisions, patients with CKD presenting with CKD ought to receive the same treatment as those without CKD.

Non-ST Elevation Myocardial Infarction (NSTEMI)

With regards to the management of NSTEMI, the guidelines recommend an early invasive strategy (angiography within 24 h) for those in the high risk category. Any one of the following factors would be sufficient to denote high risk: established NSTEMI diagnosis, GRACE score > 140, dynamic ECG changes, resuscitated cardiac arrest) [15]. While data from observational studies has suggested that an early invasive approach is beneficial in CKD patients, this has not been supported in randomised controlled trials where there has been no survival benefit between patients randomised to early intervention versus those managed conservatively [16].

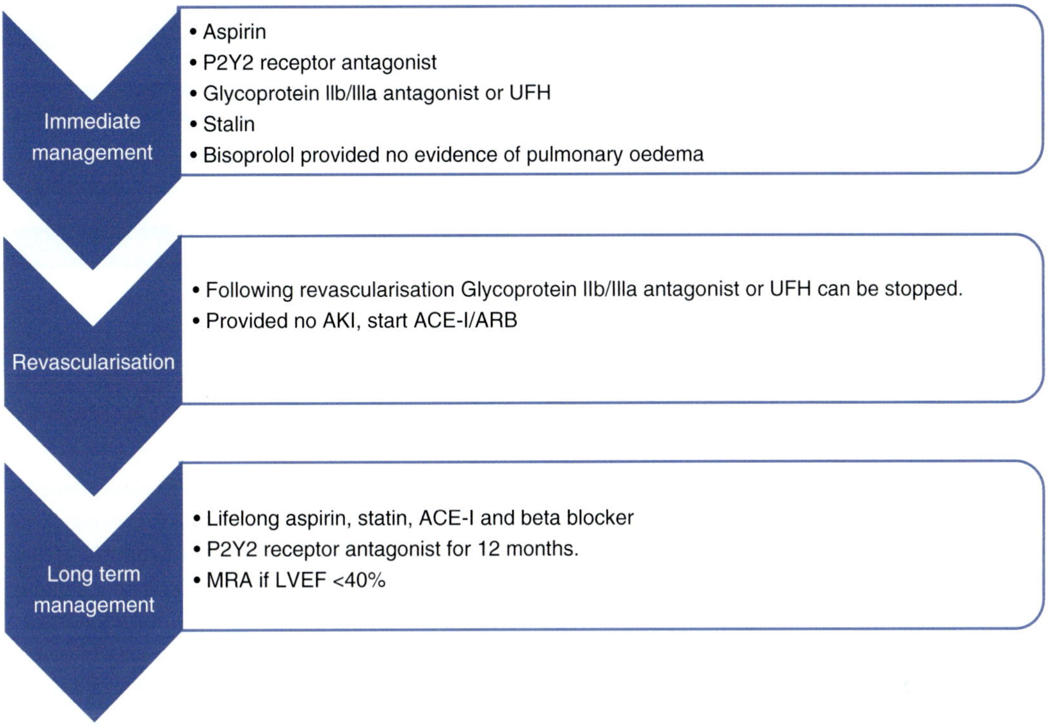

Fig. 11.6 Management of acute coronary syndromes (ACS)

Table 11.3 Medications for the treatment of acute coronary syndromes

Drug	Recommendations	Dose modification
Aspirin	All CKD patients	Not required
Oral P2Y12 receptor antagonist	Mild to moderate CKD patients only. Increased bleeding risk Prasugrel and ticagrelor preferred to clopidogrel in patients without CKD though do carry a higher bleeding risk. Neither have been tested in patients with ESKD Optimum duration of DAPT has not yet been determined	Not required
Beta blockers	All patients Shorter acting agents preferred where possible	Atenolol only requires dose reduction
Angiotensin converting enzyme (ACE) inhibitors	All patients	May be required, monitor creatinine and potassium
Statins	All patients	No dose reduction necessary
Fibrinolysis (tissue plasminogen activator tPA e.g. alteplase)	Should be considered only where PPCI not available	No dose reduction necessary
Glycoprotein IIb/IIIa antagonist e.g. tirofiban	May be considered but increases the risk of bleeding	Dose reduction necessary
Anticoagulation e.g. Fondaparinux or Unfractionated heparin (UFH)	Consider in all patients Fondaparinux not recommended if eGFR <20 mL/min/1.73 m^2	No dose reduction required

Contrast Induced AKI (CI-AKI)

The risk of contrast induced acute kidney injury is substantial and this risk increases as the eGFR falls. However, it is important that the theoretical risk of kidney injury does not prevent patients with CKD from receiving necessary investigation and treatment. The mainstay therapy for preventing CI-AKI is hydration, which should start 12 h pre-angiography and continue for a further 24 h. In some centres, targeted hydration regimens are used; whereby hydration is titrated to a haemodynamic marker, for instance central venous pressure or left ventricular end diastolic pressure. Such an approach has been shown to decrease rates of AKI when compared with standard hydration [17]. In other circumstances an automated system (such as RenalGuard®) can be employed to deliver controlled hydration with a loop diuretic-forced diuresis, again proving superior to standard hydration [18]. A large trial failed to demonstrate any benefit from sodium bicarbonate as hydration over isotonic sodium chloride, or from the use of n-acetylcysteine as prophylaxis [19]. Statins are recommended by the European Society of Cardiology having been shown to decrease the risk of CI-AKI in a large meta-analysis (Fig. 11.7) [18].

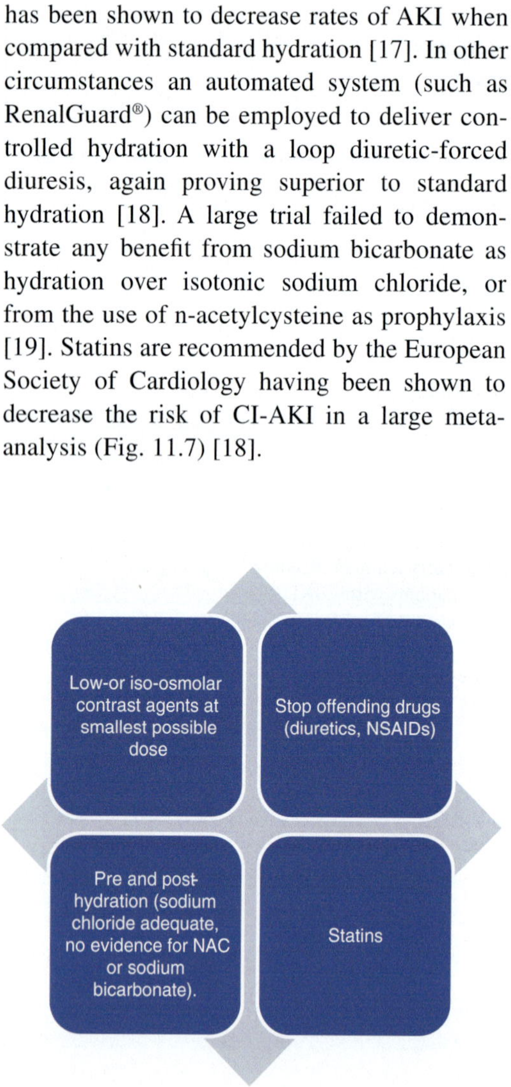

Fig. 11.7 Strategies to minimise the risk of CI-AKI in patients undergoing coronary artery revascularisation

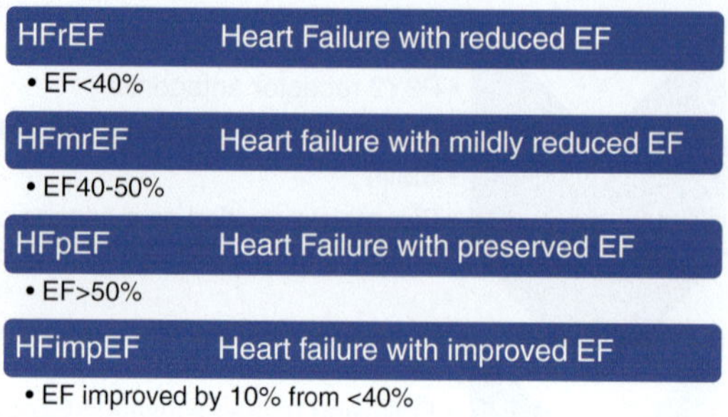

Fig. 11.8 Classification of heart failure

Heart Failure

Patients with heart failure and CKD can experience these conditions both as primary, co-existing disorders or one may engender the other. Comorbidity acts synergistically and can have an impact on symptoms and quality of life, hospital admission and mortality. To this end, prevention of heart failure is an important aspect of managing patients with CKD, this involves tight blood pressure and glycaemic control along with salt restriction, exercise and smoking cessation. The classification of heart failure is based on ejection fraction, see Fig. 11.8. Diagnosis of heart failure with preserved ejection fraction in patients with chronic kidney failure can be difficult as both conditions may present with symptoms and signs of fluid retention. The use of biomarkers such as brain natriuretic peptide (BNP) can also be difficult due to the fact that chronic kidney failure causes high BNP due to reduced clearance. Presence of diastolic dysfunction on echocardiography may help establish the diagnosis of HFpEF in kidney failure (Fig. 11.8).

Management of heart failure involves symptom control as well as the use of prognostic medications. As yet, there are no proven treatments for the management of HFpEF. There is good evidence to support the use of prognostic medications in HFrEF in patients with CKD stages 1 to 3. The majority of trials excluded patients with eGFR <30 mL/min per 1.73 m^2 and these patients are at higher risk of toxicity from recommended therapies. Hyperkalaemia for instance often limits the use of renin-angiotensin-aldosterone inhibitors. Whether the use of potassium binders such as sodium zirconium cyclosilicate improves use of these drugs and as a result, long term outcomes, is a question which remains to be answered in the literature (Fig. 11.9 and Table 11.4).

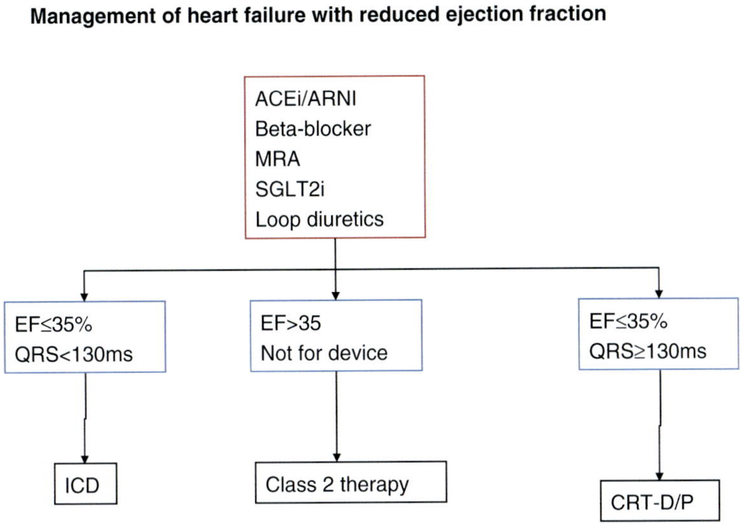

Fig. 11.9 Approach to managing chronic heart failure in the setting of CKD (Adapted from European Society of Cardiology Guideline). *ACE-I* Angiotensin converting enzyme inhibitor, *ANRI* Angiotensin receptor-neprilysin inhibitor, *BB* Beta blocker, *CRT* cardiac resynchronization therapy, *ICD* Implantable cardioverter defibrillator, *LVEF* Left ventricular ejection fraction, *MRA* mineralocorticoid antagonist, *SGLT2i* Sodium Glucose Cotransporter 2 inhibitor

Table 11.4 Prescribing prognostic heart failure drugs in patients with CKD

	Recommendations	Dosing	Monitoring	Advice to patient
ACE inhibitors/ Angiotensin receptor blockers Ramipril, candesartan	Should be used in all patients with HFrEF Contraindicated in pregnancy, bilateral renal artery stenosis	Start with lowest dose, uptitrate to maximum tolerated dose	Monitor serum potassium and creatinine (up to 30% increase in creatinine from baseline can be accepted). Hyperkalaemia and a rise in creatinine is more common CKD 4/5	Explain benefits—improved symptoms, increased survival and reduced hospitalization Can cause cough, dizziness, postural hypotension
Beta blockers Bisoprolol, metoprolol	Should be used in all patients with HFrEF Attempts should be made to reach euvolaemia prior to initiation Second degree AV block Critical limb ischaemia Asthma is relative contraindication, COPD is not	Start with low dose and uptitrate to maximum tolerated No adjustments needed	Monitor HR	Explain benefits. Symptomatic benefits make take 3–6 months or longer Temporary deterioration in symptoms may occur during initiation (tiredness, fatigue, breathlessness)
Mineralocorticoid receptor antagonists Spironolactone, eplerenone	Recommended where patient remains symptomatic or LVEF ≤35% despite treatment with ACE-I and BB Potassium ≥5.0 mmol/L	No dose adjustment required	Close monitoring potassium Spironolactone can cause gynaecomastia in men—consider switch to eplerenone	Explain long term benefits Can take weeks to months to see symptomatic benefit Advise against "low salt" food substitutes which can contain high potassium

(continued)

Table 11.4 (continued)

	Recommendations	Dosing	Monitoring	Advice to patient
Ivabradine	Recommended for symptomatic patients with LVEF ≤35% despite treatment with ACE-I and BB. Patients must be in sinus rhythm with HR >70 Can be used in lieu of BB in patients with contraindication to BB  Atrial fibrillation	No dose adjustment required. Unknown effects in those with CKD 4 and 5	Monitor HR (reduce or stop treatment if HR <50 or if symptoms of bradycardia occur) If patient develops AF then treatment should be stopped	Explain long term benefits Encourage patients to monitor their own pulse regularly Can experience transient visual phenomena, usually short lived
Hydralazine/ Isosorbide dinitrate (ISDN)	Can be considered in those unable to tolerate ACE/ARB Or Self-identified black patients with LVEF ≤35% despite treatment with ACE-I and BB  Aortic stenosis HOCM Recent MI/untreated coronary artery disease (hydralazine can cause hyperdynamic state)	Start at low dose and uptitrate in accordance to response No adjustments required		Warn patients that they may experience headache in association with ISDN Warn against combined use of PDE-5 inhibitors
Angiotensin receptor neprilysin inhibitor (ARNI) (Sacubitril/valsartan or Entresto®)	Recommended as a replacement for ACE-I or first line	Must stop ARB 36 h prior to initiation of ANRI Limited evidence in CKD 4/5. Avoid in patients with eGFR <20 mL/min/1.73 m^2	Monitor potassium and creatinine	Explain long term benefits Symptomatic hypotension is more common than with ACE-I—alert patients to symptoms
Sodium-glucose co-transporter 2 (SGLT2) inhibitors	SGLT-2 inhibitors been shown to improve outcomes in patients with HF, both in those with and without type 2 diabetes Research is ongoing regarding their potential utility in patients with HFpEF	Avoid in those with eGFR <20 mL/min/1.73 m^2		Warn patients they are at higher risk of genital/urinary tract infections Risk of hypoglycaemia in combination with other agents.

Intravenous iron should be considered in symptomatic patients with heart failure (HFrEF) and iron deficiency, with or without anaemia. In studies, iron supplementation has been shown to improve exercise capacity and quality of life in addition to reducing hospitalization [20].

Diuretic therapy is key to managing the symptoms of fluid retention and pulmonary congestion seen in CKD patients with heart failure. High doses and combination therapy are often necessary; commonly used thiazide diuretics may be ineffective and loop diuretics are the mainstay of therapy with additional use of metolazone where required. Patients require close monitoring of their weight, electrolytes and creatinine with appropriate titration of their diuretic therapy. Where oral formulations fail to achieve an adequate diuresis, inpatient admission is indicated with use of intravenous diuretics. With regards to intravenous diuretic strategies, there is no significant difference between continuous infusion versus bolus dosing [21].

A multidisciplinary approach and closer working between nephrologists, cardiologists, specialist nurses and pharmacists may help improve outcomes in the often elderly and multimorbid patients with CKD and heart failure.

Arrythmias

Patients with CKD are predisposed to heart rhythm disorders including atrial fibrillation (AF)/atrial flutter, supraventricular tachycardias, ventricular arrhythmias and sudden cardiac death [22].

Atrial Fibrillation

Patients with CKD have an increased burden of atrial fibrillation (AF), with the prevalence ranging from 16–21% in non-dialysis-dependent CKD and 15–40% in dialysis-dependent CKD [23]. The presence of AF increases the risk of incident CKD and progression to end stage kidney disease, and also increases the risk of death independent of whether patients are on dialysis [24]. The management of AF includes consideration of rate or rhythm control strategies as well as initiation of anticoagulation.

> **Practice Point 2**
>
> All patients with newly diagnosed AF require the following
>
> - Clinical assessment of symptoms
> - Full biochemical panel and thyroid function
> - 12 lead ECG
> - Echocardiogram (LV size and function, LA size, valvular disease, and right heart size and systolic function)
> - Assessment of stroke and bleeding risk

Patients with AF and CKD are at an elevated risk of thromboembolism compared to the general population with AF, however, they are also more likely to suffer from bleeding complications, particularly those on dialysis.

> **Practice Point 3**
>
> The European Society of Cardiology (ESC) recommend the 'ABC' approach to management of AF [25]
>
> - Anticoagulation/Avoid stroke
> - Better symptom control (control rate)
> - Cardiovascular risk factor and concomitant diseases

Anticoagulation/Avoid stroke

All patients must have both their risk for thromboembolism and bleeding assessed prior to the initiation of anticoagulation (Figs. 11.10 and 11.11).

Once a decision has been made to anticoagulate, the choice of anticoagulant agent will depend on the GFR (Table 11.5).

Fig. 11.10 Calculation of $CHA_2DS_2VAS_c$ score for risk of thromboembolism. https://www.mdcalc.com/cha2ds2-vasc-score-atrial-fibrillation-stroke-risk

https://www.mdcalc.com/cha2ds2-vasc-score-atrial-fibrillation-stroke-risk

	CHA_2 DS_2 VAS_c	
C	Congestive HF or LV dysfunction	1
H	Hypertension	1
A	Age ≥ 75 years	2
D	Diabetes mellitus	1
S	Stroke / TIA / Thromboembolism history	2
V	Vascular disease (known CAD, previous MI, PAD)	
A	Age 65-74 years	1
Sc	Female sex	1
	Total possible score	9

Score	Recommended Therapy
0 males **1 females**	No antithrombotic therapy
1 males **2 females**	Consider oral anticogulation
≥ 2 males **≥ 3 females**	Recommend oral anticoagulation

Fig. 11.11 Calculation of HAS-BLED score for bleeding risk. https://www.mdcalc.com/has-bled-score-major-bleeding-risk

HAS-BLED	
Hypertension (systolic blood pressure >160mmHg)	1
Abnormal renal / liver function (1 point each)	1 or 2
Stroke	1
Bleeding tendency or pre - disposition	1
Labile INR if on warfarin	1
Elderly (age >65 years)	1
Drugs (e.g. concomitant aspirin, clopidogrel or NSAIDS) or alcohol use (> 8 drinks / week) (1 point each)	1 or 2
Maximum total score	9

A HAS-BLED score ≥3 suggests that caution is warranted when prescribing oral anticoagulation and therapy should be reviewed regularly with reversible risk factors addressed.

Large trials have established the non-inferiority of the direct oral anticoagulants (DOACS) when compared with vitamin K antagonists (VKAs) and additionally they appear to be associated with fewer bleeding events. These trials included patients with an estimated creatinine clearance of 30–50 mL/min (25–50 mL/min in the case of apixaban) but data is unfortunately absent for those patients with CKD 4 and 5. Studies to date have been conflicting with regards to the benefit of VKAs as stroke prevention for patients with ESKD with one large metanalysis demonstrating a high risk of bleeding in those taking VKAs with no benefit in terms of stroke reduction [26].

Better Symptom Control

For most patients, the key to AF management is rate control. Beta blockers are the drug of choice unless there is a history of severe asthma or COPD in which case non-dihydropyridine calcium channel blockers can be used. These should

Table 11.5 Anticoagulation for atrial fibrillation in CKD

	Recommendations	Dose adjustment	Monitoring
Aspirin	Not recommended in management of AF	Not necessary	
Warfarin	Can be used in CKD 1–5, may reduce stroke risk in CKD but not in dialysis patients who are at highest risk of bleeding complications Those with CKD 5D are at risk of calciphylaxis	Variable	Monitor INR to maintain INR target of 2.5. Data suggests that time in therapeutic range is lower in CKD versus non-CKD cohorts
Apixaban	Should be considered in CKD 1–3 and used with caution in CKD 4–5	5 mg BD if eGFR >30 mL/min/1.73 m^2 Reduce to 2.5 mg BD if eGFR >30 mL/min/1.73 m^2 But age > 80 or weight < 60 kg Reduce to 2.5 mg BD if eGFR <30 mL/min/1.73 m^2 and use with caution N.B. The lower dose range may also be indicated where body weight is ≤60 kg or age >80 years	No routine anticoagulant monitoring Clinical monitoring of bleeding or anaemia
Dabigatran	Consider for CKD 1–3	110–150 mg BD if eGFR ≥30 mL/min/1.73 m^2 Avoid if eGFR <30	No routine anticoagulant monitoring Clinical monitoring of bleeding or anaemia
Edoxaban	Consider for CKD 1–4	60 mg OD if eGFR >50 mL/min/1.73 m^2 Reduce dose to 30 mg OD if eGFR 15–49 mL/min/1.73 m^2 Avoid if eGFR <15	No routine anticoagulant monitoring Clinical monitoring of bleeding or anaemia
Rivaroxaban	Consider in CKD 1–4	20 mg OD if eGFR >50 mL/min/1.73 m^2 Reduce dose to 15 mg OD if eGFR <50 mL/min/1.73 m^2 and use with caution with eGFR <15	No routine anticoagulant monitoring Clinical monitoring of bleeding or anaemia

however be used with caution in patients with concomitant heart failure given their negative inotropic effect. Studies have not shown the targeting of a lower heart rate <80 bpm to have any significant benefit than a more lenient target heart rate of <110 bpm so rate control should aim for a more lenient approach to rate control (Fig. 11.12).

Rhythm control is indicated for symptom control and quality of life improvement. Rhythm control can be either electrical DCCV (planned or emergency) or pharmacological (see Table 11.6). Where traditional rate or rhythm control fail to control symptoms catheter ablation should be considered.

Cardiovascular Risk Factors and Concomitant Diseases

A new diagnosis of atrial fibrillation should prompt a thorough review and risk assessment for the presence of other cardiovascular diseases as well as non-cardiac associated conditions such as obstructive sleep apnoea.

Ventricular Arrhythmias

Ventricular arrhythmias are common in all patients with CKD, particularly those on dialysis, and are the most frequent cause of death

tion procedure and no mortality benefit [29]. There is ongoing research into the use of external wearable defibrillators.

Practice Point 5

ICD implantation is recommended in patients with documented VF or VT with haemodynamic compromise in the absence of reversible causes who are receiving chronic optimal medical therapy and have a life expectancy of >1 year.

Valvular Heart Disease

Valvular heart disease is highly prevalent in patients with CKD and is associated with poor outcomes and significant mortality [30]. Optimal management of these patients relies on close interdisciplinary working between nephrologists, cardiologists, cardiac surgeons while keeping the patient at the centre of all decision making (Fig. 11.14).

Mitral annular and aortic valve calcifications are highly prevalent in CKD patients and these commonly progress to valvular stenosis and regurgitation (Figs. 11.15 and 11.16).

The consequences of valvular heart disease in patients with CKD are significant. The 5-year mortality rate among CKD patients with at least

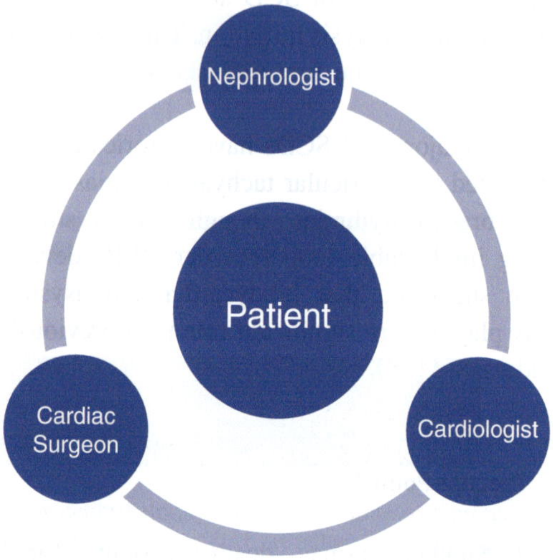

Fig. 11.14 MDT approach to VHD in CKD patients

Fig. 11.15 Prevalence of valvular calcification in the general population and in patients with kidney disease (Adapted from TH Marwick et al: CKD and valvular disease: a KDIGO conference report)

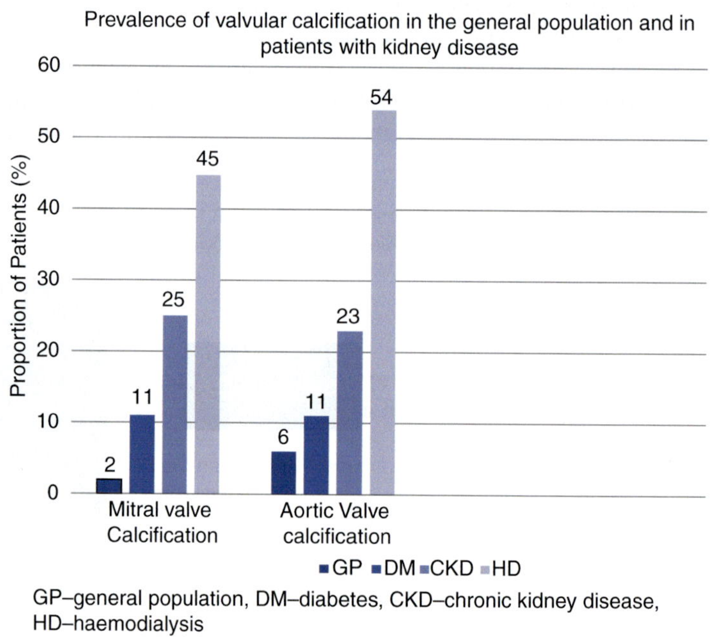

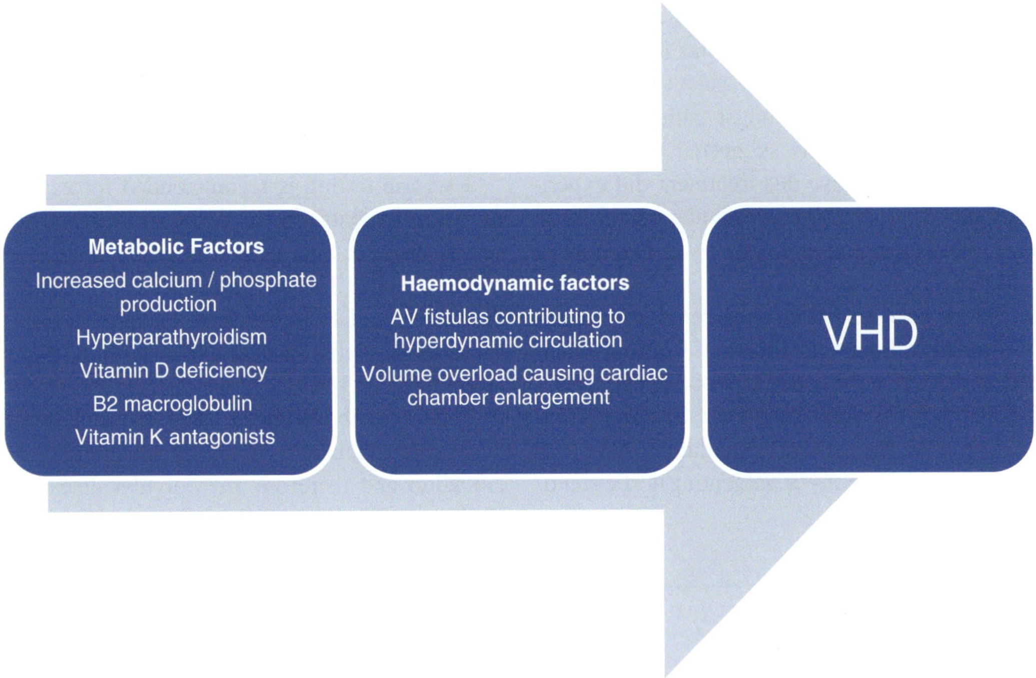

Fig. 11.16 Factors in the pathophysiology of VHD in CKD population

mild aortic stenosis or mitral regurgitation is more than 50% greater than in those without CKD [31].

> **Practice Point 6**
>
> The 5-year mortality rate among CKD patients with at least mild aortic stenosis or mitral regurgitation is more than 50% greater than in those without CKD.

Assessing VHD in CKD Patients

VHD guidelines all recognise that there is a long pre-clinical phase of disease development before a patient develops symptoms. However, even the development of symptomatic VHD can be problematic to detect and diagnose amongst the CKD population. The haemodynamic effects of CKD can confound; dyspnoea may be attributed to volume overload, muscle weakness and fatigue are established symptoms of both CKD and VHD so may not be recognised as adequately strong evidence of symptomatic VHD. Similarly, systolic murmurs can result from increased stroke volume, left ventricular hypertrophy (LVH) and volume overload so may confound or compromise the recognition of VHD. Echocardiographic evaluation is therefore essential and has much clinical relevance in the management of the CKD population. Assessment of left ventricular dysfunction, LVH and pulmonary pressures can influence non-cardiac as much as cardiac aspects of care including dialysis management and transplant candidacy [32].

Prevention of VHD

Valvular calcification is an important contributor to VHD among patients with CKD and ESKD. If measures can be put in place to delay the onset of valvular calcification this may be key to delaying the development of VHD.

Cinacalcet has been suggested as one such delaying treatment. One study has looked at the effects of cinacalcet and low dose vitamin D on vascular calcification amongst patients on haemodialysis. The results suggested that patients randomised to receive this treatment did experience slower progression of valvular calcification [33]. Further research is however required to evaluate this further.

Statins have also been considered as a means of slowing valvular calcification. Certainly their efficacy is well established in terms of preventing ischaemic cardiovascular events, but large studies amongst the general population have not shown benefit in terms of preventing aortic stenosis [31].

Aortic Stenosis

Aortic stenosis is the most common primary valve disease leading to surgery or catheter intervention in Europe and North America. Amongst patients with ESKD its prevalence is estimated to be between 6–13% and the disease progresses more rapidly than in patients without kidney disease [33]. There are 4 categories of disease which are outlined in Fig. 11.17.

Exercise testing is recommended for asymptomatic patients with echocardiographically severe disease. This should be undertaken with caution, under the supervision of experienced operators, and in a suitably equipped facility given the potential risks of exercise in this population (Fig. 11.18).

Patients with advanced CKD, particularly on dialysis are likely to have significant valvular calcification and therefore any valvular disease is likely to progress at a faster rate.

Management of Severe Aortic Stenosis

The options for intervening on the aortic valve are surgical valve replacement (SAVR) or transcath-

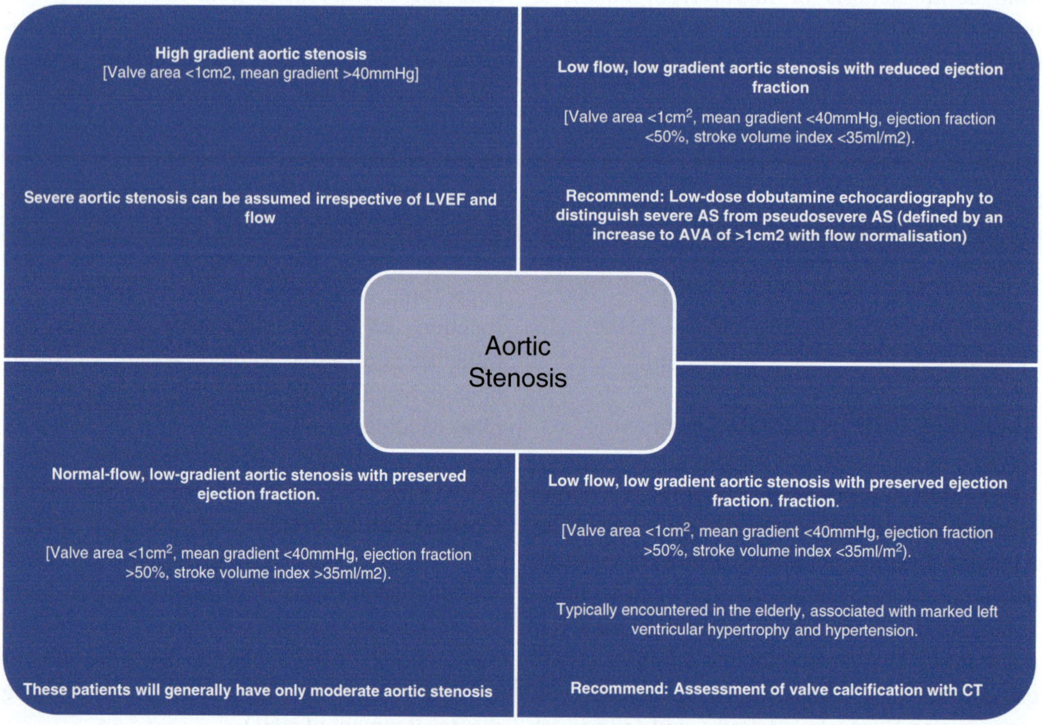

Fig. 11.17 Categorisations of severe aortic stenosis

	Severity			
	Mild		**Moderate**	**Severe**
	Minimal calcification	**Significant calcification**		
Recommended surveillance	2-3 yearly echo	Annual echo	Annual echo	6 monthly echo and re-assessment of symptoms

Fig. 11.18 Recommended surveillance of asymptomatic aortic stenosis by severity [34]

eter aortic valve replacement (TAVI). The development of the transcatheter approach has led to many more patients being considered for valve replacement who may have previously been turned down based on their age or comorbidities.

For patients with mild to moderate CKD the relative benefits and risks of intervention on the valve are comparable with the general population. Data as to which approach is most suitable for patients with advanced CKD /ESKD is however limited. The evidence that does exist has been gained from post-hoc analysis. There is no data comparing valvular intervention with conservative management in these patients.

All decisions regarding valve replacement need to be undertaken by a multidisciplinary team, taking into account patient preferences and priorities. The use of an objective scoring system for assessing surgical risk (STS or EUROSCORE II) is recommended. Figure 11.19 demonstrates the options for intervening in severe aortic stenosis.

SAVR carries with it a progressive increase in complication rates when comparing patients with moderately reduced kidney function to those without kidney disease. Similarly, the perioperative mortality increases as eGFR worsens. Limited data into TAVI suggests a similar correlation between worsening eGFR and complications/mortality. There is no robust trial evidence comparing TAVI and SAVR directly. The little data that is available would suggest that, in patients with advanced CKD, TAVI is associated with decreased mortality and fewer peri-procedure complications than SAVR (aside from pacemaker implant which is more common with TAVI) (Fig. 11.19). Patients with advanced kidney disease are at higher risk of developing an AKI requiring dialysis when undergoing SAVR [32].

Follow Up Post Valve Replacement (Transcatheter and Surgical)

Post-operative echocardiogram within 30 days post implantation, then 1 year post implantation and annually thereafter.

Mitral Regurgitation

Mitral valve regurgitation can be classified into primary and secondary disease. In primary disease one or more component of the valve is directly affected. Secondary disease, also known as “functional” mitral regurgitation refers to mitral regurgitation in the context of normal valve components. The regurgitation in these circumstances results from dilatation of the left atrium and mitral annulus, as commonly seen in relation to volume overload. Importantly, functional mitral regurgitation may be reversible with judicious management of fluid status and blood pressure.

Investigation

Echocardiography is best performed with the patient at their optimum dry weight.

Management of Severe Mitral Regurgitation

Functional mitral regurgitation is managed through control of fluid status with use of diuretics and haemofiltration, where indicated, in order to control congestive symptoms. Echocardiography can be used in such cases to

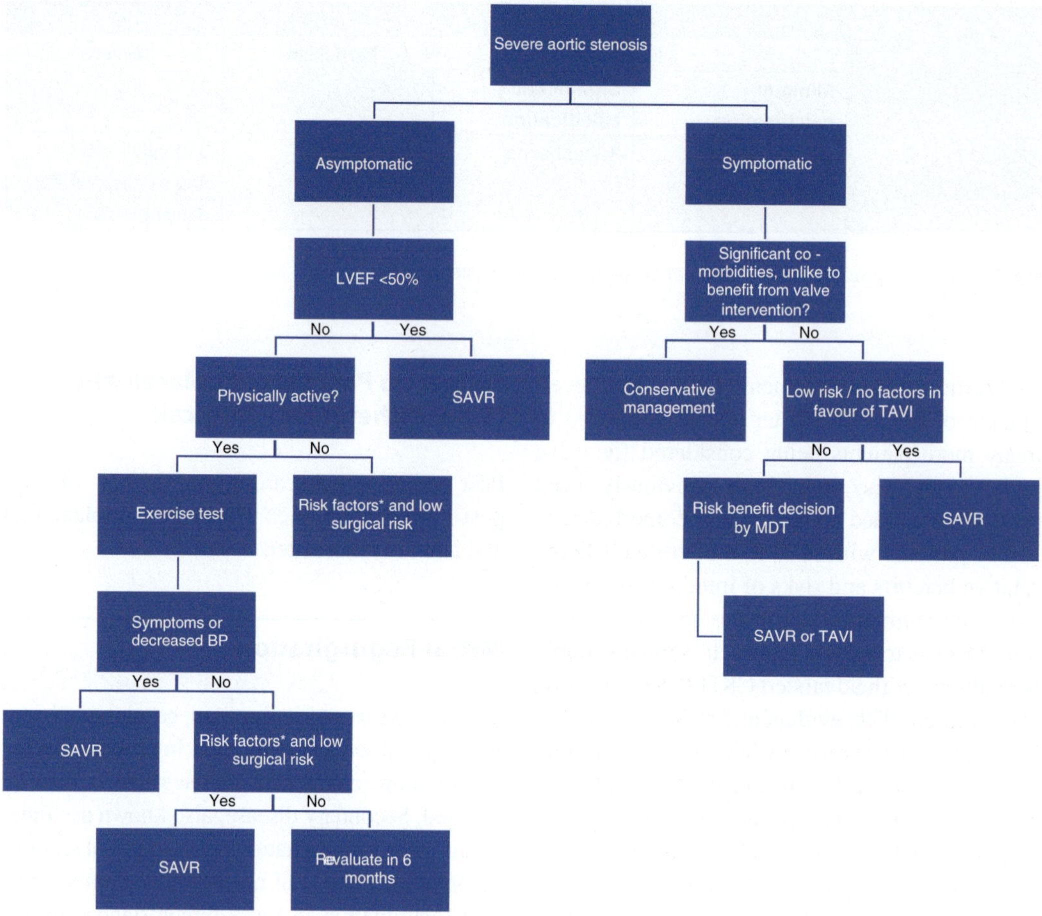

Fig. 11.19 Choice of intervention in severe aortic stenosis (adapted from ESC guidelines) [34]. *Risk factors prompting consideration of surgery: peak velocity >5.5 m/s, severe valve calcification + peak velocity progression ≥0.3 m/s/year, markedly elevated BNP levels (3× age and sex corrected normal range) without other explanation, severe pulmonary hypertension (systolic pulmonary artery pressure > 60mmHg confirmed by invasive measurement) without other explanation. *SAVR* Surgical Aortic Valve Replacement, *TAVI* Transcatheter Aortic Valve Replacement

help guide new target intravascular dry weight targets which, in some cases, may be effective at treating the regurgitation.

Surgery is indicated for acute severe mitral regurgitation and chronic severe symptomatic mitral regurgitation in the presence of symptoms or other objective markers of severity. See Fig. 11.20 for further information.

Though there has been no randomised comparison between mitral valve repair versus replacement, the former is preferred where possible. There is no reported difference in the procedural success rate between either procedure when assessed in the dialysis population. Both are associated with increased risk of side effects and mortality. For all mitral operations, 30 day mortality was 9.3% (vs 2.3% in those without CKD).

Percutaneous mitral valve repair with a MitraClip device is increasingly available as an alternative means of valve intervention, particularly for those with an unfavourable surgical risk profile. The presence of CKD correlates with poorer outcomes with MitraClip compared to those with normal kidney function [35]. Successful reduction in MR following interven-

Indications for surgery in chronic severe primary mitral regurgitation

*Presence of symptoms

*Asymptomatic but any of:

- LVEF ≤ 60% or LVESD ≥45mm
- Atrial fibrillation
- Pulmonary systolic pressure ≥50mmHg (needs invasive confirmation if sole indication for surgery)

*Asymptomatic patients with low surgical risk

- LVESD≥40mm in the presence of a flail leaflet or LA volume ≥60ml/m^2 BSA in sinus rhythm

Fig. 11.20 Indications for surgery in chronic severe MR

tion with the MitraClip device has however been shown to improve kidney function in those with moderate or severe CKD at baseline, possibly as a result of the haemodynamic ramifications of improving stroke volume [36]. Patient selection is key and further research is needed to establish which patients will benefit from MitraClip.

Choice of Prosthesis

Traditionally, guidelines have recommended the use of mechanical valve prostheses over bioprosthetic valves for patients with advanced CKD. The main basis for this recommendation was the fear of accelerated calcification, particularly in the dialysis population, which would result in failure of the replacement valve. While there have been no randomised controlled studies directly comparing bioprosthetic and mechanical valves, a retrospective study found that survival at two years was similar between the two groups [37].A smaller retrospective study found no difference in survival over 10 years between the two different valve types, though overall survival was low [38]. Bioprosthetic valves do not require systemic anticoagulation so the risk of bleeding is lower than with mechanical prostheses which may be of relevance to patients at high risk of bleeding events. KDOQI and ESC recommend that mechanical or bioprosthetic valve prostheses may be considered following individualised, patient-centred evaluation of the options [33].

Investigating the Pre-transplant Patient

Cardiovascular disease is the most common cause of death post-transplant, with patients being at particularly high risk in the early post-operative period. Given the high risk to the patient from such events combined with the need to consider a precious resource (the transplanted organ), assessment and work up for coronary artery disease prior to kidney transplant is warranted, even in the asymptomatic patient (Fig. 11.21). This enables disease to be addressed pre-emptively and aims to reduce cardiovascular events in both the immediate post-operative period and in the longer term. Despite this common approach however, there is a lack of evidence to confirm the proposed benefits and in fact, a recently published post-hoc analysis of patients included in the ISCHAEMIA-CKD trial did not demonstrate any improvement in outcome for those patients who were treated conservatively versus those who were managed invasively with coronary angiography and revascularisation [39].

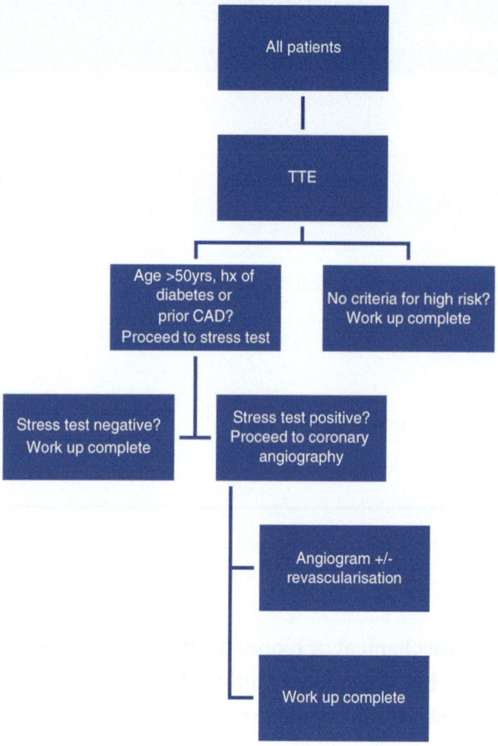

Fig. 11.21 Algorithm for pre-transplant work up

Conclusions

The management of heart failure in the 55 year old south east Asian man from the clinical scenario will require introducing life prolonging medication such as beta-blockers and renin-angiotensin-aldosterone inhibitors with careful monitoring of potassium, creatinine and sodium. He will need help from a dietician and anaemia nurse depending on his haemoglobin and ferritin. Moreover, his management will require a careful multidisciplinary approach with collaborative working between cardiologists and nephrologists.

Questions

1. A 65-year-old male with CKD stage G3aA2 is seen for the first time in the general nephrology clinic, having been referred by his primary care physician. He is known to have hypertension, for which he takes Ramipril 5 mg orally once daily. He reports several episodes of chest pain over the past year, all of which have occurred at a high level of exertion. There have been no episodes occurring at rest and he is pain free at present. An ECG performed in clinic meets voltage criteria for left ventricular hypertrophy, there are no acute indicators of ischaemia. You send blood tests and request an echocardiogram. What would be the most appropriate next line investigation?
   A. Invasive coronary angiography
   B. Coronary artery calcium score
   C. Exercise ECG
   D. Dobutamine stress echocardiogram
   E. Cardiac MRI

Answer: D. Dobutamine stress echocardiogram.

A. **Incorrect: Invasive coronary angiography**—Given the fact that his pain is produced at high levels of exertion, the risks associated with invasive coronary angiography this would not be the first line investigation of choice. If, however, he was suffering from angina symptoms at a very low level of exertion or at rest then moving straight to invasive angiography may be appropriate.

B. **Incorrect: Coronary artery calcium score**—A hypertensive 65-year-old male with CKD is very likely to have a raised coronary artery calcium score, this result would not give any further information on likely territories involved and would therefore be of limited diagnostic utility

C. **Incorrect: Exercise ECG**—An exercise ECG would be difficult to interpret due to his underlying left ventricular hypertrophy.

D. **Correct: Dobutamine stress echocardiogram**—A functional test is the test of choice for assessing coronary artery disease in patients with CKD. The presence of regional systolic dysfunction on stress testing would suggest the presence of coronary artery disease.

E. **Incorrect: Cardiac MRI**—While cardiac MRI may give some indication of underlying ischaemic damage or myocardial scarring it would not be a first line test for assessing the presence of coronary artery disease.

2. A 51-year-old gentleman with no significant past medical history is newly diagnosed with G3aA2 CKD. His eGFR is 50 mL/min/1.73 m^2. A lipid profile is as follows: LDL cholesterol 3.5 mmol/L, HDL cholesterol 0.70 mmol/L, triglycerides 2.20 mmol/L.

   What is the most appropriate management?
   A. Statin in combination with ezetimibe
   B. Fenofibrate
   C. Lifestyle advice
   D. Ezetimibe monotherapy
   E. Statin in combination with fenofibrate

Answer: A. Statin in combination with ezetimibe.

A. **Correct: Statin in combination with ezetimibe**—the non-dialysis population, patients over the age of 50 years with an eGFR of less than 60 mL/min/1.73 m^2 should receive statin and ezetimibe.

B. **Incorrect: Fenofibrate—**Fibric acid derivatives have been considered in relation to managing hypertriglyceridemia—both in terms of reducing cardiovascular risk and preventing pancreatitis. However, there is insufficient evidence of any clinical benefit and they are not recommended.

C. **Incorrect: Lifestyle advice**—Lifestyle measures typically only reduce serum cholesterol by a small margin and therefore pharmacological measures are necessary. Nonetheless, lifestyle advice should be provided in tandem given the positive impact on general health (independent of effect on lipid levels).

D. **Incorrect: Ezetimibe monotherapy**—Although ezetimibe has lipid lowering properties, only regimens which include a statin have been shown to reduce adverse cardiovascular events in patients with CKD.

E. **Incorrect: Statin in combination with fenofibrate**—The patient is over 50 years of age and given that he has an eGFR of <60 the KDIGO lipid guidelines recommend treatment with a statin or combination therapy with a statin and ezetimibe.

3. Which of the following statements is true regarding the clinical presentation of ischaemic heart disease amongst the CKD population?
   A. STEMI is more common than NSTEMI.
   B. The CKD patient presenting with an acute coronary syndrome will most commonly report central crushing chest pain radiating to the left arm.
   C. Patients tend to present with less obvious chest pain and more prominent heart failure.
   D. Patients are more present with exertional angina than an acute MI.
   E. Dyspnoea is unlikely to be associated with acute MI.

Answer: C. Patients tend to present with less obvious chest pain and more prominent heart failure.

A. **STEMI is more common than NSTEMI**: Incorrect—NSTEMI presentations are more common than STEMI in the CKD population.

B. **The CKD patient presenting with an acute coronary syndrome will most commonly report central crushing chest pain radiating to the left arm: Incorrect—**while of course patients may present with "classical" ischaemic chest pain, atypical presentations with dyspnoea and heart failure are more common.

C. **Patients tend to present with less obvious chest pain and more prominent heart failure: Correct—**Presentations of acute coronary syndromes in the CKD population are atypical, with heart failure symptoms being more obvious than chest pain.

D. **Patients are more likely to present with exertional angina than an acute MI: Incorrect**—The opposite in fact is true, patients are more likely to present with an MI than stable exertional angina.

E. **Dyspnoea is unlikely to be associated with acute MI: Incorrect—**As discussed above, ACS presentations in the CKD patient are atypical and heart failure symptoms such as dyspnoea are prominent.

4. A 79-year-old woman with a past medical history of type 2 diabetes mellitus, hypertension and G3bA2 CKD presents to the emergency department with central chest pain and breathlessness. An ECG demonstrates 2 mm ST segment depression in the lateral chest leads. Blood results reveal the following: Urea 14.2 mmol/L, Creatinine 148 mmol/L, eGFR 36 mL/min/1.73 m^2. Her initial troponin is 72 ng/L rising to 280 ng/L at 3 h. She is diagnosed with a non-ST elevation MI and loaded with dual antiplatelets. The cardiology team contact you for a nephrology opinion with regards to planning invasive coronary angiography. Which of the following statements best reflects your advice for minimising the risk of contrast associated AKI:

   A. The volume of contrast during angiography should be minimised as far as possible and the patient should receive intravenous 0.9% sodium chloride both pre and post angiography.
   B. Oral acetylcysteine should be commenced on the day of angiography and continued for 4 further days post angiography.
   C. Intravenous acetylcysteine should be administered pre- and post-angiography.
   D. The patient should be given 0.9% sodium chloride 6 h pre-angiography and 24 h post-angiography along with a 5-day course of oral acetylcysteine.
   E. Use of intravenous 1.26% sodium bicarbonate has been shown to be superior to 0.9% sodium chloride for reducing contrast associated AKI when combined with other measures such as reducing the volume of contrast administered and stopping nephrotoxic drugs.

Answer: A. The volume of contrast during angiography should be minimised as far as possible and the patient should receive intravenous 0.9% sodium chloride both pre- and post-angiography.

A. **Correct: The volume of contrast during angiography should be minimised as far as possible and the patient should receive intravenous 0.9% sodium chloride both pre- and post-angiography.** Standard measures such as minimising the contrast load and suspending nephrotoxic medications are recommended, along with adequate pre- and post-angiography hydration. Studies have shown that 0.9% sodium chloride is non-inferior to the use of sodium bicarbonate.
B. **Incorrect: Oral acetylcysteine should be commenced on the day of angiography and continued for 4 further days post angiography.** There is no evidence to support the use of acetylcysteine, it is therefore not recommended.
C. **Incorrect: Intravenous acetylcysteine should be administered pre- and post-angiography.** There is no evidence to support the use of acetylcysteine, it is therefore not recommended.
D. **Incorrect: The patient should be given 0.9% sodium chloride 6 hours pre-angiography and 24 hours post-angiography along with a 5-day course of oral acetylcysteine.** While fluids such as 0.9% sodium chloride should be given pre- and post-angiography there is no evidence for acetylcysteine.
E. **Incorrect: Use of intravenous 1.26% sodium bicarbonate has been shown to be superior to 0.9% sodium chloride for reducing contrast associated AKI when combined with other measures such as reducing the volume of contrast administered and stopping nephrotoxic drugs.** The large PRESERVE RCT evaluated patients at high risk of renal complications undergoing coronary and non-coronary angiography and found no benefit of intravenous bicarbonate over intravenous sodium chloride or of

oral acetylcysteine over placebo for the prevention of contrast associated acute kidney injury. As such, in tandem with stopping nephrotoxic medications and minimising the contrast load the most appropriate means of minimising AKI is through administration of IV 0.9% sodium chloride.

5. An 81-year-old gentleman is seen in the outpatient's department. He has a background of CKD G2A2, hypertension, atrial fibrillation and heart failure with an ejection fraction of 30% on his most recent echocardiogram. He has been troubled by breathlessness which has been progressively worsening over the preceding 6 months despite up-titration of his regular furosemide. A recent 24 h holter monitor has demonstrated that his atrial fibrillation is rate controlled. His regular medications include ramipril 10 mg OD, bisoprolol 7.5 mg OD, eplerenone 25 mg OD, apixaban 2.5 mg BD and atorvastatin 80 mg OD. You send some routine bloods from clinic. Which of the following would be the most appropriate next line management?
   A. Perform an ECG and initiate ivabradine if the heart rate is above 70 bpm.
   B. Commence digoxin with regular monitoring of levels.
   C. Refer for implantation of a CRT device if the ECG shows a QRS duration of >120 ms.
   D. Stop the ramipril and switch to an ANRI.
   E. Up-titrate the eplerenone to 50 mg OD if the serum potassium allows.

Answer: E. Up-titrate the eplerenone to 50 mg OD if the serum potassium allows.
   A. **Incorrect: Perform an ECG and initiate ivabradine if the heart rate is above 70 bpm.** Ivabradine is only indicated if the patient is in sinus rhythm, the patient in our case has atrial fibrillation so would not derive benefit from ivabradine.
   B. **Incorrect: Commence digoxin with regular monitoring of levels.** Digoxin could be considered for its positive inotropy but would not be the next line choice as per the ECS Guidelines.
   C. **Incorrect: Refer for implantation of a CRT device if the ECG shows a QRS duration of >120 ms.** A CRT is indicated in the presence of left bundle branch block and QRS >130 ms, not >120 ms. An ECG would be required prior to referral for CRT.
   D. **Incorrect: Stop the ramipril and switch to an ANRI.** This would be a reasonable next step once his other prognostic medications had been up-titrated to the maximum dose. There is still scope to increase the eplerenone prior to ANRI initiation.
   E. **Correct: Up-titrate the eplerenone to 50 mg OD if the serum potassium allows.** All medications should be up-titrated to the maximum tolerated dose prior to drug measures being added, given that there is scope to increase the eplerenone this should be the next step in managing this patient's heart failure.

6. A 45-year-old with a renal transplant is seen in the transplant clinic where he reports a 1 week history of palpitations. An ECG confirms atrial fibrillation with a ventricular rate of 115 beats per minute. His blood pressure is 128/77 and other observations are within normal limits. The underlying aetiology of his renal failure is APCKD, his transplant was from a live-related donor 2 years ago and the kidney is functioning well with an eGFR of 60. His other past medical history includes hypertension and asthma and he has been admitted to hospital twice in the past 3 years with asthma exacerbations. What is the most appropriate management of his new atrial fibrillation?
   A. Load with oral amiodarone, counsel regarding anticoagulation, check blood tests including thyroid function, book transthoracic echo
   B. Commence bisoprolol, counsel regarding anticoagulation, check blood tests including thyroid function, book transthoracic echo.

Document Group. 2017 ESC guidelines for the management of acute myocardial infarction in patients presenting with ST-segment elevation: the task force for the management of acute myocardial infarction in patients presenting with ST-segment elevation of the European Society of Cardiology (ESC). Eur Heart J. 2018;39(2):119–77.

15. Collet J-P, Thiele H, Barbato E, Barthélémy O, Bauersachs J, Bhatt DL, Dendale P, Dorobantu M, Edvardsen T, Folliguet T, Gale CP, Gilard M, Jobs A, Jüni P, Lambrinou E, Lewis BS, Mehilli J, Meliga E, Merkely B, Mueller C, Roffi M, Rutten FH, Sibbing D, Siontis GCM, ESC Scientific Document Group. 2020 ESC guidelines for the management of acute coronary syndromes in patients presenting without persistent ST-segment elevation: the task force for the management of acute coronary syndromes in patients presenting without persistent ST-segment elevation of the European Society of Cardiology (ESC). Eur Heart J. 2021;42(14):1289–136.
16. Charytan DM, Wallentin L, Lagerqvist B, Spacek R, De Winter RJ, Stern NM, Braunwald E, Cannon CP, Choudhry NK. Early angiography in patients with chronic kidney disease: a collaborative systematic review. Clin J Am Soc Nephrol. 2009;4(6): 1032–43.
17. Brar SS, Aharonian V, Mansukhani P, Moore N, Shen AY, Jorgensen M, Dua A, Short L, Kane K. Haemodynamic-guided fluid administration for the prevention of contrast-induced acute kidney injury: the POSEIDON randomised controlled trial. Lancet. 2014;383(9931):1814–23.
18. Neumann F-J, Sousa-Uva M, Ahlsson A, Alfonso F, Banning AP, Benedetto U, Byrne RA, Collet J-P, Falk V, Head SJ, Jüni P, Kastrati A, Koller A, Kristensen SD, Niebauer J, Richter DJ, Seferović PM, Sibbing D, Stefanini GG, Windecker S, Yadav R, Zembala MO, ESC Scientific Document Group. 2018 ESC/EACTS guidelines on myocardial revascularization. Eur Heart J. 2019;40(2):87–165.
19. Weisbord SD, Gallagher M, Jneid H, Garcia S, Cass A, Thwin SS, Conner TA, Chertow GM, Bhatt DL, Shunk K, Parikh CR, McFalls EO, Brophy M, Ferguson R, Wu H, Androsenko M, Myles J, Kaufman J, Palevsky PM, PRESERVE Trial Group. Outcomes after angiography with sodium bicarbonate and acetylcysteine. N Engl J Med. 2018;378(7):603–14.
20. Anker SD, Kirwan BA, van Veldhuisen DJ, Filippatos G, Comin-Colet J, Ruschitzka F, Lüscher TF, Arutyunov GP, Motro M, Mori C, Roubert B, Pocock SJ, Ponikowski P. Effects of ferric carboxymaltose on hospitalisations and mortality rates in iron-deficient heart failure patients: an individual patient data meta-analysis. Eur J Heart Fail. 2018;20(1):125–33.
21. Felker GM, Lee KL, Bull DA, Redfield MM, Stevenson LW, Goldsmith SR, LeWinter MM, Deswal A, Rouleau JL, Ofili EO, Anstrom KJ, Hernandez AF, McNulty SE, Velazquez EJ, Kfoury AG, Chen HH, Givertz MM, Semigran MJ, Bart BA, Mascette AM, Braunwald E, O'Connor CM, NHLBI Heart Failure Clinical Research Network. Diuretic strategies in patients with acute decompensated heart failure. N Engl J Med. 2011;364(9):797–805.
22. Wanner C, Herzog CA, Turakhia MP, Committee CS. Chronic kidney disease and arrhythmias: highlights from a kidney disease: improving global outcomes (KDIGO) controversies conference. Kidney Int. 2018;94:231–4.
23. Turakhia MP, Blankestijn PJ, Carrero JJ, Clase CM, Deo R, Herzog CA, Kasner SE, Passman RS, Pecoits-Filho R, Reinecke H, Shroff GR, Zareba W, Cheung M, Wheeler DC, Winkelmayer WC, Wanner C, Conference Participants. Chronic kidney disease and arrhythmias: conclusions from a kidney disease: improving global outcomes (KDIGO) controversies conference. Eur Heart J. 2018;39(24):2314–25.
24. Tan J, Liu S, Segal JB, Alexander GC, McAdams-DeMarco M. Warfarin use and stroke, bleeding and mortality risk in patients with end stage renal disease and atrial fibrillation: a systematic review and meta-analysis. BMC Nephrol. 2016;17:157.
25. Hindricks G, Potpara T, Dagres N, Arbelo E, Bax JJ, Blomström-Lundqvist C, Boriani G, Castella M, Dan GA, Dilaveris PE, Fauchier L, Filippatos G, Kalman JM, La Meir M, Lane DA, Lebeau JP, Lettino M, Lip GYH, Pinto FJ, Thomas GN, Valgimigli M, Van Gelder IC, Van Putte BP, Watkins CL, ESC Scientific Document Group. 2020 ESC guidelines for the diagnosis and management of atrial fibrillation developed in collaboration with the European Association for Cardio-Thoracic Surgery (EACTS): the task force for the diagnosis and management of atrial fibrillation of the European Society of Cardiology (ESC) developed with the special contribution of the European Heart Rhythm Association (EHRA) of the ESC. Eur Heart J. 2021;42(5):373–498.
26. United States Renal Data System. 2020 USRDS annual data report: epidemiology of kidney disease in the United States. Bethesda: National Institutes of Health, National Institute of Diabetes and Digestive and Kidney Diseases; 2020.
27. Bleyer AJ, Russell GB, Satko SG. Sudden and cardiac death rates in hemodialysis patients. Kidney Int. 1999;55(4):1553–9.
28. Wong MCG, Kalman JM, Pedagogos E, Toussaint N, Vohra JK, Sparks PB, Sanders P, Kistler PM, Halloran K, Lee G, Joseph SA, Morton JB. Bradycardia and asystole is the predominant mechanism of sudden cardiac death in patients with chronic kidney disease. J Am Coll Cardiol. 2015;65(12):1263–5.
29. Jukema JW, Timal RJ, Rotmans JI, Hensen LCR, Buiten MS, de Bie MK, Putter H, Zwinderman AH, van Erven L, Krol-van Straaten MJ, Hommes N, Gabreëls B, van Dorp W, van Dam B, Herzog CA, Schalij MJ, Rabelink TJ, ICD2 Trial Investigators. Prophylactic use of implantable cardioverter-defibrillators in the prevention of sudden cardiac death in dialysis patients. Circulation. 2019;139(23):2628–38.

30. Samad Z, et al. Prevalence and outcomes of left-sided valvular heart disease associated with chronic kidney disease. J Am Heart Assoc. 2017;6(10):e006044.
31. Marwick TH, Amann K, Bangalore S, Cavalcante JL, Charytan DM, Craig JC, Gill JS, Hlatky MA, Jardine AG, Landmesser U, Newby LK, Herzog CA, Cheung M, Wheeler DC, Winkelmayer WC, Sarnak MJ, Conference Participants. Chronic kidney disease and valvular heart disease: conclusions from a kidney disease: improving global outcomes (KDIGO) controversies conference. Kidney Int. 2019;96(4):836–49.
32. Vahanian A, Beyersdorf F, Praz F, Milojevic M, Baldus S, Bauersachs J, Capodanno D, Conradi L, De Bonis M, De Paulis R, Delgado V, Freemantle N, Gilard M, Haugaa KH, Jeppsson A, Jüni P, Pierard L, Prendergast BD, Sádaba JR, Tribouilloy C, Wojakowski W. ESC/EACTS Scientific Document Group, ESC National Cardiac Societies,2021 ESC/EACTS Guidelines for the management of valvular heart disease: Developed by the Task Force for the management of valvular heart disease of the European Society of Cardiology (ESC) and the European Association for Cardio-Thoracic Surgery (EACTS), Euro Heart J. 2022;43(7):561–632. https://doi.org/10.1093/eurheartj/ehab395
33. Raggi P, Chertow GM, Torres PU, et al. The ADVANCE study: a randomized study to evaluate the effects of cinacalcet plus low-dose vitamin D on vascular calcification in patients on hemodialysis. Nephrol Dial Transplant. 2011;26:1327–39.
34. Lo KB, Dayanand S, Ram P, Dayanand P, Slipczuk LN, Figueredo VM, Rangaswami J. Interrelationship between kidney function and percutaneous mitral valve interventions: a comprehensive review. Curr Cardiol Rev. 2019;15(2):76–82.
35. Wang A, Sangli C, Lim S, Ailawadi G, Kar S, Herrmann HC, Grayburn P, Foster E, Weissman NJ, Glower D, Feldman T. Evaluation of renal function before and after percutaneous mitral valve repair. Circ Cardiovasc Interv. 2015;8(1):e001349.
36. Herzog CA, Ma JZ, Collins AJ. Long-term survival of dialysis patients in the United States with prosthetic heart valves: should ACC/AHA practice guidelines on valve selection be modified? Circulation. 2002;105(11):1336–41.
37. Williams ML, Bavaria JE, Acker MA, Desai ND, Vallabhajosyula P, Hargrove WC, Atluri P, Szeto WY. Valve selection in end-stage renal disease: should it always be biological? Ann Thorac Surg. 2016;102(5):1531–5.
38. K/DOQI Workgroup. K/DOQI clinical practice guidelines for cardiovascular disease in dialysis patients. Am J Kidney Dis. 2005;45(4 Suppl 3):S1–S153.
39. Herzog CA, Simegn MA, Xu Y, Costa SP, Mathew RO, El-Hajjar MC, Gulati S, Maldonado RA, Daugas E, Madero M, Fleg JL, Anthopolos R, Stone GW, Sidhu MS, Maron DJ, Hochman JS, Bangalore S. Kidney transplant list status and outcomes in the ISCHEMIA-CKD trial. J Am Coll Cardiol. 2021;78(4):348–61.

Further Reading

Banerjee D, Rosano G, Herzog CA. Management of heart failure patient with CKD. Clin J Am Soc Nephrol. 2021;16(7):1131–9. https://doi.org/10.2215/CJN.14180920. Epub ahead of print. PMID: 33495289.

Bangalore S, Maron DJ, O'Brien SM, Fleg JL, Kretov EI, Briguori C, Kaul U, Reynolds HR, Mazurek T, Sidhu MS, Berger JS, Mathew RO, Bockeria O, Broderick S, Pracon R, Herzog CA, Huang Z, Stone GW, Boden WE, Newman JD, Ali ZA, Mark DB, Spertus JA, Alexander KP, Chaitman BR, Chertow GM, Hochman JS, ISCHEMIA-CKD Research Group. Management of coronary disease in patients with advanced kidney disease. N Engl J Med. 2020;382(17):1608–18. https://doi.org/10.1056/NEJMoa1915925. Epub 2020 Mar 30. PMID: 32227756; PMCID: PMC7274537.

Marwick TH, Amann K, Bangalore S, Cavalcante JL, Charytan DM, Craig JC, Gill JS, Hlatky MA, Jardine AG, Landmesser U, Newby LK, Herzog CA, Cheung M, Wheeler DC, Winkelmayer WC, Sarnak MJ, Conference Participants. Chronic kidney disease and valvular heart disease: conclusions from a kidney disease: improving global outcomes (KDIGO) controversies conference. Kidney Int. 2019;96(4):836–49. https://doi.org/10.1016/j.kint.2019.06.025. PMID: 31543156.

Sarnak MJ, Amann K, Bangalore S, Cavalcante JL, Charytan DM, Craig JC, Gill JS, Hlatky MA, Jardine AG, Landmesser U, Newby LK, Herzog CA, Cheung M, Wheeler DC, Winkelmayer WC, Marwick TH, Conference Participants. Chronic kidney disease and coronary artery disease: JACC state-of-the-art review. J Am Coll Cardiol. 2019;74(14):1823–38. https://doi.org/10.1016/j.jacc.2019.08.1017. PMID: 31582143.

Turakhia MP, Blankestijn PJ, Carrero JJ, Clase CM, Deo R, Herzog CA, Kasner SE, Passman RS, Pecoits-Filho R, Reinecke H, Shroff GR, Zareba W, Cheung M, Wheeler DC, Winkelmayer WC, Wanner C, Conference Participants. Chronic kidney disease and arrhythmias: conclusions from a kidney disease: improving global outcomes (KDIGO) controversies conference. Eur Heart J. 2018;39(24):2314–25. https://doi.org/10.1093/eurheartj/ehy060. PMID: 29522134; PMCID: PMC6012907.

12 Primary Glomerular Disease

Raja Ramachandran and Neil Sheerin

Introduction

Glomerular diseases are classified as primary and secondary. They are primary when the pathology remains confined to the kidney, with no systemic disease, and the aetiology is idiopathic or unknown. We classify the clinical syndromes of glomerular disease according to combinations of features like proteinuria, haematuria, oliguria, reduction in glomerular filtration rate, hypertension, and salt & water retention. Specific glomerular diseases produce characteristic syndromes (Table 12.1), but different glomerular diseases can present with the same syndrome. The diagnosis of glomerular disease requires recognition of one of these syndromes, followed by laboratory, and histopathological evaluation where appropriate.

The primary glomerular diseases include minimal change disease (MCD), focal segmental glomerulosclerosis (FSGS), primary membranous nephropathy (PMN), IgA nephropathy (IgAN), membranoproliferative glomerulonephritis (MPGN) and acute post-streptococcal glomerulonephritis (PSGN).

R. Ramachandran
Postgraduate Institute of Medical Education and Research (PGIMER), Chandigarh, India

N. Sheerin (✉)
Newcastle University, Newcastle upon Tyne, UK
e-mail: neil.sheerin@ncl.ac.uk

Minimal Change Disease

Clinical Scenario
A 25-year-old software professional presented with leg oedema and anasarca of 2 months' duration. On evaluation, he had a protein excretion rate (PER) of 4.3 g/day (urine for albumin 4+, with no erythrocytes or leucocytes) and serum albumin and creatinine of 1.9 g/dL and 1.2 mg/dL, respectively. His blood pressure was 110/76 mmHg. He underwent a kidney biopsy, which revealed MCD. The patient was commenced on oral prednisolone (1 mg/kg), and achieved clinical remission within 2 weeks of commencing therapy. He remains in remission, without further medications.

Introduction

MCD is the commonest cause (up to 90%) of nephrotic syndrome in children. MCD is a disease of the glomerular podocyte, and lacks glomerular immune deposits: there may be a role for circulating permeability factors in disease aetiopathogenesis.

D. Banerjee et al. (eds.), *Management of Kidney Diseases*,
https://doi.org/10.1007/978-3-031-09131-5_12

Table 12.1 Clinical syndromes and commonly associated primary glomerular diseases

Acute kidney injury (AKI) (acute glomerulonephritis):	PSGN
Rapidly progressive kidney failure (Rapidly progressive glomerulonephritis/RPGN) or acute kidney disease (AKD)	IgAN, PIGN, MPGN
Asymptomatic urinary abnormalities: *asymptomatic proteinuria, asymptomatic microscopic haematuria, recurrent gross haematuria*	FSGS; PMN; IgAN
Nephrotic syndrome	MCD; FSGS; PMN
Chronic kidney disease (glomerulonephritis)	IgAN; FSGS; PMN

PSGN Post-streptococcal glomerulonephritis, *IgAN* IgA nephropathy, *PIGN* post-infection-related glomerulonephritis, *MPGN* membranoproliferative glomerulonephritis, *FSGS* focal segmental glomerulonephritis, *PMN* primary membranous nephropathy, *MCD* minimal change disease

Table 12.2 Secondary causes of MCD

Autoimmune disorders	Systemic lupus erythematosus, Coeliac disease, Myasthenia gravis
Infections	Viral, Parasitic, *Mycoplasma infection*
Allergy	Pollen, Bee sting, food allergens (milk, eggs)
Neoplasms	Hodgkin's disease, Non-Hodgkin's disease, Leukaemia, Multiple Myeloma, Kimura disease
Drugs	NSAIDs, lithium, IFN

NSAIDs Non-steroidal anti-inflammatory drugs, *IFN* Interferon

Epidemiology and Aetiopathogenesis

Approximately three quarters of patients are younger than 6 years old at the time of diagnosis. It also occurs in adults, in whom it accounts for 15–20% of all nephrotic syndrome. Almost all cases are idiopathic, but a minority may have an identifiable cause, such as non-steroidal anti-inflammatory drugs (NSAIDs) or Hodgkin's lymphoma (Table 12.2). The exact aetiopathogenesis of MCD is unclear, although scientists worldwide have variously proposed a role for regulatory T-cell dysfunction, podocyte proteins CD80 or angiopoietin-like protein 4 in the pathophysiology of MCD in adults and children [1].

Clinical Presentation and Laboratory Findings

There is a male preponderance in children (2:1), whereas amongst adult patients, males and females are equally affected. The onset of nephrotic syndrome is acute, and oedema/anasarca is a typical presentation. Up to one-quarter of patients may have kidney dysfunction at presentation, primarily attributable to intravascular volume contraction. A history of upper respiratory infection and atopy may be present in children. Proteinuria and hypoalbuminemia may cause malnutrition, and be implicated in an increased susceptibility to infection. Almost all patients have nephrotic syndrome, and proteinuria is selective (Immunoglobulin G/Transferrin clearance ratio is <0.1). Both hypertension and microscopic haematuria are rare in MCD. The steroid responsiveness in children confirms the diagnosis of MCD; however, considering the epidemiological trend, both adolescents and adults require a kidney biopsy to diagnose MCD.

Pathology

The glomeruli appear normal on light microscopy. Immunofluorescence reveals no immune deposits of immunoglobulins or complement proteins in the glomeruli. Electron microscopy suggests diffuse podocyte foot process effacement with obliteration of slit pores without electron dense deposits.

Treatment

General Measures

- Diuretics: Diuretics, mainly loop-diuretics, are the first-line therapy for the management of oedema.
- Lipid-lowering: Experts do not recommend specific agents for managing hypercholesteremia in patients with MCD, as it normalises with remission in proteinuria.

Immunosuppressive Therapy

- Steroids given in high dose [1 mg/kg/day, max 80 mg/day, for 4–16 weeks] orally are the mainstay of treatment in both adults and children. The vast majority of MCD is steroid responsive.
- The duration of therapy varies between adults and children. We taper the steroids after 2 weeks post remission, to stop over 24 weeks.
- There is an emerging role of calcineurin inhibitors [2] and mycophenolate mofetil [1000 mg BD for a year] [3] for steroid avoidance or minimisation to achieve remission in adult MCD patients.
- The disease relapses in three quarters of children and one-third of adults. Experts recommend using oral cyclophosphamide [2–2.5 mg/kg/day for 8 weeks], levamisole (children only), calcineurin inhibitors (CNIs) [tacrolimus 0.5–1 mg/kg/day for 1–2 years maintaining levels 4–7 ng/mL or rituximab [1 g two doses 2 weeks apart] as steroid-sparing agents in frequently relapsing or steroid-dependent MCD.
- Patients with steroid-resistant MCD need evaluation for unsampled FSGS.
- The prognosis is excellent, with 25 years' survival in the vast majority.

Focal Segmental Glomerulosclerosis

Clinical Scenario

A 22-year-old non-diabetic, hypertensive homemaker presented with oedema of 5-month's duration. The patient was hypertensive (blood pressure 160/90 mm Hg) with pitting oedema of both lower limbs on evaluation. Investigation revealed albuminuria (4+) with PER, serum albumin and creatinine of 6.7 g/day, 2.3 mg/dL and 1.2 mg/dL. The patient was commenced on oral prednisolone, but showed no response to therapy. Genetic testing for candidate genes revealed a pathogenic mutation in the ACTN gene. The patient was continued on telmisartan, atorvastatin and diuretic therapy.

Introduction

FSGS is a common cause of nephrotic syndrome in adults. The FSGS is because of an injury that is inherent or targeted to podocytes.

Epidemiology and Aetiopathogenesis

The incidence of FSGS has increased over the last decade. FSGS accounts for one-third of idiopathic nephrotic syndrome in adults. FSGS [4] is an insult to the network of the glomeruli's visceral and parietal epithelial cells by either the immune system, a genetic defect [5] or hyperfiltration. FSGS may be primary or secondary (Table 12.3) to a variety of causes.

Clinical Presentation and Laboratory Findings

FSGS is three times more common in males. The onset of FSGS is typically insidious. Nephrotic syndrome is the commonest clinical presentation; less than a third of patients with FSGS present with sub-nephrotic proteinuria. One-fifth of FSGS patients are hypertensive at presentation, and 50% have microscopic haematuria at diagno-

Table 12.3 Secondary causes of FSGS

Reduced number of functioning nephrons	Low birth weight and renal dysplasia
Hyperfiltration	Obesity, reflux nephropathy, high-protein diet, sickle cell disease
Viral infections	HIV, CMV, EBV, HCV
Drugs	mTOR inhibitors, heroin(adulterants), CNIs, lithium, IFN, anabolic steroids
Genetic causes	

CMV cytomegalovirus, *EBV* Epstein-Barr virus, *HCV* Hepatitis C virus, *CNIs* calcineurin inhibitors, *mTOR* mechanistic target of rapamycin, *IFN* interferon

sis. Proteinuria is typically non-selective. Kidney function is usually normal in early stages. Serum complement levels are normal. Some patients may have proximal tubular defects manifesting as glycosuria and aminoaciduria.

Pathology

FSGS is characterised by focal (less than 50% of total glomeruli) and segmental (<50% of each glomerulus) solidification of the glomerular tuft because of the accumulation of cellular matrix and hyaline deposits. The initial lesions of FSGS appear in the juxtamedullary cortex. To date, authors describe five morphological variants of FSGS: [1] collapsing variant; (2) cellular variant; (3) tip variant; (4) perihilar variant; (5) FSGS-not otherwise specified [6]. Direct immunofluorescence reveals no immune deposits of immunoglobulins or complement proteins in the non-sclerotic glomeruli; often, we find granular deposits of IgM and C3 in the sclerotic areas. On electron microscopy, based on the aetiology, glomeruli show segmental (some in secondary) or diffuse (mostly in primary) foot process effacement.

Treatment

General Measures

- Diuretics: Diuretics, mainly loop-diuretics, are the first-line therapy for the management of oedema. In a patient with an unsatisfactory response to loop-diuretics, we may add spironolactone or thiazide diuretics.
- Anti-proteinuric treatment: All patients with nephrotic or sub-nephrotic range proteinuria need therapy with a maximal tolerable dose of angiotensin-converting enzyme inhibitor (ACEi) or angiotensin receptor blockers (ARBs). ACEi or ARBs may be started in normotensive patients, with utmost care to avoid symptomatic hypotension.
- Lipid-lowering: We treat all patients with persisting nephrotic syndrome or chronic kidney disease (CKD) with statin therapy.

Immunosuppressive Therapy

- Steroids are the mainstay of treatment in both adults and children. Over two-thirds of FSGS is steroid responsive. Steroid responsiveness remains the most reliable determinant of long-term prognosis. Usual dose is 1 mg/kg of prednisolone (max 80 mg) or alternate day 2 mg/kg (max 120 mg) for 4 weeks or up to maximum 16 weeks. After remission, taper prednisolone by 5 mg every 1–2 weeks to complete a total duration of 6 months' therapy. Calcineurin inhibitors (CNIs) are alternatives if steroids are not tolerated or contraindicated.

- The duration of steroid therapy varies among adults and children. We taper the steroids to stop after achieving clinical remission.
- CNIs are the first-line therapy to manage steroid-resistant FSGS. Typical doses are Tacrolimus 0.05–0.1 mg/kg/day in two divided doses with target tough level 5–10 ng/L OR ciclosporin 3–5 mg/kg/day in two divided doses with trough level 100–175 ng/mL—to be continued for at least 6 months before considering resistance to therapy. Continue therapy for 12 months and then taper over 6–12 months.
- Experts recommend genetic testing to identify a mutation in the candidate genes in a patient with steroid-resistant (and/or calcineurin inhibitor (CNI)-resistant) FSGS [4]. Up to 60% of patients with steroid-resistant FSGS have a genetic mutation in podocyte or non-podocyte genes [5].
- The management of frequently relapsing or steroid-dependent FSGS is like MCD.
- Patients with steroid-resistant MCD need evaluation for unsampled FSGS.

Membranous Nephropathy

Clinical Scenario

A 55-year-old non-diabetic/hypertensive nursing officer presented with complaints of disturbing pedal oedema of 4-month duration. On evaluation, the patient had nephrotic syndrome (PER 8.2 g/day, serum albumin 1.85 g/dL and serum creatinine 90 μmol/L). The patient underwent a kidney biopsy, which showed membranous nephropathy (PMN). The patient was commenced on ARBs, atorvastatin and a vitamin K antagonist. The patient had a spontaneous remission of her nephrotic syndrome within 3 months.

Introduction

Primary membranous nephropathy (PMN) is the commonest causes of nephrotic syndrome in the middle-aged, accounting for one-third of cases. PMN is a renal-limited autoimmune disease.

Epidemiology and Aetiopathogenesis

Autoantibodies to the podocyte antigen M-type Phospholipase A2 receptor have been identified in two-thirds of PMN cases [7]. The remaining one-third have autoantibodies to either Thrombospondin type-1 domain-containing 7A (THSD7A), Exostosin (EXT) 1 and 2, Neural epidermal growth factor-like 1 protein (NELL-1), Semaphorin 3B or Protocadherin 7. Membranous nephropathy before adulthood or after 60 years of age has an association with secondary causes. In adults, systemic lupus erythematosus is the commonest cause, while in children, hepatitis B is the commonest cause of secondary MN. The secondary causes are mentioned in Table 12.4. The male-to-female ratio is 2:1, with a peak incidence in the fourth and fifth decade of life.

Table 12.4 Secondary causes of PMN

Infections	Viral (Hepatitis B/C), Parasitic infections (Schistosomiasis, Plasmodium Malaria and Filariasis)
Drugs	gold salts, penicillamine, Captopril, NSAIDs, Adalimumab
Cow's milk	
Neoplasms	solid tumours such as lung, gastrointestinal, and prostate and uterus carcinoma
Hematopoietic stem cell transplant	
Rheumatological disorders	Lupus nephropathy, Rheumatoid arthritis, Sjogren's syndrome, IgG4-related disease, Sarcoidosis

NSAIDs Non-steroidal anti-inflammatory drugs, *IgG* Immunoglobulin G

Inconsistencies in the reporting of M and endocapillary cellularity (E) lesions have been reported. A large study has also shown that E lesions are predictive of outcome in children and adults, but only in those without immunosuppression [8].

Treatment

General Measures

- The general guidelines and anti-proteinuric treatment are as mentioned in the FSGS section, with ACEi/ARB in patients with PER >0.5 g/day, and BP target 120–130 mmHg systolic
- The role of fish oil (omega-3 fatty acid) is controversial
- The prognosis is dependent of proteinuria, age, biopsy results and blood pressure at biopsy and can be calculated by an online tool at: International IgAN Prediction Tool—Adults|QxMD.

Immunosuppressive Therapy

- Currently, there is no cure for IgAN.
- Although it usually follows a relatively benign course, ESKD occurs in 15–20% of patients within 10 years.
- The role of steroids in IgAN is controversial.
- However, a six-month course of oral steroids may be considered in those with proteinuria >1 g/day despite 3–6 months of ACEi/ARB therapy and GFR >50 mL/min/1.73 m^2.
- Patients with crescentic glomerulonephritis can be treated like those with idiopathic RPGN by using intravenous pulsed methylprednisone followed by oral prednisone and cyclophosphamide.
- Poor prognostic factors are male gender, older age, hypertension, kidney insufficiency at presentation, nephrotic range proteinuria, and a diffuse proliferative lesion associated with crescents, tubular, atrophy and interstitial fibrosis on biopsy.

Membranoproliferative Glomerulonephritis

Clinical Scenario

An 18-year-old college student presented with swelling of both lower limbs. Urinalysis was positive for proteinuria (4.2 g/day) and haematuria. A kidney biopsy showed MPGN.

Introduction

MPGN is a pattern of glomerular injury, characterised by glomerular hypercellularity and thickening of the glomerular basement membrane. A previous classification for MPGN was based on the location of deposits identified on electron microscopy. This has since been superseded by a classification based on the pathogenesis of the disease. This has re-positioned the histological diagnosis of an MPGN pattern as the starting point for an exploration to identify its most likely cause.

Epidemiology and Aetiopathogenesis

Immune-complex-mediated MPGN (IC-MPGN): Is a result of chronic circulating immune-complex or antigenaemia secondary to chronic infection, monoclonal gammopathies or autoimmune disease. In the vast majority, the cause is unidentified and labelled as idiopathic. The disease may affect all age groups, but is rare in children (<5 years) and peaks at the second and third decade of life. Chronic infections, autoimmune disease and neoplasms account for most of the IC-MPGN.

Complement-mediated MPGN: complement-mediated MPGN or C3 glomerulopathy is a rare glomerular disease, including discrete entities: C3 glomerulonephritis (C3GN) and dense deposit disease (DDD) [9]. Autoantibodies (C3 nephritic factor (C3Nef) and anti-complement Factor I/B/H autoantibodies) and genetic alteration in complement regulatory proteins (factor H/I, complement factor H-related protein

(CFHR) 1–5 and membrane cofactor protein (MCP)) result in a persistent state of complement activation in the soluble phase resulting in C3 glomerulopathy. Monoclonal gammopathies are associated with both IC- and complement-mediated MPGN.

MPGN can also be a presentation, when negative for deposits of immunoglobulin and C3 in anti-phospholipid syndrome, TMA/HUS, Sickle cell disease or polycythaemia (Table 12.5).

Table 12.5 Mechanism of MPGN-type injury, according to presence of immunoglobulin/complement deposition, and the type of injury

IgG ± C3 deposit	Ig or IC mediated	Infection
		Autoimmune
		Monoclonal gammopathy
		Idiopathic
Complement deposit	Complement-mediated	C3 GN C3DDD
		C4 GN or C4DDD
No Ig or Complement deposits		HUS/TTP

Clinical Presentation and Laboratory Findings

Patients with either IC- or complement-mediated MPGN may present as asymptomatic urinary abnormalities (proteinuria and microscopic haematuria), nephrotic syndrome, nephritic syndrome, RPRF or AKD or as a combination nephritic-nephrotic syndrome. Both the frequency and degree of hypertension are variable in patients with MPGN. Hypocomplementemia is a dominant feature in patients with MPGN. Urine examination reveals microscopic haematuria and proteinuria. Experts recommend testing for complement levels (C3 and 4), C3Nef, autoantibodies to complement proteins (CFH, I, B) and genetic testing for complement proteins.

Pathology

On light microscopy, glomeruli are enlarged and hypercellular, with an increase in mesangial cellularity and matrix. The mesangial expansion leads to lobular accentuation. Immunofluorescence microscopy in patients with immune-complex mediated MPGN have C3 deposits in a granular pattern along the capillary walls and mesangium with IgG and IgM deposits. In C3 glomerulopathy, patients have C3 deposition along the capillary walls and mesangium with no significant immunoglobulin deposition. EM shows mainly subendothelial and mesangial deposits in C3GN and immune-complex MPGN and intramembranous deposits in DDD.

Treatment

- The optimal treatment of both IC- and complement-mediated MPGN is not precise
- The underlying cause of secondary forms of MPGN should be treated
- A combination of mycophenolate mofetil (MMF) and steroids induces remission and retards progression to ESKD

Post Streptococcal Glomerulonephritis

Clinical Scenario

A 6-year-old boy presented with complaints of swelling of both his lower limbs, decreased urine output and passing high-coloured urine. Urine examination was positive for protein and blood. Investigations reveals a serum creatinine of 200 μmol/L and hypocomplementemia (C3 55 mg/dL and C4 8 mg/dL).

Introduction

Infections with nephritogenic strains of group A (β-haemolytic) streptococci (GAS) causes PSGN. These include skin infection with streptococci M types 2,49,55,57 and 60 and throat infection with streptococci M types 1,3,4,12,18 and 25. Subclinical episodes occur more commonly than a clinical disease. PSGN can occur sporadically or as part of an epidemic. During epidemics, the incidence of PSGN is nearly 10%.

Epidemiology and Aetiopathogenesis

PSGN is the most common cause of acute nephritis worldwide. It is commoner in developing countries. PSGN is frequent in children and has a male predisposition. The incidence of PSGN is increasing in older (>60 years) patients. PSGN is an immune-complex disease and follows infection with specific nephritogenic strains of group A (β-haemolytic) streptococci. These include skin infection with streptococci M types 2, 49, 55, 57 and 60 and throat infection with streptococci M types 1, 3, 4, 12, 18 and 25. The exact pathogenesis is unclear, and various hypotheses include deposition of immune-complex in the kidneys or in-situ formation of immune-complex because of molecular mimicry of glomerular components to Streptococcal antigen. The two putative antigens include Nephritis-associated plasmin receptor (NAPlr) and Streptococcal pyrogenic exotoxin B (SPE-B).

Clinical Presentation and Laboratory Findings

The clinical presentation ranges from asymptomatic to microscopic haematuria and classic acute nephritic syndrome (oedema, gross haematuria and hypertension). Rapidly progressive glomerulonephritis (RPGN) is rare as a clinical presentation. Kidney function at presentation is variable; although dialysis-requiring AKI is rare. A preceding history of a GAS throat or skin infection, with a typical latent period varying from 1 to 3 weeks. Subclinical presentation is common during epidemics, and may present with microscopic haematuria alone. Rarely, a patient can have hypertensive encephalopathy, and magnetic resonance imaging (MRI) shows posterior reversible leukoencephalopathy: these patients need urgent control of their blood pressure. Urine examination on a freshly voided sample typically reveals haematuria, with or without erythrocyte casts, with varying, often sub-nephrotic proteinuria. Complement levels (C3 and C4) are low during the first 2–4 weeks, and levels normalise within 4–8 weeks. The yield of a throat or skin culture in isolating GAS is relatively low. An increase in antibody titre to GAS antigens suggests recent infection, and the best markers are anti-SPE-B and NAPlr. Streptozyme test (anti-streptolysin (ASOT), anti-streptokinase (ASKase), anti-hyaluronidase (AHase), anti-nicotinamide-adenine dinucleotidase (anti-NAD) and anti-DNase B antibodies) a combination of antibodies to 5 GAS antigens is positive in 95% of patients with pharyngitis and 80% of patients with skin infections.

Pathology

PSGN is a clinical diagnosis, and kidney biopsy is only performed for patients with advanced kidney failure, or persistent hypocomplementemia at 1-month of illness. The kidney biopsy reveals diffuse proliferative glomerulonephritis on light microscopy, and IF shows IgG and C3 deposits in a 'starry-sky' or 'garland' pattern.

Treatment

The treatment of PSGN is mainly supportive and focused on managing fluid overload with salt and fluid restriction, along with loop diuretics. Patients with severe hypertension, refractory fluid overload and advanced kidney failure are indications for referral to a centre with expertise.

Practice Points

- The cause of primary glomerular disease is often possible to predict according to the clinical presentation
- A definitive diagnosis by kidney biopsy is most frequently required in adults, except where PSGN is clinically most likely, in the absence of kidney dysfunction
- Patients with steroid-resistant MCD should be evaluated for unsampled FSGS
- All patients with significant proteinuria should be treated with a maximum tolerable dose of ACEi or ARB therapy

Anti-glomerular Basement Membrane (GBM) Antibody Glomerulonephritis

Anti-glomerular basement membrane (GBM) antibody glomerulonephritis is rare disease, with an incidence of <1 per million population, caused by autoantibodies against the Non-collagenous domain of the a3 chain of type IV collagen.

Anti-GBM glomerulonephritis may present either as an isolated kidney disease with rapidly progressive crescentic glomerulonephritis or as a pulmonary–renal syndrome (Goodpasture's syndrome) with alveolar haemorrhage.

Diagnostic work-up includes anti-GBM antibodies, kidney function, urine for blood and protein, Chest X-ray or CT for lung haemorrhage, kidney biopsy for crescentic glomerulonephritis.

Management of Anti-glomerular Basement Membrane (GBM) Antibody Glomerulonephritis

The treatment should be prompt, particularly when associated with alveolar haemorrhage and the details are as follows

Plasma exchange: 40–50 mL/kg ideal body weight against 5% albumin. Use fresh frozen plasma at the end of plasma exchange in patients with alveolar haemorrhage and after kidney biopsy. Plasma exchange till anti-GBM antibodies are undetectable.

Cyclophosphamide: 2–3 mg/kg orally (2 mg/kg if >55years), reduce dose if neutropenia. If cyclophos is not tolerated give rituximab or mycophenolate for 3 months.

Glucocorticoids: Methyl prednisolone upto 1000 mg daily for 3 days followed by prednisolone 1 mg/kg reduce to 20 mg/day by 6 weeks. Treat for 6 months.

Treatment should be stopped at 6 months, smoking should be discouraged.

Conclusions

The presentation of primary glomerulonephritis may be with nephrotic syndrome, as seen in the 25 year old software engineer in case 1, who had MCD. Minimal change disease responds well to immunosuppression. Similar presentations may however be due to FSGS, which does not respond treatment that well. Kidney biopsy is necessary to establish the diagnosis. Advances in our understanding of the underlying pathophysiology for conditions such as PLA2R positive primary membranous nephropathy (PMN) has helped us in determining disease prognosis, appropriate management, and monitoring for this, and several other primary glomerulonephritides.

Questions

1. Which of the following statements is **true** regarding minimal change disease?
   A. The most common cause of nephrotic syndrome in adults.
   B. Immunofluorescence shows deposition of complements and immunoglobulins.
   C. Hypertension and hematuria are common manifestations.
   D. Glucocorticoids are the mainstay of treatment of MCD.
   E. The disease rarely relapses in children.

Answer: D, steroids are the mainstay of treatment of MCD.

2. Concerning focal segmental glomerular diseases (FSGS), which of the following is **false**?
   A. Nephrotic syndrome is the most common clinical presentation.
   B. Proteinuria is typically selective.
   C. Proximal tubular defects seen in some patients.
   D. Calcineurin inhibitors are the first-line treatment for steroid-resistant cases
   E. FSGS is more common in males

Answer: B, proteinuria in FSGS is non-selective.

3. Following auto-antibodies are implicated in cases of membranous nephropathy, **except**-
   A. Anti-PLA2R
   B. Thrombospondin type 1 domain-containing 7a
   C. Exostosin 1 and 2
   D. NELL- 1
   E. Angiopoietin-like protein 4

Answer: E, angiopoietin-like protein 4 is implicated in MCD.

4. Following are true about IgA nephropathy, **except**
   A. Most common primary glomerular disease
   B. Complement levels are decreased
   C. ESKD occurs in 15–20% patients within 10 years
   D. Asymptomatic gross hematuria is the most common presentation
   E. Serum IgA levels are increased in up to 50% patients

Answer: B, complement levels remain normal in IgA nephropathy.

5. Patients with MPGN **have**
   A. Hypocomplementemia
   B. Peak incidence in second and third decade of life
   C. Monoclonal gammopathies may be associated
   D. Mycophenolate and steroids have been tried as a treatment
   E. All of the above

Answer: E, all of the above.

6. The putative antigens implicated in the pathogenesis of PSGN are
   A. Nephritis associated plasmin receptor
   B. Streptococcal pyrogenic exotoxin B
   C. Soluble urokinase plasminogen receptor
   D. Both a & c
   E. None of the above

Answer: D, Both A & C.

7. 8-year-old male child, following 7–10 days of cough and sore throat, developed cola-coloured urine and anasarca. On evaluation, the boy had elevated BP records of 160/100 mm Hg. His investigations revealed many erythrocytes in urine and 2+ for albumin with a serum creatinine of 4.8 mg/dL and low complement levels (C3 = 46, C4 = 6), which is the most **probable** diagnosis?
   A. MCD
   B. FSGS
   C. PMN
   D. PSGN
   E. Amyloidosis

Answer: D, PSGN.

8. A 26-year-old male presented with anasarca and raised BP records. He was found to have deranged serum creatinine (3.2 mg/dL) with urine showing 3+ albumin and 40–50 erythrocytes on further evaluation. He tested positive for anti-HCV. He underwent a renal biopsy, light microscopy showed lobular accentuation, with double contouring of GBM, immunofluorescence was positive for complements and immunoglobulins while EM showed no dense deposits.

   What is the **pattern** of kidney biopsy?
   A. MPGN
   B. Membranous glomerulonephritis
   C. Podocytopathy only
   D. Mesangial-proliferative glomerulonephritis
   E. FSGS

Answer: A, MPGN pattern.

9. A 35-year-old man presented with oedema and anasarca of 2 month duration. On evaluation, he had proteinuria of 4.3 g/day (urine for albumin 4+, with no erythrocyte or leucocyte) and serum albumin and creatinine of 1.9 g/dL and 0.7 mg/dL, respectively. His blood pressure was 110/76 mm of Hg. He underwent a kidney biopsy, light microscopy section had 28 glomeruli, all were grossly normal, with normal tubulointerstitial compartment and immunofluorescence was negative for complements, whereas electron microscopy showed diffuse podocytes effacement. What is the most **probable diagnosis**?
   A. FSGS
   B. MCD

C. Mesangioproliferative glomerulonephritis
D. MPGN
E. PMN

Answer: B, MCD.

10. Pathological **classification** of FSGS into tip, perihilar, cellular, collapsing and NOS is-
    A. Oxford classification
    B. Columbia classification
    C. Banff classification
    D. Berden Classification
    E. Mayo classification

Answer: B, Columbia classification.

Test your learning and check your understanding of this book's contents: use the "Springer Nature Flashcards" app to access questions using https://sn.pub/cz9Cok. To use the app, please follow the instructions in Chap. 1.

References

1. Hogan J, Radhakrishnan J. The treatment of minimal change disease in adults. J Am Soc Nephrol. 2013;24(5):702–11.
2. Chin HJ, Chae DW, Kim YC, An WS, Ihm C, Jin DC, et al. Comparison of the efficacy and safety of tacrolimus and low-dose corticosteroid with high-dose corticosteroid for minimal change nephrotic syndrome in adults. J Am Soc Nephrol. 2021;32(1):199–210.
3. Remy P, Audard V, Natella PA, Pelle G, Dussol B, Leray-Moragues H, et al. An open-label randomized controlled trial of low-dose corticosteroid plus enteric-coated mycophenolate sodium versus standard corticosteroid treatment for minimal change nephrotic syndrome in adults (MSN study). Kidney Int. 2018;94(6):1217–26.
4. De Vriese AS, Sethi S, Nath KA, Glassock RJ, Fervenza FC. Differentiating primary, genetic, and secondary FSGS in adults: a clinicopathologic approach. J Am Soc Nephrol. 2018;29(3):759–74.
5. Landini S, Mazzinghi B, Becherucci F, Allinovi M, Provenzano A, Palazzo V, et al. Reverse phenotyping after whole-exome sequencing in steroid-resistant nephrotic syndrome. Clin J Am Soc Nephrol. 2020;15(1):89–100.
6. D'Agati VD, Fogo AB, Bruijn JA, Jennette JC. Pathologic classification of focal segmental glomerulosclerosis: a working proposal. Am J Kidney Dis. 2004;43(2):368–82.
7. Beck LH Jr, Bonegio RG, Lambeau G, Beck DM, Powell DW, Cummins TD, et al. M-type phospholipase A2 receptor as target antigen in idiopathic membranous nephropathy. N Engl J Med. 2009;361(1):11–21.
8. Trimarchi H, Barratt J, Cattran DC, Cook HT, Coppo R, Haas M, Liu ZH, Roberts IS, Yuzawa Y, Zhang H, Feehally J, IgAN Classification Working Group of the International IgA Nephropathy Network and the Renal Pathology Society; Conference Participants. Oxford classification of IgA nephropathy 2016: an update from the IgA Nephropathy Classification Working Group. Kidney Int. 2017;91(5):1014–21. https://doi.org/10.1016/j.kint.2017.02.003. Epub 2017 Mar 22. PMID: 28341274.
9. Smith RJH, Appel GB, Blom AM, Cook HT, D'Agati VD, Fakhouri F, et al. C3 glomerulopathy—understanding a rare complement-driven renal disease. Nat Rev Nephrol. 2019;15(3):129–43.

Secondary Glomerular Disease and Renal Vasculitis

13

Neil Sheerin and Raja Ramachandran

Introduction

In this chapter each condition including ANCA associated vasculitis, lupus nephritis, cryoglobulinemia, protein deposition diseases, thrombotic microangiopathies is introduced separately with a typical case which is followed by epidemiology, clinical presentation investigations and management. The typical presentations and histological features of primary glomerulonephritis are presented in Chap. 12.

Anti-Neutrophil Cytoplasmic Antibody (ANCA) Associated Vasculitis

Clinical Scenario

A 67-year-old man presents with a 2 month history of fatigue, weight loss and myalgia. On examination he had a temperature of 37.7 °C, was pale and there was evidence of non-blanching, petechial rash on the dorsum of his feet. Urinalysis was positive for blood (+++) and protein (++). He had evidence of acute kidney injury with a serum Creatinine (Cr) of 387 μmol/L, having been normal 12 months previously. He was anaemic (Haemoglobin 97 g/L), with a raised white cell count (13.4×10^9/L) and CRP of 87 mg/L. He was referred to nephrology for assessment of his AKI.

Introduction

ANCA associated vasculitis (AAV) refers to a group of systemic autoimmune diseases with a wide range of clinical presentations. Vasculitis with kidney involvement typically causes a pauci-immune necrotising glomerulonephritis with crescent formation. There are several subtypes of AAV including; microscopic polyangiitis (MPA), granulomatosis with polyangiitis (GPA) and eosinophilic GPA (EGPA) [1]. Although each subtype has distinct features there is significant overlap in clinical presentations, investigation and treatment.

Epidemiology and Causes

The incidence of AAV is approximately 15–20 per million population per year, increasing with age, peaking in the seventh–eighth decade of life with a male predominance. AAV is less common in African populations and there is also geographical variation in the subtypes with GPA

N. Sheerin (✉)
Newcastle University, Newcastle upon Tyne, UK
e-mail: neil.sheerin@ncl.ac.uk

R. Ramachandran
Postgraduate Institute of Medical Education and Research (PGIMER), Chandigarh, India

D. Banerjee et al. (eds.), *Management of Kidney Diseases*,
https://doi.org/10.1007/978-3-031-09131-5_13

more common in Northern Europe and MPA more common in Southern Europe and Asia, probably reflecting both environmental and genetic factors.

Defects in immune regulation lead to the development of autoantibodies again constituents of neutrophil primary granules due to a combination of environmental triggers in people with a genetic predisposition.

Clinical Presentation

Previously the AAV subtypes were classified according to clinical features, with GPA more commonly involving the lungs and upper respiratory tract. However, there is significant overlap in clinical presentation and renal limited disease can occur in the absence of other features of systemic disease. Classification of the disease on the basis of ANCA type may be better than the traditional clinical classification. Table 13.1 summarises the main clinical features of the two main subtypes of AAV.

EGPA is associated with asthma and eosinophilia. ANCA positivity is less common as is renal involvement (20%).

Relapse is common affecting 30–50% of patients in the 5 years after diagnosis. Risk factors for relapse include younger age, PR3-ANCA (and persistent positivity), GPA phenotype, lower cumulative cyclophosphamide dose and discontinuation of therapy. Recurrence can occur after transplantation in approximately 15–20% of cases.

Investigations

Patients will often have evidence of systemic inflammation with a raised WCC and CRP. ANCA is detected in the majority of cases. Immunofluorescence on neutrophils detects two patterns, cytoplasmic (cANCA) and perinuclear (pANCA). The antigens detected are two constituents of neutrophil primary granules, Proteinase 3 and Myeloperoxidase respectively. Further assessment is usually performed by antigen specific ELISA, which has now replaced immunofluorescence in many laboratories. ANCA can also be found in other inflammatory conditions and is therefore not specific for AAV. Also some patients with vasculitis are ANCA negative, but their clinical presentation and response to treatment are similar to ANCA positive cases. Table 13.2 summarises the prevalence of ANCA in different forms of vasculitis.

Kidney biopsy shows necrotising glomerulonephritis with crescent formation. Immune complex deposition is not seen on immunofluorescence microscopy. Tubulointerstitial inflammation may also be present.

Table 13.1 Clinical features of AAV

	MPA (MPO-ANCA)	GPA (PR3-ANCA)
Age	60–80 years	50–70 years
Pathology	Necrotising vasculitis	Necrotising vasculitis with granulomas
Systemic features (fatigue, myalgia, fever)	Common	Common
Renal involvement	Can present with AKI or CKD	Common with rapidly progressive glomerulonephritis
Upper respiratory tract involvement	Uncommon	Common with destructive granulomatous lesions (nasal collapse), sinusitis, otitis media, nose bleeds
Lung	Pulmonary haemorrhage. Pulmonary fibrosis can occur.	Cavitating, destructive lesions
Skin	Common, leukocytoclastic vasculitis	Common, leukocytoclastic vasculitis
Response to treatment	Worse outcomes, particularly if evidence of chronicity	More likely to relapse responds better to therapy with Rituximab
Risk of relapse	Lower	Higher

Differential Diagnosis

It is important to exclude infection as patients have evidence of systemic inflammation and require immunosuppressive treatment. Also, ANCA can be positive in some chronic infections, for example endocarditis. Testing for ANCA and kidney biopsy will differentiate from other forms of rapidly progressive glomerulonephritis.

Table 13.2 ANCA in vasculitis

	MPO-ANCA (pANCA)	PR3-ANCA (cANCA)	ANCA negative
MPA	60%	30%	10%
GPA	20%	75%	5%
EGPA	45%	5%	50%
Kidney-limited vasculitis	80%	10%	10%

Management

With typical clinical presentation of small vessel vasculitis, rapidly progressive disease and positive MPO or PR3 ANCA serology waiting for kidney biopsy or biopsy results should not delay treatment.

Management of AAV should be considered in two phases; induction and maintenance. Induction treatment involves the first 3–6 months of therapy and aims to reduce inflammation quickly. It is usually with a combination of corticosteroids with either cyclophosphamide or rituximab. If disease is resistant to one induction treatment switching to the alternative approach is recommended. It is important to tailor treatment regimens to patients as a significant proportion of the morbidity and mortality from AAV is treatment related. Relapse requires a further course of induction treatment. Table 13.3 summarises

Table 13.3 Induction treatment in ANCA associated vasculitis

	Rationale	Dose
Induction		
Corticosteroids	Anti-inflammatory	In severe disease (rapidly progressive GN or lung involvement) usually pulsed intravenous treatment (3 doses of methylprednisolone), followed by oral taper starting a 1 mg/kg prednisolone and reducing to maintenance dose by 3–6 months. Emerging evidence that lower doses of corticosteroid may be equally effective and safer [2]. See Table 13.4
Cyclophosphamide	Immunosuppressive action reducing lymphocyte proliferation	Used in combination with steroids. Can be given orally (2 mg/kg) or intravenously (15 mg/kg every 2–3 weeks). Intravenous treatment uses a lower cumulative dose and is associated with less marrow suppression but a higher relapse rate. Preferred with high or rising creatinine (>354 μmol/L)
Anti-CD20 monoclonal antibody (Rituximab)	B cell depletion	Used as an alternative to cyclophosphamide with evidence of non-inferiority for remission induction. Dosed either weekly 375 mg/m^2 or 1000 mg every 2 weeks. May be superior to cyclophosphamide in patients with PR3-ANCA. Removed by plasma exchange. It is may be preferred in children, adolescents, frail adults, premenopausal women, men concerned about fertility
Mycophenolic acid	Anti-proliferative. Suppression of lymphocyte responses	Can be used as an alternative to cyclophosphamide for induction for patients with less severe disease - 2000–3000 mg/day. Higher relapse rate
C5a Receptor antagonist (Avacopan)	Anti-inflammatory action by blocking the anaphylotoxin C5a	Can be used to reduce or avoid the use of corticosteroids as part of an induction regime

Table 13.7 ISN/RPS classification of LN

	Histological features
Class I	Minimal mesangial changes. Normal light microscopy mesangial with immune deposits
Class II	Mesangial hypercellularity or matrix expansion with mesangial IC deposition
Class III	Focal segmental or global endocapillary or extracapillary glomerulonephritis involving <50% of glomeruli, typically with focal subendothelial immune deposits. Includes assessment of active (A) or chronic (C) lesions
Class IV	Diffuse segmental or global endocapillary or extracapillary glomerulonephritis involving >50% of glomeruli, typically with difffuse subendothelial immune deposits. Includes assessment of active (A) or chronic (C) lesions
Class V	Membranous lupus nephritis with global or segmental immune deposits
Class VI	Advanced sclerosing LN (>90% glomerular sclerosis)

Other results including anaemia, thrombocytopenia and low white cell count are also typical and may correlate with disease activity. Proteinuria indicates renal involvement and should be part of the assessment of all patients with SLE.

Kidney biopsy is important in the assessment of LN. There is significant diversity in glomerular findings, between patients and histology can change in an individual patient over time and in response to treatment. Biopsy findings are classified according to the International Society of Nephrology/Renal Pathology Society classification (Table 13.7) [4] and the class of disease predicts prognosis and is used to determine the treatment required.

The detection of immune deposits by immunofluorescence and electron microscopy is a common feature in LN. Deposits will usually contain IgG but also IgM, IgA, C3 and C1q. When all are seen, this pattern is highly suggestive of LN.

Differential Diagnosis

Clinically other connective tissue disease can mimic SLE. Diagnosis is made from the pattern of symptoms and testing for autoantibodies.

Management

The treatment of LN is dependent on the class of disease and is aimed at preventing progressive kidney injury. Standard treatment includes the use of ACE inhibitors or angiotensin receptor blockers and hydroxychloroquine. Subsequent treatment is then determined by the class of LN.

Class I and II

This is associated with a good prognosis and therapy is directed to extra-renal involvement. Class I and II LN can evolve into more aggressive disease, so long-term monitoring is required.

Class III

Milder forms of class III LN with infrequent proliferative lesions, no necrotising lesions or crescents can be treated with a short course of immunosuppression, often corticosteroids. More severe class III LN should be treated a Class IV.

Class IV

There is no universally accepted treatment for Class IV LN and treatment has to be varied depending on a patient's clinical condition and previous treatment exposure. Corticosteroids in combination with another agent is the most commonly used treatment as corticosteroids alone are insufficient to control disease. Current European recommendations are for initial intravenous methylprednisolone [0.25–0.5 g/day for 1–3 days] followed by oral steroids starting at 0.3–0.5 mg/kg (reduced dose) for 4 weeks [or 0.6–1 mg/kg/day] then tapered over 3 months [5].

Steroids are combined with cyclophosphamide, usually administered intravenously, or mycophenolate mofetil (MMF) / mycophenolate sodium which have similar efficacy, with MMF potentially being better in black patients. The dose of MMF should be 2–3 g/day (MPA 1.44–2.16 g/day) and cyclophosphamide dosing should usually follow the low dose Euro-Lupus regime [0.6 g every 2 weeks, 6 doses] which has equivalent long-term outcomes compared to higher dose regimes [0.5–1 g/m^2/month for 6 months] [6].

Calcineurin inhibition with either cyclosporine or tacrolimus [trough level 5.5 ng/L] has been used either as monotherapy or in combination (for example with MMF). Although there are some promising results, further data is required before this can be recommended as a first line treatment. Voclosporin 23.5 mg BD can be used with MPA for 52 weeks in patients with eGFR > 45 mL/min/1.73 m^2.

In patients with refractory disease switching to an alternative treatment regime should be considered. The addition of anti-CD20 (Rituximab or Obinutuzumab) or anti-BLyS (Belimumab 10 mg/kg every 2 week for 6 weeks and every 4 week with MPA or cyclo) monoclonal antibody treatment can also be considered.

Class V

MMF/MPA with glucocorticoid is the usual first choice treatment with calcineurin inhibition, either alone or in combination with MMF/MPA) is an alternative option. There is some evidence for Rituximab in patients who have not responded to first line treatment.

Rapid and complete remission, with proteinuria <0.5 g/day, is associated with better long-term outcomes. However, relapse occurs in approximately 50% of patients and requires further induction treatment. Relapse can be predicted by rising anti-dsDNA titres and falling complement (C3 and C4) concentrations.

Once remission is achieved patients should remain on maintenance treatment for a period of at least 5 years. MMF/MPA [1–2 g/day] or azathioprine [1.5–2 mg/kg/day] can be used with current the recommendation to continue MMF/MPA if remission was induced by these agents and to use either MMF/MPA or azathioprine if remission was induced by cyclophosphamide.

Antiphospholipid Syndrome

Antiphospholipid (APL) antibody syndrome (APS) is associated with IgG or IgM autoantibodies to plasma proteins containing phospholipids including anticardiolipin and anti-β_2-glycoprotein I antibodies and lupus anticoagulant activity. Diagnostic criteria includes: a positive antibody test on two occasions at least 12 weeks apart, episodes of venous or arterial thrombosis and fetal loss. APS occurs in the absence of another autoimmune disease in 50% of cases (primary). Approximately 30–50% of patients with SLE have detectable APL antibodies although a majority do not develop features of APS.

Renal involvement with APS (APL nephropathy) relates to vascular thrombosis ranging from the main renal artery or vein to glomerular capillaries and occurs in 25% of patients with APS. Vascular thrombosis is associated with an inflammatory, proliferative response. Other patterns of glomerular disease have also been reported. Thrombotic lesions on kidney biopsy can be seen in 10% of patients with SLE and is significantly higher in patients who have anti-APL antibodies.

Patients can present with hypertension, proteinuria and progressive renal dysfunction. Acute reduction in renal function can occur in the context of major vessel thrombosis and rapidly progressive GN has also been reported.

For patients with clinical features of APS warfarin treatment, aiming to maintain INR > 3, is the first line therapy. The role of immunosuppression, other than for the treatment of co-existing SLE, is uncertain.

Cryoglobulinaemia

Clinical Scenario

A 37 year old male intravenous drug user presents with a purpuric rash over his feet and lower part of his legs. He was noted to have non-visible haematuria and a Cr of 192 μmol/L. His liver functions tests were abnormal and he was found to be Hep C IgG positive. Complement C4 (0.04 mg/mL) and C3 (0.65 mg/mL) were both low.

Introduction

Cryoglobulins are circulating immunoglobulins that precipitate in the cold. They usually occur in the presence of underlying infection, autoim-

Table 13.8 Classification and cause of cryoglobulinaemia

	Immunoglobulin type	Cause
Type 1	Monoclonal (IgM > IgG)	Monoclonal gammopathy of renal significance, Waldenström macroglobulinaemia, multiple myleoma
Type 2	Monoclonal (IgMκ 90%) directed against polyclonal immunoglobulin	Hepatitis C, autoimmune disease and other infections
Type 3	Polyclonal IgG/IgM directed against polyclonal immunoglobulin	Hepatitis C, autoimmune disease and other infections

mune disease (particularly Sjögren's syndrome) or lymphoproliferative disease and are classified according to the type(s) or immunoglobulin involved (Table 13.8). Cryoglobulins can cause either hyperviscosity (particularly type 1) or a systemic vasculitic illness with skin, kidney and neurological involvement.

Epidemiology and Causes

Cryoglobulinaemia is an uncommon disease with kidney involvement in approximately 25–50% of cases. In the majority of cases an underlying cause can be identified. Type 1 is associated with a monoclonal immunoglobulin only whereas type 2 and 3 involve different types of immunoglobulin (mixed cryoglobulinaemia), with one component possessing Rheumatoid factor like activity.

Clinical Presentation

Systemic symptoms include malaise, Raynaud phenomenon, arthralgia, hepatosplenomegaly, peripheral neuropathy, skin involvement (common) with levido reticularis, purpuric rash and ulceration and gangrene (Type 1>2 and 3). Renal disease is present in approximately 50% of cases and typically leads to haematuria, proteinuria, hypertension and renal insufficiency. Nephrotic syndrome or rapidly progressive disease can occur.

Investigations

Detection of cryoglobulins can be difficult and requires careful handling of samples to maintain a constant temperature and prevent precipitation. A precipitate is seen on cooling of serum to 4 °C. Rheumatoid factor is positive in mixed cryoglobulinaemia. Liver function is often abnormal (>50% of cases) and complement C4 levels are often suppressed. A screen for an underlying cause will most frequently identify Hepatitis C infection in patients with mixed cryoglobulinaemia.

Kidney biopsy shows endocapillary proliferation with large subendothelial deposits which can fill the capillary lumen. Immunofluorescence is positive for IgG and IgM (with IgM often dominant) and also C3 and C1q.

Differential Diagnosis

There can be features of other systemic autoimmune disease and systemic vasculitis. The presence of cryoglobulins and the renal biopsy appearance are diagnostic of cryoglobulinaemia.

Management

Treatment is usually targeted at the underlying condition, either hepatitis, other infection, lymphoproliferative disease or autoimmune disease. A combination of corticosteroids with a cytotoxic agent or rituximab can be used in idiopathic disease. In severe cases with ulcerative skin involvement, peripheral gangrene or rapidly progressive GN plasma exchange, in addition to corticosteroids and cytotoxics should be considered.

Protein Deposition Diseases

Clinical Scenario

A 72 year old man presents with increasing ankle oedema. He has no other symptoms and other than peripheral oedema clinical examination is normal. He has significant proteinuria with an ACR of 128 mg/mmol and a serum albumin of 26 mg/L. His creatinine is normal. A kidney biopsy shows deposition of hyaline material in the mesangium and capillary walls which shows apple green birefringence under polarised light on Congo red staining.

Introduction

Amyloid describes the deposition of protein fibrils in various organs. Approximately 25 proteins can form amyloid fibrils in association with Serum Amyloid P component and all demonstrate characteristic apple green birefringence under polarised light on Congo red staining.

Epidemiology and Causes

Renal amyloid is uncommon affecting approximately 10 per million population per year and is found in approximately 2% of kidney biopsies. AA and AL are the most common renal amyloidoses accounting for >80% of cases the remainder being due to hereditary amyloidoses. AL amyloid is caused by the deposition of a proportion of an immunoglobulin light chain ($\lambda > \kappa$, 12:1) produced by a clonal population of plasma cells. AA amyloid is due to the deposition Serum Amyloid A protein in chronic inflammatory conditions. The reason that amyloid fibrils form only in some patients is not known. Genetic variants in Fibrinogen A, transthyretin, apolipoproteins and leukocyte chemotactic factor 2 (LECT2) and other proteins can cause renal amyloid.

Clinical Presentation

AL amyloid usually involves the kidney and most patients will develop kidney disease at some point. The median age of presentation is 60 years with men affected twice as frequently as women. Patients present with oedema, fatigue, weight loss or painful neuropathy. Renal involvement is most common and is the only organ involved in 30% of cases. Most patients have proteinuria and 25% have nephrotic syndrome. A reduced GFR and hypertension are common. Cardiac (40%), peripheral nerve (25%), lymph node, liver and spleen (hepatosplenomegaly) involvement can occur. Multiple myeloma occurs in about 20% of patients with AL amyloid.

AA amyloid occurs in the context of chronic inflammation, due to chronic infection, inflammatory arthropathy or periodic fever syndromes. Renal involvement causes proteinuria and progressive decline in GFR. The presentation of hereditary amyloidosis is similar, and they can be difficult to distinguish form AL or AA amyloid.

Investigations

Renal amyloid is typically diagnosed in a biopsy from a patient being investigated for proteinuria although amyloid can be diagnosed on liver biopsy or less invasively on skin, fat pad or rectal biopsy. In patients with AL amyloid serum or urinary electrophoresis and immunofixation may show a monoclonal band and serum free light chains will show excess of either λ or κ light chain (monoclonal gammopathy of renal significance).

The injection of radiolabelled SAP (SAP scintigraphy) allows the extent of amyloid deposition to be determined. Genetic screening is required if hereditary amyloid is suspected.

Kidney biopsy demonstrates deposition of acellular hyaline material in the mesangium and capillary walls, which can be nodular, but is not stained by silver stain. Amyloid stains orange with Congo red and has a typical apple green birefringence under polarised light. Immunofluorescence for light λ or κ chains will stain AL amyloid deposits. In all types of amyloid electron microscopy typically shows 8–12 nm-wide fibrils.

Differential Diagnosis

Renal amyloidosis should be considered in older patients presenting with proteinuria. In some cases, there will be systemic symptoms to suggest amyloidosis but biopsy will often be required t distinguish renal amyloid from other proteinuric diseases.

Management

AL amyloid has a poor prognosis without treatment (median survival <2 years) with cardiac or renal involvement predicting a poor outcome. Prognosis has improved with the introduction of new treatments. If the patient is fit enough autologous stem cell transplantation (ASCT) should be considered otherwise chemotherapy (for example melphalan and corticosteroids) are effective. A response to treatment and reduction in light chain production (monitored by serum free light chain measurements) can lead to regression of deposits and good long-term outcomes. Bortezomib can also be used, often in combination with chemotherapy. The anti-CD38 monoclonal antibody, daratumumab, has shown promising results in the treatment of AL amyloid.

AA amyloid treatment is targeted at the underlying inflammatory disease. If inflammation can be suppressed with control of SAA protein concentration the prognosis is good (median survival >10 years) and amyloid deposits can regress.

In patients with ESKD due to amyloid transplantation can be considered if inflammation or the plasma cell clone is suppressed (usually after ASCT).

Other Forms of Protein Deposition Disease

Fibrillary glomerulonephritis, with 20 nm fibrils containing the chaperone protein DNAJB9 and IgG, can be idiopathic or occur in association with monoclonal gammopathies and malignancy. *Fibronectin nephropathy* is an autosomal dominant inherited disease that has a similar fibrillary structure, but the deposits contain fibronectin.

Immunotactoid glomerulonephritis is associated with larger (30–50 nm) hollow microtubules containing immunoglobulin which is commonly monoclonal. This disease has a poor prognosis, progresses rapidly to ESKD and is often associated with a lymphoproliferative disorder.

Monoclonal immunoglobulin deposition disease (MIDD) describes a group of diseases characterised by light chain, heavy chain or light and heavy chain deposition. *Light chain deposition disease* is most common, with granular, non-amyloid deposits of light chain (usually the constant region of κ). The median age of presentation is 50–60 years and an abnormal serum free light chain can usually be identified. On biopsy immunofluorescence for the abnormal immunoglobulin fragment is usually positive. Treatment is the same as for AL amyloid.

Thrombotic Microangiopathies (TMAs)

Clinical Scenario

A 12 year old girl presents with breathlessness and fatigue. She also reported passing 'coca-cola' coloured urine. Ten days previously she had 5 days of abdominal pain and diarrhoea which had resolved by the time she presented. On examination mucosal membranes were pale and blood pressure was raised at 148/108 mmHg. Urinalysis was positive for blood. Haematology screen showed a severe anaemia (Hb 54 g/L) and thrombocytopenia (Platelets 32 × 10^9/L). The blood film showed evidence of fragmentation. She had AKI with a Cr of 292 μmol/L.

Introduction

The thrombotic microangiopathies (TMAs) are a group of diseases characterised by microangiopathic haemolytic anaemia (MAHA), thrombocytopenia and end organ damage due to small vessel thrombosis. Classically TMA was divided into two diseases depending upon the clinical presentation; Thrombotic Thrombocytopenic Purpura (TTP) in which neurological manifestations predominated and Haemolytic Uraemic Syndrome (HUS) in which kidney involvement was more common. However, there is significant overlap in clinical presentation and therefore it is more appropriate to consider TMAs according to their aetiology. Both TTP and HUS can be inherited or acquired.

Epidemiology and Causes

TTP is due to inherited (very rare) or acquired deficiency in a circulating enzyme, ADAMTS13 which is responsible for the breakdown of large multimers of von Willebrand factor. Reduced breakdown leads to activation of coagulation and thrombus formation. Acquired disease effect 5–10 per million population per year and is due to an inhibitory autoantibody.

HUS is most commonly due to infection with a shiga toxin producing enteropathogen, either *Escherichia coli* (STEC) or *Shigella,* which occurs after consumption of contaminated food. The toxin impairs endothelial function leading to thrombus formation. STEC HUS has an incidence of 20 per million population, most common affects children and can occur in localised outbreaks. STEC HUS accounts for 90% of HUS cases. The remaining cases, termed atypical HUS, are most commonly due to a defect in complement regulation leading to excessive activation and endothelial injury. A TMA can develop in response to a defined trigger including infection (HIV), drugs (anti-VEGF, calcineurin inhibitors, mitomycin, gemcitabine), after bone marrow transplantation or malignancy. HUS can also follow infection with *Streptococcus pneumonia* (pneumococcal HUS).

TMA occurring after a transplant can be complement mediated atypical HUS particularly if atypical HUS was the cause of ESKD, but can also be CNI toxicity or an infective or alloimmune process.

Clinical Presentation

TMAs and present with a range of symptoms and should be considered in any patient with unexplained anaemia [with fragmented red cells] and thrombocytopenia. Serum LDH can be elevated with low haptoglobin and negative coombs test. TTP typically presents with neurological involvement (>80%) but renal involvement is seen in 30% and systemic features including fever and other organ involvement (heart, pancreas) are common (25–50%). Very low platelet counts and raised inflammatory markers is typically evident. Without treatment TTP has a poor prognosis with a mortality of >50% which can occur rapidly (hours) after presentation.

Symptoms of STEC infection typically develop 3 days after infection with diarrhoea (bloody in 60%) and abdominal pain. This resolves after 5–7 days. Only about 15% of patients with STEC infection then go onto develop HUS. Anaemia can be severe and AKI is almost always present and 60% of patients require dialysis. Neurological involvement is reported in 20–50% of cases. Recovery occurs in most cases, although death can occur (<5%) and CKD and hypertension can develop.

Atypical HUS usually causes AKI but other organ involvement is common, including abdominal pain and diarrhoea. An environmental trigger (e.g. pregnancy) can be identified. The presentation of secondary forms of HUS will be defined by the underlying cause.

Differential Diagnosis

Other diseases that can present with features similar to a TMA with thrombocytopenia and MAHA include sepsis with disseminated intravascular coagulation (abnormal coagulation and low fibrinogen) and autoimmune disease particularly SLE and APS (prolonged PT and APL antibodies). Malignant hypertension, causing endothelial injury, can cause thrombocytopenia, MAHA and AKI and is difficult to differentiate from other causes of TMA which can cause hypertension.

Investigation and Management

It is important to diagnose a TMA in a patient as prompt initiation of treatment is important particularly for TTP. There are no reliable clinical features to distinguish between the causes of TMA although certain features, for example presence of bloody diarrhoea 1 week before presentation in a patient with STEC, will suggest the cause. The investigation and management of TMA are summarised (Fig. 13.1).

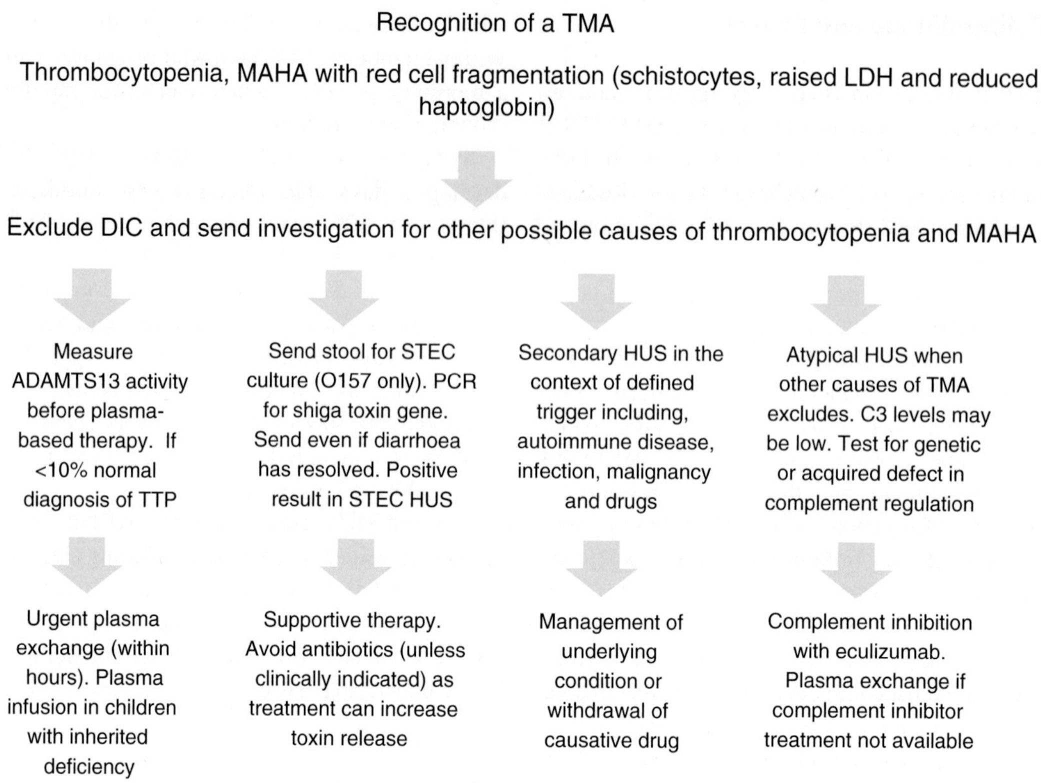

Fig. 13.1 Investigation and management of a TMA

Plasma exchange should be started as soon as the diagnosis of TMA is made until TTP has been excluded by assessing ADAMTS13 activity. The diagnosis of STEC HUS may be suggested by the history of colitic symptoms, but these are not always present (approximately 10%) and diarrhoea will usually have stopped by the time HUS develops. There may be evidence of an inflammatory response with high WCC and CRP. It is important to send stool for culture and PCR even if diarrhoea has stopped.

Atypical HUS is a diagnosis of exclusion and if suspected the patient should be assessed for abnormalities in complement regulation including genetic loss of function variants in complement factor H, factor I and CD46. Gain of function variants in the complement pathway proteins C3 and factor B can also occur. Approximately 10% (or higher in some countries) of cases of atypical HUS are due to acquired autoantibodies to factor H.

The management depends on the cause of TMA. TTP requires urgent plasma exchange which should be started until TTP has been excluded. Although, many different therapies have been tested in STEC HUS there is no evidence for anything other than supportive care including dialysis if required. Complement inhibition with eculizumab, if available, is effective in atypical HUS otherwise plasma exchange should be considered.

If a kidney biopsy is performed there is evidence of thrombi in the glomerular capillaries and small and medium sized arteries. Other features include mesangiolysis, microaneurysm formation and necrosis in blood vessel walls.

Practice Points

- Clinical assessment, including serological testing and kidney biopsy, are important to diagnose secondary glomerular diseases.
- Most secondary glomerular diseases are treatable. Treatment is determined by the diagnosis, severity of kidney involvement and extra-renal disease manifestations.
- Treatment will often involve a combination of drugs the use of which is associated with significant risk and therefore treatment should be supervised by an experienced clinician.
- Secondary glomerular diseases can relapse so long-term monitoring is important.

Conclusions

The presentation of secondary glomerulonephritis present with haematuria, proteinuria, increase creatinine and hypertension. Extrarenal features such as skin rash, joint pains, oral ulcers may be helpful like the 67-year-old man with ANCA-associated vasculitis. However the diagnosis largely depends on serological findings and kidney biopsy. Immunosuppressive treatment has improved outcomes over the last four decades. Better understanding of the pathophysiology and drug development has helped us with newer therapies.

Questions

1. In a patient who is diagnosed with PR3-ANCA associated with a GPA phenotype which of the following are correct:
   A. The PR3 ANCA detects proteinase 3 in a perinuclear distribution by immunofluorescence
   B. The risk of relapse after induction is lower than in a patient who is MPO-ANCA positive
   C. Higher cumulative dose of corticosteroids is associated with increased mortality
   D. C5aR inhibition can replace cyclophosphamide as part of the induction regime
   E. Rituximab is only indicated if induction with cyclophosphamide has been unsuccessful

   Answer: C (Difficult)

   A significant proportion of mortality in AAV is attributed to treatment. Lower doses of corticosteroids appear to be equally effective with a better side effect profile and associated with lower mortality rates. The other answers are incorrect.
2. In the clinical TMA clinical case which of the following is true:
   A. The presence of AKI excludes a diagnosis of TTP
   B. STEC HUS is unlikely because the diarrhoea has stopped
   C. STEC HUS can be excluded by a negative stool culture
   D. Close contacts should be screened for STEC infection
   E. STEC is likely so neurological disease will not occur

   Answer: D (Difficult)

   The likely diagnosis is STEC HUS. This can be passed from person to person and outbreaks can occur. Close household contacts should be screened. The presence of AKI does not exclude TTP, but the preceding history and age of the patient make TTP unlikely. STEC HUS typically develops after diarrhoea has stopped and neurological disease can occur. A negative culture does not exclude STEC HUS, particularly in the stool sample is sent after antibiotics. PCR is more sensitive and can remain positive when culture is negative.
3. For a 24 year woman with a new diagnosis of SLE, proteinuria (2 g/day), a Cr of 138 μmol/L and a kidney biopsy demonstrating Class IV LN which of the following treatment option should be advised:
   A. Pulse methylprednisolone followed by oral steroids
   B. Pulse methylprednisolone followed by oral steroids and azathioprine
   C. Pulse methylprednisolone followed by oral steroids and plasma exchange

D. Pulse methylprednisolone followed by oral steroids and MMF
E. Pulse methylprednisolone followed by oral steroids and oral cyclophosphamide

Answer: D (Easy)

The only first line treatment is steroids and MMF. Cyclophosphamide is given intravenously for the treatment of LN.

4. A 60-year-old man presented with a 5 day history of abdominal pain. He is drowsy and hypertensive (BP 188/108 mmHg) but otherwise examination was normal. He was anaemic (Hb 94 g/L) with a platelet count of 16×10^9/L. He has evidence of AKI with a Cr of 316 μmol/L. Which is the most important next step.
   A. Haemodialysis
   B. Plasma exchange
   C. Platelet transfusion
   D. Plasma infusion
   E. Blood pressure control

Answer: B (Easy)

This could be TTP with a reduced level of consciousness and very low platelet count. It is a medical emergency and should be treated urgently with plasma exchange until ADAMTS13 activity is known. In this age group an inhibitor of ADAMTS13 is more likely so plasma infusion is insufficient.

5. In the protein deposition clinical case which is the most likely diagnosis:
   A. AL amyloid due to a polyclonal plasma cell disorder
   B. AA amyloid due to an undiagnosed chronic infection
   C. AL amyloid due to an undiagnosed chronic infection
   D. AA amyloid due to monoclonal plasma cell disorder
   E. AL amyloid due to monoclonal plasma cell disorder

Answer: E (Easy)

AL amyloid is more likely that AA amyloid and is use to an abnormal plasma cell clone (not polyclonal). AA amyloid is associated with chronic infection.

6. In the cryoglobulinaemia clinical case the low level of C4 suggests:
   A. A likely association with SLE
   B. Activation of the alternative pathway of complement
   C. Reduced hepatic synthesis of C4 due to liver disease
   D. The presence of C1q binding immune complexes
   E. An underlying defect in complement regulation resulting in excessive activation

Answer: D (Difficult)

The formation of immune complexes in cryoglobulinaemis will activate the classical pathway of complement due to C1q binding the Fc position of IgG and IgM. This leads to the low C4 which is typically found in croglobulinaemia in the absence of any other autoimmune disease.

7. In which of the following protein deposition diseases is not associated with immunoglobulin fragment deposition:
   A. Light chain deposition disease
   B. AA Amyloid
   C. AL Amyoid
   D. Fibrillary glomerulonephritis
   E. Immunotactoid glomerulonephritis

Answer: B (Easy)

AA amyloid is due to deposition of Serum Amyloid A protein. The other diseases are due to deposition of immunoglobulin (or a fragment of immunoglobulin).

8. In the AAV case a biopsy was performed which showed a necrotising glomerulonephritis with crescents in 35% of glomeruli. Which of the following is the most appropriate treatment:
   A. High dose corticosteroids
   B. High dose corticosteroids and azathioprine
   C. High dose corticosteroids and cyclophosphamide
   D. High dose corticosteroids, cyclophosphamide and plasma exchange
   E. Delay immunosuppression because of concerns about infection

Answer: C (Easy)

The presence of fever raised white cell count and CRP are consistent with a diagnosis of vasculitis and should not delay treatment. A combination of corticosteroids with cyclophosphamide is the most appropriate treatment. There is no benefit of adding plasma exchange.

9. In the SLE clinical scenario which of the following statements about investigation is most appropriate:
   A. Provided kidney function does not decline further a biopsy is not required
   B. ANA titers are specific for a diagnosis of SLE
   C. Anti-Sm antibodies will be positive in most cases of lupus nephritis
   D. Low serum C3 concentration reflects urinary protein loss
   E. Anti-dsDNA antibody titres are associated with disease activity

Answer: E (difficult)

Anti dsDNa antibody titres do reflect disease activity. A kidney biopsy is required to assess class of lupus nephritis. ANA titres are found in a range of autoimmune disease unlike anti-Sm which is specific to SLE but only found in a minority of cases. Low C3 levels are due to complement activation and consumption.

10. In a patient with mixed croglobulinaemia which antibodies could be found in the precipitate from serum on cooling:
   A. Monoclonal IgM binding polyclonal IgG
   B. Polyclonal IgG binding monoclonal IgM
   C. Polyclonal IgM binding to monoclonal IgG
   D. Polyclonal IgG binding monoclonal IgG
   E. Monoclonal IgM binding monoclonal IgM

Answer: A (Difficult)

In most cases of mixed cryoglobulinaemia type 2 a monoclonal immunoglobulin (usually IgM) with Rheumatoid factor activity will bind to polyclonal IgG and IgM.

Test your learning and check your understanding of this book's contents: use the "Springer Nature Flashcards" app to access questions using https://www.sn.pub/cz9Cok. To use the app, please follow the instructions in Chap. 1.

References

1. Jennette JC, Falk RJ, Bacon PA, Basu N, Cid MC, Ferrario F, Flores-Suarez LF, Gross WL, Guillevin L, Hagen EC, et al. 2012 revised international Chapel Hill consensus conference nomenclature of vasculitides. Arthritis Rheum. 2013;65(1):1–11.
2. Walsh M, Merkel PA, Peh CA, Szpirt WM, Puechal X, Fujimoto S, Hawley CM, Khalidi N, Flossmann O, Wald R, et al. Plasma exchange and glucocorticoids in severe ANCA-associated vasculitis. N Engl J Med. 2020;382(7):622–31.
3. Aringer M, Costenbader K, Daikh D, Brinks R, Mosca M, Ramsey-Goldman R, Smolen JS, Wofsy D, Boumpas DT, Kamen DL, et al. 2019 European League Against Rheumatism/American College of Rheumatology classification criteria for systemic lupus erythematosus. Ann Rheum Dis. 2019;78(9):1151–9.
4. Weening JJ, D'Agati VD, Schwartz MM, Seshan SV, Alpers CE, Appel GB, Balow JE, Bruijn JA, Cook T, Ferrario F, et al. The classification of glomerulonephritis in systemic lupus erythematosus revisited. Kidney Int. 2004;65(2):521–30.
5. Fanouriakis A, Kostopoulou M, Cheema K, Anders HJ, Aringer M, Bajema I, Boletis J, Frangou E, Houssiau FA, Hollis J, et al. 2019 update of the joint European League Against Rheumatism and European Renal Association-European Dialysis and Transplant Association (EULAR/ERA-EDTA) recommendations for the management of lupus nephritis. Ann Rheum Dis. 2020;79(6):713–23.
6. Tamirou F, D'Cruz D, Sangle S, Remy P, Vasconcelos C, Fiehn C, del Mar Ayala Guttierez M, Gilboe IM, Tektonidou M, Blockmans D, et al. Long-term follow-up of the MAINTAIN nephritis trial, comparing azathioprine and mycophenolate mofetil as maintenance therapy of lupus nephritis. Ann Rheum Dis. 2016;75(3):526–31.

Infections and the Kidney

14

Saraladevi Naicker, John B. Eastwood,
Gloria Ashuntantang, and Ifeoma Ulasi

Clinical Scenario 1

A 71-year old woman with end-stage kidney disease (ESKD) secondary to diabetic nephropathy, maintained on twice-weekly haemodialysis (HD), was admitted for management of profuse rectal bleeding secondary to diverticulitis. She was catheterised and transfused with a unit of packed red cells. A week into her admission, she started vomiting and became listless. Her temperature and vital signs were normal. Urinalysis revealed a positive leukocyte esterase, and her urine bag and tubing acquired a purple colour (Fig. 14.1a). Urine samples obtained from the urine bag and urethral catheter did not have the purple coloration (Fig. 14.1b and c). The urethral catheter was removed and her urine cultured, yielding. *Escherichia coli* sensitive to Ceftazidime. She was treated with intravenous ceftazidime, with resolution of her symptoms, and a negative urine culture thereafter.

Clinical Scenario 2

An 11-year-old female, presented to the emergency department (ED) with a 2-week history of fever. For the previous 6 days, she had noted that her urine had become brown (sometimes referred to as "coke-coloured") followed by a reduced urine output, and generalized body swelling. Two days before admission she had become short of breath, and a few hours before she attended the ED she had suffered a seizure. She had had a skin infection 3 weeks prior to her symptoms. On examination, she was pale, febrile, in respiratory distress, with an impaired state of consciousness, with a Glasgow coma score of 8/15. Her temperature was 37.8 °C, her respiratory rate 38 breaths/min, BP 160/110 mmHg, and pulse 110/min. She had significant bilateral pitting leg oedema. It was also noted that she had multiple bilateral hyperpigmented macular skin lesions. She had demonstrable ascites and fine bilateral crepitations. Catheterization revealed the brown urine, with a urine flow rate of 0.3 mL/kg/h. Urinalysis showed blood, protein, leukocytes, and microscopy revealed red cell casts. Blood results: Sodium: 122 mmol/L, potassium: 5.6 mmol/L, HCO_3 12.4 mmol/L, chloride: 84.4, iCa: 1.01, BUN: 63.3 mmol/L, creatinine: 884 μmol/L, hae-

S. Naicker (✉)
Department of Internal Medicine, School of Clinical Medicine, University of the Witwatersrand, Johannesburg, South Africa
e-mail: saraladevi.naicker@wits.ac.za

J. B. Eastwood
Department of Renal Medicine, Institute of Medical and Biomedical Education, St. George's University of London, London, UK
e-mail: jbeastwo@sgul.ac.uk

G. Ashuntantang
Department of Internal Medicine and Specialties, Faculty of Medicine and Biomedical Sciences, University of Yaoundé, Yaoundé, Cameroon

I. Ulasi
Department of Medicine, University of Nigeria, Ituku-Ozalla, Enugu, Nigeria and Federal Teaching Hospital, Abakaliki, Nigeria
e-mail: ifeoma.ulasi@unn.edu.ng

D. Banerjee et al. (eds.), *Management of Kidney Diseases*,
https://doi.org/10.1007/978-3-031-09131-5_14

Table 14.2 (continued)

Category	Complicated UTI	Recurrent UTIs: relapse/reinfection	Sepsis/urosepsis
Treatment and Follow-up	**EAU Guidelines 2019** [7]: Patients with systemic symptoms requiring hospital admission should be initially treated with an IV antimicrobial regimen: aminoglycoside with/without amoxicillin, or a second or third generation cephalosporin, or an *Extended-spectrum beta-lactamase* with or without an aminoglycoside Choice should be based on local resistance data and susceptibility results. Considering current resistance percentages of amoxicillin, co-amoxicillin/clavulanic acid, TMP and TMP-SMX, they should not be used for treatment of all complicated UTIs **NICE Guidance: 2018 Update** [10] Ceftolozane/tazobactam 1 g/0.5 g IV 8 hourly (very expensive compared to other antibiotics); Levofloxacin 500 mg (up to 750 mg IV daily); Piperacillin/tazobactam 4 g/0.5 g IV 8 hourly; Cefotaxime 2–12 g IV daily in divided doses; Cefuroxime 1.5 g IV 8 hourly; Ceftazidime 1–2 g IV 8 or 12 hourly; Ceftriaxone 1–2 g IV daily; Ciprofloxacin IV 400 mg 8 or 12 hourly or oral 500 mg 12 hourly; Meropenem 0.5–1 g IV 8 hourly; Gentamicin IV 3–6 mg/kg in divided doses or 160 mg once daily Duration of treatment: 10–14 days; closely related to the treatment of the underlying abnormality Follow-up urine cultures should be performed post treatment	Figure 14.3 shows an algorithm for management approach.) [12] for management Antibiotic prophylaxis [13]: Choose antibiotics depending on recent culture and susceptibility results. Select a different antibiotic for prophylaxis if treating an acute UTI **First choice:** TMP 200 mg single dose when exposed to a trigger, **or** 100 mg at night Nitrofurantoin (if eGFR ≥45 mL/min) 100 mg single dose when exposed to a trigger, **or** 50–100 mg at night **Second choice:** Cefalexin 500 mg single dose when exposed to a trigger, **or** 125 mg at night For those who have urological anomaly, correct surgically if possible **Correctable abnormalities** include: Infected stones, chronic bacterial prostatitis Infected atrophic kidneys, ectopic/duplex ureters Foreign bodies, etc.	**EAU Guidelines 2019** [7]: Commence intravenous antibiotics promptly to eliminate the infection Supportive care: Institute measures to prevent further injury (avoid nephrotoxic agents) Stabilize and maintain effective intravascular volume and renal perfusion Adopt early goal-directed therapy using volume and vasopressor support (fluid, vasopressors, blood products, and inotropes) to achieve and maintain a mean arterial pressure of 65 mmHg and a central venous pressure of 8–12 mmHg **Antibiotics for 7–10 days or longer:** Cefotaxime 2 g 8 hourly; Ceftazidime 1–2 g 8 hourly; Ceftriaxone 1–2 g daily; Cefepime 2 g 12 hourly; Piperacillin/tazobactam 4.5 g 8 hourly; Ceftolozane/tazobactam 1.5 g 8 hourly Ceftazidime/avibactam 2.5 g 8 hourly/5 mg/kg daily; Ertapenem 1 g daily; Imipenem/cilastatin 0.5 g 8 hourly; Meropenem 1 g 8 hourly

CT computerized tomography, *IV* intravenous, *IVU* intra-venous urogram, *MSU* mid stream urine microscopy, *MC&S* microscopy, culture and sensitivities, *TMP* trimethoprim, *TMP-SMX* trimethoprim-sulfamethoxazole

Table 14.3 Investigations and management of chronic tubulo-interstitial nephritis (TIN), genitourinary TB and leptospirosis

Category	Chronic TIN/chronic kidney disease (CKD)	Genitourinary TB	Leptospirosis
Investigations	Urinalysis: microscopy and dipsticks MSU MC&S Blood culture Imaging studies	Diagnosis of UGTB requires high index of suspicion. Patients who have insidious onset, non-specific symptoms with culture-negative pyuria in endemic regions must be evaluated for UGTB. Imaging studies (abdominal x-ray, MRI) may help diagnosis Confirm diagnosis with urine: at least 6 (preferably >9) specimens of urine, prostatic secretion or ejaculate cultured in Lowenstein–Jensen, Finn–II, and Middlebrook 7H9-12 media [13]. Detection of AAFB from samples by microscopy using Ziehl-Nielsen acid fast stain is unreliable, as M. smegmatis are acid-fast too [14] Histopathological examination is the gold standard, PCR has sensitivity and specificity of 87.5% and 86.7% respectively [13]. GeneXpert MTB/RIF outperforms AFB smear and culture for the detection of mycobacterium in urine samples [15]. Ultrasound-guided fine needle aspiration of the abscess/masses may show histologic evidence of UGTB. Other investigations: tuberculin provocation test with 20, 50 or 100 units injected subcutaneously; cystoscopy and ureteroscopy; bladder biopsy	Based on clinical and epidemiologic data and confirmed through Microscopic Agglutination Test (MAT) for serology identification and PCR amplification of DNA of the spirochete from blood [16]. However, MAT is most widely performed using 2 blood samples collected 2 weeks apart

(continued)

Table 14.3 (continued)

Category	Chronic TIN/chronic kidney disease (CKD)	Genitourinary TB	Leptospirosis
Treatment and Follow-up	Treat existing infection; Prevent future infections; Preserve renal function Institute conservative CKD management: Restrict dietary protein intake Aggressive BP control using antihypertensives like ACEi Commence kidney replacement therapy at end-stage	EAU Guidelines for UGTB [14] *First 2 months:* Isoniazid (INH) 300 mg daily; Rifampicin 600 mg daily; Ethambutol 1200 mg daily; Pyrazinamide 2000 mg daily; Pyridoxine 20 mg daily or 50 mg alt daily *Continuation phase (4 months):* Isoniazid (INH) 300 mg daily; Rifampicin 600 mg daily; Pyridoxine 20 mg daily or 50 mg alt daily *Dosage Calculation:* [14] *Anti-TB drug—dose mg/kg (body weight–daily dose)* *Isoniazid—5 mg/kg (300 mg)* *Rifampicin—10 mg/kg (<50 kg–450 mg; >50 kg–600 mg)* *Pyrazinamide—25–35 (<50 kg–1.5 g; >50 kg–2.0 g; >75 kg–2.5 g)* *Streptomycin—15–20 (<50 kg–0.75 g; >50 kg−1.0 g)* *Ethambutol—25 (2.0 g; 0.8–2.0 g)* *Ethionamide—5–15 (0.5–1.0 g)* Surgery includes: Abscess drainage, total or partial nephrectomy, epididymectomy, correction of ureteral strictures, etc.	Appropriate antibiotics such as penicillin or tetracycline are effective for leptospiral nephropathy [17]

AAFB alcohol & acid-fast bacilli, *ACEi* angiotensin converting enzyme inhibitors, *BP* blood pressure, *CKD* chronic kidney diease, *DNA* deoxy-ribonucleic acid, *EAU* European Association of Urology, *INH* isoniazid, *MAT* microscopic agglutination test, *MC&S* microscopy culture & sensitivities, *MSU* mid-stream urine, *PCR* polymerase-chain reaction, *TB* tuberculosis, *TIN* tubule-interstitial nephritis, *UGTB* uro-genital tuberculosis

Asymptomatic bacteriuria: Is defined as significant bacteriuria in a midstream urine (MSU) specimen in people with no relevant genitourinary symptoms, with uro-pathogens $>10^5$ CFU/mL in two consecutive samples in females, or a single sample in males [6, 7].

Uncomplicated UTIs: Consist of community-acquired cystitis (lower urinary tract infection with symptoms of dysuria, frequent and urgent urination and suprapubic pain) and pyelonephritis (infection of the renal parenchyma and pelvi-calyceal system with symptoms of fever and flank pain). Figure 14.2 and Table 14.1 outline an algorithm for management of uncomplicated UTIs [9].

Complicated UTIs: Infection associated with a structural/functional genitourinary tract anomaly or underlying diseases that increase risk of worse outcome [8]; such as: indwelling urinary catheters, urinary obstruction, anatomical abnor-

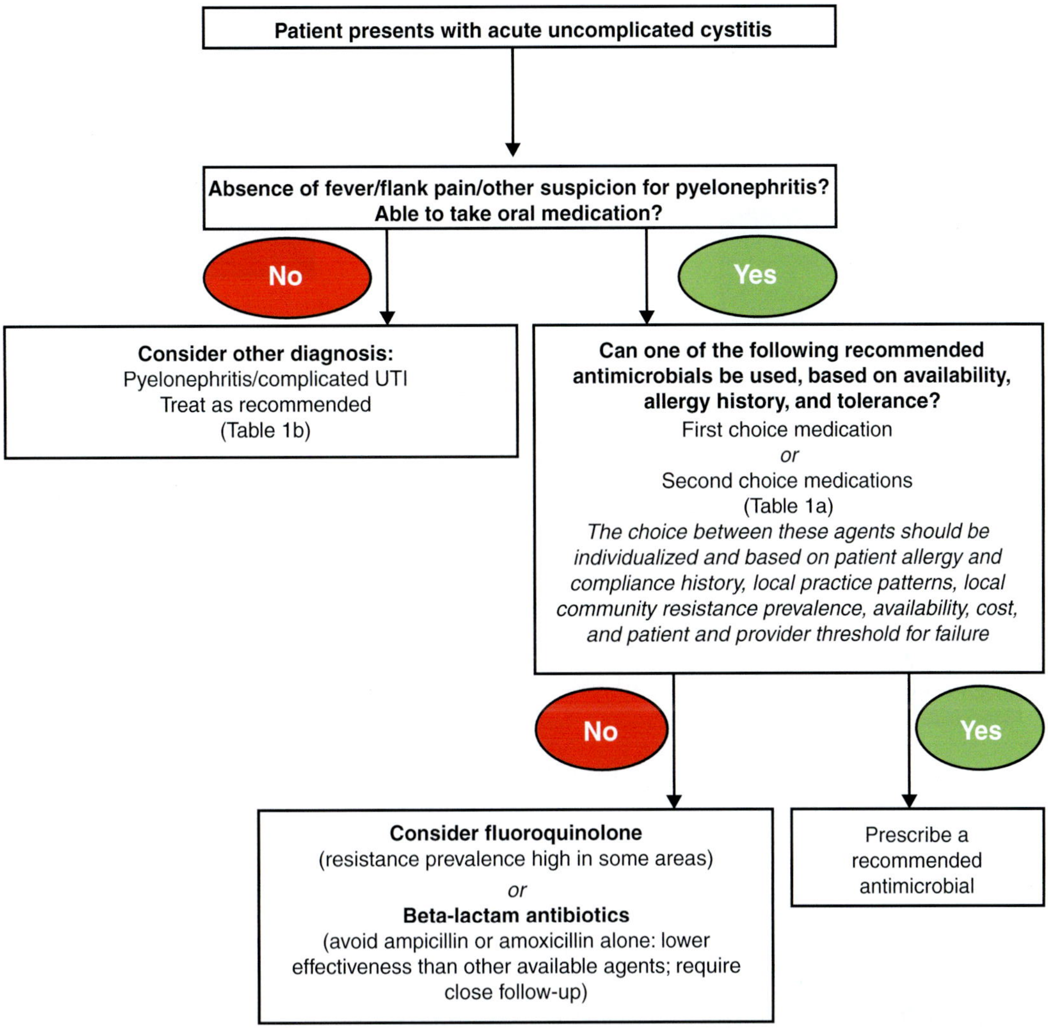

Fig. 14.2 Algorithm for the approach to management of acute uncomplicated cystitis (adapted from IDSA Guidelines [9]). *UTI* urinary tract infection

malities, peri-operative urinary tract infections, including kidney transplantation (Table 14.2).

Recurrent UTIs: Defined as at least three episodes of uncomplicated infection confirmed by urine culture over a 12-month period or 2 episodes over 6 months. They include lower and upper UTIs. The two types of recurrent UTI are:

Relapse—defined as recurrent UTI involving the same organism(s) after adequate therapy; and

Reinfection—defined as recurrent UTI caused by an infection that has been treated and subsequent repeat infection with the original bacteria or a second or new isolate [6]. Figure 14.3 illustrates an algorithm for management of recurrent UTIs [11].

Complications of UTIs include:

Urosepsis: Complicated and severe UTI occurring in the setting of a systemic inflammatory response syndrome (SIRS). It causes multiple organ dysfunction (acute respiratory distress syndrome, acute kidney injury (AKI), and disseminated intravascular coagulopathy (DIC)). In 20–30% of patients with sepsis, the urinary tract is the source; the estimated global mortality rate

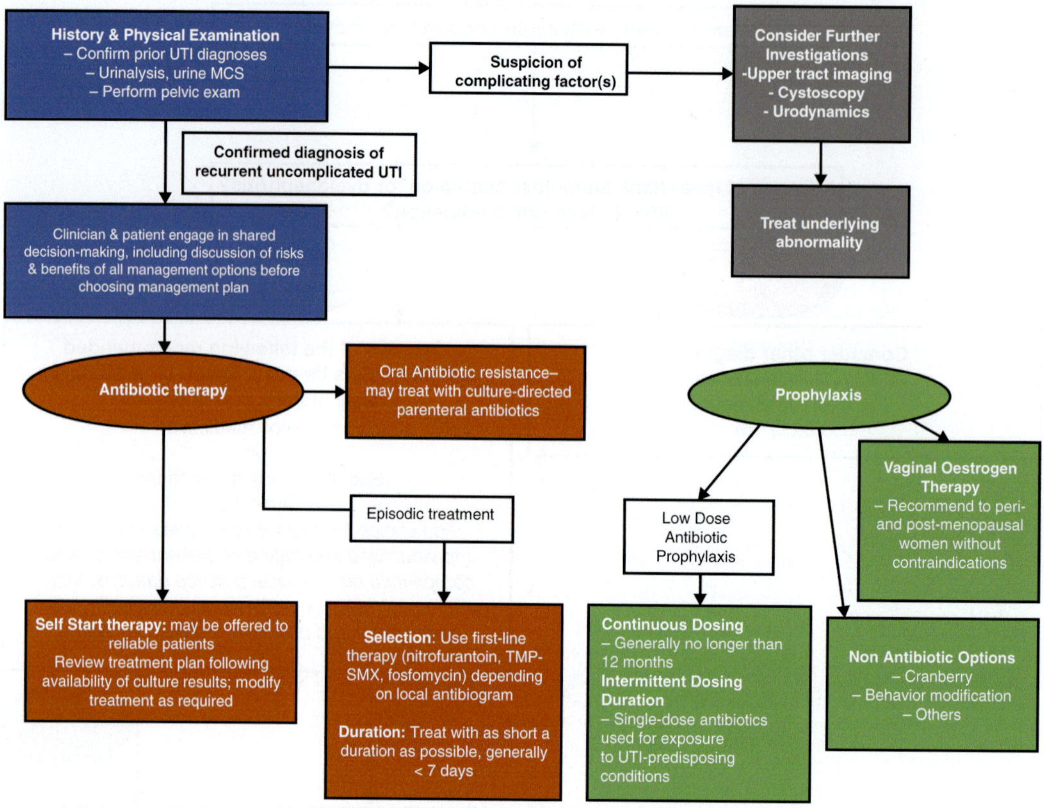

Fig. 14.3 Algorithm for management of recurrent uncomplicated urinary tract infections [11]. The target patient group is of otherwise healthy adult females with recurrent uncomplicated UTIs; Patients with complicating factors such as listed below are outside the scope of the pathway: (1) Anatomic or functional abnormality of the urinary tract, (2) Immunocompromised host, (3) Multi-drug resistant bacteria. *MCS* microscopy, culture & sensitivities, *TMP-SMX* trimethoprim-sulfamethoxazole, *UTI* urinary tract infection

for sepsis is about 30–40% [18]. The management of urosepsis is outlined in Table 14.2. Predisposing factors include urological anomalies, stones, urinary tract obstruction and, in male children, posterior urethral valves.

Other complications of UTI include kidney abscess, perinephric abscess, infected hydronephrosis/pyonephrosis, acute focal bacterial nephritis, emphysematous and xanthogranulomatous pyelonephritis, and malakoplakia.

Reflux Nephropathy

Reflux nephropathy has replaced the term 'Chronic pyelonephritis', a term that has become obsolete.

Aetiology

Reflux nephropathy is a result of an abnormality at the uretero-vesical junction. The musculature of the lowermost part of the normal ureter prevents reflux of urine from the bladder into the ureter. Failure at the vesico-ureteric junction means that urine passes up the ureter on bladder emptying, and in some patients there is free reflux, even when the bladder is not contracting. This is known as vesico-ureteric reflux (VUR).

Background

Until the 1970s, reflux nephropathy was known as 'chronic pyelonephritis', and was thought to be a chronic progressive condition. It was also thought that each urinary infection was capable of producing a scar, and furthermore that reflux nephropathy caused hypertension. In the 1970s, Dr. Jean Smellie challenged the nephrological world to show that new scars could arise in adulthood: no such developing scars were found. It became clear that the scarring process took place mainly in the first 5 years of life, and that the change in kidney shape and the 'development of scars' during teenage years was simply the result of normal growth of the unaffected kidney tissue, thereby making the existing scarred elements more prominent.

Clinical Management

The abnormality is sometimes first detected *in utero,* when urine may be seen entering the foetal ureter during micturition. This will enable the neonatologist to take appropriate measures to prevent urinary infection in the neo-natal period.

A proportion of young children will present with a febrile illness that may not be recognised initially as a urinary tract infection. It is important to establish such a diagnosis, so that measures can be implemented to keep the urine sterile; this involves keeping the bladder empty. If a significant volume of urine refluxes up the ureter(s), there will inevitably be urine in the bladder after micturition (residual urine). One method in older children is to advise double micturition: the volume passed on the second occasion will give some idea of the scale of the reflux. If necessary, the bladder can be emptied again to be sure that the bladder is empty.

Investigations

VUR is diagnosed by the demonstration of backflow of urine into the upper renal tract(s). Historically, the diagnosis has been made by micturating cystourethrography, which provides good anatomical detail, but does require bladder catheterisation. For older children, indirect radionuclide cystography is preferable, as it does not require catheterisation.

Clinical Features in Adults

Typically in adults, the signs of reflux nephropathy will be found as an incidental finding on abdominal imaging: there will be one or more cortical scars overlying an anatomically distorted calyx, involving one kidney or both. In most cases the vesico-ureteric reflux will have remitted, and the urine will be sterile. In the absence of other factors (such as hypertension), the kidney function will remain relatively stable, and the number of adults requiring kidney replacement therapy (KRT) is small. Chronic kidney disease in this setting tends to progress when there is significant proteinuria (secondary FSGS), when hypertension is not well controlled, or when UTIs continue to recur.

Practice Point 1 Congenital Abnormalities of the Kidneys and Urinary Tract [CAKUT]

CAKUT encapsulates the various congenital urinary tract abnormalities that—although arising in childhood—sometimes present in adulthood, including vesicoureteric reflux. They include duplex pelvicalyceal systems, horseshoe kidney, pelvic kidney, mega-ureter, posterior urethral valves and a number of other uncommon disorders [19]

Mycobacterial Infections

Tuberculosis

Tuberculosis (TB) has a world-wide distribution, but is especially common in developing countries. The highest incidence rates are in sub-Saharan Africa and in the region stretching from the Indian subcontinent to South-East Asia and the Western Pacific (Fig. 14.4). In 2018, ten million people became ill with TB; 1.5 million of them died [21]. The emergence of multi-drug resistant TB as a co-infection with HIV/AIDs has made TB a major public health challenge. Extra-pulmonary TB (ETB) is estimated to occur in 10–34% of patients who do not have HIV, compared to about 50–70% in patients with HIV/AIDs [22].

Kidney involvement occurs as part of a disseminated infection, or as localized genitourinary disease. The disease causes extensive papillary necrosis and cavities, destroying the kidney parenchyma, and extending to the collecting sys-

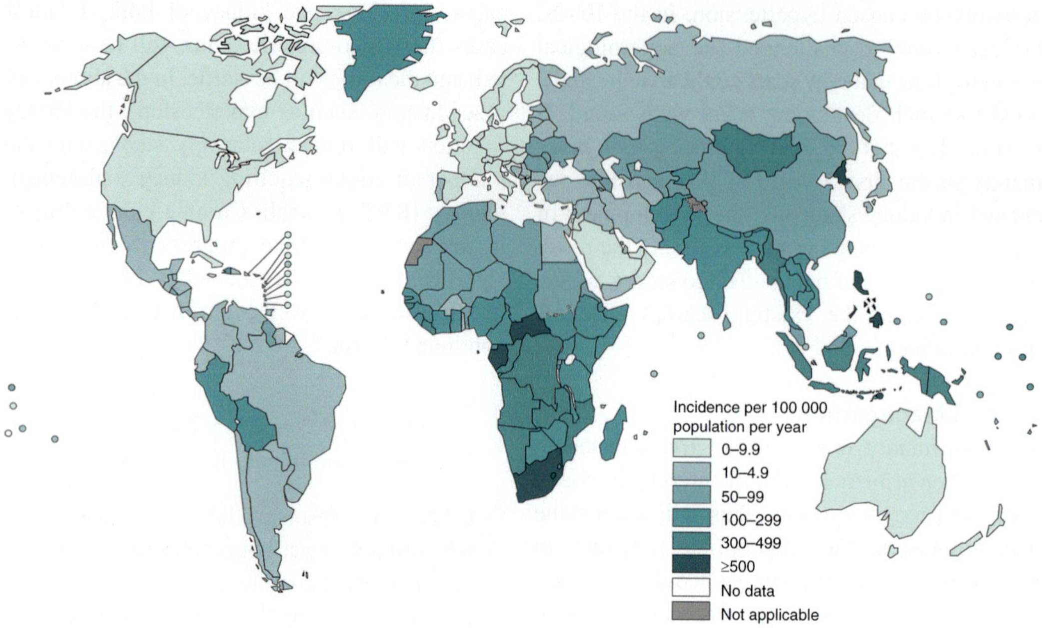

Fig. 14.4 Global Incidence of Tuberculosis in 2020; reproduced with permission from the World Health Organisation (WHO) [20]

tem, causing obstructive uropathy and kidney impairment. Management of genitourinary TB is outlined in Table 14.3. Glomerulopathy (like focal proliferative glomerulonephritis) and amyloidosis can occur from TB occurring in any part of the body [23]. Patients on KRT (haemodialysis, peritoneal dialysis and following kidney transplantation), and those on immunosuppressive therapy are particularly prone to TB infection.

Classical Uro-Genital Tuberculosis (UGTB)

Clinical Features

Uro-genital tuberculosis (UGTB), which is estimated to affect 6–8% of patients with TB, is easy to overlook. Systemic symptoms are uncommon. Often, lower urinary symptoms draw attention to the urinary tract, and typically there is pyuria, but no growth on culture using standard media—a so-called 'sterile' pyuria. Other reasons for the finding of a sterile pyuria are listed in Table 14.4.

The suspicion of TB may be aroused when the symptoms are not relieved by conventional antibiotics, however, there are sometimes suggestive symptoms - back, flank and suprapubic pain, macroscopic haematuria, frequency, and nocturia. Unlike newly-presenting TB, fever, weight loss and night sweats are unusual, and only a third of patients have an abnormal chest X-ray.

Table 14.4 Causes of a 'sterile' pyuria

• Tuberculosis of the uro-genital tract (UGTB)
• *Chlamydia trachomatis, Mycoplasma, Ureaplasma* infection
• Chemically-induced cystitis
• Kidney calculi, prostatitis
• Coliform [or other pathogen] UTI in the presence of antibiotic (inhibiting culture growth)
• Failure to realize that low numbers of organisms can indicate infection
• WBC from outside urinary tract, e.g. from foreskin or vulva
• Kidney parenchymal cause—e.g. acute TIN, glomerular disease

TIN tubulo-interstitial nephropathy, *UGTB* uro-genital tract tuberculosis, *UTI* urinary tract infection, *WBC* white blood cells

Investigations

Abdominal X-ray may show calcification, and urinary tract ultrasound is likely to show focal fibrosis and/or scarring—sometimes severe—as well as calcification in kidneys and bladder (thimble bladder).

Treatment

For newly presenting TB, the World Health Organisation (WHO) recommends oral treatment for 6 months, commencing with 4 drugs, that should include rifampicin and isoniazid (Table 14.3). In patients with kidney dysfunction, careful attention needs to be taken regarding the dosing of the drugs prescribed.

Tuberculous Interstitial Nephritis

There have been a number of reports of interstitial nephritis with granuloma formation, and there has been a suspicion that TB has been responsible. Some patients have had TB elsewhere and hypersensitivity to tuberculin. An early report described three such patients [24]. More recently, it has become clear that such patients cannot reliably be distinguished from sarcoidosis, and it has been suggested that a trial of anti-tuberculous drugs can be justified [25].

End-Stage Kidney Disease

Once TB is recognized and treated, it is likely that kidney replacement therapy (KRT) can be avoided. There are very few data on the frequency of TB as a cause of end-stage kidney disease (ESKD), but there is one report using data from the European Dialysis and Transplant Registry. Analysis of data from 5 years between 1984 and 1991 showed that the primary kidney diagnosis was classified as kidney TB [code 91] in 0.5–1.0% of patients starting KRT [26].

Leprosy

The incidence and prevalence of leprosy has been falling slowly over recent years but there has been little change in the global extent of the disease. It remains more or less confined to middle- and low-income countries, especially Brazil and the countries of the Indian sub-continent (Fig. 14.5).

Clinical Features

Kidney involvement is common in leprosy, and it is now clear that it is the multi-bacillary (lepromatous) form that is most closely associated with kidney disease. A study of 199 autopsies from Brazil showed that 144 [72%] had kidney lesions. Sixty-one of the 144 (42.4%) showed amyloidosis [28]. This included 36% of the lepromatous group but only 5% of the tuberculoid and

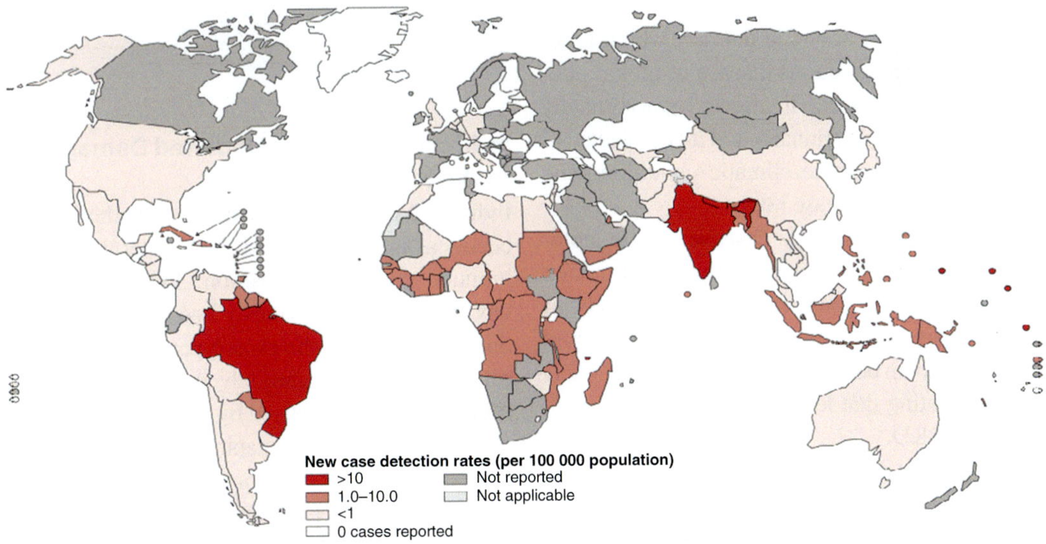

Fig. 14.5 Leprosy new case detection rates 2016 reproduced with permission from the World Health Organisation (WHO) [27]

borderline cases. It was noted that during flare-ups of erythema nodosa leprosum, the serum creatinine would tend to rise.

Silva et al. reported on 16 studies of kidney disease in patients with leprosy [29]. Excluding 10 studies where there was either no biopsy or fewer than five patients, there were 354 biopsies in 6 studies. All six mentioned amyloidosis as the prominent diagnosis; many of the patients described had proteinuria.

There are a few reports of glomerulonephritis among patients with leprosy but there is no consistent pattern, and such associations are as yet unproven.

Treatment

The WHO recommends a 3-drug regimen for multi-bacillary [lepromatous] leprosy - rifampicin, clofazamine and dapsone. The recommendation for pauci-bacillary leprosy [tuberculoid] is a 2-drug regimen - rifampicin and dapsone. Rifampicin and dapsone do not require dose reduction in patients with reduced GFR; for Clofazimine, the UK British National Formulary (BNF) states “Use with caution”.

Leptospirosis

Leptospirosis is a zoonotic disease, which is re-emerging as an infectious disease of global public health importance. It affects approximately 1.03 million people annually and it is projected to rise further as extreme climatic conditions and global warming increase [30].

Leptospirosis Kidney Disease: Acute leptospirosis causes multiple organ dysfunction including AKI. A long-term follow-up study of leptospirosis AKI patients in Sri Lanka found that 9% of them developed an early stage of CKD [31], indicating that leptospirosis AKI can result in CKD/ESKD.

Asymptomatic carriers harbor the Leptospira spirochaete in the kidney where they colonize the proximal tubule resulting in chronic tubulointerstitial nephritis and fibrosis causing insidious progression to CKD. It is thus suggested that asymptomatic exposure to leptospira infection carries the risk for CKD. Histologic findings in leptospirosis kidney disease are tubulointerstitial nephritis, interstitial fibrosis, and tubular atrophy. Proximal tubule dysfunction and hypokalaemia are seen also in adult male patients with leptospirosis. These bear a characteristic similarity to findings in CKD of unknown aetiology (CKDu), a form of CKD that clusters amongst farmers who work in hot dry climates. Table 14.3 outlines the diagnosis and management of leptospirosis.

Practice Point 2 Leptospirosis Kidney Disease and CKDu Overlap

Leptospirosis kidney disease and CKDu tend to affect similar populations in similar geographical regions. The similarity of their kidney pathologies has put leptospirosis as a priority candidate for some patients with CKDu. It is postulated that secondary injury from heat stress and dehydration worsens the kidney injury. Thus, leptospira infection causes primary kidney disease or acts as a CKD susceptibility factor.

Indirect or Immune-Mediated Damage to the Kidney

Indirect bacteria-related damage to the kidney occurs as inflammation of the glomerulus due to immune complex deposition. Infection related GN (IRGN) was previously known as postinfectious GN (PIGN); the prototype, poststreptococcal GN (PSGN) commonly occurs in children. PIGNs are mainly caused by streptococcal infections (28–47%), while staphylococcal and gram-negative infections account for 12–24% and 22%, respectively [32]. Other infections, such as bacterial endocarditis and shunt infections can also cause a PIGN.

Bacterial Infection-Related Glomerulonephritis (B-IRGN)

B-IRGN is described as kidney dysfunction from glomerular inflammation, with evidence of ongoing bacterial infection, unlike PSGN which occurs weeks after the infection. The incidence of IRGN, though decreasing, constitutes about 5% of all glomerular diseases [33]. It occurs more frequently in developing countries. It is commoner in adults, with much higher rates in the elderly and patients with diabetes. Other risk factors include malignancy, malnutrition, chronic infections (HIV and TB), and prosthetic heart valves. IRGN can result from infections occurring in any part of the body (skin, upper and lower respiratory tract, heart, urinary tract, bone). Many bacterial species can be involved, but staphylococcal species are more common in adults and the elderly.

The most common presentation is an acute nephritic syndrome, with or without impaired kidney function. B- IRGN has poorer prognosis than PSGN, and also has a poorer prognosis in adults than in children [32, 33]. Early detection and treatment of infections can prevent kidney involvement (Table 14.5).

Post-streptococcal GN (PSGN)

PSGN is diagnosed in a patient with antecedent streptococcal infection who presents with acute GN; for streptococcal sore-throat, the nephritis follows 7–15 days afterwards, while for skin infections 4–6 weeks after (see Clinical Scenario 2). PSGN is an immune-mediated GN triggered by immune-complex deposits in the subendothelium and mesangium comprising of bacterial antigens (glyceraldehyde-3-phosphate dehydrogenase and streptococcal pyrogenic exotoxin B).

The most common clinical manifestation is acute nephritic syndrome which lasts <2 weeks. Other less common manifestations are asymptomatic proteinuria, nephrotic syndrome or rapidly progressive GN. The prognosis in children is excellent, but in the elderly, there is an associated mortality of up to 20% [32]. The long-term prognosis is worse in patients who have persistent proteinuria >6 months. Clinical Scenario 2 illustrates a typical presentation of severe PSGN, in a patient in Nigeria, although many patients are seen with a less severe presentation. The management of PSGN is outlined in Table 14.5.

Kidney Injury as Part of Ongoing Sepsis

One of the commonest ways by which bacterial infections cause kidney dysfunction is through AKI, which occurs as part of multi-organ dysfunction following sepsis from any focus. About 20% of very ill patients have irreversible kidney injury from acute cortical necrosis and many more (40%) progress to CKD following incomplete recovery [34]. Often, these patients have pre-existing mild-moderate CKD from diverse causes. AKI incidence increases according to severity of sepsis, from 4.2% in mild sepsis to 22.7% in severe sepsis and rising to 52.8% in septic shock [35]. Table 14.3 outlines the management of sepsis/urosepsis.

Nephrotoxic Damage from Medications, Used in Patients with Infection

Drugs commonly cause kidney damage and drug-induced nephrotoxicity (DIN) occurs in 14%–26% and 16% of AKI in adult and paediatric populations respectively [36]. It is commoner in older patients, who are more likely to have diabetes and cardiovascular disease and are consequently exposed to several medications and diagnostic procedures that can harm the kidney. Antibiotics and other medications like non-steroidal anti-inflammatory drugs (NSAIDs) useful in treatment of bacterial infections are known to be nephrotoxic. Table 14.6 shows the common mechanisms leading to drug-induced nephropathy and some implicated medications.

Factors that increase the risk of nephrotoxicity include intravascular volume contraction, age > 60 years, diabetes, use of multiple nephrotoxins, heart failure, sepsis, underlying kidney impairment.

Prevention, vigilance, recognition and early intervention are key to successful outcome [37].

Table 14.5 Investigations and management of other bacterial infection-related kidney diseases: bacterial infection-related glomerulonephritis (B-IRGN), post-streptococcal glomerulonephritis (PSGN) and nephrotoxic damage

Category	Bacterial infection-related GN	Post-streptococcal GN	Nephrotoxic damage
Investigations	Histological findings: membranoproliferative GN, diffuse proliferative GN, or mesangioprolifertive GN with or without crescents	Urinalysis ASO titre Kidney function tests—creatinine, urea/blood urea nitrogen (BUN) C3 complement Kidney biopsy is not indicated except when diagnosis is in doubt. Histology demonstrates acute endocapillary GN with mesangial and capillary granular immune deposition	Urinalysis Complete blood count Kidney function tests Liver function tests
Treatment and Follow-up	Identify and eradicate the infection using appropriate antibiotics Manage complications Immunosuppression is not recommended	Early antibiotic therapy (penicillin, or erythromycin) to help resolve infection Hypertension and oedema respond to diuresis. Admit patients who have severe hypertension or congestive heart failure Serum C3 should normalize in 8–10 weeks; if hypocomplementaemia persists beyond 3 months, perform kidney biopsy Proteinuria persisting beyond 6 months, use ACE-I or ARBs Patients who have extensive glomerular crescents/RPGN should receive pulses of intravenous methylprednisolone Note: antibiotics do not reverse GN	Prevention is crucial: Institute measures to prevent nephrotoxicity: Estimate patient's baseline renal function before prescribing medications (where appropriate monitor blood levels). Avoid combining nephrotoxic agents Check and correct risk factors for nephrotoxicity before initiating therapy Ensure adequate hydration before and during therapy or diagnostic procedures Vigilance, recognition and early intervention are key to successful outcome At first sign of nephrotoxicity, withdraw offending medication Support blood pressure and maintain adequate hydration

Table 14.6 Mechanisms of drug-induced nephropathy

Mechanism of kidney damage	Medications
Disruption of intra-glomerular haemodynamics	ACEIs; ARBs; Cyclosporine
Hypersensitivity	Beta-lactams; Quinolones; Rifampicin; Sulfonamides; Vancomycin
Inflammation	NSAIDs
Tubular cell toxicity	Aminoglycosides; Amphotericin B; Tenofovir
Crystal nephropathy	Ampicillin; Ciprofloxacin; Sulfonamides
Rhabdomyolysis/Haemolysis	Triamterene
Thrombotic microangiopathy	Benzodiazepines; Statins; Clopidogrel; Cyclosporine

ACEIs Angiotensin converting enzyme inhibitors, *ARBs* Angiotensin receptor blockers, *NSAIDs* non-steroidal anti-inflammatory drugs

Awdishu and Mehta proposed the 6R approach (Risk assessment, early Recognition, targeted Response, timely Renal support and Rehabilitation coupled with Research) for management of DIN [38]. Table 14.5 outlines the investigations and management of infection-related kidney damage due to nephrotoxic damage.

Viral Infections and the Kidney

Viral infections can cause kidney damage through direct viral invation, immune mediated damage, haemodynamic instability, haemolysis, rhabdomyolysis, and cytokine storm, amongst other mechanisms. Table 14.7 summarises the viruses associated with kidney damage, the mechanism of injury, typical kidney involvement and management of the condition.

Dengue Virus

Dengue virus (DV) infection causes widespread capillary leakage, dengue haemorrhagic fever (DHF) and dengue shock syndrome (DSS) resulting in ischaemic acute tubular necrosis. Direct viral cytopathic effects, and immune complex injury, haemolysis and rhabdomyolysis are other mechanisms of kidney disease [39]. Clinical manifestations vary from asymptomatic urinary abnormalities to severe acute kidney injury(AKI) in native and allograft kidneys [40]. Proteinuria occurs in over 70%, whereas haematuria is less frequent in DHF. Kidney involvement occurs during acute infection, with detectable anti-DV antibodies and viral nucleic acid in plasma. AKI is more frequent in DHF and DSS and is associated high mortality. Kidney biopsy may reveal acute tubular necrosis, interstitial nephritis and various immune complex GN, as shown in Table 14.7. DV antigen may be detected in tubular epithelial cells [41]. Management is supportive with fluid resuscitation, control of metabolic derangements and management of coagulopathies. Kidney outcomes are good; however, proteinuria and haematuria may persist after recovery of AKI [42].

Hantavirus

Hantavirus(HV) infection is associated with increased vascular permeability and haemorrhage leading to organ dysfunction, with kidney involvement reported in 30–60% of cases, especially in hantavirus haemorrhagic fever with renal syndrome(HFRS) [43]. Kidney disease occurs in the course of active infection from direct viral invasion of tubular epithelial cells, glomerular endothelial cells and podocytes [44]. Systemic inflammatory and immune complex deposition may also contribute to kidney disease. Oliguric AKI with haematuria and sub-nephrotic proteinuria, followed by polyuria is the usual clinical presentation in HFRS. Milder forms of kidney dysfunction may be seen in the other Hanta virus syndromes. Kidney histopathology shows acute haemorrhagic interstitial nephritis with mononuclear cell infiltrates (CD8+ T-lymphocytes and macrophages), tubular necrosis and congestion of peritubular capillaries, especially in the outer medulla [45]. Glomerular lesions have also occasionally been reported; (see Table 14.7). Management is mainly supportive with antipyretics, fluid resuscitation, control of electrolyte disorders, vasopressors and KRT when indicated. Kidney recovery is usual; however, hypertension, cardiovascular disease, hypopituitarism and chronic kidney disease of unknown aetiology have been reported in those who recover [46, 47].

Ebola Virus

Ebola infection is marked by uncontrolled viral replication, which results in excessive proinflammatory responses, endothelial dysfunction, and dysregulation of the coagulation cascade, haemorrhage and subsequently severe organ dysfunction. Viral invasion of tubular and endothelial cells, systemic complications of the infection, and bacterial and malarial super infection result in kidney involvement [48]. Acute kidney injury is the main manifestation in 20–50% of cases. AKI is multifactorial, as outlined in Table 14.7. Kidney biopsy is not

Table 14.7 Kidney involvement in viral infections

Virus	Mechanism of kidney injury	Kidney involvement	Management
Acute			
Dengue	Direct viral invasion Immune-mediated, haemodynamic instability, haemolysis, rhabdomyolysis	ATN, ICGN, MesPGN TMA, AIN, IgA, pre-renal azotaemia	Supportive care, fluid resuscitation
Hantavirus HFRS	Direct viral invasion Immune-mediated haemolysis, rhabdomyolysis, volume depletion	ATN, MesPGN, AIN, pre-renal azotaemia	Supportive treatment, fluid resuscitation, dialysis without heparin
Ebola	Direct viral invasion, haemodynamic instability, Cytokine storm, coinfection with malaria, gram negative septicaemia	ATN, DIC, pre-renal azotaemia	Supportive treatment, fluid resuscitation, dialysis without heparin
Varicella-zoster	Immune-mediated Direct invasion	DPGN, TMA, HSP, MPGN, microscopic polyangiitis, AIN ATN, RPGN	IV Acyclovir 10 mg–20 mg/kg bodyweight for 2 weeks, then orally for 3 months in renal allograft recipients Supportive care
Parvovirus	Direct viral invasion Immune-mediated	ICGN, PAN, TMA, HSP, microscopic polyangiitis, TIN acute renal allograft rejection	Supportive care
Hepatitis A	Immune-mediated	ICGN, mesPGN, ATN, Pre-renal azotaemia	Supportive care, fluid resuscitation,
Hepatitis E	Direct viral invasion	ATN, Pre-renal azotaemia	Supportive care, fluid resuscitation.
Hepatitis B	Immune-mediated Systemic effects of infection	MN, MPGN, IgA, ATN, DPGN, RPGN	NAs, pegylated interferon, supportive care **RPGN**: NA + corticosteroids + cyclophospamide/ rituximab
Cytomegalovirus	Direct viral invasion Immune complex	cFSGS, MN, IgA, HSP, ICGN, MPGN, TMA, RPGN	Valganciclovir 900 mg/12 hourly per os; IV Ganciclovir 5 mg/kg/12 hourly for 14–28 days or for refractory disease; forscanet 90 mg/kg/12 h; IV immunoglobulins; or cidofovir. Prophylactic valganciclovir 900 mg/daily for a further 30 days

ATN acute tubular necrosis, *ICGN* immune complex glomerulonephritis, *MesPGN* mesangial proliferative glomerulonephritis, *DPGN* diffuse proliferative glomerulonephritis, *cFSGS* collapsing focal glomeruloscleroses, *ncFSGS* non-collapsing focal segmental glomeruloscleroses, *MN* membranous nephropathy, *IgA* Immunoglobulin A, *HSP* Henoch Schoenlein purpura, *HFRS* hemorrhagic fever and renal syndrome, *MPGN* membranoproliferative glomerulonephritis, *MC* mixed cryoglobulinemia, *TMA* thrombotic microangiopathy, *DIC* disseminated intravascular coagulopathy, *HIVAN* HIV-associated nephropathy, *HIVICK* HIV immune complex disease of the kidney, *PAN* polyarteritis nodosa, *RPGN* rapidly progressive glomerulonephritis, *UTI* urinary tract infection, *DAAs* direct acting antivirals, *IS* immunosuppressive agents, *IV Ig* intravenous immunoglobulins, *cART* combined antiretroviral therapy, *RAAS* renin angiotensin aldosterone system, *SARS-CoV-2* severe acute respiratory syndrome-coronavirus-2, *MGRS* monoclonal gammopathy of renal significance, *TIN* tubulo-interstitial nephritis, *AIN* acute interstitial nephritis, *DILS* diffuse infiltrative lymphocytic syndrome, *IRIS* immune reconstitution syndrome, *NA* nucleos(t)ide analogs (Lamivudine, telbivudine, tenofovir, adefovir)

routine for diagnosis; however, acute tubular necrosis and degeneration with interstitial oedema and mild cellular infiltrates have been reported on kidney histology [49]. Aggressive fluid resuscitation and usual care for AKI, including KRT is the mainstay of management, with particular consideration of staff safety [50].

Parvovirus

Symptomatic parvovirus B(PVB) infection occurs in 2–12% of patients in the first year of kidney transplantation, with 10% of these developing allograft dysfunction [51]. PVB kidney disease may also occur in native kidneys of immunocompetent individuals. Direct invasion of kidney tissue and immune-mediated kidney injury are the main disease mechanisms [52]. Acute nephritic syndrome with hypocomplementaemia, following a prodrome of rash, fever, and arthritis is frequent. Nephrotic syndrome or chronic kidney disease is seen in sub-acute infection; and aplastic crisis may follow the nephrotic syndrome in patients with sickle cell disease [53]. Endocapillary and mesangial proliferation with subendothelial deposits of C3 and IgG, suggestive of acute post-infectious glomerulonephritis is frequent on kidney histopathology [54]. Other histological lesions seen on kidney biopsy are shown in Table 14.7. Viral antigens are often present in blood and may be detectable in kidney tissue. Management is supportive; and is often combined with reduction of immunosuppression and administration of intravenous immunoglobulins in transplant recipients with persistent infection [55].

Polyoma Virus

Polyoma virus nephropathy (PVN), caused mainly by the BK virus, occurs in 1–10% of kidney transplants, causing graft loss in about 50% of these cases [56]. PVN is rare in native kidneys of non-kidney organ recipients. Viral replication in the kidney epithelium causes a tubulointerstitial nephritis [57]. The major risk factor for PVN is intense immunosuppression; however, patient, organ, viral and other immunity-related risk factors may play a role. Nephropathy follows viraemia, resulting from latent viruria [58]. PVN often presents as asymptomatic worsening of kidney function, and/or chronic graft dysfunction in the first year of transplantation. The diagnosis of PVN requires urine cytology, urine and plasma BK viral load and kidney biopsy. Viral inclusion bearing epithelial cells called 'decoy cells' may be present on urine cytology. Decoy cells $\geq$10/cytospin [59], a urine BK viral load >10^7 copies/mL and a plasma BK viral load >10^4 copies/mL [60, 61] are indicative of a presumptive diagnosis of PVN. Kidney biopsy remains the diagnostic gold standard. Three histological patterns of patchy tubulo-interstitial nephritis with varying degrees of viral cytopathic changes, interstitial inflammation, and in late stages, tubular atrophy and interstitial fibrosis are observed [62]. Three classes of PVN based on tissue replication load, and interstitial fibrosis(ci) score have been described [63]. Reduction of immunosuppression (IS) is the mainstay of management, with addition of antiviral agents in refractory cases. Various algorithms of stepwise and careful reduction of antimetabolites and calcineurin inhibitors are in use. Some antiviral agents, and fluoroquinolones and intravenous immunoglobulins may be useful in refractory PVN. Re-transplantation is possible after graft loss when the viral load becomes undetectable [64, 65].

Cytomegalovirus

Cytomegalovirus (CMV) nephropathy occurs in both immunocompetent and immunocompromised individuals, and results from viral replication in kidney cells and immune complex mediated injury [66]. CMV infection is common after kidney transplantation, where it adversely affects graft and patient survival [67]; however, CMV nephropathy is rare, occurring in <1% of transplanted patients [68]. Kidney disease often occurs during acute systemic CMV illness, following reactivation of latent infection in the setting of intense immunosuppression, or less often during primary infection. The usual clinical manifestation is acute kidney injury with or without haematuria, and varying degrees of proteinuria. Nephrotic syndrome is infrequent. Diagnosis is based on the presence of viral cytopathic changes in kidney tissue, usually in the presence of CMV viraemia. A high viral load of >10,000 copies/mL seems to correlate with CMV nephropathy [69]. Kidney histopathology shows patchy acute or chronic peritubular pleomorphic mononuclear interstitial infiltrates with tubulitis; tubular epithelial cells are markedly enlarged with characteristic intranuclear eosinophilic inclusions ('owl eye' type inclusions). Viral particles may be seen in both the nuclei and cytoplasm of infected cells, and CMV is present on immunostaining [70]. Glomerular and vascular lesions may occur either in coexistence with tubulo-interstitial disease or in isolation (Table 14.7). Management of CMV nephritis in kidney allografts involves the use of antiviral agents, reduction of immunosuppression and use of immunomodulators [71] (Table 14.7). CMV nephritis is usually mild and self-limiting in immunocompetent patients.

Varicella Infections

Kidney involvement in varicella zoster virus (VZV) infection is rare and occurs essentially during primary infection in both native and allograft kidneys [72, 73]. Kidney disease is mediated through viral immune complex injury and dysregulation of complement activity [74, 75]. Clinical manifestations include acute glomerulonephritis syndromes, nephrotic syndrome, atypical haemolytic uraemic syndrome, vasculitis and acute kidney injury. Kidney biopsy findings are shown in Table 14.7. Acyclovir, together with supportive care for kidney syndromes is usual care.

Hepatitis E Virus

Kidney disease, essentially glomerulonephritis (GN) is association with acute and chronic hepatitis E virus (HEV) infection in both immunocompetent and immunocompromised individuals [76]. Immune- mediated mechanisms and direct viral cytopathic effects may contribute to kidney damage [77]. A monoclonal gammopathy of renal significance presenting as light chain cast nephropathy was recently reported [78]. Acute kidney failure and the nephrotic syndrome are the usual clinical presentation. In kidney allograft recipients, HEV is associated with proteinuria and a decline in glomerular filtration rate [79]. The spectrum of lesions reported on kidney biopsy are shown in Table 14.7. Treatment is supportive, however in kidney allograft recipients, reduction in immunosuppression and use of ribavirin for 3–6 months are the mainstay of treatment.

Hepatitis A

Hepatitis A virus (HAV)-associated kidney disease occurs in both non-fulminant and fulminant disease, manifesting essentially as AKI with acute tubular necrosis as the main mechanism [80]. Immune-complex-mediated injury, and direct viral cytopathic effects are other suggested mechanisms of kidney pathology [81]. The diagnosis is based on laboratory evidence of infection, in the presence of clinical features consistent with any of the kidney syndromes. Kidney biopsy is rarely required for diagnosis, except with an atypical presentation**.** Oher mechanisms of AKI and histopathological findings are shown in Table 14.7. Management is supportive and aimed at improving kidney perfusion, and treating complications of kidney syndromes. Kidney recovery is frequent, even in dialysis-requiring AKI.

Hepatitis B Virus

Hepatitis B virus (HBV)-associated nephropathy remains frequent in HBV endemic zones, and occurs mainly with chronic HBV infection. Glomerulonephritis (GN) and polyarteritis nodosa (PAN) from immune-mediated and possible direct viral effects are the main presentations [82]. Consequences of severe liver disease may cause AKI [83]. GN may present with proteinuria, nephrotic syndrome, microscopic haematuria, hypertension or kidney impairment, with the latter unusual in children. HBV DNA, and serological markers of HBV infections are often present in serum, however HBV GN has been reported in HBsAg seronegative patients [84]. Hypocomplementaemia may exist with MPGN and PAN, whereas mixed cryoglobulinaemia is rare. MN, MPGN and MesPGN are the main histological patterns. MN is common in children whereas MesPGN is common in adults and may coexist with MN. Sub-epithelial, sub-endothelial and mesangial deposits of IgG with C3, IgA, IgM and C1q are frequent and immune complexes may contain HBsAg and HBeAg and HBcAg. Other forms of GNs have been reported in adults [85] (Table 14.7). Treatment is with antiviral nucleos(t)ide analogs(NAs). Immunosuppressive agents, pegylated interferon and plasma exchange maybe added to NAs in PAN and rapidly progressive GN [86], as shown in Fig. 14.6. Spontaneous remission is frequent in children with clearance of HBeAg whereas about a third of adults with HBV GN eventually develop chronic kidney failure [85].

Hepatitis C Virus

Hepatitis C virus (HCV) nephropathy is essentially immune complex mediated GN and vasculitis [87]. The pathological hallmark of HCV-GN is type I MGPN with or without type 2 mixed cryoglobuinaemia [33]. HCV GN presents as an acute nephritic syndrome, varying degrees of albuminuria or rapidly progressive GN, with presence of viral RNA and anti-HCV antibodies in serum. Cryoglobulinaemia occurs in 50–70% and it is associated will low early complement components (C4, C1q, CH50). Kidney histology typically shows MPGN with mononuclear, polymorphonuclear leucocyte infiltrates, and subendothelial deposits of IgG, IgM and C3 [88]. Other glomerular lesions and vascular lesions have

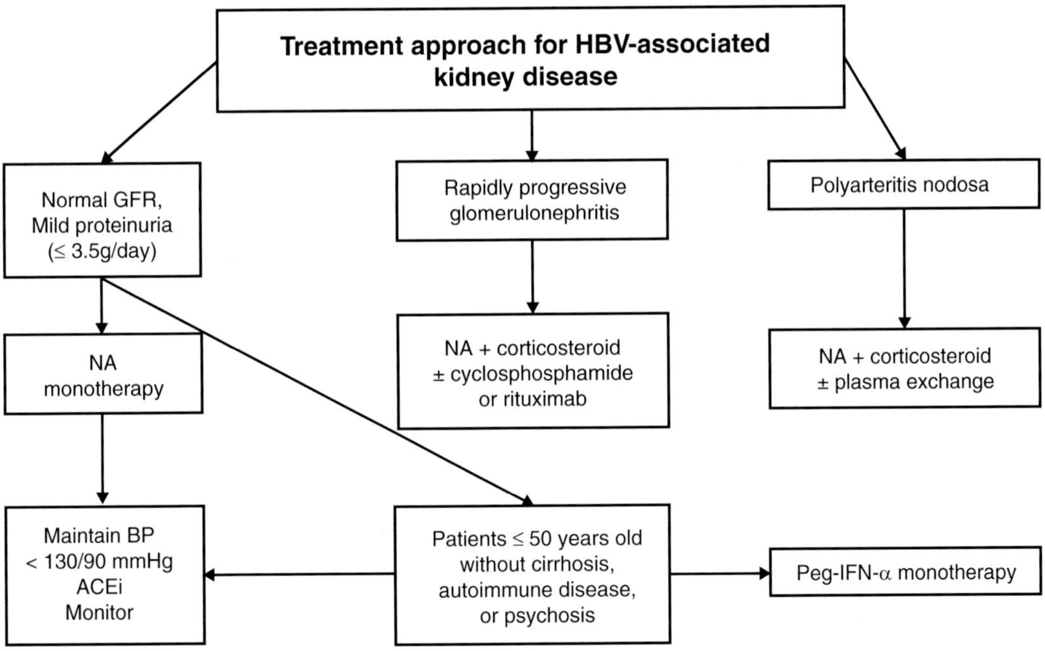

Fig. 14.6 Algorithm showing treatment approach to Hepatitis B-associated kidney disease. [*BP* blood pressure, *GFR* glomerular filtration rate, *HBV* Hepatitis B virus, *NA* Nucleotide/Nucleoside antagonist, *ACEi* angiotensin converting enzyme inhibitor, *Peg-IFN-α* pegylated interferon-alfa]

been reported (Table 14.7). KDIGO has recommended the use of direct acting antivirals (DAAs) for HCV kidney disease, with the choice, dosage and duration of DAAs therapy based on HCV genotype, glomerular filtration rate, virologic response and possible drug interactions, as shown in Fig. 14.7 [89]. In addition to DAAs, it recommends the use of immunosuppressive agents (IS) with or without plasma exchange in case of a cryoglobulinaemic flare or nephrotic syndrome, with rituximab as first line IS for cryoglobulinaemic kidney disease.

Kidney function	HCV genotype	Recommended regimen(s)	strength of evidence	Alternate regimen(s)	Strength of evidence
CKD G4–G5 (GFR < 30 ml/min per 1.73 m^2) including HD, KTR[b]	1a	Grazoprevir/elbasvir	1B	Ritonavir-boosted paritaprevir, ombitasvir, and dasabuvir (also known as PrOD or 3D regmien) with ribavirin	2D
		Glecaprevir/pibrentasvir	1B	Dactatasvir/asunaprevir	2C
	1b	Grazoprevir/elbasvir	1B	Ritonavir-boosted paritaprevir, ombitasvir, and dasabuvir (also known as ProD or 3D regimen)	2D
		Glecaprevir/pibrentasvir	1B	Daclatasvir/asunaprevir	2C
	2,3	Glecaprevir/pibrentasvir	1B		
	4	Grazoprevir/elbasvir	2D		
		Glecaprevir/pibrentasvir	1B		
	5,6	Glecaprevir/pibrentasvlr	2D		
CKD G5 PD	n/a (reasonable to follow proposed regimens for HD)				
KTR (GFR ≥ 30 ml/min per 1.73 m^2)	1a	Sofosbuvir with ledipasvir, daclatasvir or simeprevir	1B	Sofosbuvir/ribavirin	2D
		Glecaprevir/pibrentasvir[c]	1C		
	1b	Solosbuvir with ledipasvir, daclatasvir or simeprevir	1B		
		Glecaprevir/pibrentasvir[c]	1C		
	2,3,5, 6	Glecaprevir/pibrentasvir[c]	1D	Sofosbuvir/daclatasvir/ribavirin[d]	2D
	4	Sofosbuvir with ledipasvir, daclatasvir or simeprevir	1D		
		Glecaprevir/pibrentasvir[c]	1D		

Fig. 14.7 Recommendation grades (1–2) and strength of evidence (**a–d**) are listed for each recommended treatment regimen and HCV genotype. (**a**) Recommended Hepatitis C virus (HCV) direct-acting antiviral (DAA) treatment regimens for patients with CKD G1-G5D and kidney transplant recipients (KTRs), by hepatitis C virus (HCV) genotype. (**b**) Treatment scheme for CKD stages G1-G5D patients with confirmed Hepatitis C infection. (**c**) Treatment algorithm for Kidney Transplant Recipients with confirmed Hepatitis C infection, by GFR and HCV genotype. *CKD* chronic kidney disease, *DAA* direct-acting antiviral, *GFR* glomerular filtration rate, *HCV* Hepatitis C virus, *NAT* nucleic acid testing

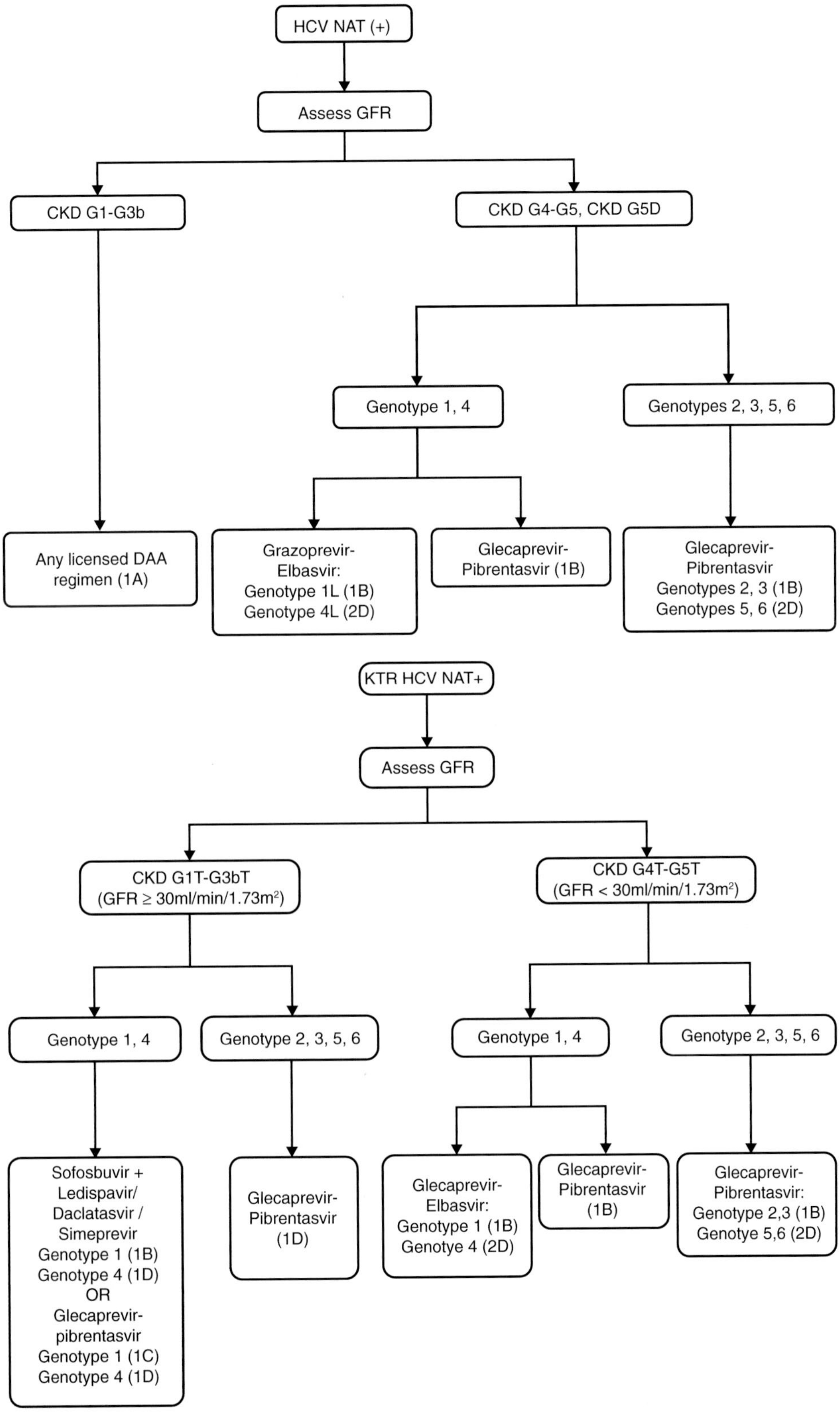

Fig. 14.7 (continued)

HIV

Both acute and chronic kidney disease are common in the course of HIV infection. Mechanisms of kidney injury in the course of HIV infection vary from direct viral cytopathic effects, immune complex disease, and systemic complications of immunodepression and infection or their therapies [90, 91]. The diagnosis of kidney disease in an HIV-positive patient must therefore consider whether patient is combination anti-retroviral therapy (cART)-naïve or not, and whether there is an ongoing co-infection. HIV-associated nephropathy (HIVAN), focal segmental glomerulosclerosis (FSGS) and HIV immune complex disease (HIVICK) are the main kidney manifestations of HIV infection. HIVAN, the most frequent cause of kidney disease in HIV-positive individuals of African descent, results from the cytopathic effects of the virus on visceral and parietal epithelial cells [92]. cART-naïve African blacks with apolipoprotein-1 (APOL-1) G1/G2 variants are especially at risk [93, 94]. The lifetime risk of developing HIVAN in an untreated HIV-positive black patient is 2–10%, but the risk rises to 50% if the patient is homozygous for APOL-I variants [95]. HIVAN typically presents with varying degrees of proteinuria or the nephrotic syndrome with progressive kidney failure. Histologically, classic HIVAN is characterized by collapsing glomerulopathy and attendant tubulointerstitial disease including tubular microcyst formation, interstitial inflammation and tubular injury [91]. HIVICK represents a heterogenous group of proliferative immune-complex mediated GN occurring in a patient with active HIV infection without other possible aetiologies. HIVICK usually manifests as a nephritic or nephrotic-nephritic syndrome in the absence of coinfections such as HBV or HCV. Various proliferative GNs are seen on kidney histology in HIVICK with a post-infectious GN histological pattern observed in about 50% of cases [96]. Other podocytopathies, tubulointerstitial and vascular diseases have been reported in the setting of HIV infection, as shown in Table 14.7. Management involves viral suppression with cART, and measures to slow progression of chronic kidney disease. Recommendations on the screening, management and monitoring of kidney disease in HIV-positive individuals were published recently [91].

Severe Acute Respiratory Syndrome Coronavirus-2 [SARS-CoV-2]

The global pandemic of coronavirus disease 2019 (COVID-19) caused by SARS-CoV-2 has affected millions of people around the world, and kidney disease is increasingly recognized as one of its serious complications. A study of 710 hospitalized patients in Wuhan, China with COVID-19 showed that 44% had proteinuria and haematuria, and 26.7% had haematuria on admission. The prevalence of elevated serum creatinine and blood urea nitrogen was 15.5% and 14.1%, respectively. AKI occurred in 5.1% and was associated with a four-fold increase in mortality [97]. A systematic review reported the incidence of AKI to be 8.9% in 6945 COVID-19 patients [98]. There was a higher risk of mortality (RR 3.08–4.19) in severe AKI (AKI Stage 3, or requiring KRT) was reported in a meta-analysis [99]. The proposed mechanisms of kidney injury are diverse, and include direct viral infection, effects on the renin-angiotensin-aldosterone system, haemodynamic instability, coagulopathy and cytokine storm [100]. Histology of native and allograft kidney biopsies in 17 patients in New York, 15 of whom presented with AKI, and 9 with nephrotic range proteinuria, showed that 5/14 native kidneys had collapsing glomerulonephritis (cGN); 2 with membranous GN; one each with minimal change disease, lupus nephritis with crescents, anti-GBM nephritis; and 4 with acute tubular injury (Table 14.7). The 3 allograft biopsies showed acute T-cell mediated rejection, cortical infarction and acute tubular injury. Three patients with cGN (labelled as "COVAN") and one with minimal change disease were shown to have *APOL1* high-risk genotype [101]. In a study of 114 chronic haemodialysis patients from New York, intensive care unit (ICU) admission was required in 13.2% and 16.7% required mechanical ventilation with an overall mortality of 28%; of 86.7% of those requiring ICU, nearly 100% required mechanical ventilation [102].

Kidney transplant recipients appear to be at increased risk of severe COVID-19 disease and mortality rate of 28% was reported in one centre [103]. Treatment is supportive with supplemental oxygen, anticoagulation and dexamethasone for those requiring oxygen, with various agents under clinical trial (including remisidivir, tocilizumab). The vaccines against SARS Cov-2 have reduced the infection rates, severe infection, hospitalization and mortality. Randomised controlled trials to date have shown benefits of dexamethasone, tocilizumab, neutralizing antibodies, and remdesivir.

Protozoal and Parasitic Infections and the Kidney

Malaria

The World Health Organization (WHO) reported 228 million cases of malaria worldwide in 2018, 93% in Africa; 405,000 deaths were reported, 94% of which occurred in Africa [104]. Figure 14.8 shows the distribution of malaria

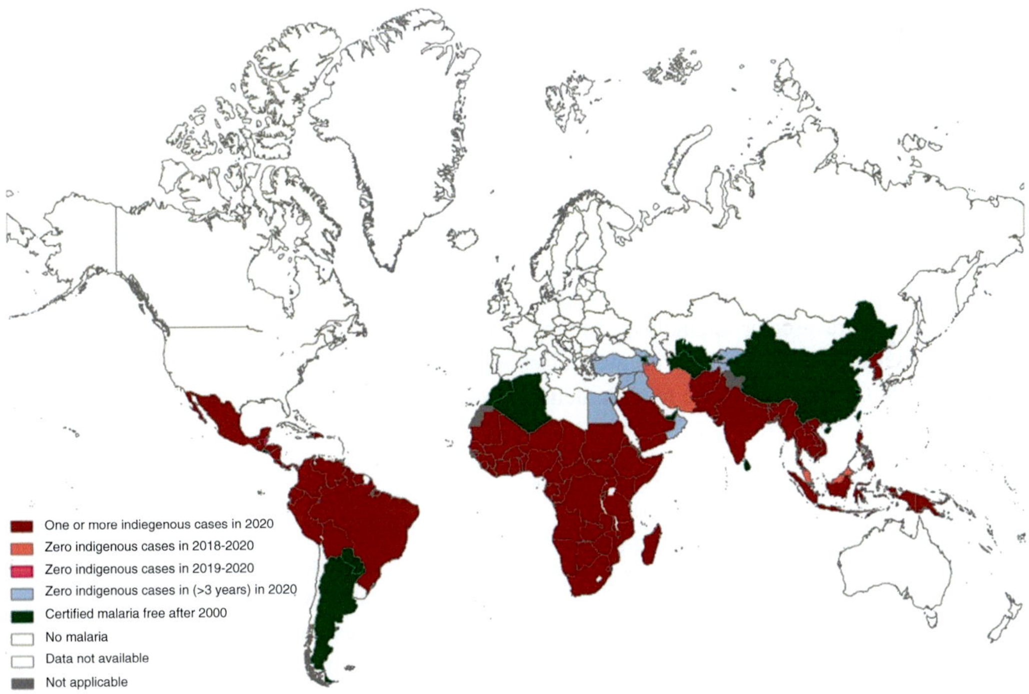

Fig. 14.8 Countries with indigenous cases in 2000 and their status by 2020: Countries with zero indigenous cases for at least three consecutive years are considered to have eliminated malaria. In 2020, the Islamic Republic of Iran and Malaysia reported zero indigenous cases for the third consecutive year, and Belize and Cabo Verde reported zero indigenous cases for the second time. China and El Salvador were certified malaria free in 2021, following 4 years of zero malaria cases. (Reproduced with permission from the World Health Organisation (WHO) [105])

worldwide [106]. The most vulnerable groups are young children, who have not yet developed immunity to malaria, and pregnant women, whose immunity has decreased with pregnancy. Malaria is transmitted by the bite of an infected *Anopheles* mosquito. There are four pathogenic species of malaria: *Plasmodium falciparum, P. vivax, P. ovale, P. malariae; P. falciparum* causes the most severe disease with heaviest parasitaemia. The clinical presentation of severe disease is dehydration with hypotension, oliguria, severe anaemia and jaundice.

Kidney Disease with Malaria

Malarial nephropathies are reported in endemic areas, such as Southeast Asia, India, and Sub-Saharan Africa [107–109]. Histologic evidence shows the presence of acute tubular necrosis, interstitial nephritis and glomerulonephritis [110–113] (Table 14.8).

Acute kidney injury (AKI) occurs in severe malaria in less than 4.8% of cases, with clinical presentation of hypotension, oliguria, severe anaemia, jaundice, and hepatosplenomegaly and a high risk of mortality (15–45%) [107–109]. Risk factors for malarial AKI include delayed diagnosis, heavy parasitaemia, volume depletion, hyperbilirubinaemia, intravascular haemolysis, kidney ischaemia, sepsis, disseminated intravascular coagulation (DIC), cytoadherence to endothelial cells, and microvascular sequestration [114]. Endothelial activation leads to the release of several cytokines, including thromboxane, catecholamines, endothelin and other inflammatory mediators, that are also implicated in the pathogenesis of malaria-associated kidney injury [114].

Table 14.8 Kidney disease with different malaria species

Kidney disease	Malaria species
Acute kidney injury Acute tubular necrosis Acute interstitial nephritis	*P. falciparum; P. vivax; P.ovale; P.malariae* (less commonly)
Renal cortical necrosis	*P. falciparum; P. vivax (rarely)* [111, 112]
Glomerular disease	*P. falciparum; P. malariae; P. vivax* (rarely) [113]

Immune system activation in malaria involves Th1 and Th2 responses [110]. When the Th2 response prevails (especially with infection by *P. malariae*), complement activation occurs, with immune complex deposition leading to glomerulonephritis. When Th1 response is predominant, acute interstitial nephritis and acute glomerulonephritis occur. Renal cortical necrosis has also been described in malaria, characterizing more severe kidney injury and is generally associated with non-recovery of kidney function and development of end-stage kidney disease (ESKD) [112]. Hepatic dysfunction also contributes to kidney disease in malaria: hyperbilirubinemia can lead to cast nephropathy, and AKI, and liver disease and its complications can also cause AKI (hepato-renal syndrome (HRS)) [111, 113, 115–117]. The principal pathogenic mechanisms of kidney disease in malaria are depicted in Fig. 14.9.

Diagnosis

Microscopy is the gold standard and preferred option for diagnosing malaria. In nearly all cases, examination of thick and thin blood films will reveal malaria parasites. Thick films are more sensitive than thin films for detecting low levels of parasitaemia.

Rapid diagnostic tests (RDT) are useful for diagnostic purposes, especially for diagnosing malaria in patients who have recently received antimalarial treatment and in whom blood films are transiently negative for malaria parasites. Commonly targeted antigens are histidine-rich protein 2 (HRP2), which is specific for P. falciparum, and plasmodium lactate dehydrogenase (pLDH), which is present in all Plasmodium species [115, 116].

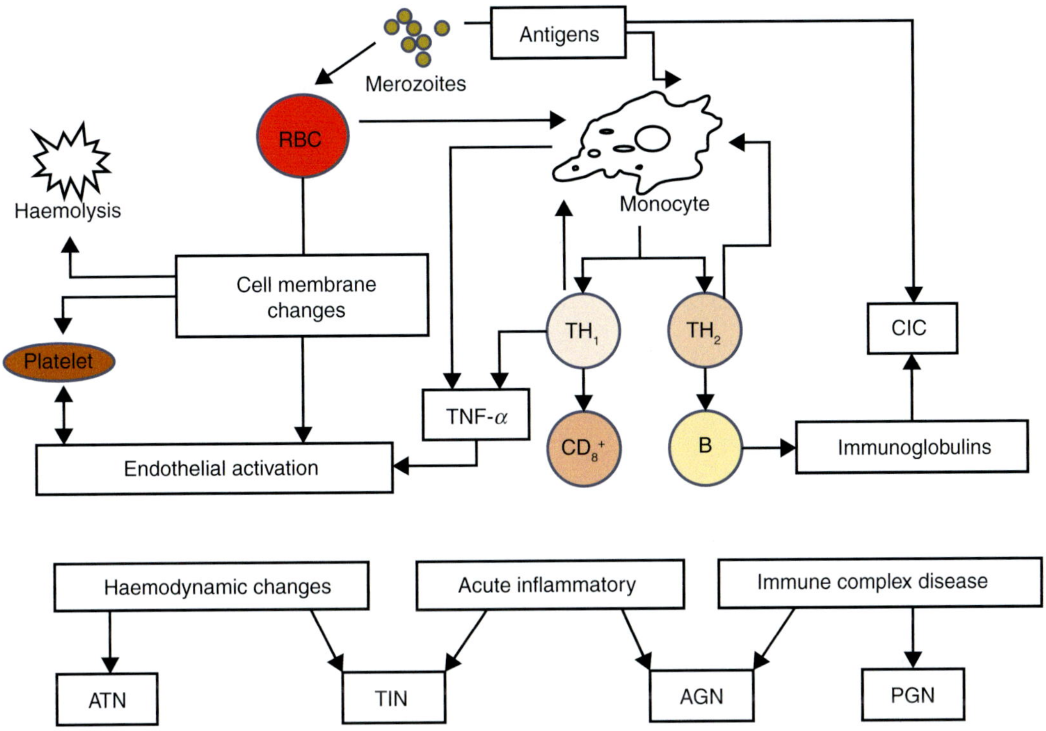

Fig. 14.9 Mechanisms of kidney disease with malaria (adapted from Barsoum RS, 1998) [110]. *ATN* acute tubular necrosis, *TIN* tululo-interstitial nephritis, *AGN* acute glomerulonephritis, *PGN* progressive glomerulonephritis, *CIC* circulating immune complexes, *RBC* red blood cell

Treatment

The control and eradication of malaria demands a multifaceted approach, including insecticide spraying and insecticide-treated bed nets.

Close monitoring with rehydration, correction of hypoglycaemia (if present) and control of any seizures are important. If the patient remains oliguric after adequate rehydration, and kidney function continues to decline, then KRT (haemofiltration or haemodialysis, and if neither is available, peritoneal dialysis) should be implemented, especially for severe disease. Haemofiltration is more efficient, and is associated with a significantly lower mortality than peritoneal dialysis. When possible, refer the patient to a dialysis unit.

The current WHO-recommended first-line treatment for the majority of malaria cases is artemisinin-based combination therapy (ACT) (Table 14.9).

Table 14.9 Treatment of severe malaria [117]

Drug	Treatment schedule
Pre-referral treatment Artesunate rectally Artesunate IMI Artemether IMI Quinine IMI	Given if delay in receiving definitive Rx for >6 h 10 mg/kg OR 2.4 mg/kg OR 3.3 mg/kg OR 20 mg/kg (10 mg/kg into each thigh)
Artesunate	2.4 mg/kg body weight (BW) IVI or IMI on admission, and then 12 hourly × 24 h (until oral intake is possible) OR
Artemether	3.2 mg/kg BW IMI on admission, then 1.6 mg/kg BW daily OR
Quinine HCl	20 mg/kg loading dose on admission, then 10 mg/kg 8 hourly as IV infusion over 2–4 h in 10 mL/kg BW isotonic fluid OR IMI in 2 sites. Duration X 24 h (minimum)
Follow-up oral Rx: Artemether + Lumefantrine Artesunate + Amodiaquine Artesunate + Mefloquine[a] Artesunate + sulfadoxine-pyrimethamine Dihydroartemisinin + Piperaquine	Full course for to be given when able to take oral medication

[a]Avoid in presence of cerebral malaria due to risk of neuropsychiatric side effects

Schistosomiasis

Approximately 240 million people worldwide, living in poor communities without potable water and inadequate sanitation, are affected by schistosomiasis, which is prevalent in tropical and sub-tropical areas of the world (Fig. 14.10) [118], with 90% living in Africa. It is estimated that more than 200,000 deaths per year are due to schistosomiasis in sub-Saharan Africa. Table 14.10 depicts the geographical distribution of the different schistosomal species [119].

Clinical Features

The incubation period for patients with acute schistosomiasis is usually 2–12 weeks; many people are asymptomatic and have subclinical disease during both acute and chronic stages of infection. Acute infection (Katayama syndrome) may present with rash, fever, headache, myalgia, and respiratory symptoms. Eosinophilia is often present with hepato- and/or splenomegaly [120].

Clinical manifestations of chronic disease result from host immune responses to schistosomal ova. *S. mansoni* and *S. japonicum* ova most commonly lodge in the blood vessels of the liver or intestine and can cause diarrhoea, constipation, and blood in the stool. Chronic inflammation can lead to bowel ulceration, hyperplasia, and polyposis; and with heavy infections, may result in liver fibrosis and portal hypertension. *S. haematobium* ova tend to lodge in the urinary tract causing dysuria and haematuria. Chronic infections may increase the risk of bladder cancer. *S. haematobium* ova deposition has also been associated with damage to the female genital tract, causing female genital schistosomiasis. Central nervous system lesions are rare and due to ectopic deposition of ova in the spinal cord (*S. mansoni* or *S. haematobium*) or brain (*S. japonicum*) forming granulomas that act as space occupying lesions [121].

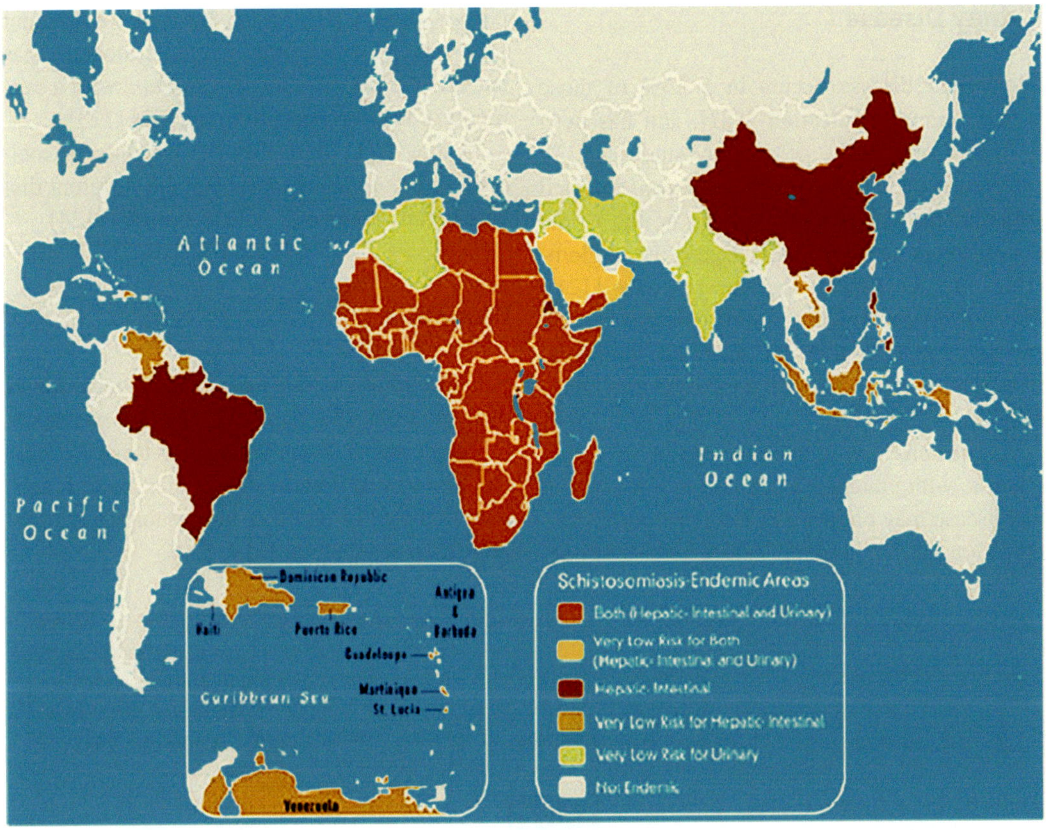

Fig. 14.10 World-wide Prevalence of Schistosomiasis [118]. (Reproduced with permission from the authors of Ismail et al., 2016 [118])

Table 14.10 Geographical distribution of the different types of Schistosomes [119]

	Species	Geographical distribution
Intestinal schistosomiasis	*Schistosoma mansoni*	Africa, the Middle East, the Caribbean, Brazil, Venezuela and Suriname
	Schistosoma japonicum	China, Indonesia, the Philippines
	Schistosoma mekongi	Several districts of Cambodia and the Lao People's Democratic Republic
	Schistosoma guineensis and related *S. intercalatum*	Rain forest areas of central Africa
Urogenital schistosomiasis	*Schistosoma haematobium*	Africa, the Middle East

Kidney Disease

Glomerular disease occurs in 5–15% of those with *S. mansoni* infection [122], and has been described in 10–12% of autopsy studies [123]; proteinuria occurs in 20% of *S. mansoni*-infected patients [124]. Glomerular injury is due to the deposition of schistosomal antigens in the glomerulus and subsequent immune response [121]. The histopathological patterns described are mesangial proliferative GN, membranoproliferative GN, FSGS, proliferative GN and amyloidosis [122].

S. haematobium infections present with haematuria, with granuloma formation; if untreated, the disease may progress to bladder fibrosis, calcification, vesico-ureteric reflux and hydronephrosis, and CKD [120]; the risk of bladder cancer is increased. Rarely, glomerulopathy has been described with *S. haematobium*, with a case report of membranoproliferative GN [123].

Figure 14.11 describes the timelines associated with the pathogenesis and the different disease manifestations of schistosomiasis [124].

Diagnosis

Schistosomiasis is diagnosed by the detection of ova in stool (*S. mansoni*, *S. japonicum*, *S. mekongi*, and *S. intercalatum*) or urine (*S. haematobium)* specimens. Antibodies and/or antigens detected in blood or urine samples are also indicative of infection [119, 120].

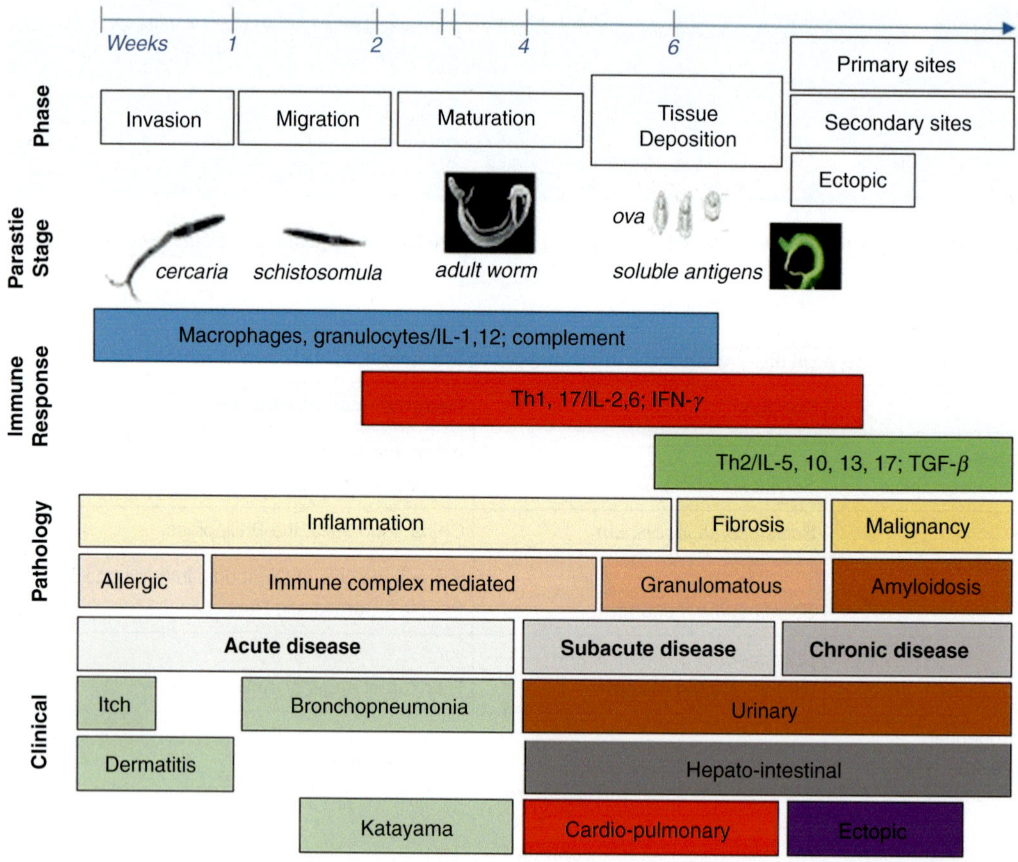

Fig. 14.11 Timelines, Clinical features and Pathogenesis of Schistosomal Disease (adapted from Barsoum R et al., 2013 [124])

Table 14.11 Treatment schedule for Schistosomiasis by *Schistosoma* species infection

Schistosoma species infection	Praziquantel dose and duration
S. mansoni, S. haematobium, S. intercalatum	40 mg/kg per day orally in two divided doses for one day
S. japonicum, S. mekongi	60 mg/kg per day orally in three divided doses for one day

Treatment

Infections with all major *Schistosoma* species can be treated with praziquantel (Table 14.11). Although a single course of treatment is usually curative, repeat treatment may be needed after 2 to 4 weeks to increase effectiveness [119].

Prevention and Control

The control of schistosomiasis is based on large-scale treatment of at-risk population groups, access to safe water, improved sanitation, education, and snail control. Preventive measures include avoiding contact with freshwater in disease-endemic countries.

The WHO strategy for schistosomiasis control focuses on reducing disease by periodic, targeted treatment with praziquantel of all at-risk population groups [119].

Fungal Infections and Kidney Disease

Fungal infections occur more commonly in hospitalized or immunocompromised patients; Table 14.12 outlines the major risk factors for fungal infections of the kidney. Most common organisms are Candida species [125]; less common fungi are filamentous fungi (Mucor, Aspergillus, Penicillium); and rare are endemic fungi (Blastomycosis, Histoplasmosis, Coccidioidomycosis). Patients who are symptomatic usually have urinary tract obstruction from masses of fungal elements (fungal balls). Angio-invasion by fungi may lead to numerous micro-abscesses in the kidney, and extensive kidney infarcts, leading to kidney dysfunction. Treatment with systemic antifungal agents, and surgical removal of the obstructing mass is usually required [126]. In extensive disease, mortality remains very high, especially with angio-invasive fungal infection with mucormycosis and aspergillus infections [127].

Table 14.12 Major risk factors for fungal infections of the kidney

Major risk factors for fungal infections of the kidney
Older age
Female gender
Prolonged antibiotic use
Indwelling catheter
Prior surgical procedures
Mechanical ventilation
Parenteral nutrition
Diabetes mellitus
Immunocompromised state (including post kidney transplantation)

Conclusions

Kidney and urinary tract infections are associated with significant morbidity—and amongst vulnerable groups, mortality. The first clinical case describes a bacterial infection with *E. Coli*, and illustrates how clinical presentations with urinary tract infection may be unusual, but with appropriate clinical awareness, affected patients can be commenced on appropriate antibiotics early, and hence offered the best chance of a full recovery. The second clinical scenario illustrates the reversible nature of infection-related immune-mediated glomerulonephritis, which may present in a young female who is very unwell, confused and dialysis dependent.

Questions

1. A 55 year old man presented to the emergency room with fever, non-productive cough, anosmia, muscle aches and fatigue for one day and sore throat for 3 days. He had been to his local pub 5 days previously. His

temperature was 38.3 °C, BP 124/76, respiratory rate 28/min and oxygen saturation 88%. Chest radiograph was suggestive of bilateral lower lobe interstitial pneumonitis. Laboratory results revealed haemoglobin 13.3 g/dL; white cell count 4.1 × 10^9/L; lymphocyte count 1.3 × 10^9/L; blood glucose 12.2 mmol/L; serum creatinine 98 μmol/L; CRP 185 mg/L. Three days after admission he was breathless and transferred to ITU, his creatinine increased to 210 μmol/L.

What is the most likely cause of his illness?

A. COVID-19
B. Cytomegalovirus infection
C. Staphylococcus infection
D. Pneumococcus infection
E. Malaria

Answer: A

A nasal swab PCR confirmed the diagnosis of COVID-19. He was admitted to the intensive care unit and commenced on intravenous fluids, high flow oxygen via a nasal cannula, enoxaparin 20 mg subcutaneously, dexamethasone 6 mg daily intravenously and insulin adjusted according to glucometer readings. He was transferred out of ICU after 5 days and continued to improve in hospital.

2. A 30 year old black woman, recipient of a deceased donor kidney transplant 3 months previously, was noted to have a decline in her baseline kidney function at a clinic visit. She had received antithymocyte globulin, high dose steroid induction therapy and was being maintained on tacrolimus, mycophenolate mofetil (MMF) and prednisolone. She had been noted to be CMV IgG positive while on dialysis. Her BP was130/60 mmHg, pulse 78/min and temperature 39 °C. Laboratory tests: haemoglobin 11.8 g/dL; WCC 3.1 × 10^9/L; platelet count 130,000; serum creatinine 180 μmol/L from a previous baseline of 110 μmol/L. Urine examination revealed 50 red cells/HPF and proteinuria of 0.5 g/day. Tacrolimus levels were between 5 and 15 ng/mL. She underwent a kidney biopsy.

Histology of the allograft biopsy showed a peritubular mononuclear interstitial infiltrate; some tubular cells had intranuclear inclusions.

What is the most likely diagnosis?

A. Acute cellular rejection
B. Acute antibody mediated rejection
C. BK virus infection
D. Cytomegalovirus infection
E. Tacrolimus toxicity

Answer: D

CMV viral load was 15,000 copies/mL. She was treated with intravenous ganciclovir 5 mg/kg every 12 h for 14 days, and thereafter maintained on valganciclovir 900 mg daily for 30 days. MMF was discontinued, tacrolimus dose was optimized according to blood levels, and she continued with low dose prednisolone. Her serum creatinine stabilized at 125 μmol/L.

3. An 18-year old boy, recipient of a second (deceased donor) kidney transplant was noted to have an asymptomatic rise in his serum creatinine during a routine clinic visit 12 months after transplantation. He had received antithymocyte globulin, high dose steroid induction therapy and was being maintained on tacrolimus, mycophenolate mofetil (MMF) and prednisolone. He had been noted to be CMV IgG positive previously. He was noted to have haemoglobin 12.8 g/dL; WCC 5.1 × 10^9/L; platelet count 230,000; serum creatinine 220 μmol/L from a previous baseline of 120 μmol/L. Urine cytology showed epithelial cells with viral inclusions 'decoy cells', Allograft biopsy showed mononuclear interstitial inflammation, and some degree of tubulitis with basophilic changes of the tubular epithelium.

What is the most likely diagnosis?

A. Acute cellular rejection
B. Acute antibody mediated rejection
C. BK virus infection
D. Cytomegalovirus infection
E. Tacrolimus toxicity

Answer: C

He had a urine BK load of 11^7 copies/mL and a serum BK viral load of 10^5 copies/mL. His MMF dose was halved, and tacrolimus trough levels lowered and he was treated with leflunomide 100 mg daily for 5 days and 40 mg daily thereafter until the virus was cleared. His kidney function gradually stabilized to around his baseline levels and surveillance for BKV is carried out on a monthly basis.

4. A 45 year old black man was recently diagnosed with HIV infection and referred to a Renal Clinic with proteinuria and renal dysfunction. He had minimal ankle oedema, BP 126/82 and had 3 g proteinuria/day. His serum albumin was 25 g/L, serum cholesterol 4.1 mmol/L, serum creatinine 188 μmol/L, eGFR 42.1 mL/min/1.73 m^2, CD4 count 180 cells/mL, viral load 125,000 copies/mL. He underwent a kidney biopsy.

   What is the most likely biopsy diagnosis?

   A. Crescentic glomerulonephritis
   B. Focal segmental glomerulonephritis
   C. Membranous glomerulonephritis
   D. Membranoproliferative glomerulonephritis
   E. Minimal change disease

   Answer: B

   His kidney biopsy showed typical HIV associated nephropathy, with glomerular collapse, microcystic tubular dilatation and interstitial inflammation. He was commenced on Losartan 50 mg daily, and Abacavir 300 mg BD, Lamuvidine (3TC) 150 mg daily and Dolutegravir 50 mg daily. Avoid fixed dose combinations if GFR < 50 mL/min, and tenofovir if possible. His APOL1 genotype was not available.

5. A 25 year old man was admitted to the emergency room with a fever of 39.1 °C, and dehydration. He had been on a beach vacation in Mozambique 2 weeks previously. He was noted to have tachycardia of 100/min, BP 96/60 and was pale and had a 2 cm splenomegaly. His haemoglobin was 10.1 g/dL; white cell count 4.1 × 10^9/L; platelets 92,000; serum bilirubin 35 mmol/L; blood urea 32 mmol/L; serum creatinine 220 μmol/L.

   What is the most likely cause of his acute kidney injury?

   A. Cytomegalovirus infection
   B. Epstein barr virus infection
   C. Malaria
   D. Pneumococcal infection
   E. Staphylococcus infection

   Answer: C

   A thin smear revealed the presence of tropozoites of P falciparum. He was commenced on intravenous fluids and therapy with artesunate 2.4 mg/kg intravenously immediately and 12 hourly for 24 h and thereafter switched to oral treatment with artemether-lumefantrine for 3 days. A blood smear at 72 h demonstrated that the parasitaemia had been eradicated and he made a a full recovery.

6. A 45 year old man, a visitor from Egypt, was hospitalized with abdominal distension. He had been an agricultural worker. He was noted to have hepatosplenomegly. Investigations showed dipstick proteinuria of 3+, and was measured to be 2.9 g/24 h; serum albumin 35 g/L; serum globulins 50 g/L; haemoglobin was 10.8 g/dL; white cell count 4.1 × 10^9/L; platelets 112,000; serum bilirubin 10 mmol/L; blood urea 5 mmol/L; serum creatinine 88 μmol/L. Ultrasound of the liver was suggestive of hepatic fibrosis, and was confirmed by fibroscan. A kidney biopsy showed membranoproliferative glomerulonephritis.

   What is the cause of the renal disease?

   A. Cytomegalovirus infection
   B. Hepatitis B infection
   C. HIV infection
   D. Malaria
   E. Schistosomiasis

   Answer: E

   A stool specimen showed the presence of schistosoma mansoni. He was treated with praziquantel and advised to avoid future schistosomal infection, and to return to his physician for review.

7. A 25 year old forest worker in the Democratic Republic of the Congo presented to the Emergency Department with 3 day history of headache, fever, shivering at night, muscle ache and joint pains. The headache was worst behind the eyes and he also mentioned shivering at night. His temperature was 40.0 °C

with a BP of 100/60 and regular tachycardia of 120/min. By Day 4 he had developed a maculo-papular rash with patches of purpura. Haemoglobin 13.0 g/dL, WBC 4.0×10^9/L, platelets 80×10^9/L [normal: 150–400]. Creatinine 350 µmol/L with urea 40 mmol/L, eGFR 24 mL/min/1.73 m^2. There was proteinuria 0.6 g/L and RBC 50–100/µL. Renal biopsy was not considered as it was felt that it would not influence treatment; furthermore it would add an unnecessary hazard for someone already at risk of bleeding.

What is the most likely diagnosis?

A. COVID 19 infection
B. Dengue fever
C. Ebola virus infection
D. Malaria
E. Tuberculosis infection

Answer: B

He was diagnosed with Dengue fever and managed with supportive treatment and scrupulous attention to clinical signs, pulse, blood pressure and urine output replacing fluid as necessary but avoiding overload. There is unfortunately no specific treatment for dengue virus and as yet no vaccine.

8. An 18 year-old female presented with history of fever for 2 weeks, and the passage of brown urine for 6 days, generalized body swelling for 5 days followed by reduced urine output and breathlessness for 2 days. She had a seizure episode a few hours before presentation. She had noted skin infections 3 weeks preceding the above symptoms. On presentation, she had impaired consciousness (GCS 8/15) but recovered within a few hours. She was pale, with bilateral pitting leg oedema temperature of 37.8 °C, respiratory rate 38 breaths/min, pulse 110 bpm and BP 160/110 mmHg. Urinalysis showed blood, protein, and microscopy revealed red cell casts. Her blood tests showed sodium: 122 mmol/L, potassium: 5.6 mmol/L, HCO_3: 12.4 mmol/L, chloride: 84.4, iCa: 1.01, BUN: 63.3 mmol/L, creatinine: 884 µmol/L, haemoglobin: 8.3 g/dL, leukocytosis with neutrophila of 78%.

What is the most likeley investigation which will help with diagnosis?

A. ASO titre
B. ANCA
C. Hepatitis B serology
D. Kidney biopsy
E. Serum immunoglobulin

Answer: A

Her ESR was 125 mm/hr and qualitative ASO titre: elevated/positive

9. An 18 year-old female presented with history of fever for 2 weeks, red-brown coloured urine for 6 days, generalized body swelling for 5 days followed by reduced urine output and breathlessness for 2 days. She had a seizure episode a few hours before presentation. She had noted skin infections 3 weeks preceding the above symptoms. On presentation, she had impaired consciousness (GCS 8/15) but recovered within a few hours. She was pale, with bilateral pitting leg oedema temperature of 37.8 °C, respiratory rate 38 breaths/min, pulse 110 bpm and BP 160/110 mmHg. Urinalysis showed blood, protein, and microscopy revealed red cell casts. Her blood tests showed sodium: 122 mmol/L, potassium: 5.6 mmol/L, HCO_3: 12.4 mmol/L, chloride: 84.4, iCa: 1.01, BUN: 63.3 mmol/L, creatinine: 884 µmol/L, haemoglobin: 8.3 g/dL, leukocytosis with neutrophila of 78%.

What is the most likely diagnosis?

A. Haemolytic uraemic syndrome
B. IgA nephritis
C. Lupus nephritis
D. Post infectious glomerulonephritis
E. Polyarteritis nodosa

Answer: D

Her ESR was 125 mm/hr and qualitative ASO titre: elevated/positive

10. A 42 year old rural drainage engineer, living in Sao Paulo state in southern Brazil, presented to the Dermatology clinic giving a history of intermittent skin rash sometimes associated with a change in pigmentation. He was found to have heavy proteinuria and referred to the nephrologist. In recent months he had been feeling more tired than usual. He

had a pale complexion. There was mild oedema of the ankles. Temperature: 36.5 °C, Haemoglobin 100 g/L, sodium 140 mmol/L, Potassium 5.3 mmol/L, bicarbonate 22 mmol/L, creatinine 216 μmol/L, albumin 23 g/L. Urine protein amounted to 10.5 g/24 h. An MSU revealed neither cells nor blood or glucose; the urine was sterile on culture. A repeat of the investigations a week later gave similar results.

What is the most likely diagnosis?

A. Leptospirosis
B. Systemic lupus erythematosus
C. Nephropathy of tuberculoid leprosy
D. Amyloidosis secondary to lepromatous leprosy
E. Falciparum malaria

Answer: D Amyloidosis secondary to lepromatous leprosy

A. Leptospirosis	Incorrect	Lack of fever, and no active urinary sediment
B. Systemic lupus erythematosus	Incorrect	No joint pain, no fever, no significant urinary sediment
C. Nephropathy of tuberculoid leprosy	Incorrect	Nephrotic syndrome not common in the tuberculoid form of leprosy
D. Amyloidosis secondary to lepromatous leprosy with nephrotic syndrome	Correct	Frequency of amyloidosis in leprosy types: lepromatous [36%], tuberculoid and borderline [5%]. The nephrotic syndrome is a consequence of the amyloidosis.
E. Falciparum malaria	Incorrect	No fever or other evidence of malaria

Test your learning and check your understanding of this book's contents: use the "Springer Nature Flashcards" app to access questions using https://sn.pub/cz9Cok. To use the app, please follow the instructions in Chap. 1.

References

1. Ndulue C, Jisike-Onuigbo N, Anyanor A, Ozuemba B, Osakwe A, Oguejiofor N, et al. SAT-459 purple urine bag syndrome in a Nigerian with gastrointestinal bleeding. Kidney Int Rep. 2020;5(3):S191–2.
2. Godaly G, Ambite I, Svanborg C. Innate immunity and genetic determinants of urinary tract infection susceptibility. Curr Opin Infect Dis. 2015;28:88–96.
3. Medina M, Castillo-Pino E. An introduction to the epidemiology and burden of urinary tract infections. Ther Adv Urol. 2019;11:3–7.
4. Tan CW, Chlebicki MP. Urinary tract infections in adults. Singap Med J. 2016;57(9):485–90.
5. Tandogdu Z, Wagenlehner FM. Global epidemiology of urinary tract infections. Curr Opin Infect Dis. 2016;29:73–9.
6. NICE Guideline: urinary tract infection (lower): antimicrobial prescribing. www.nice.org.uk/guidance/ng109. Accessed 20 Apr 2020.
7. EAU Guidelines. Edn. Presented at the EAU annual congress Barcelona 2019. isbn:978-94-92671-04-2.
8. Smelov V, Naber K, Bjerklund Johansen KE. Improved classification of urinary tract infection: future considerations. Eur Urol Suppl. 2016;5:71–80.
9. Gupta K, Hooton TM, Naber KG, Wullt B, Colgan R, Miller LG, et al. International clinical practice guidelines for the treatment of acute uncomplicated cystitis and pyelonephritis in women: a 2010 update by the Infectious Diseases Society of America and the European Society for Microbiology and Infectious Diseases. Clin Infect Dis. 2011;52(5):e103–20.
10. Rubin RH, Shapiro ED, Andriole VT, Davis RJ, Stamm WE. Evaluation of new anti-infective drugs for the treatment of urinary tract infection. Infectious Diseases Society of America and the Food and Drug Administration. Clin Infect Dis. 1992;15(suppl 1):S216–27.
11. Anger J, Lee U, Ackerman AL, Chou R, Chughtai B, Clemens JQ, et al. Recurrent uncomplicated urinary tract infections in women: AUA/CUA/SUFU guideline. J Urol. 2019;202:282–9.
12. NICE Guidance—Complicated urinary tract infections: ceftolozane/tazobactam. BJU Int. 2018;121:825–834.
13. NICE guideline: urinary tract infection (recurrent): antimicrobial prescribing. www.nice.org.uk/guidance/ng112. Accessed 20 Apr 2020.
14. Kulchavenya E. Best practice in the diagnosis and management of urogenital tuberculosis. Ther Adv Urol. 2013;5:143–51.
15. Pang Y, Shang Y, Lu J, Liang Q, Dong L, Li Y, et al. GeneXpert MTB/RIF assay in the diagnosis of urinary tuberculosis from urine specimens. Sci Rep. 2017;7:6181. https://doi.org/10.1038/s41598-017-06517-0.

16. Cek M, Lenk S, Naber KG, Bishop MC, Johansen TEB, Botto H, et al. EAU guidelines for the management of genitourinary tuberculosis. Eur Urol. 2005;48:353–62.
17. Yang C-W. Leptospirosis renal disease: emerging culprit of chronic kidney disease unknown etiology. Nephron. 2018;138:129–36.
18. Qiang XH, Yu TO, Li YN, Zhou LX. Prognosis risk of urosepsis in critical care medicine: a prospective observational study. Biomed Res Int. 2016;2016:9028924, 5 pages. https://doi.org/10.1155/2016/9028924.
19. Neild GH, Thomson G, Nitsch D, et al. Renal outcome in adults with renal insufficiency and irregular asymmetrical kidneys. BMC Nephrol. 2004;5:12.
20. Global tuberculosis report 2021. Geneva: World Health Organization; 2021. Licence: CC BY-NC-SA 3.0 IGO.
21. World Health Organization. Global tuberculosis report 2019. https://www.who.int/tb/publications/global_report/en/. Accessed 20 Apr 2020.
22. Gonzalez OY, Teeter LD, Thanh BT, Musser JM, Graviss EA. Extrathoracic tuberculosis lymphadenitis in adult HIV seronegative patients: a population-based analysis in Houston, Texas, USA. Int J Tuberc Lung Dis. 2003;7:987–93.
23. Daher EF, Silva Junior GB, Guardao Barros EJ. Review: renal tuberculosis in the modern era. Am J Trop Med Hyg. 2013;88(1):54–64.
24. Mallinson WJW, Fuller RW, Levison DA, et al. Diffuse interstitial renal tuberculosis. An unusual cause of renal failure. QJM. 1981;198:137–48.
25. Oliveira B, Jayawardene S, Shah S. Single centre experience of granulomatous interstitial nephropathy; time for a new approach? Clin Kidney J. 2017;10:249–54.
26. Eastwood JB, Zaidi M, Maxwell JD, et al. Tuberculosis as primary renal diagnosis in end-stage uremia. J Nephrol. 1994;7:290–3.
27. Global leprosy update, 2016: accelerating reduction of disease burden. WHO Weekly Epidemiological Record. 2017;92(35):501–520.
28. Nakayama EE, Ura S, Fleury RN, Soares V. Renal lesions in leprosy: a retrospective study of 199 autopsies. Am J Kidney Dis. 2001;38(1):26–30.
29. Silva Junior GB, Daher EF, Pires Neto RJ, et al. Leprosy nephropathy: a review of clinical and histopathological features. Rev Inst Med Trop Sao Paulo. 2015;57:15–20.
30. Torgerson PR, Hagan JE, Costa F, Calcagno J, Kane M, Martinez-Silveira MS, et al. Global burden of leptospirosis: estimated in terms of disability adjusted life years. PLoS Negl Trop Dis. 2015;9:e0004122.
31. Herath NJ, Kularatne SA, Weerakoon KG, Wazil A, Subasinghe N, Ratnatunga NV. Long term outcome of acute kidney injury due to leptospirosis? A longitudinal study in Sri Lanka. BMC Res Notes. 2014;7:398.
32. Kidney Disease: Improving Global Outcomes (KDIGO) Glomerulonephritis Work Group. KDIGO clinical practice guideline for glomerulonephritis. Kidney Int Suppl. 2012;2:139–274.
33. Prasad N, Patel MR. Infection-induced kidney diseases. Front Med. 2018;5:327. https://doi.org/10.3389/fmed.2018.00327.
34. Schiffl H. Renal recovery from acute tubular necrosis requiring renal replacement therapy: a prospective study in critically ill patients. Nephrol Dial Transplant. 2006;21:1248–52. https://doi.org/10.1093/ndt/gfk069.
35. Lopes JA, Jorge S, Resina C, Santos C, Pereira A, Neves J, et al. Acute kidney injury in patients with sepsis: a contemporary analysis. Int J Infect Dis. 2009;13:176–81.
36. Hoste EA, Bagshaw SM, Bellomo R, Cely CM, Colman R, Cruz DN, et al. Epidemiology of acute kidney injury in critically ill patients: the multinational AKI-EPI study. Intensive Care Med. 2015;41:1411–23.
37. Naughton CA. Drug-induced nephrotoxicity. Am Fam Physician. 2008;78(6):743–50.
38. Awdishu L, Mehta RL. The 6R's of drug induced nephrotoxicity. BMC Nephrol. 2017;18:124. https://doi.org/10.1186/s12882-017-0536-3.
39. Lizarraga KJ, Nayer A. Dengue-associated kidney disease. J Nephropathol. 2014;3(2):57–62.
40. Nasim A, Anis S, Baqi S, Akhtar SF, Baig-Ansari N. Clinical presentation and outcome of dengue viral infection in live-related renal transplant recipients in Karachi, Pakistan. Transplant Infect Dis. 2013;5(15):516–25.
41. Jessie K, Fong MY, Devi S, Lam SK, Wong KT. Localization of dengue virus in naturally infected human tissues, by immunohistochemistry and in situ hybridization. J Infect Dis. 2004;189(8):1411–8.
42. Méndez A, González G. [Dengue haemorrhagic fever in children: ten years of clinical experience]. Biomedica. 2003;23(2):180–193.
43. Jonsson CB, Figueiredo LTM, Vapalahti O. A global perspective on hantavirus ecology, epidemiology, and disease. Clin Microbiol Rev. 2010;23(2):412–41.
44. Krautkrämer E, Grouls S, Stein N, Reiser J, Zeier M. Pathogenic old world hantaviruses infect renal glomerular and tubular cells and induce disassembling of cell-to-cell contacts. J Virol. 2011;85(19):9811–23.
45. Ferluga D, Vizjak A. Hantavirus nephropathy. JASN. 2008;19(9):1653–8.
46. Miettinen MH, Mäkelä SM, Ala-Houhala IO, Huhtala HSA, Kööbi T, Vaheri AI, et al. Ten-year prognosis of Puumala hantavirus-induced acute interstitial nephritis. Kidney Int. 2006;69(11):2043–8.
47. Gamage CD, Sarathkumara YD. Chronic kidney disease of uncertain etiology in Sri Lanka: are lepto-

spirosis and Hantaviral infection likely causes? Med Hypotheses. 2016;91:16–9.
48. Prasad N, Novak JE, Patel MR. Kidney diseases associated with parvovirus B19, Hanta, Ebola, and dengue virus infection: a brief review. Adv Chronic Kidney Dis. 2019;26(3):207–19.
49. Baseler L, Chertow DS, Johnson KM, Feldmann H, Morens DM. The pathogenesis of Ebola virus disease. Annu Rev Pathol. 2017;12:387–418.
50. Uyeki TM, Mehta AK, Davey RT, Liddell AM, Wolf T, Vetter P, et al. Clinical management of Ebola virus disease in the United States and Europe. N Engl J Med. 2016;374(7):636–46.
51. Zolnourian ZR, Curran MD, Rima BK, Coyle PV, O'Neill HJ, Middleton D. Parvovirus B19 in kidney transplant patients. Transplantation. 2000;69(10):2198–202.
52. Waldman M, Kopp JB. Parvovirus B19 and the kidney. Clin J Am Soc Nephrol. 2007;2(Suppl 1):S47–56.
53. Wierenga KJ, Pattison JR, Brink N, Griffiths M, Miller M, Shah DJ, et al. Glomerulonephritis after human parvovirus infection in homozygous sickle-cell disease. Lancet. 1995;346(8973):475–6.
54. Leiri N, Hotta O, Taguma Y. Characteristics of acute glomerulonephritis associated with human parvovirus B19 infection. Clin Nephrol. 2005;64(4):249–57.
55. Liefeldt L, Buhl M, Schweickert B, Engelmann E, Sezer O, Laschinski P, et al. Eradication of parvovirus B19 infection after renal transplantation requires reduction of immunosuppression and high-dose immunoglobulin therapy. Nephrol Dial Transplant. 2002;17(10):1840–2.
56. Hirsch HH, Knowles W, Dickenmann M, Passweg J, Klimkait T, Mihatsch MJ, et al. Prospective study of polyomavirus type BK replication and nephropathy in renal-transplant recipients. N Engl J Med. 2002;347(7):488–96.
57. Randhawa PS, Finkelstein S, Scantlebury V, Shapiro R, Vivas C, Jordan M, et al. Human polyoma virus-associated interstitial nephritis in the allograft kidney. Transplantation. 1999;67(1):103–9.
58. Hirsch HH, Brennan DC, Drachenberg CB, Ginevri F, Gordon J, Limaye AP, et al. Polyomavirus-associated nephropathy in renal transplantation: interdisciplinary analyses and recommendations. Transplantation. 2005;79(10):1277–86.
59. Drachenberg CB, Beskow CO, Papadimitriou JC, Cangro CB, Rocca M, Klassen DK, et al. Human polyoma virus infected cells (PoVIC): incidence in renal biopsies (BX), urine cytology and correlation with clinical presentation. Transplantation. 1999;67(7):S217.
60. Hirsch HH. Human polyomavirus and papillomavirus infection and disease posttransplant. In: Transplant infections. Springer; 2016. p. 631–652.
61. Nankivell BJ, Renthawa J, Jeoffreys N, Kable K, O'Connell PJ, Chapman JR, et al. Clinical utility of urinary cytology to detect BK viral nephropathy. Transplantation. 2015;99(8):1715–22.
62. Drachenberg CB, Papadimitriou JC, Chaudhry MR, Ugarte R, Mavanur M, Thomas B, et al. Histological evolution of BK virus–associated nephropathy: importance of integrating clinical and pathological findings. Am J Transplant. 2017;17(8):2078–91.
63. Nickeleit V, Singh HK, Randhawa P, Drachenberg CB, Bhatnagar R, Bracamonte E, et al. The Banff working group classification of definitive polyomavirus nephropathy: morphologic definitions and clinical correlations. J Am Soc Nephrol. 2018;29(2):680–93.
64. Sawinski D, Goral S. BK virus infection: an update on diagnosis and treatment. Nephrol Dial Transplant. 2015;30(2):209–17.
65. Hirsch HH, Randhawa P, AST Infectious Diseases Community of Practice. BK polyomavirus in solid organ transplantation. Am J Transplant. 2013r;13(Suppl 4):179–88.
66. Cummins NW, Sohail MR. Cytomegalovirus, BK, and other viral infections of the kidney. In: Core concepts in parenchymal kidney disease. Springer; 2014. p. 229–240.
67. Helanterä I, Koskinen P, Finne P, Loginov R, Kyllönen L, Salmela K, et al. Persistent cytomegalovirus infection in kidney allografts is associated with inferior graft function and survival. Transpl Int. 2006;19(11):893–900.
68. Agrawal V, Gupta RK, Jain M, Prasad N, Sharma RK. Polyomavirus nephropathy and cytomegalovirus nephritis in renal allograft recipients. Indian J Pathol Microbiol. 2010;53(4):672–5.
69. Posadas Salas MA, Thompson J, Kadian M, Ngo T, Bruner E, Self S. Cytomegalovirus renal infection: rare manifestation of a common post-transplant viral infection-a case series. Transpl Infect Dis. 2019;21(6):e13169.
70. Fogo A. Cytomegalovirus infection. Am J Kidney Dis. 2000;36(2):E7–8.
71. Ferreira AC, Navarro D. Cytomegalovirus nephropathy in the transplant patient. Nephrol Dial Transplant. 2021;36:777–8. https://doi.org/10.1093/ndt/gfz194.
72. Kole AK, Roy R, Kole DC. An observational study of complications in chickenpox with special reference to unusual complications in an apex infectious disease hospital, Kolkata, India. J Postgrad Med. 2013;59(2):93–7.
73. Os I, Ström EH, Stenehjem A, Gudmundsdottir H, Langberg H, Draganov B, et al. Varicella infection in a renal transplant recipient associated with abdominal pain, hepatitis, and glomerulonephritis. Scand J Urol Nephrol. 2001;35(4):330–3.
74. Zaki S, Bhongade S, Shanbag P. Acute glomerulonephritis following varicella infection. Indian J Nephrol. 2012;22(1):64. https://doi.org/10.4103/0971-4065.83753.
75. Condom P, Mansuy J-M, Decramer S, Izopet J, Mengelle C. Atypical hemolytic uremic syndrome triggered by varicella infection. ID Cases. 2017;9:89–90.

76. Bazerbachi F, Haffar S, Garg SK, Lake JR. Extra-hepatic manifestations associated with hepatitis E virus infection: a comprehensive review of the literature. Gastroenterol Rep (Oxf). 2016;4(1):1–15.
77. Pischke S, Hartl J, Pas SD, Lohse AW, Jacobs BC, Van der Eijk AA. Hepatitis E virus: infection beyond the liver? J Hepatol. 2017;66(5):1082–95.
78. Agrawal P, Kumar V, Kumar A, Sachdeva MUS, Malhotra P, Nada R. Monoclonal Gammopathy of renal significance triggered by viral E hepatitis. Indian J Nephrol. 2019;29(1):50–2.
79. Kamar N, Rostaing L, Izopet J. Hepatitis E virus infection in immunosuppressed patients: natural history and therapy. In: Seminars in liver disease. New York: Thieme Medical Publishers; 2013. p. 62–70.
80. Andrievskaya M, Lenhart A, Uduman J. Emerging threat: changing epidemiology of hepatitis A and acute kidney injury. Adv Chronic Kidney Dis. 2019;26(3):171–8.
81. Fan P-C, Chen Y-C, Tian Y-C, Chang C-H, Fang J-T, Yang C-W. Acute renal failure associated with acute non-fulminant hepatitis A: a case report and review of literature. Ren Fail. 2009;31(8):756–64.
82. Bhimma R, Coovadia HM. Hepatitis B virus-associated nephropathy. Am J Nephrol. 2004;24(2):198–211.
83. Kamimura H, Setsu T, Kimura N, Yokoo T, Sakamaki A, Kamimura K, et al. Renal impairment in chronic hepatitis B: a review. Diseases. 2018;6(2):52. https://doi.org/10.3390/diseases6020052.
84. Li D, Gao G, Jiang H, Tang Z, Yu Y, Zang G. Hepatitis B virus-associated glomerulonephritis in HBsAg serological-negative patients. Eur J Gastroenterol Hepatol. 2015;27(1):65–9.
85. Lai K. Hepatitis-related renal disease. Futur Virol. 2011;6:1361–76.
86. Pipili C, Papatheodoridis G, Cholongitas E. Treatment of hepatitis B in patients with chronic kidney disease. Kidney Int. 2013;84:880–5.
87. Gill K, Ghazinian H, Manch R, Gish R. Hepatitis C virus as a systemic disease: reaching beyond the liver. Hepatol Int. 2016;3(10):415–23.
88. Meyers CM, Seeff LB, Stehman-Breen CO, Hoofnagle JH. Hepatitis C and renal disease: an update 1. Am J Kidney Dis. 2003;42(4):631–57.
89. Kidney Disease: Improving Global Outcomes HCV Work Group. KDIGO 2018 clinical practice guideline for the prevention, diagnosis, evaluation, and treatment of hepatitis C in chronic kidney disease. Kidney Int Suppl. 2018;8(3):91–165.
90. Jotwani V, Atta MG, Estrella MM. Kidney disease in HIV: moving beyond HIV-associated nephropathy. JASN. 2017;28(11):3142–54.
91. Swanepoel CR, Atta MG, D'Agati VD, Estrella MM, Fogo AB, Naicker S, et al. Kidney disease in the setting of HIV infection: conclusions from a kidney disease: improving global outcomes (KDIGO) controversies conference. Kidney Int. 2018;93(3):545–59.
92. Fabian J, Naicker S. HIV and kidney disease in sub-Saharan Africa. Nat Rev Nephrol. 2009;5(10):591–8. https://doi.org/10.1038/nrneph.2009.141.
93. Kasembeli AN, Duarte R, Ramsay M, Mosiane P, Dickens C, Dix-Peek T, et al. APOL1 risk variants are strongly associated with HIV-associated nephropathy in black South Africans. JASN. 2015;26(11):2882–90.
94. Dummer PD, Limou S, Rosenberg AZ, Heymann J, Nelson G, Winkler CA, et al. APOL1 kidney disease risk variants: an evolving landscape. Semin Nephrol. 2015;35(3):222–36.
95. Kopp JB, Nelson GW, Sampath K, Johnson RC, Genovese G, An P, et al. APOL1 genetic variants in focal segmental glomerulosclerosis and HIV-associated nephropathy. J Am Soc Nephrol. 2011;22(11):2129–37.
96. Nobakht E, Cohen SD, Rosenberg AZ, Kimmel PL. HIV-associated immune complex kidney disease. Nat Rev Nephrol. 2016;12(5):291–300.
97. Cheng Y, Luo R, Wang K, et al. Kidney disease is associated with in-hospital death of COVID-19 patients. Kidney Int. 2020;97:829–38. https://doi.org/10.1016/kint.2020.03.005.
98. Chen YT, Shao SC, Hsu CK, et al. Incidence of acute kidney injury in COVID-19 infection: a systematic review and metanalysis. Crit Care. 2020;24:346. https://doi.org/10.1186/s13054-020-03009-y.
99. Ali H, Daoud A, Mohamed MM, Salim SA, Yessayan L, Baharani J, et al. Survival rate in acute kidney injury superimposed COVID-19 patients: a systematic review and meta-analysis. Ren Fail. 2020;42:393–7. https://doi.org/10.1080/0886022x2020.17.
100. Batlle D, Soler MJ, Sparks MA, Hiremath S, South AM, Welling PA, et al., on behalf of the COVID-19 and ACE2 in Cardiovascular, Lung, and Kidney Working Group. Acute kidney injury in COVID-19: emerging evidence of a distinct pathophysiology. JASN. 2020;31:1380–1383. https://doi.org/10.1681/ASN.2020040419.
101. Kudose S, Batal I, Santoriello D, Xu K, Barasch J, Peleg Y, et al. Kidney biopsy findings in patients with COVID-19. JASN. 2020;31(9):2158–67. https://doi.org/10.1681/ASN.2020050744.
102. Fisher M, Yunes M, Mokrzycki MH, et al. Chronic hemodialysis patients hospitalized with COVID-19—short-term outcomes in Bronx, New York. Kidney360. 2020;1(8):755–62. https://doi.org/10.34067/KID.0003672020.
103. Akalin E, Azzi Y, Bartash R, et al. Covid-19 and kidney transplantation. N Engl J Med. 2020;382:2475–7. https://doi.org/10.1056/NEJMc2011117.
104. https://www.who.int/malaria/en/. Accessed 30 Apr 2020.

105. World malaria report 2021. Geneva: World Health Organization; 2021. Licence: CC BY-NC-SA 3.0 IGO.
106. Global distribution of Malaria in 2018—CDC 'Heat' Map. https://www.cdc.gov/malaria/travellers/country_table/a.html
107. Barsoum RS. Malarial acute renal failure. J Am Soc Nephrol. 2000;11:2147–54.
108. Das BS. Renal failure in malaria. J Vector Borne Dis. 2008;45:83–97.
109. Manan JA, Ali H, Lal M. Acute renal failure associated with malaria. J Ayub Med Coll Abbottabad. 2006;4:47–52.
110. Barsoum RS. Malarial nephropathies. Nephrol Dial Transplant. 1998;13:1588–97.
111. Kute VB, Trivedi HL, Vanikar AV, Shah PR, Gumber MR, Patel HV, et al. Plasmodium vivax malaria–associated acute kidney injury, India, 2010–2011. Emerg Infect Dis. 2012;18:842–5.
112. Naqvi R. Plasmodium vivax causing acute kidney injury: a foe less addressed. Pak J Med Sci. 2015;31:1472–5.
113. Bircan Z, Kervancioglu M, Soran M, Gonlusen G, Tuncer I. Two cases of nephrotic syndrome and tertian malaria in South-Eastern Anatolia. Pediatr Nephrol. 1997;11(1):78–9.
114. da Silva Junior GB, Pinto JR, Barros EJG, Geysa Farias GMN, De Francesco DE. Kidney involvement in malaria: an update. Rev Inst Med Trop São Paulo. 2017;59:e53. https://doi.org/10.1590/S1678-9946201759053.
115. Poti KE, Sullivan DJ, Dondorp AM, Woodrow CJ. HRP2: transforming malaria diagnosis, but with caveats. Trends Parasitol. 2020;36(2):112–26. https://doi.org/10.1016/j.pt.2019.12.004.
116. Plucinski MM, Candrinho B, Dimene M, Colborn J, Lu A, Nace D, et al. Assessing performance of HRP2 antigen detection for malaria diagnosis in Mozambique. J Clin Microbiol. 2019;57(9):e00875–919. https://doi.org/10.1128/JCM.00875-19.
117. WHO Malaria Publications. Management of severe malaria. In: A practical handbook. 3rd ed. 2012. isbn:978-92-4-154852-6. https://www.who.int/malaria/publications/atoz/9789241548526/en/
118. Ismail SA, Kamal W, Salem HK. Schistosoma prevalence world-wide. In: Schistosomiasis. 2016. isbn:978-1-944685-64-5. http://www.smgebooks.com/schistosomiasis/index.php#
119. World Health Organization. https://www.who.int/schistosomiasis/epidemiology/table3/en/. Accessed 2 May 2020.
120. CDC. www.cdc.gov/parasites/schistosomiasis. Accessed 2 May 2020.
121. da Silva Junior GB, Duarte DB, Barros EJ, De Francesco DE. Schistosomiasis-associated kidney disease: a review. Asian Pac J Trop Dis. 2013;3(1):79–84.
122. Barsoum RS. Schistosomal glomerulopathies. Kidney Int. 1993;44:1–12.
123. Seck SM, Sarr ML, Dial MC, Ka EF. Schistosoma hematobium-associated glomerulopathy. Indian J Nephrol. 2011;21(3):201–3. https://doi.org/10.4103/0971-4065.78076.
124. Barsoum RS, Esmat G, El-Baz T. Human schistosomiasis: clinical perspective. J Adv Res. 2013;4(5):433–44.
125. Fraser VJ, Jones M, Dunkel J, Storfer S, Medoff G, Dunagan WC. Candidemia in a tertiary care hospital: epidemiology, risk factors, and predictors of mortality. Clin Infect Dis. 1992;15:414–21. https://doi.org/10.1093/clind/15.3.414.
126. Singh N. Trends in the epidemiology of opportunistic fungal infections: predisposing factors and the impact of antimicrobial use practices. Clin Infect Dis. 2001;33:1692–6. https://doi.org/10.1086/323895.
127. Badiee P, Hashemizadeh Z. Opportunistic invasive fungal infections: diagnosis & clinical management. Indian J Med Res. 2014;139:195.

15 Genetic Kidney Diseases

Radaa G. Sritharan, Jill Vanmassenhove, Anand K. Saggar, J. Christopher Kingswood, and Nicholas M. P. Annear

Clinical Scenario

A 19-year-old male presents to his primary care doctor with a 6-week history of intermittent abdominal pain. He has no significant past medical history. On examination, his blood pressure is 124/76 mmHg, and his pulse 64 beats per minute, and regular. His abdominal examination is unremarkable. His urinalysis reveals 1+ haematuria only. An ultrasound of his abdomen and urinary tract demonstrates multiple cortical renal cysts bilaterally. His blood tests show a serum creatinine of 75 μmol/L (eGFR >90 mL/min/1.73 m^2).

On further questioning, there is a family history of 'chronic kidney disease' in his father and paternal grandmother. His family pedigree is represented in Fig. 15.1.

R. G. Sritharan · A. K. Saggar
St George's University Hospitals NHS Foundation Trust, London, UK
e-mail: radaagowrry.sritharan@stgeorges.nhs.uk; a.saggar@nhs.net

J. Vanmassenhove
Department of Internal Medicine, Renal Division, Ghent University Hospital, Ghent, Belgium
e-mail: jill.vanmassenhove@ugent.be

J. C. Kingswood
Brighton & Sussex Renal Unit, Brighton, UK

St George's University of London, London, UK

N. M. P. Annear (✉)
St George's University Hospitals NHS Foundation Trust, London, UK

St George's University of London, London, UK
e-mail: nannear@sgul.ac.uk

D. Banerjee et al. (eds.), *Management of Kidney Diseases*,
https://doi.org/10.1007/978-3-031-09131-5_15

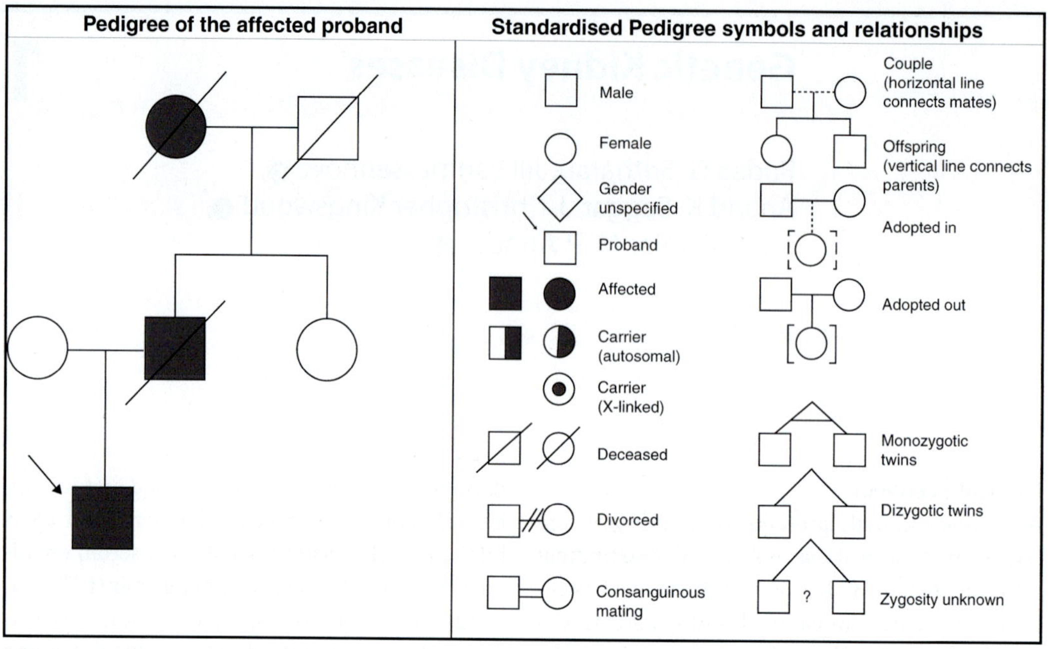

Fig. 15.1 Pedigree of the affected proband (the individual being studied), with key of standardised pedigree symbols and relationships

Introduction

Genetic kidney disorders are caused by mutations in genes that code for proteins including receptors, channels and transporters, enzymes, transcription factors, and structural components, that play a role in normal kidney function, and may also play a role in the normal function of other organs, including the brain, bones, eyes and skin [1].

Inherited single-gene (monogenic) kidney diseases, such as autosomal dominant polycystic kidney disease (ADPKD) or Alport syndrome, are the fifth commonest cause of end stage kidney disease (ESKD) worldwide, accounting for over 10% of adults, and nearly all children who progress to dialysis or transplantation. Moreover, since the early stages of CKD are often clinically silent, patients may not present until they are at or near ESKD. Advances in kidney replacement therapy (KRT) mean that—despite progressive disease, these patients can live for many years. The impact of both complications from the underlying genetic condition and ESKD on the healthcare system, and on their quality of life, can nevertheless be very significant, often necessitating the input of multiple specialties to facilitate optimal patient care [1].

In addition to recognised hereditary conditions, there is compelling evidence for a genetic contribution across many other forms of kidney disease, where no one causative gene has been implicated, including diabetes mellitus and CKD: The heritability of glomerular filtration rate (GFR) is estimated to be around 30–60% in the general population; other parameters such as tubular transport of electrolytes also show substantial hereditability [2].

Furthermore, the cause of CKD is classified as unknown in more than ten percent of patients with ESKD, a proportion of whom may have an underlying genetic cause: earlier and more specific diagnoses may enable the delivery of more effective care, and hence help to prevent or limit progression to ESKD [2].

Classically, the diagnostic journey for patients with suspected inherited kidney disease involves multiple clinical visits and complex investigations, often including a kidney biopsy. Bringing the results of these investigations together allows the clinician to identify the most likely aetiology, and select one or a few associated genes for sequencing, and confirm the genetic diagnosis. The recent adoption in many countries of newer genetic technologies such as chromosomal microarray (CMA) and next-generation sequencing (NGS) to clinical cases reflects a revolution in the work-up of suspected genetic disorders in clinical medicine, wherein genome-wide testing approaches are used to identify the aetiology of disease in a patient, and the genetic variant(s) identified used to guide their clinical care. This approach to testing may help overcome the diagnostic challenges posed by the genetic and phenotypic heterogeneity displayed in many inherited kidney diseases [2].

Ensuring that the approach to genetic testing developed at well-resourced, specialist tertiary care centres can also be adopted in less-resource-intensive settings is an important consideration that underpins the ongoing development of best practice guidelines for diagnosis and treatment of these rare inherited kidney disorders. Equally important are educational drives to support clinicians, patients, and society—as this information becomes more widely available. These efforts are supported by numerous network and initiatives, including organisations such as the National Organisations of Rare Disorders (NORD) in the USA, and Orphanet and ERKNet in Europe [1].

Practice Point 1: Key Questions When Designing Pathways for Genetic Testing in Kidney Disease

- In which patient cohort(s) is genetic testing indicated?
- How is the most appropriate genetic test identified?
- How is the genetic test interpreted and communicated?
- How are the genetic findings translated into personalised care?
- What are the ethical, legal and social implications of genetic testing?

Monogenic and Polygenic Kidney Disease

In monogenic (single-gene) disorders, the genetic mutation itself represents the primary cause of the disease. In general, these disease-causing genes are rare, exert strong causality on the disease phenotype with nearly full penetrance, manifest in early life, and leave little room for environmental influences. Detection is by classical targeted gene sequencing, or gene panel testing. The wider adoption of genetic screening has led to a growing awareness that genetic penetrance is rather more variable: many patients display a milder disease phenotype, and yet retain the same genetic variation [3] (Table 15.1).

The main modes of inheritance in monogenic disorders are autosomal dominant (AD), autosomal recessive (AR), X-linked recessive (XR), and X-linked dominant (XD) (Table 15.2):

Many of the commonest health disorders, such as diabetes mellitus, appear to be caused by the interplay of multiple genetic and environmental factors: These conditions are not likely to follow a simple pattern of inheritance, but rather may show a clustering in a family of several people with the condition. This inheritance pattern is referred to as 'multifactorial' or 'polygenic' inheritance. In these circumstances, we can rarely accurately estimate the chance that a particular family member will inherit the condition. Genetic information is therefore based on data obtained from observing whole populations. In general, polygenic disorders are more common, manifest in adulthood, exert weak causality on the disease phenotype, manifest later in life, leave more room for environmental influences, and are usually detected by genome-wide associated studies

Table 15.1 Benefits of Identifying a Monogenic disease-causing variant

Identification of a single disease-causing genetic variant provides the following opportunities for diagnostics, therapy, and insights into pathogenesis [3]:
• Unequivocal molecular genetic test may negate the need for invasive procedures e.g. *the diagnosis of nephronophthisis can be made without the necessity for kidney biopsy* • Prenatal diagnosis is possible *e.g. diagnosis of the perinatal-lethal Meckel-Gruber syndrome (MKS)* • Specific prognostic outcomes can be delineated for specific mutations *e.g. PKD1 and PKD2 mutations are associated with earlier or later onset of autosomal dominant polycystic kidney disease (ADPKD), respectively* • Subgroups of diseases may be classified for differential therapy *e.g. in mutations in NPHS2, which convey resistance to steroid treatment in nephrotic syndrome* • Disease mechanisms can be studied in related monogenic animal models *e.g. mouse models have offered important insights into how kidney cysts develop*

Table 15.2 Modes of Inheritance (MOI) in monogenic disorders

	Autosomal dominant (AD)	**Autosomal recessive (AR)**	**X-Linked recessive (XR)**	**X-Linked dominant (XD)**
Definition	One copy of mutated gene causes genetic condition	Mutations present on both alleles (copies) of a given gene causes genetic condition	Gene mutations on X chromosome Males carrying a single XR mutation affected	Gene mutations on X chromosome Sons and daughters of an affected parent may also be affected
Main Features	M & F equally affected >1 generation affected M & F can both pass condition to sons & daughters	M & F equally affected Individuals affected with the condition are in one sibship in one generation More likely in consanguineous families	Mostly males affected Gene mutation transmitted from female carriers to sons Affected males cannot pass condition to sons Females rarely affected (second unaltered copy of gene on other X chromosome)	M & F affected Rare MOI Affected males cannot pass condition to sons, but daughters will be affected
Genogram	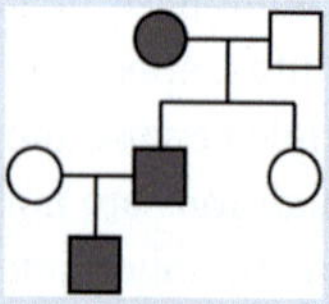	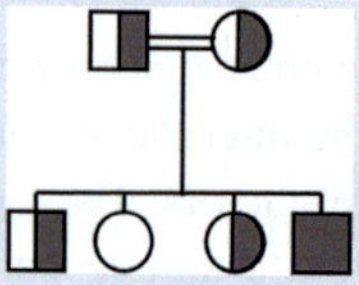	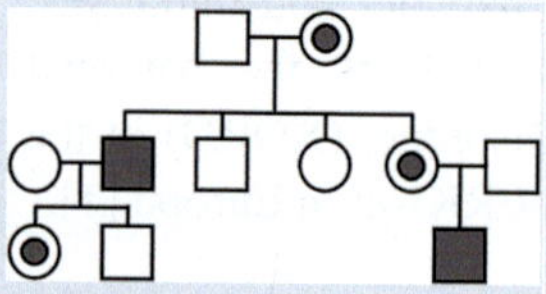	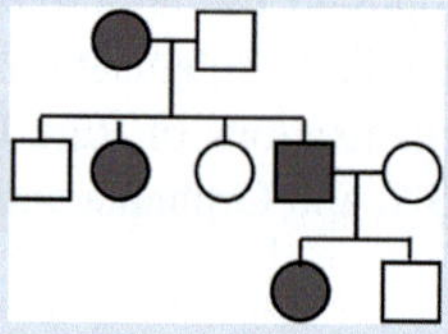
Chance of inheritance (in each pregnancy)	50% chance affected child 50% chance unaffected child	25% chance affected child 50% chance carrier child 25% chance non-carrier child	**XR in a Female** 25% chance affected son 25% chance carrier daughter 25% chance non-carrier son 25% chance non-carrier daughter **XR in a Male** All daughters affected Sons unaffected	**XD in a Female** 50% chance affected child **XD in a Male** All daughters affected Sons unaffected

Abbreviations: AD Autosomal dominant, *AR* Autosomal recessive, *F* Female, *M* Male, *MOI* Mode of inheritance, *XD* X-linked dominant, *XR* X-linked recessive

Table 15.3 The Threshold model for polygenic and multifactorial inheritance

The Threshold model for polygenic and multifactorial inheritance
Many genes and environmental factors influence the liability to develop disease, each having a small effect: The Threshold model may help explain the expression of a disease phenotype, bringing together a collection of factors that form a 'liability' to develop a multifactorial disease, such as diabetes mellitus or hypertension. The liability across a population follows a normal (bell-shaped) distribution, and a disease threshold, where individuals whose liability is greater than the disease threshold have/will develop the disease. This is illustrated in the figure below: Two thresholds for developing a disease are shown—a lower one for males, and a higher one for females.

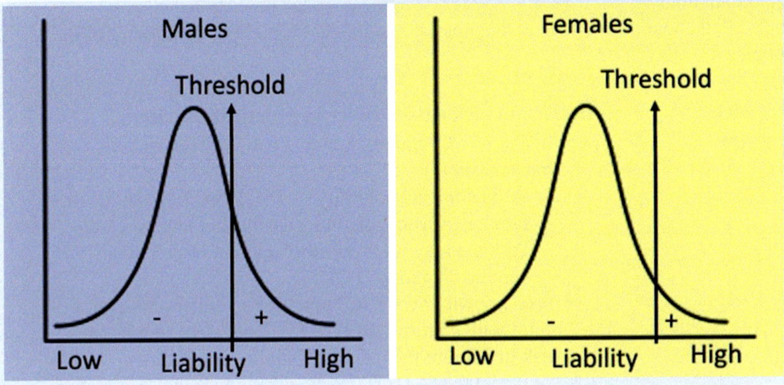

(GWAS), and now, next-generation sequencing (NGS) technologies [3] (Table 15.3).

Practice Point 2: Risk Alleles in Polygenic and Multifactorial Disease

The genetic variants that cause susceptibility to common complex kidney phenotypes, such as low GFR (CKD), have small effect sizes, and therefore need to be common to be detected. Interestingly, some variants display both a strong effect size and high frequency, for example:

- Identification of *APOL1* variants, found to be associated with an increased risk for focal segmental glomerulosclerosis (FSGS) and CKD amongst African American patients
- Identification of *PLA2R* variants, associated with susceptibility to idiopathic membranous nephropathy [3, 4]

Genetic Testing

A key part of genetic testing is counselling the patient, and their families where this is appropriate, about the process, its benefits and risks, to help them understand the full potential impact of testing (Practice points 3 & 4), whether these are diagnostic or not. Part of this process must be initiated before testing is done, and part of the more detailed information—particularly regarding reproductive options and cascade testing—may be the focus of onward referral to Genetic counselling services, once the genetic diagnosis has been made.

Practice Point 3: Benefits & Risks of Genetic Testing

Benefits	Risks
• Family planning and reproductive choice • Early detection and treatment of disease complications • Selection of unaffected family members for living donor transplantation	• Possible discrimination in terms of insurance and employment • Psychological effects of living with a disease without effective treatment • Unexpected unrelated findings from WES

Practice Point 4: Genetic Counselling [5]

- Clinicians must be an advocate for the patient and their children
- Respect patient's religious & cultural beliefs, and autonomy in decision making
- Patients with any genetic diagnosis should be counselled about reproductive options, including natural conception, germ cell donation, prenatal diagnosis, and preimplantation genetic diagnosis (PGD)
- Nephrologists should collaborate with clinical Geneticists and Genetic Counsellors to provide information and recommendations
- Patients should be counselled about how a genetic diagnosis could hinder their ability to obtain health or other types of insurance

Examples [6]:

Disease	**MOI**	**Important elements to cover in genetic counselling**
Tuberous Sclerosis Complex (TSC)	AD	• If *TSC1/TSC2* mutation in one partner, 50% risk of transmission – Wide clinical variability of *TSC1/TSC2* mutations in families: severe outcome possible but unpredictable – Partners may want pre-implantation or prenatal genetic diagnosis (PGD) • If no known *TSC1/TSC2* mutation in either parent of a child with confirmed *TSC1/TSC2* mutation, predicting risk in a future pregnancy difficult: – Parental *TSC1/TSC2* mosaicism (germinal ± somatic) possible – *De novo* mutation after fertilization/in later development (*de novo* mosaicism) more common Pre-implantation/prenatal genetic diagnosis possible
Autosomal Recessive Polycystic Kidney Disease (ARPKD)	AR	• If parents have a child with ARPKD, risk of future children – Being a carrier = 50% – Being affected = 25% (variable disease severity) • Identification of *PKHD1* mutation allows prenatal diagnosis
X-linked Alport Syndrome	XR	• Transmission by father: – no father to son transmission – all females will be heterozygous • Transmission by mother: – 50% of girls will be heterozygous for the mutation – 50% of boys will be affected • Heterozygous females have haematuria, may develop CKD • Affected boys reach ESKD aged 15–60 years • Prenatal genetic testing based on gender determination and identification of causative *COL4A5* mutation

Abbreviations: AD Autosomal dominant, *AR* Autosomal recessive, *XR* X-linked recessive, *MOI* Mode of inheritance

Table 15.4 Types of genetic testing

Targeted Gene sequencing/ Panel testing (specific genes known to cause condition)	Chromosomal Microarray (CMA)	Whole Exome Sequencing (WES) (coding region)	Whole Genome Sequencing (WGS) (entire genome)
• Analysis restricted to known gene associations • Likelihood of a variant being pathogenic greatly increased	• Enables detection of small and large copy number variants. • CMAs cannot detect balanced chromosomal rearrangements/low-grademosaicism. • Limited sensitivity to detect changes in certain regions, e.g. • pseudogenes and repetitive elements	• The exome is the portion of the genome containing the protein-coding regions of genes (exons). • Less comprehensive analysis (1-2% ofgenome) than WGS High diagnostic yield (most variants associated with hereditary conditions are located within exons, or flanking regions). • Analysis not restricted to genes known to cause a givencondition	• Examines nearly all coding and non-coding DNA. • Analysis not restricted to those genes known to cause given condition. • The most comprehensive analysis of the genome available
• Cost-effective	• Cost-effective	• Cheaper than WGS	• Most expensive of current NGS technologies
• Fewer variants detected Data easier to interpret	• Fewer variants detected than with WESor WGS • Increased risk of incidental findings over targeted panel	• Fewer variants detected than WGS and but increased risk of identifying incidental findings over targeted panel	• Greater risk of incidental findings and variants of unknown significance (VUS)
• Very deep sequencing - Increases chance of mosaicism being detected	• Less able to detect mosaicism	• Deep sequencing increases sensitivity and detection of mosaicism	• Shallow sequencing (fewer reads per gene) : less sensitive; less able to detect mosaicism
• Used when monogenic disorder suspected, e.g. ADPKD	• First line diagnostic tool amongst patients with syndromic CAKUT or paediatric nephropathy	• Disorders with high genetic and/or phenotypic heterogeneity such as nephronophthisis-related ciliopathies	

Next generation sequencing (NGS) technologies have opened up a large number of cost-effective approaches to genetic testing. Four key approaches to NGS genetic testing are outlined in Table 15.4:

An Approach to Genetic Testing

In adult kidney patients, genetic testing is recommended for those who are strongly suspected to have a known form of hereditary nephropathy, or a phenotype of kidney disease that may have a strong genetic basis, as outlined in Fig. 15.2. Other clinical situations may warrant genetic testing: where diagnostic findings would negate the need for kidney biopsy (e.g. in suspected nephronophthisis); or prevent patients receiving ineffective treatments with risk of adverse effects (e.g. steroid therapy in hereditary steroid-resistant nephrotic syndrome (SRNS)), also in females with clinical features and/or a history suggestive of a monogenic X-linked nephropathy, such as X-linked Alport syndrome or Fabry disease, because although female carriers of these diseases generally display a milder (often subclinical) phenotype than that seen in males, they can nevertheless develop severe disease.

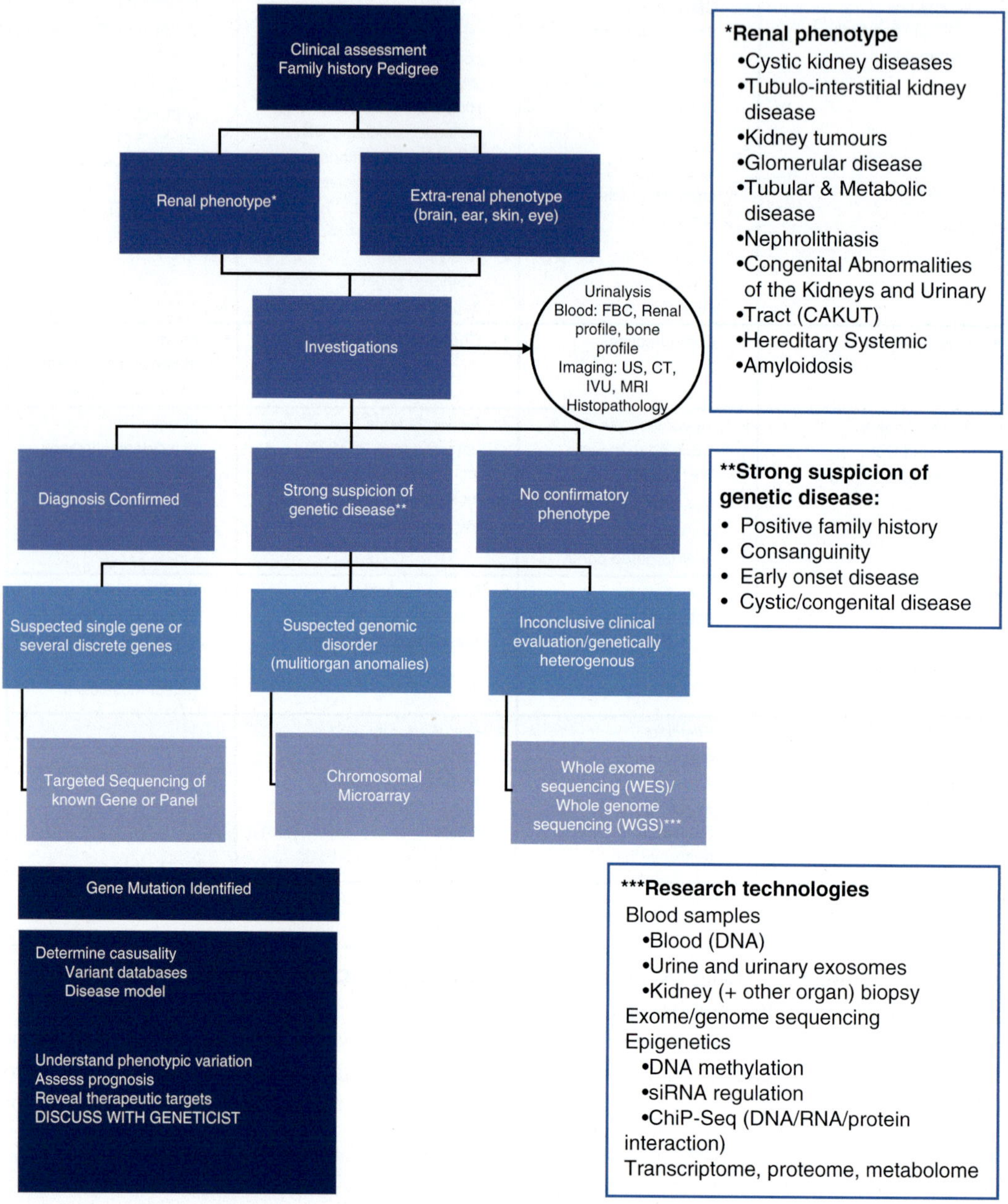

Fig. 15.2 An approach to Genetic Testing in suspected Genetic Kidney Disease [2]

Genetic testing has also been recommended in the evaluation of potential living kidney donors, with donation contraindicated amongst those found to have autosomal dominant forms of inherited kidney disease such as ADPKD or who share genetic susceptibility factors for atypical haemolytic uraemic syndrome (aHUS) [2].

Carriers of autosomal recessive disorders have generally been deemed suitable kidney donors, since individuals who are heterozygous for a recessive causal allele are classically not expected to develop the disease. Reports of milder, subclinical disease phenotypes amongst such carriers may instead suggest that these individuals are at a higher risk of developing kidney disease than previously thought, and therefore may warrant specialist surveillance [2].

Classification of Genetic Kidney Diseases

The approach to Genetic Kidney Disease may be simplified by classifying presentations into the phenotypes summarised in Fig. 15.3. There are many conditions and syndromes, which may

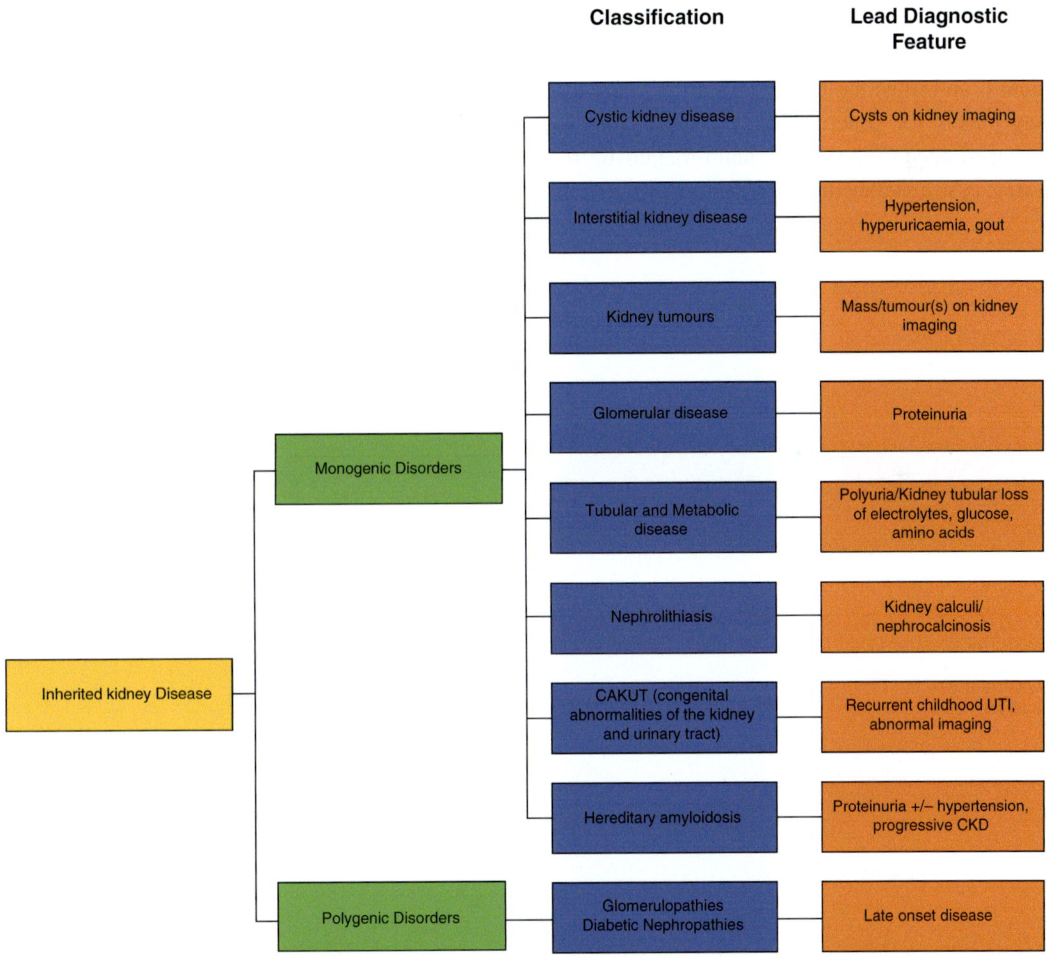

Fig. 15.3 Classification of Genetic Kidney Disease

cross classifications, e.g. Bardet-Biedl syndrome: in this multisystem disorder, the kidney phenotype is highly variable, and includes structural anomalies, cysts, ciliopathies and urine concentrating defects.

Monogenic Kidney Diseases

The strong correlation between genotype and phenotype in the monogenic kidney diseases enables mutation analysis to offer a definitive diagnosis, allow prognostication, and where appropriate, the opportunity to offer prenatal diagnostic testing. The following tables provide an overview of most of the monogenic kidney diseases for which a molecular genetic diagnosis can be made. To aid in the selection of target genes, and illustrate the rationale for many testing panels for genetic kidney disease, they are grouped according to their main diagnostic features: cystic kidney disease (Table 15.5); interstitial kidney disease (Table 15.8); tumorous kidney diseases (Table 15.10); glomerular disease (Table 15.12); tubular and metabolic disease (Table 15.15); nephrolithiasis (Table 15.19); congenital abnormalities of the kidney and urinary tract (CAKUT) (Table 15.23) and hereditary amyloidosis (Table 15.24). Additional tables offer a focus on the diagnosis and management of some of the commoner genetic kidney conditions, or those for which international consensus diagnostic and management guidelines are available.

Cystic Kidney Disease

Genetic causes of cystic kidney disease are described in Table 15.5, and the diagnosis and management of Autosomal Dominant Polycystic Kidney Disease (ADPKD) summarised in Table 15.6, and that of Autosomal Recessive Polycystic Kidney Disease (ARPKD) in Table 15.7.

Table 15.5 Cystic kidney disease [3, 7]. In addition to the genetic diseases listed, the differential for cystic kidney disease should also include non-genetic cause—simple renal cysts are common, increase in number and size with age, but are associated with otherwise normal-sized kidneys and normal kidney function; acquired cystic kidney disease (ACKD) is common in patients with CKD or ESKD, is characterised by multiple cysts, and associated with normal- or small-sized kidneys

Genetic Disorder	MOI	Characteristic signs and features	Gene symbol(s): Gene product(s)	Management
ADPKD* Types 1 & 2	AD	Type 1: Polycystic kidneys; liver cysts; brain aneurysms; CKD Type 2: Polycystic kidneys; CKD	Type 1: *PKD1*: polycystin 1 Type 2: *PKD2*: polycystin 2	See table 5.6
ARPKD**	AR	Incidence ~1:20,000; Neonatal death (30%); Potter's phenotype; Biliary dysgenesis	*PKHD1*: fibrocystin/ polyductin	See table 5.7
Meckel-Gruber syndrome (MKS)	AR	Polycystic kidneys; multi-organ dysplasia; occipital encephalocele; postaxial polydactyly, perinatally lethal	*MKS1*; *MKS3*: meckelin (also allelic with NPHP genes)	Cardiac repair/neurosurgical intervention for encephalocele Mortality rate 100%
Bardet-Biedl syndrome	AR	Hypertension; tubular dysfunction: (diabetes insipidus, acidosis); abnormal calyces; communicating cysts; foetal lobulation; interstitial nephritis; glomerular scarring; CKD; retinal degeneration; polydactyly; obesity; short stature; developmental delay; hypogonadism	*BBS1-BBS19*: BBS proteins	ophthalmic evaluation; control hypertension; dietary assessment for obesity & diabetes; growth hormone; ECG & ECHO for cardiac function; developmental evaluation
Short rib polydactyly syndrome (Jeune's syndrome)	AR	Polycystic kidneys; polydactyly; short rib; dysplasia; narrow thorax	*IFT80 / DYNC2H1 / WDR19 / IFT140 / TTC21B*	symptomatic treatment; Risk of severe respiratory complications: mechanical ventilation & surgical intervention may be required KRT: dialysis/transplant
Renal cysts and diabetes (RCAD) syndrome	AD	Kidney cysts/malformation (90%); diabetes mellitus (45%); hypomagnesaemia (40%); genital tract abnormalities (20%); hyperuricaemia (20%); elevated liver enzymes (15%) FHx: 50% de novo mutations	*HNF1B (TCF2)*; hepatocyte nuclear factor-β (transcription factor 2)	See table 15.23
Tuberous Sclerosis Complex (TSC)§	AD	FHx: absent in 2/3 Brain (90% - LD, SEGA, epilepsy); Skin >90% (ash leaf spots, angiofibromas, shagreen patches); Lung (LAM); Kidney (50-70% - AML, cysts); Eyes (50% - retinal hamartomas	*TSC1*: hamartin *TSC2*: tuberin	See tables 15.10 & 15.11
PKD1-TSC2 contiguous gene syndrome	AD	FHx: frequently spontaneous presentation Early presentation with severe ADPKD: polycystic kidneys & AMLs; Frequently present after first year of age;	*PKD1 / TSC2* (contiguous gene mutation)	See table 15.10

(continued)

Table 15.5 (continued)

von Hippel-Lindau (VHL) disease	AD	FHx: 20% de novo mutations Incidence ~1 in 36,000 CNS: Cerebellar and spinal haemangioblastoma; Eyes: retinal angiomas; Pancreas: serous cystadenomas and neuroendocrine pancreatic tumours Abdomen: phaeochromocytoma Kidneys: RCC, kidney cysts GU: epididymal cystadenoma	*VHL:* pVHL tumor suppressor gene	See table 10
ADTKD***	AD	Family history rare Slowly progressive kidney disease; medullary cysts	*UMOD/MUC1/ REN/HNF1B*	See tables 15.8 & 15.9
Medullary sponge kidney (MSK)	(AD)	FHx: familial clustering reported Haematuria; medullary nephrocalcinosis; nephrolithiasis; urolithiasis; UTI; metabolic acidosis	*GDNF: Glial-derived neurotrophic factor*	See table 19

Abbreviations: ACEi Angiotensin converting enzyme inhibitor, *AD* Autosomal dominant, *ADPKD* Autosomal dominant polycystic kidney disease, *ADTKD* Autosomal dominant tubulointerstitial kidney disease, *AML* Angiomyolipoma, *AR* Autosomal recessive, *ARPKD* Autosomal recessive polycystic kidney disease, *ESKD* End-stage kidney disease, *IVP* Intravenous pyelogram, *MODY5* Maturity onset diabetes mellitus of the young type 5

* See Table 15.6

** See Table 15.7

*** See Table 15.8 and 15.9

Table 15.6 Diagnosis & Management of Autosomal Dominant Polycystic Kidney Disease (ADPKD)* [7, 8]

Autosomal Dominant Polycystic Kidney Disease (ADPKD)[8,23]

Clinical Presentation

- 12.5 million people affected worldwide, from all ethnic groups,
- Accounts for around 10% of patients at ESKD
- Multisystemic disorder involving cardiac, CNS, GI, GU and Lung complications:

System	Manifestation (Percentage affected)
Cardiac	Valve abnormalities: mitral valve prolapse (25%); Pericardiac effusion (35%)
CNS	Extracranial Aneurysms; Arachnoid Cysts (8-12%); Spinal meningeal cysts (2%)
GI	Pancreatic cysts (10%); Diverticular disease (20-50% in ESKD); Abdominal Hernias; CHF rare
GU	Seminal vesicle cysts (40%); Male infertility
Lung	Bronchiectasis

- Despite continuous destruction of renal parenchyma, compensatory hyperfiltration in surviving glomeruli maintains kidney function within normal range for decades.
- Only once majority of nephrons are destroyed does kidney function decline, typically after age 30 years, with progression toward ESKD
- Performance of ultrasound-based unified criteria for diagnosis or exclusion of ADPKD:

Age (yrs)		PKD1	PKD2	Unknown gene type
Diagnostic confirmation				
15-29	Total >3 cysts[a]	PPV 100%; SEN 94.3%	PPV 100%; SEN 69.5%	PPV 100%; SEN 81.7%
30-39	Total >3 cysts[a]	PPV 100%; SEN 96.6%	PPV 100%; SEN 94.9%	PPV 100%; SEN 95.5%
40-59	> 2 cysts/kidney	PPV 100%; SEN 92.6%	PPV 100%; SEN 88.8%	PPV 100%; SEN 90%
Disease exclusion				
15-29	No renal cyst	NPV 99.1%; SPEC 97.6%	NPV 83.5%; SPEC 96.6%	NPV 90.8%; SPEC 97.1%
30-39	No renal cyst	NPV 100%; SPEC 96%	NPV 96.8%; SPEC 93.8%	NPV 98.3%; SPEC 94.8%
40-59	No renal cyst	NPV 100%; SPEC 93.9%	NPV 100%; SPEC 93.7%	NPV 100%; SPEC 93.9%

NPV, negative predictive value; PPV, positive predictive value; SEN, sensitivity; SPEC, specificity;
[a]Unilateral or bilateral

Genetic Diagnosis

- Mutations in *PKD1* (polycystin 1); and *PKD2*: (polycystin 2) account for most ADPKD cases
- PKD1 associated with more severe disease & greater likelihood of progression to ESKD

Management

Baseline Assessments

Cyst size

- Baseline cross-sectional imaging (CT/MRI) is recommended to evaluate: maximum kidney length, width and depth, and estimate TKV. Tools such as the Mayo classification tool may help with prognostication[24]
- Average rates of increase of TKV in adult ADPKD patients are 5-6%/year
- Repeated assessment can be used to assess progression/response to treatment

Kidney function

- Baseline estimation of GFR using CKD-EPI and MDRD eGFR are
- Measured GFR (mGFR) using inulin, iothalamate, DTPA or iohexol clearance may be warranted, e.g. where patient's muscle mass renders eGFR unreliable for timing of KRT
- Elevated TKV, together with age and kidney function, identifies those at highest risk of progression toward ESKD

Hypertension

- Lifestyle modification and medical treatment
- First line anti-hypertensives: RAAS blockade
- No consensus on second-line antihypertensives

Kidney Cysts

- Increased cAMP, driven by AVP in kidney cysts, mediate cyst growth in the kidney
- Suppressing AVP through increased oral water intake
- Vasopressin V_2-receptor antagonists – (Tolvaptan) reduce intracellular cAMP in kidney cysts, and shown to reduce rate of growth of TKV, and rate of eGFR decline

(continued)

Table 15.6 (continued)

	• **Indications:** rapidly progressing CKD stages 1-3 in adult ADPKD patients aged < 50 yrs • **Contraindications:** elevated liver enzymes, volume depletion, hypernatraemia, pregnancy, breast feeding, hypersensitivity, patients who cannot respond to thirst • **Side-effects:** idiosyncratic hepatic toxicity (increased ALT/AST, bilirubin), dehydration, fluid and electrolyte disturbance, anaphylaxis (rare), diabetes mellitus, uric acid increases, reversible reduction in GFR
	Haematuria and cyst haemorrhage • Usually self-limiting • If symptoms >1week, exclude neoplasm • Extensive bleeding requires admission • Consider withholding RAAS inhibitors & diuretics to avoid AKI during an episode of acute cyst hemorrhage
	Nephrolithiasis • There are three stone forming conditions associated with ADPKD: • i) uric acid nephrolithiasis, ii) hypocitraturic calcium oxalate nephrolithiasis, and iii) distal acidification defects • Potassium citrate is the treatment of choice for each of these stone-forming conditions • ECSWL and percutaneous nephrostolithotomy may be used
	Cyst Infection • Blood and urine cultures may be negative • cyst aspiration for culture should be considered if complex cyst identified in setting of refractory/recurrent infection • Lipid-permeable anti-microbial agents such as the fluoroquinolones or trimethoprim-sulfamethoxazole, depending on antimicrobial sensitivities (where available) are standard treatment for cyst infections • Once antibiotic therapy has been initiated, the precise duration of treatment and indications/timing of percutaneous/surgical drainage vary considerably • extended antibiotic therapy is often warranted • Cyst infection may recur even after adequate periods of antibiotic therapy
	Chronic Pain • MDT pain team approach • Percutaneous cyst aspiration may help determine whether definitive interventions e.g. cyst sclerosis/laparoscopic cyst fenestration is worth pursuing • Coeliac plexus blockade/radiofrequency ablation/spinal cord stimulation may be useful
	Reproductive issues • Pre-emptive discontinuation of RAAS inhibitors necessary due to teratogenicity & risk of inducing AKI in developing foetus • Referral to a high-risk obstetric medicine team recommended, especially in patients with hypertension or elevated creatinine level: *ADPKD pregnancies associated with enhanced frequency of new onset hypertension, pre-eclampsia, intrauterine growth retardation and premature delivery*
	ESKD Management • Kidney transplantation is the optimal choice for KRT in appropriate ADPKD patients • HD or PD are both suitable KRT modalities (although kidney cyst size may complicate or preclude PD) for those awaiting transplantation, or where transplant not possible
	Intracranial Aneurysm • ADPKD patients with a family history of ICA or a personal history of ICA rupture should be screened for asymptomatic ICA • Patients with no or unknown family history should be counselled about risk of ICA associated with ADPKD, as well as pros and cons of pre-symptomatic screening • Screening should be considered in individuals with high-risk professions • Management of UIA should be discussed with in a neurovascular MDT • Endovascular procedures have lower associated morbidity and mortality compared with neurosurgical approaches
	Polycystic Liver Disease • Conservative Management • Surgical: aspiration & sclerotherapy, fenestration, partial or segmental liver resection; more rarely combined liver & kidney transplantation • Medical: Somastatin analogues (in clinical trial setting)

Abbreviations: AD Autosomal dominant, *ALT* Alanine aminotransferase, *AST* Aspartate aminotransferase, *AVP* Arginine vasopressin, *cAMP* Cyclic adenosine monophosphate, *CHF* Congenital hepatic fibrosis, *CNS* Central nervous system, *DTPA* Diethylenetriaminepentaacetic acid, *ECSWL* Extracorporeal shock wave lithotripsy, *eGFR* Estimated glomerular filtration rate, *ESKD* End stage kidney disease, *GI* Gastrointestinal, *GU* Genito-urinary, *HD* Haemodialysis, *KRT* Kidney replacement therapy, *ICA* Intracranial aneurysm, *MDT* Multi-disciplinary team, *PD* peritoneal dialysis, *RAAS* Renin-angiotensin-aldosterone system, *TKV* Total kidney volume, *UIA* Unruptured intracranial aneurysm

*See Table 15.5

Table 15.7 Diagnosis & Management of Autosomal Recessive Polycystic Kidney Disease (ARPKD)** [10]

Autosomal Recessive Polycystic Kidney Disease (ARPKD) [10]	
Clinical Presentation	• Severe, early-onset cystic disease involving kidneys and biliary tract • Variable phenotype and age at presentation • Non-renal manifestations can be life-threatening • Ultrasound imaging with typical clinical features usually sufficient for postnatal diagnosis of ARPKD • May be phenotypic overlay with ADPKD and other hepatorenal fibrocystic disease. • Genetic testing may facilitate the diagnosis in patients with suspected ARPKD
Genetic Diagnosis	• Identification of biallelic mutations in *PKHD1* (encodes fibrocystin/ polyductin)
Management	**General Principles** • Optimal clinical management directed by multidisciplinary care team: • Perinatologists, neonatologists, nephrologists, hepatologists, geneticists, and behavioural specialists coordinate patient care from perinatally to adulthood
	Hypertension • Mainstay of current treatment is RAAS blockade • Combined ACEi/ARB not recommended
	Hyponatraemia • In euvolemia/hypervolemia, minimise fluid intake without compromising nutrition • Supplementation with NaCl likely to worsen HTN: avoid unless hypovolemic
	CHF • Screening for liver disease, especially complications of CHF vital in ARPKD children • Portal hypertension defined by splenomegaly, thrombocytopenia, varices, ascites, hepatopulmonary syndrome • Variceal haemorrhage or cholangitis can be life threatening: • Haematemesis, haematochezia, and/or melena require immediate medical attention

Abbreviations: ACEi Angiotensin converting enzyme inhibitor, *ARB* Angiotensin receptor blocker, *RAAS* Renin-angiotensin-aldosterone system, *cAMP* Cyclic adenosine monophosphate, *CHF* Congenital hepatic fibrosis, *NaCl* Sodium chloride, *HTN* Hypertension

**is a shorthand reference to where management of ARPKD is referenced elsewhere in other tables

Interstitial Kidney Diseases

Genetic causes of interstitial kidney disease are described in Table 15.8, and the diagnosis and management of Autosomal Dominant Tubulointerstitial Kidney Disease (ADTKD) summarised in Table 15.9.

Table 15.8 Interstitial Kidney Disease [3]

Genetic Disorder	MOI	Characteristic signs and features	Gene symbol(s): Gene product(s)	Management
Nephro-nophthisis types 1–16	AR	Early onset; polyuria; polydipsia; anaemia; CKD; ESKD	*NPHP1*-*NPHP9*: Nephro-cystin 1–9	manage CKD: correct hypovolaemia; treat anaemia - ESA KRT: kidney transplant (no disease recurrence in transplanted kidney)
Joubert Syndrome	AR (XR)	polycystic kidney disease; nephronophthisis; CNS abnormalities (molar tooth sign); ataxia; hyperpnoea; eye abnormalities	*CEP290; KIF7; NPHP1; OFD1* (>30 genes)	supportive and symptomatic treatment
Cranio-ectodermal dysplasia	AR	nephronophthisis; metabolic acidosis; CKD; hepatic fibrosis, ectodermal defects; ocular anomalies	*IFT122; IFT43; WDR19; WDR35;*	NaCl supplementation monitor kidney function KRT: kidney transplant surgical and orthopaedic care
Renal-Hepatic Pancreatic Dysplasia (RHPD1)	AR	cystic dysplasia; pancreatic fibrosis; hepatic dysgenesis	*NPHP3*: Nephro-cystin 3 *NEK8*: NIMA-related kinase 8	combined kidney and liver transplant
ADTKD* **	AD	Adolescent/adult presentation Early gout; Occasional cortical kidney cysts; Hyperuricemia; Low fractional urate excretion (<5%); Low urinary excretion of uromodulin; defect in urinary concentration; bland urinary sediment Progressive CKD Histology: Intracellular uromodulin deposits in TAL profiles	*UMOD*: Uro-modulin	See table 9
	AD	No characteristic findings, Occasional cortical kidney cysts Adult onset Progressive loss of kidney function Histology: Intracellular accumulation of MUC1-fs in distal tubules	*MUC1*: Mucin-1	See table 9
	AD	Mild hypotension; Increased risk of AKI; childhood anaemia; Hyperuricemia; hyperkalaemia; low urinary excretion of uromodulin; Progressive loss of kidney function Histology: Reduced renin staining in cells of the JGA	*REN*: Renin	See table 9
	AD	Usually presents in childhood/prenatal US; MODY5; few bilateral kidney cysts; genital abnormalities; pancreatic atrophy; Hypomagnesemia; hypokalemia; LFT abnormalities Progressive loss of kidney function	*HNF1B*: Hepato-cyte nuclear factor 1-β	See table 9

Abbreviations: AD Autosomal dominant, *CKD* Chronic kidney disease, *CNS* Central nervous system, *ESA* Erythropoietin-stimulating agents, *ESKD* End stage kidney disease, *JGA* Juxtaglomerular apparatus, *KRT* Kidney replacement therapy, *MOI* Mode of inheritance, *NaCl* Sodium chloride, *NSAIDs* Non-steroidal anti-inflammatory drugs, *RAAS* Renin-angiotensin-aldosterone system, *T2DM* Type 2 diabetes mellitus, *US* Ultrasound

[a]See Table 15.9 for diagnosis & management

Table 15.9 Diagnosis & Management of Autosomal Dominant Tubulointerstitial Kidney Disease (ADTKD)*** [11]

<table>
<tr><th colspan="2">Autosomal Dominant Tubulointerstitial Kidney Disease (ADTKD)[9]</th></tr>
<tr><td>Clinical Presentation</td><td>Clinical:
• AD inheritance
• Progressive loss of kidney function
• Bland urinary sediment
• No severe hypertension during early stages
• No drug exposure potentially causing tubulointerstitial nephritis
• Normal/small-sized kidneys on US
• Nocturia or enuresis in children (owing to loss of renal concentration ability)
• Progresses to ESKD; Age at ESKD requiring KRT varies widely within and between families: usually 20-80 yrs - most require KRT at 30-50 yrs
Histology:
• Interstitial fibrosis; Tubular atrophy; Thickening & lamellation of tubular basement membranes; Tubular dilatation (microcysts)
• No significant glomerular pathology
• Negative immunofluorescence for complement and immunoglobulins</td></tr>
<tr><td>Genetic Diagnosis</td><td><table>
<tr><th>Suspected diagnosis</th><th>Confirmed diagnosis</th></tr>
<tr><td>• Family history of AD inheritance of CKD; Clinical characteristics consistent with ADTKD</td><td>- Compatible family history (minimum 1 first degree relative), and
- Compatible kidney biopsy in one affected individual</td></tr>
<tr><td>• No compatible family history;
• Compatible histology on kidney biopsy, or
• Compatible extra-renal manifestations e.g. Gout/Diabetes</td><td>- Demonstrated mutation in one of the 4 ADTKD-associated genes: MUC1, UMOD, HNF1B or REN</td></tr>
</table>
• Genetic testing is only way of definitively diagnosing ADTKD and subtypes, and excluding disease in affected family members
• Testing of minors not generally recommended due to lack of disease-specific therapeutic options
• Failure to identify a mutation does not exclude the diagnosis of ADTKD: not all pathogenic genes have yet been identified</td></tr>
<tr><td rowspan="5">Management</td><td>Principles of Management
• No specific therapies yet available for different types of ADTKD:
• Treatment options for minors at risk for UMOD or MUC1 related diseases are few, and the need for treatment is infrequent
• children with HNF1B and REN related disease are likely to benefit from early management, so children at risk should be referred to a paediatric nephrologist</td></tr>
<tr><td>Control of Risk factors
• Potentially affected family members should be well-controlled for other risk factors that aggravate or cause CKD</td></tr>
<tr><td>Monitoring of Kidney function
• Kidney function should be tested annually
• MDT approach for monitoring in asymptomatic minors</td></tr>
<tr><td>Management of CKD
• Treatment according to established CKD guidelines.
• No evidence of RAAS blockade on CKD progression. If these agents are used, those with hyperuricemia should be treated with
• losartan, as it is the only agent that lowers serum urate levels
• owing to increased urinary urate excretion.</td></tr>
<tr><td>Allopurinol
• Patients with UMOD-associated disease who develop gout
• will likely have further episodes.</td></tr>
</table>

(continued)

Table 15.9 (continued)

	• Patients should therefore be started on allopurinol or febuxostat (when allopurinol cannot be tolerated) after the first attack of gout has resolved. • NB. Allopurinol should also be stopped before pregnancy, as it has been associated with cleft palate and other facial anomalies.
	Diuretics • Diuretics should be used with caution in all patients with ADTKD, as they may aggravate hyperuricemia and volume depletion.
	High fluid intake • Liberal water intake is recommended to compensate for possible urinary concentration defects. • A low-salt diet frequently prescribed in CKD is NOT recommended for ADTKD-*UMOD* (may aggravate hyperuricemia) and ADTKD-*REN* (may cause volume depletion)
	Erythropoiesis-stimulating agents • Used for the treatment of anaemia in ADTKD-*REN*
	Fludrocortisone • Used for the treatment of symptomatic hypotension in ADTKD-*REN* patients. However, possible beneficial effects of fludrocortisone on symptoms and disease progression need to be balanced against the possible risk of aggravating interstitial fibrosis. • Fludrocortisone should not be used in those with declining kidney function, hypertension, hyperkalaemia, or oedema.
	Avoid NSAIDs • NSAIDs should be avoided in all patients with ADTKD; in particular patients with *REN* mutations are at high risk of AKI
	Kidney Transplant • Kidney transplantation is the treatment of choice for ESKD due to ADTKD, as the disease does not recur in the graft. In *HNF1B* patients with diabetes mellitus, combined kidney/pancreas transplantation should be considered.

Abbreviations: AD Autosomal dominant, *CKD* Chronic kidney disease, *ESKD* End stage kidney disease, *KRT* Kidney replacement therapy, *NSAIDs* Non-steroidal anti-inflammatory drugs, *US* Ultrasound

***is a shorthand for where management of ADTKD is referred to in other tables in this chapter

Tumourous Kidney Diseases

Genetic causes of kidney masses (Tumourous Kidney Disease) are described in Table 15.10, and the diagnosis and management of Tuberous Sclerosis Complex (TSC) summarised in Table 15.11.

Table 15.10 Tumourous Kidney Diseases [3]

Genetic Disorder	MOI	Characteristic signs and features	Gene symbol(s): Gene product(s)	Management
Tuberous Sclerosis Complex (TSC)[§]	AD	FHx: absent in 2/3 Brain (90% - LD, SEGA, epilepsy); Skin >90% (ash leaf spots, angiofibromas, shagreen patches); Lung (LAM); Kidney (50-70% - AML, cysts); Eyes (50% - retinal hamartomas)	*TSC1*: hamartin *TSC2*: tuberin	See table 15.11
PKD1-TSC contiguous gene syndrome	AD	Presentation of severe ADPKD at an early age, with polycystic kidneys with renal angiomyolipomas frequently present after the first year of age.	*PKD1* & *TSC2*: polycystin and tuberin	Address CKD risk factors; Active surveillance: brain/ chest/ abdominal imaging as for TSC (see table 15.11); Associated with more rapid progression to ESKD
von Hippel-Lindau (VHL) disease	AD	FHx: 20% de novo mutations Incidence ~1 in 36,000 CNS: Cerebellar and spinal haemangioblastoma; Eyes: retinal angiomas; Pancreas: serous cystadenomas and neuroendocrine pancreatic tumours Abdomen: phaeochromocytoma Kidneys: RCC, kidney cysts GU: epididymal cystadenoma	*VHL*: pVHL tumor suppressor gene	Active surveillance: CT/MRI[12] NSS: cryotherapy / radiofrequency / microwave ablation KRT TKIs; HIF2-α antagonists (currently at Phase 2 clinical trial)
WAGR syndrome	AD	Wilms tumour, aniridia, growth retardation (WAGR); Associated with syndromes such as BWS	*WT1*: WT suppressor gene	Treatment dependent on age, staging, histology, unilateral or bilateral disease, IVC involvement and metastases. Preoperative chemotherapy, (vincristine, dactomycin) Surgical resection/nephrectomy, post-op chemotherapy, radiotherapy
Hereditary Papillary renal carcinoma (HPRC)	AD	Haematuria; kidney tumours; Types 1 & 2; Type 1 commoner & better prognosis	*MET* protooncogene (HGFR): cMet	Limited treatment options, Surgery, NSS TKI, Molecular targeted therapy – clinical trial
HLRCC	AD	Cutaneous Leiomyomas, early onset uterine leiomyomas (symptomatic requiring surgery), early onset Type 2 papillary renal cell cancer Aggressive kidney cancer, high risk dissemination	*FH*: fumarate hydratase	Limited treatment options Immediate Surgical excision with wide margins, possible retroperitoneal lymph node dissection. Surveillance abdominal MRI
Birt-Hogg-Dubé	AD	Fibrofolliculomas; pulmonary cysts; recurrent spontaneous pneumothoraces; kidney tumours;	*FLCN*: folliculin	Screening MRI, NSS, delayed surgery, imaging intervals based on tumour type, size and growth rate
SDH-RCC	AD	Haematuria; kidney tumours;	*SDH*: succinate dehydrogenase	Surgery, NSS

Abbreviations: AD Autosomal dominant, *AML* Angiomyolipoma, *BP* Blood pressure, *BWS* Beckwith-Wiedeman syndrome, *CT* Computerised tomography, *GU* Genito-urinary, *HIF-2α* Hypoxia inducible factor 2-alpha, *HLRCC* Hereditary leiomyomatosis and renal cell carcinoma, *LAM* Lymphangioleiomyomatosis, *LD* Learning disability, *MRI* Magnetic resonance imaging, *MOI* Mode of inheritance, *mTOR* Mechanistic target of rapamycin, *NSS* Nephron-sparing surgery, *SDH-RCC* Succinate dehydrogenase-renal cell cancer, *SEGA* Subependymal giant cell astrocytoma, *TKI* Tyrosine kinase inhibitor, *TSC* Tuberous sclerosis complex, *VHL RCC* Renal cell carcinoma, *TAND* TSC-associated neuropsychiatric disorders, *WAGR* Wilms tumour/aniridia/growth retardation

[§]See Table 15.11

Table 15.11 Diagnosis & Management of Tuberous Sclerosis Complex (TSC)[§] [13, 14]

<table>
<tr><th colspan="2">Tuberous Sclerosis Complex (TSC)[10,11]</th></tr>
<tr><td>Clinical Presentation</td><td>
• TSC is a genetic disorder affecting every organ system, but disease manifestations vary significantly among affected individuals
• Kidney AMLs in TSC are also associated with the development of pulmonary LAM, a progressive cystic disease of the lungs affecting women almost exclusively
<table>
<tr><th>MAJOR FEATURES</th><th>MINOR FEATURES</th></tr>
<tr><td>Hypomelanotic macules (≥3; at least 5mm diameter)</td><td>"Confetti" skin lesions</td></tr>
<tr><td>Angiofibroma (≥3) or fibrous cephalic plaque</td><td>Dental enamel pits (>3)</td></tr>
<tr><td>Ungual fibromas (≥2)</td><td>Intraoral fibromas (≥2)</td></tr>
<tr><td>Shagreen patch</td><td>Retinal achromatic patch</td></tr>
<tr><td>Multiple retinal hamartomas</td><td>Multiple kidney cysts</td></tr>
<tr><td>Multiple cortical tubers and/or radial migration lines[$]</td><td>Nonrenal hamartomas</td></tr>
<tr><td>Subependymal nodule (SEN) (≥2)</td><td>Sclerotic bone lesions</td></tr>
<tr><td>Subependymal giant cell astrocytoma (SEGA)</td><td></td></tr>
<tr><td>Cardiac rhabdomyoma</td><td></td></tr>
<tr><td>Lymphangioleiomyomatosis (LAM)[$$]</td><td></td></tr>
<tr><td>Kidney angiomyolipomas (AMLs) (>2)[$$]</td><td></td></tr>
<tr><td colspan="2">Definite TSC: 2 major features or 1 major feature with 2 minor features.
Possible TSC: either 1 major feature or ≥2 minor features.
[$] includes tubers and cerebral white matter radial migration lines.
[$$] a combination of the 2 Major clinical features LAM and AMLs without other features does not meet criteria for a definite diagnosis.</td></tr>
</table>
</td></tr>
<tr><td>Genetic Diagnosis</td><td>
• A definite clinical diagnosis requires two major features or one major feature with at least 2 minor features, from the table above
• A pathogenic mutation in TSC1 or TSC2 is sufficient for the diagnosis or prediction of TSC, regardless of the clinical findings
• 10–25% of TSC patients have no mutation identified by conventional genetic testing. Therefore, a normal result does not exclude TSC
</td></tr>
<tr><td rowspan="4">Management</td><td>
General principles
• Surveillance for complications
• Targeted therapy: mTOR inhibitors represent the first systemic approach to treating the underlying pathophysiology of TSC disease by blocking activation of the mTOR pathway
• Two oral mTOR inhibitors - sirolimus and everolimus have been widely approved for treatment of TSC-associated SEGA, refractory epilepsy, pulmonary LAM, and growing kidney AMLs
</td></tr>
<tr><td>
Genetics:
• Offer genetic counselling for patient & family when TSC suspected
</td></tr>
<tr><td>
Brain
• MRI to assess for presence of tubers, SEGA or other lesions and regular monitoring if identified
• Evaluate for TAND and epilepsy with education on infantile spasms – consider EEG or 24 hour EEG for subclinical seizures
• Either surgical resection or medical treatment (mTOR) inhibitors may be used for growing but otherwise asymptomatic SEGA
• Surgical resection should be performed for acutely symptomatic SEGA
</td></tr>
<tr><td>
Kidney
• Assess kidney function and blood pressure
• MRI abdomen to assess for presence or progression of AMLs & kidney cysts (annual if present)
• mTOR inhibition with sirolimus/everolimus has been shown to reduce AML size & vascularity, and reduce the risk of acute haemorrhage
Indications
</td></tr>
</table>

Table 15.11 (continued)

	- mTOR inhibitor therapy is now first line treatment for asymptomatic, growing kidney AMLs > 3 cm in diameter; Selective embolization or kidney-sparing resection are acceptable second-line therapy for asymptomatic angiomyolipoma **Contraindications** - acute haemorrhage: Embolization followed by corticosteroids is first-line therapy for angiomyolipoma presenting with acute haemorrhage. Nephrectomy should be avoided **Side-effects** - mouth ulcers, gastrointestinal upset, menstrual disturbance, hypercholesterolaemia, acne, immune-suppression related infection
	Lungs - Screen for LAM symptoms, perform lung function, monitoring HRCT in asymptomatic individuals at risk of LAM - Counsel regarding smoking and oestrogen use - Individuals with lung cysts on HRCT should have annual Lung Function testing and HRCT - mTOR inhibitors may be used to treat LAM with moderate to severe lung disease or rapid progression - TSC patients with LAM are candidates for lung transplantation but TSC comorbidities may impact transplant suitability
	Skin • Rapidly changing, disfiguring, or symptomatic TSC-associated skin lesions should be treated as appropriate for the lesion and clinical context, using approaches such as surgical excision, laser(s), or possibly topical mTOR inhibitor
	Dental • Symptomatic/deforming dental lesions, oral fibromas, and bony jaw lesions should be treated with surgical excision or curettage
	Cardiac • ECG for asymptomatic patients of all ages to monitor for conduction defects; advanced diagnostics for symptomatic patients • Echocardiogram every 1-3 yrs in asymptomatic children with cardiac rhabdomyomas until documented regression
	Eyes • Annual ophthalmologic evaluation in patients with previously identified ophthalmologic lesions/visual symptoms at baseline evaluation

Abbreviations: AD Autosomal dominant, *AML* Angiomyolipoma, *ECG* Electrocardiogram, *EEG* Electroencephalogram, *HRCT* High resolution computerised tomogram, *LAM* Lymphangioleimyomatosis, *MRI* Magnetic resonance imaging, *mTOR* Mechanistic target of rapamycin, *SEGA* Subependymal giant cell astrocytoma, *TAND* TSC-associated neuropsychiatric disorders, *TSC* Tuberous sclerosis complex

Glomerular Diseases

Multiple genetic disorders cause glomerular diseases, as illustrated in Fig. 15.4 and Table 15.12. The diagnosis and management of atypical HUS and C3 Glomerulopathy is summarised in Table 15.13, and that of Fabry Disease in Table 15.14.

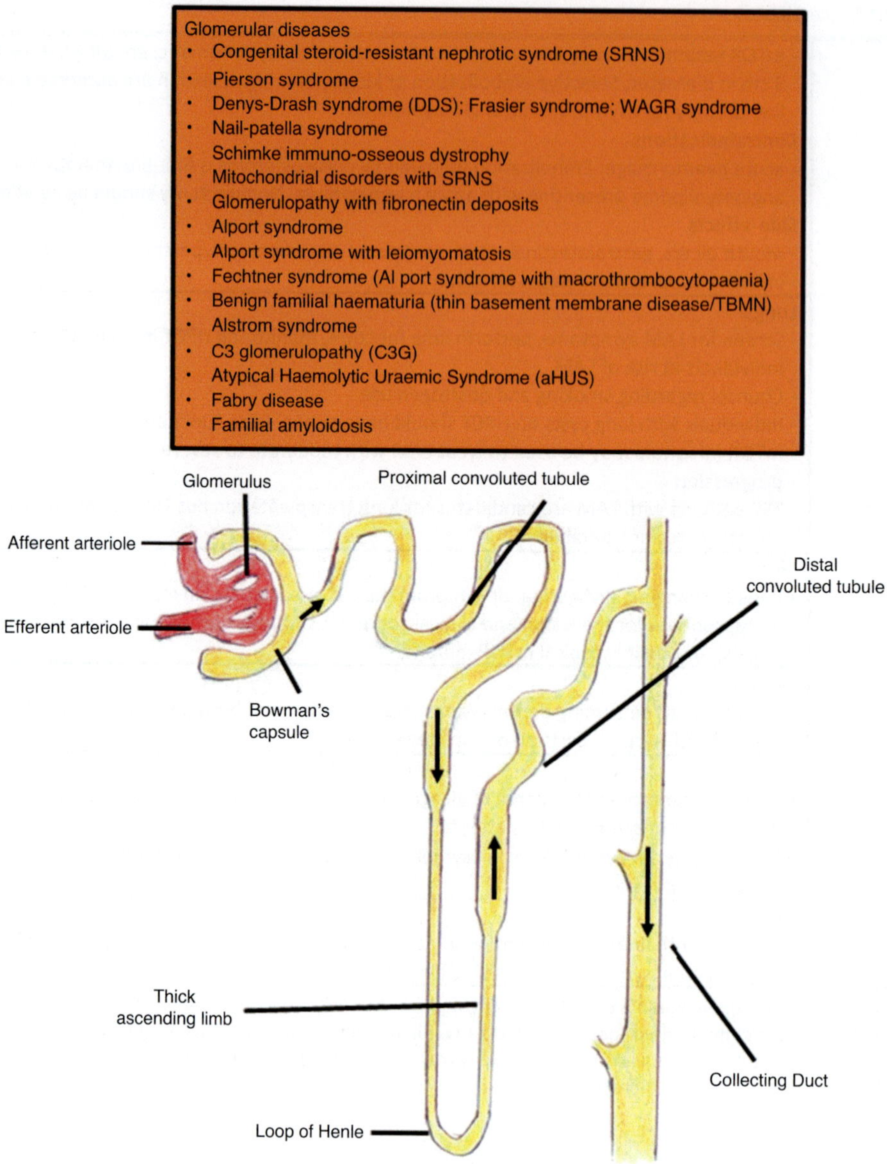

Fig. 15.4 Glomerular Diseases

Table 15.12 Glomerular disorders [3]

Genetic Disorder	MOI	Characteristic signs and features	Gene symbol(s), Gene product(s)	Management
Steroid resistant nephrotic syndrome (SRNS)	AR AD Mt	Proteinuria, hypoalbuminaemia, oedema; Kidney biopsy: MCD/FSGS/DMS on LM, podocyte foot process effacement on EM; Multi-drug resistant; Progresses to ESKD; Low risk of recurrence after transplantation Mitochondrial SRNS patients may also present +/- encephalomyopathy	>60 genes associated *NPHS1: (AR)* *NPHS2: (AR)* *INF2: (AD)* *WT1: (AD)* *COQ8B: (AR)* *Also:* *ARHGDIA; CUBN; PLCE1;* *COQ2; COQ6; ADCK4; PDSS2*: (Mt)	- RAASi - >8 week trial of CS in children recommended to define steroid resistance[13] - CNI recommended as initial therapy for children with SRNS - In children who fail to achieve remission with CNI therapy: trial MMF, high-dose CS/ combination. - CP **NOT** for children with SRNS. - If SRNS relapse after complete remission, restart therapy with one of: oral CS/return to previous successful immune suppressive agent/ alternative immune suppressive agent to minimize cumulative toxicity - *ARHGDIA*: eplerenone - *COQ2; COQ6; ADCK4; PDSS2*: experimental treatment with coenzyme Q10 - *PLCE1:* CS/CYA - *CUBN:* Vit. B12 - KRT for ESKD; low risk of recurrence after transplant
Pierson syndrome	AR	SRNS and microcoria	*LAMB2*: laminin-β2	Conservative management; KRT: Kidney transplant
Denys-Drash Syndrome (DDS); Frasier syndrome; WAGR syndrome	AD	Wilms tumour; ambiguous genitalia; gonadal dysgenesis; nephrotic syndrome; WAGR – Aniridia	*WT1*: WT suppressor gene	Conservative management; KRT at ESKD/post bilateral nephrectomy + chemotherapy for Wilms tumour; Kidney transplant
Nail-Patella syndrome	AD	• SRNS: FSGS with specific ultrastructural GBM changes; • Absent/dysplastic/hypo plastic nails and patella; elbow dysplasia; • eye disease; • sensorineural hearing loss	*LMX1B*: LIM homeo-domain protein	ACEi Manage ESKD Kidney transplantation Orthopaedic input Ophthalmology input
Schimke immuno-osseous dystrophy	AR	Short stature, Bone dysplasia, T-cell deficiency, SRNS	*SMARCAL1*: HepA-related protein (HARP)	As per treatment of SRNS Manage ESKD Kidney Transplantation
Mito-chondrial disorders with SRNS	Mt	SRNS +/– encephelomyopathy	*COQ2, COQ6, PDSS2, MTTL1*	Coenzyme Q10 supplementation
Glomerulo-pathy with	AD	Proteinuria, renal tubular acidosis, microscopic	*FN1*: fibronectin-1	Manage Hypertension: RAASi; Manage ESKD

Table 15.12 (continued)

fibronectin deposits		haematuria, hypertension, oedema		Kidney Transplantation
Alport syndrome	XD AR AD	Microscopic hematuria (constant)±episodes of gross haematuria; increasing proteinuria±nephrotic range, progressive CKD – with early ESKD in most males. Sensorineural hearing loss; anterior lenticonus and other eye anomalies	*COL4A5*, (XD): α5(IV)-collagen *COL4A3*, (AR/AD): α3(IV)-collagen, *COL4A4*, (AR/AD): α4(IV)-collagen	Management of hypertension, proteinuria & dyslipidemia: RAASi KRT: Kidney transplantation
Alport syndrome with leio-myomatosis	XD	(glomerular nephropathy, sensorineural deafness and ocular anomalies) and benign proliferation of visceral smooth muscle cells along the gastrointestinal, respiratory, and female genital tracts	*COL4A6*: α6(IV)-collagen,	Treat microalbuminuria/ proteinuria or hypertension with RAASi CKD management KRT: either pre-emptive transplantation or dialysis. Surgical intervention required for symptomatic leiomyomas.
Benign familial haematuria (TBMN)	AD	Microscopic Haematuria, minimal proteinuria, low prevalence of progressive CKD	*COL4A3*: α3(IV)-collagen	Good prognosis RAASi if proteinuric Monitor for HTN/proteinuria/ progressive CKD
Alstrom Syndrome	AR	Proteinuria, T2DM, renal failure, insulin resistance, vision abnormalities, progressive SND, dilated cardiomyopathy	*ALMS1*	Symptomatic treatment MDT approach Oral anti-diabetic treatments or insulin RAASi for proteinuria KRT, Kidney Transplantation
C3 Glomerulo-pathy (C3G)[##]	AR AD	Haematuria, proteinuria, GN, retinal drusen, acquired partial lipodystrophy DDD or C3GN Diagnosis made on immunofluorescence	*C3, CFH, CFI, CFB, CFHR-5, MLPA*	See table 13
aHUS[##]	AR AD	Thrombocytopenia, haemolytic anaemia, acute renal failure C3, CD46 (*MCP*), CFB, CFH, CF HR1, CFHR3, CFHR4, CFI, D GKE, and THBD	*CFH*: complement factor H; *CFHR1*; *CFHR3*; *MCP*; *ADAMTS13* (AD)	See table 13
Fabry disease[###]	XR	Mostly men: proteinuria, progressive CKD; sometimes tubular dysfunction (polyuria, Fanconi syndrome), kidney parapelvic cysts; kidney biopsy: glycolipid accumulation on LM/EM. Pain (acromyalgia), skin (angiokeratomas, anhydrosis), eye (corneal	*GLA:* α-galactosidase A	See table 14

(continued)

Table 15.12 (continued)

		verticillata), heart (LVH, conduction & valve anomalies, angina), strokes (hearing loss, ataxia, vascular dementia)		

Abbreviations: ACEi Angiotensin converting enzyme inhibitor, *AD* Autosomal dominant, *aHUS* Atypical Haemolytic uremic syndrome, *AR* Autosomal recessive, *CKD* Chronic kidney disease, *CNI* Calcineurin inhibitor, *CP* Cyclophosphamide, *CYA* Cyclosporin, *CS* Corticosteroids, *DDS* Denys-Drash Syndrome, *DMS* Diffuse mesangial sclerosis, *EM* Electron microscopy, *ESKD* End stage kidney disease, *FSGS* Focal segmental glomerulosclerosis, *GBM* Glomerular basement membrane, *LVH* Left ventricular hypertrophym, *LM* Light microscopy, *MCD* Minimal change disease, *MMF* Mycophenolate mofetil, *Mt* Mitochondrial inheritance, *RAASi* Renin-angiotensin-aldosterone system inhibition, *SRNS* Steroid resistant nephrotic syndrome, *TBMN* Thin basement membrane nephropathy, *WAGR* Wilms tumour/aniridia/genitourinary problems

Table 15.13 Diagnosis & Management of atypical haemolytic uremic syndrome (aHUS) and C3 glomerulopathy# [16]

Atypical haemolytic uraemic syndrome (aHUS) and C3 glomerulopathy (C3G)[14]			
Clinical Presentation	**aHUS** • Ultra-rare; characterised by AKI, thrombocytopenia & MAHA • >50% of aHUS patients have underlying inherited and/or acquired complement abnormality • Eculizumab (a humanized anti-C5 mAb) enables control of aHUS, preventing progression to ESKD (plasma exchange therapy can be used where eculizumab unavailable) • Triggers include autoimmune conditions, transplants, pregnancy, infections, drugs and metabolic conditions • Although time course & persistence not well understood, many patients appear at life-long risk for recurrent acute presentations[14] **C3G** • C3G characterised by uncontrolled activation of complement cascade, leading to glomerular C3 deposition • Dysregulation of C3 convertase driven by genetic and/or acquired defects • Majority of C3G patients follow a chronic, indolent course with persistent alternative pathway activation, resulting in a 10-year kidneysurvival of around50%[14]		
Genetic Diagnosis		**aHUS**	**C3G**
	Laboratory Analysis	- Measure ADAMTS13 activity to diagnose or exclude TTP - Investigate for STEC-HUS - Measure serum/plasma complement levels	- Measure serum/plasma complement levels ; - Test complement activity: required to define type/degree of complement deregulation
	Genetic Testing	- Genetic testing recommended for patients in whom discontinuation of eculizimab is being considered	- Benefit of genetic analysis in C3G currently unclear since our understanding of genetic basis for C3G remains incomplete
		- Minimum gene panel that should be screened in aHUS & C3G includes *CFH, CD46, CFI, C3, CFB, THBD, CFHR1, CFHR5, and DGKE* - Because of frequent concurrence of genetic risk factors in aHUS, analysis should include genotyping for risk haplotypes *CFH-H3* and *MCP* - Genetic analysis essential in live-related kidney donor transplantation	
Management	**Treatment approach in aHUS**[14]		

Table 15.13 (continued)

Management

Treatment approach inaHUS[14]

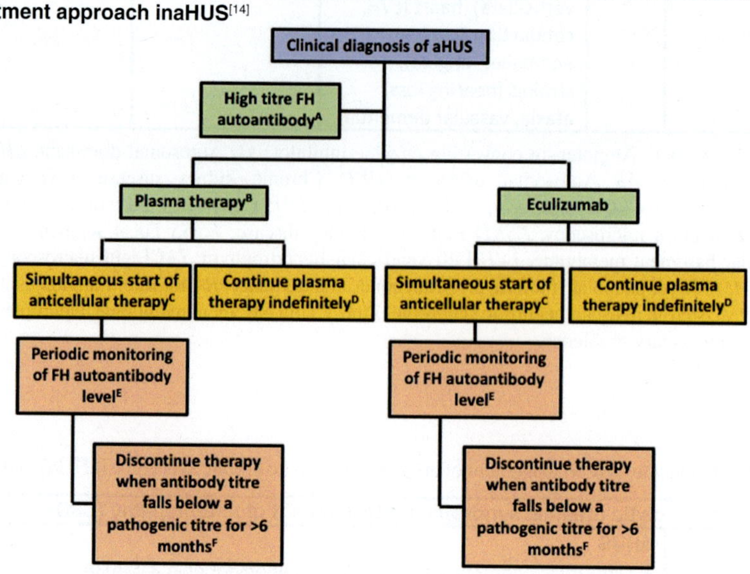

[A]abnormal titre depends on the testing laboratory
[B]decision to use plasma therapy vs. eculizumab based on patient age and local resource availability
[C]cyclophosphamide, rituximab or mycophenolate mofetil
[D]decision to continue anti-complement therapy indefinitely is not informed by data
[E]interval may be monthly or quarterly, based on local resources
[F]recommendation based on limited retrospective case reviews

Transplant considerations aHUS

Recurrence Risk	Treatment Regimen
HIGH RISK (50-100%) • Previous early recurrence • Pathogenic Mutation • Gain-of-function mutation	Prophylactic eculizumab NB. Start on day of transplantation due to potential severe recurrence and limited recovery of function in kidney allografts compared with native kidneys
MODERATE RISK • No mutation identified • Isolated CFI mutations • Complement gene mutation of unknown significance • Persistent low titre FH autoantibody	Prophylactic eculizumab or plasma exchange
LOW RISK (<10)% • Isolated *MCP* mutations • Persistently negative FH autoantibodies	No prophylaxis

Treatment approach in C3G

All patients	• Optimal BP control: ACEi/ARBs • Optimal nutrition • Lipid control
Moderate disease	**Description** • Urine protein >500mg/24h despite supportive therapy, or • Moderate inflammation on kidney biopsy, or • Recent increase in serum creatinine suggesting risk of progressive disease **Recommendation** • Prednisolone – short course (2-3 months) for anti-inflammatory effect • Mycophenolate mofetil

(continued)

Table 15.13 (continued)

Severe disease	**Description** • Urine protein >2000mg/24h despite immunosuppression and supportive therapy, or • Severe inflammation presented by marked endo- or extra-capillary proliferation with/without crescent formation despite immunosuppression and supportive therapy, or • Increased serum creatinine suggesting risk of progressive disease at onset despite immunosuppression and supportive therapy **Recommendation** • Limited success of anti-cellular immune suppressants and methylprednisolone pulse dosing in rapidly progressive disease • Data insufficient to recommend eculizumab as first-line treatment of rapidly progressive disease

Transplant considerations in C3G

Recurrence Risk	Treatment Regimen
Timing	• Avoid transplantation during acute period of renal loss • Avoid transplantation during acute inflammation • NO data to support association between specific complement abnormalities (e.g. high titre C3NeF/low C3/high soluble C5b-9) & increased risk of relapse
Donor Selection	• No specific recommendation can be made on donor choice • When considering living donors, high risk of recurrence should be weighed against presumed risk of waiting on deceased donor list
Risk reduction	• Histological recurrence of C3G is as high as 90% • Limited data suggests that rapid progression to ESKD in the native kidneys increases risk of recurrence • No known strategies to reduce risk of recurrence • Clinical recurrence should drive the decision to treat • In the absence of a clinical trial, the use of anti-complement therapy is based solely on a small open-label trial and positive case reports • C3G-associated with monoclonal gammopathy has a high rate of recurrence

Liver transplantation can be considered for kidney transplant recipients with liver-derived complement protein abnormalities, uncontrolled disease activity despite eculizumab therapy, or financial considerations regarding cost of long-term eculizumab therapy[[14]

Abbreviations: ACEi Angiotensin converting enzyme inhibitors, *AKI* Acute kidney injury, *ARB* Angiotensin receptor blocker, *BP* Blood pressure, *C3NeF* C3 nephritic factor, *ESKD* End stage kidney disease, *mAb* Monoclonal antibody, *MAHA* Microangiopathic haemolytic anaemia, *STEC-HUS* Shiga toxin *E. coli*-associated haemolytic uraemic syndrome, *TTP* Thrombotic thrombocytopenic purpura

[#]is shorthand reference for where aHUS and C3G are referenced in other tables in this chapter

Table 15.14 Diagnosis & Management of Fabry Disease (FD)### [17]

Fabry Disease (FD) [17]	
Clinical Presentation	• FD is an X-linked recessive lysosomal storage disorder • Though X-linked, both males and females can be affected • Deficient activity of α-galactosidase A results in accumulation of glycosphingolipids with terminal α-D-galactosyl residue, particularly globotriaosylceramide (GL-3, Gb3, CTH) and globotriaosylsphingosine (Lyso-GL-3, lyso-Gb3) • Lipids progressively accumulate in the circulation, all cell types and organs, resulting in multisystem involvement • Type 1 "classic" males: little or no functional α-Gal A enzymatic activity (<3% of normal mean activity). • Major symptoms in childhood/adolescence: acroparaesthesias; angiokeratomas; anhidrosis/hypohidrosis; gastrointestinal symptoms (abdominal pain, cramping, frequent bowel movements); star-burst pattern corneal dystrophy on slit-lamp examination (vision unaffected); Cardiac deposition leads to arrhythmias, LVH, and HCM; kidney deposition: progressive proteinuria, CKD, ESKD; Cerebrovascular deposition: TIAs, strokes • Incidence of Type 1 disease is around 1:18,000 to 1:95,000 • Heterozygous females from Type 1 families display variable phenotype, due to random X-chromosomal inactivation: ranges from asymptomatic to as severe as Type 1 males; around 90% have classic star-burst pattern corneal dystrophy • Type 2 "later-onset" males: residual α-Gal A activity, lack GL-3/Gb3 accumulation in capillaries and small blood vessels. • Normal childhood & adolescence, typically present with kidney/cardiac disease in third to seventh decades • Most Type 2 patients identified by enzyme screening of patients in cardiac, haemodialysis, kidney transplant, stroke clinics, and by newborn screening • Incidence of Type 2 disease is around 5–10 times more frequent than that of type 1 males • Heterozygous females from Type 2 families may be asymptomatic or develop kidney or cardiac manifestations later in life; Lack corneal or other early type 1 manifestation, typically display less frequent and less severe disease than Type 2 male relatives
Genetic Diagnosis	• Diagnosis established in males by α-galactosidase A–specific activity <25–30% of control in peripheral white blood cells • *GLA* mutations on X-chromosome • Wide phenotypic variability, even amongst patients with same mutation • FD should be considered and tested in patients with CKD, with no definitive cause of nephropathy, especially familial cases
Management	**General principles** • ERT with recombinant human α-galactosidase A (agalsidase) is only currently available therapy aimed at the aetiology of FD • Development of signs or symptoms related to FD is an indication to start ERT: • implies development of CKD, if ERT not already commenced for non-kidney manifestations e.g. pain [17] • ERT slows the progression of CKD in FD and reduces progression of HCM, especially when commenced prior to established fibrosis [17] • Individual FD patients should follow the general guidelines for management of CKD, including BP optimisation, smoking cessation, dietary salt restriction, and management of hyperlipidaemia [17]

Abbreviations: BP Blood pressure, *CKD* Chronic kidney disease, *ERT* Enzyme replacement therapy, *ESKD* End stage kidney disease, *HCM* Hypertrophic cardiomyopathy, *LVH* Left ventricular hypertrophy, *TIA* Transient ischaemic attack

Kidney Tubular and Metabolic Diseases

In primary kidney tubulopathies, the primary genetic defect causes loss of function of a specific kidney transport protein or signalling molecule. As certain transport systems are expressed in those tubule segments (Causes of genetic kidney tubular and metabolic diseases are summarised in Fig. 15.5 and Table 15.15). The diagnosis and management of X-linked hypophosphataemia is detailed in Table 15.16, that of Gitelman Syndrome (GS) in Table 15.17, and that of Cystinosis is detailed in Table 15.18. In

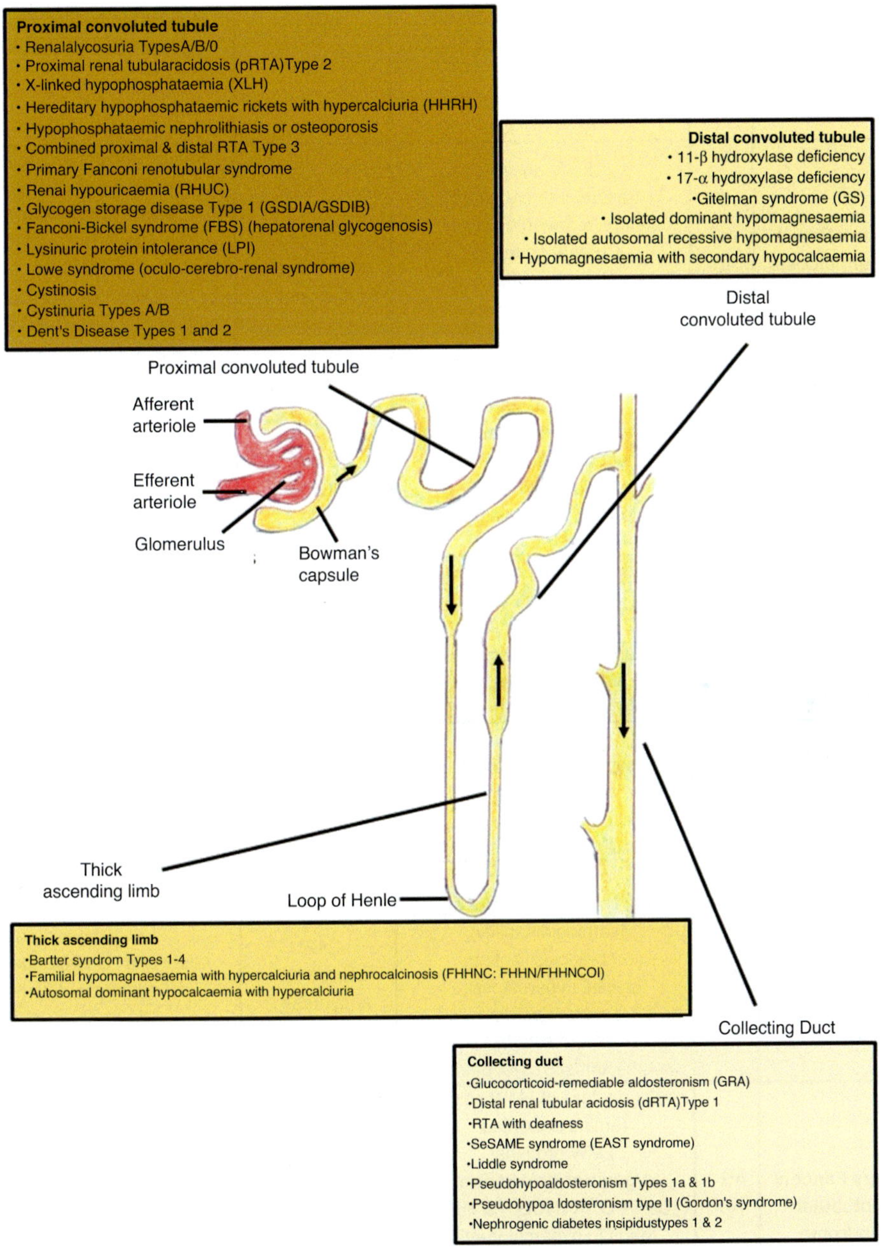

Fig. 15.5 Kidney Tubular and Metabolic diseases

Table 15.15 Kidney Tubular and Metabolic Diseases [3]

Genetic Disorder	MOI	Characteristic signs and features	Gene symbol, (gene product)	Management
Proximal Convoluted Tubule (PCT)				
Renal glycosuria **Type A** **Type B** **Type O**	AR AD	Asymptomatic in most; polyuria, polydipsia; **Type A:** low threshold for glucose excretion + reduced TmG; **Type B:** low threshold for glucose excretion + normal TmG; **Type O:** no tubular glucose reabsorption	*SLC5A2*: SGLT2	no treatment required for most patients Monitor for development of type 2 diabetes mellitus
Proximal renal tubular acidosis (pRTA) Type 2	AR AD	Early onset; Failure to thrive (short stature, learning disability); Corneal opacities; Severe acidosis, hyperchloraemia, mild hypokalaemia; Rickets, osteomalacia	*SLC4A4*: $NaHCO_3$ co-transporter 1	Prevent growth abnormalities Life-long bicarbonate replacement therapy Diuretics e.g. amiloride (reduce K^+ loss) Thiazide/loop diuretics (reduce HCO_3 loss - **BUT**may aggravate hypokalaemia) Vit. D_3 & PO_4 supplementation
X-linked hypo-phosphataemia (XLH)[±]	XD	Vit. D resistant rickets/osteomalacia; hypophosphataemia; hypocalciuria; urinary PO_4 wasting; normal Vit. D/Ca^{2+}	*PHEX*: FGF23	See table 16
Hereditary hypo-phosphataemic rickets with hypercalciuria (HHRH)	AR	hypophosphataemic rickets; short stature; hypercalciuria; urinary PO_4 wasting; nephrocalcinosis; elevated 1,25(OH) Vit. D	*SLC34A3*: Na^+/PO_4 co-transporter 2C	Oral PO_4 supplements **AVOID** active Vit. D analogs (may worsen hypercalciuria)
Hyposphataemic nephrolithiasis or osteoporosis	AD	Adult onset; hypophosphataemia; hypercalciuria; recurrent urolithiasis; osteoporosis/fractures	*SLC34A1*: NP2a *SLC9A3R1*: NHERF1	phosphate supplementation low-dose Vit. D supplementation
Combined Proximal & Distal RTA Type 3	AR	Very rare; mild metabolic acidosis; learning disability; cerebral calcification; cranial hyperostosis; malocclusion; short stature; osteosclerosis; osteopetrosis	*CA2*: carbonic anhydrase 2	Na^+ or K^+ bicarbonate K^+ supplementation
Primary Fanconi renotubular syndrome	AR AD	polyuria: loss of LMW solutes (amino acids/Glu/ LMW proteins/ organic acids/carnitine/ $Ca^{2+}/PO^{4-}/K^+/HCO^{3-}$) & H_2O - leads to hyperchloremic metabolic acidosis; failure to thrive; rickets; normoglycemic glycosuria;	*SLC34A1: (AR)* NP2a *GATM: (AD)* glycine amidino-transferase *EHHADH: (AD)* LBFP	symptomatic treatment; fluid, electrolyte & nutrient supplementation; KRT; kidney transplant

Table 15.15 (continued)

		nephrocalcinosis & nephrolithiasis less common.		
Renal Hypouricaemia (RHUC)	AR	impaired proximal tubular urate reabsorption: low serum uric acid; high urinary urate; urate nephrolithiasis; haematuria; pyelonephritis; nephrocalcinosis; exercise-induced AKI	*SLC22A12*: URAT1 *SLC2A9*: GLUT9	Increased fluid intake urine alkalization xanthine oxidoreductase inhibitors may protect from EIAKI
Glycogen Storage Disease Type 1 (GSDI) **Type 1A (GSDIA)** **Type 1B (GSDIB)**	AR	Hypoglycaemia; Fanconi-like syndrome; nephrocalcinosis; hyperuricaemia; hepatomegaly; hyperlipidaemia; lactic acidosis; early: enlarged kidneys; late: glomerular hyper-filtration; proteinuria, progressive CKD; growth retardation; osteopenia; round face; platelet ± neutrophil dysfunction; enteropathy; hepatic adenoma/carcinoma GSDIB: neutropaenia	*G6PC*: glucose-6-phosphatase **(GSDIA)** *SLC37A4*: Glucose-6-Phosphate Transporter **(GSDIB)**	Frequent meals, NG feeding, raw starch (to avoid hypoglycemia); Oral $NaHCO_3$ **AVOID** fructose/galactose (to correct acidosis) additional medication & organ transplant may be necessary GCSF for neutropenia (GSDIB)
Fanconi Bickel syndrome (FBS) (hepatorenal glycogenosis)	AR	glycogen storage disease: liver & kidney accumulation; kidney tubular dysfunction; hypoglycaemia; failure to thrive; polyuria; rickets; hepatosplenomegaly	*SLC2A2*: GLUT2	replace fluid and electrolytes Vit. D and PO_4 supplementation Small, frequent meals Fructose-predominant, Galactose-restricted diet
Lysinuric protein intolerance (LPI)	AR	Nausea & vomiting after protein-rich meal; Lethargy/coma; failure to thrive; muscle weakness; metabolic acidosis Fanconi syndrome; hypophophataemia; hypercalciuria; nephrocalcinosis; hyperammonaemia; osteoporosis; hepatosplenomegaly; pulmonary alveolar proteinosis; CKD	*SLC7A7*: y+L amino acid transporter 1	Patients unable to metabolise lysine, arginine or ornithine: protein-restricted diet ammonia scavenging therapy
Thick Ascending Limb (TAL)				
Bartter syndrome types 1–4	AR XR	salt-losing tubulopathy with secondary hyperaldosteronism: hypokalaemic alkalosis; hypercalciuria, (hypocalciuria in Type 3); high renin; alkalosis; polyuria; failure to thrive; Types 1 & 2: antenatal polyhydramnios, dehydration,	*SLC12A1*: (Type 1) *KCNJ1*: (Type 2) *CLCNKB*: (Type 3) *BSND* (Type 4A) *CLCNKA & CLCNKB:*	aggressive Na^+ & K^+ replacement; aldosterone antagonists, spironolactone, ACEi: counteract effects of AII/aldosterone; NSAIDs: Indomethacin/ Ibuprofen – to decrease prostaglandin excretion; growth hormone

(continued)

Table 15.15 (continued)

		failure to thrive Type 4: deafness	(Type 4B) *MAGED2*: (Type 5), XR	
Hypo-magnesaemia with hypercalciuria and nephrocalcinosis (FHHNC)	AR	Median age of onset 1-8 years Hypomagnaesemia; hypercalciuria; nephrocalcinosis; progressive CKD/ESKD; seizures; Ocular involvement with *CLDN19* mutations, termed FHHNCOI	*CLDN16*: claudin 16 (FHHN) *CLDN 19*: claudin 19 (FHHNCOI)	Supportive management Mg^{2+} replacement check for hypokalaemia/ hypocalcaemia thiazide diuretics manage CKD/ESKD KRT: kidney transplant Lens implants for FHHNCOI
Autosomal dominant hypocalcaemia with hypercalciuria	AD	Pseudo-Bartter syndrome; Hypocalcaemia: tetany, seizures; low PTH; hypercalciuria: nephrocalcinosis; ectopic and/or basal ganglia calcification	*CASR*: Calcium sensing receptor *GNA11*: G-protein subunit α-11	Ca^{2+} supplementation Low dose Vit. D (can increase urine Ca^{2+} & risk of nephrocalcinosis)
Distal Convoluted Tubule (DCT)				
11-βhydroxylase deficiency	AR	suppressed aldosterone; hypokalaemia; elevated androgen levels; virilisation	*CYP11B1*: 11-β hydroxylase	Glucocorticoid replacement therapy; Treat hypertension; MDT approach; Surgical reconstruction of ambiguous genitalia; prenatal dexamethasone
17-αhydroxylase deficiency	AR	suppressed aldosterone; hypokalaemia; primary amenorrhoea; sexual infantilism	*CYP17A1*: 17-α hydroxylase	Glucocorticoid replacement therapy; Treat hypertension with mineralocorticoid antagonist Hormone replacement; Address bone health
Gitelman syndrome (GS)[±±]	AR	Hypocalciuria; hypomagnesemia; hypotension; hypokalaemia; hypocalciuria; alkalosis; weakness & tetany	*SLC12A3*: thiazide-sensitive NaCl-co-transporter	See table 17
Isolated autosomal dominant hypo-magnesaemia (IADHG)	AD	Onset in infancy Hypomagnesaemia; normal K+/Ca^{2+}; normal/low urinary Ca^{2+}/ normal urinary Mg^{2+}; muscle cramps, weakness; tetany; tremor; seizures	*KCNA1*: Kv1.1	Mg^{2+} replacement
Isolated recessive hypo-magnesaemia (IRH)	AR	Onset in infancy Low Mg^{2+}; normal Ca^{2+}; High urinary Ca^{2+}/Mg^{2+}; nephrocalcinosis; stones; progressive CKD; recurrent UTIs; polyuria, polydipsia; failure to thrive; muscle cramps, weakness; tetany; tremor; seizures	*CLDN16*: claudin-16 *EGF*: epidermal growth factor *CLDN19*: claudin-19	Mg^{2+} replacement
Hypo-magnesaemia with secondary hypocalcaemia	AR	Low Mg^{2+}; Low Ca^{2+} Tetany; muscle spasms; developmental delay	*TRPM6*: HOMG	Mg^{2+} replacement

Table 15.15 (continued)

Collecting Duct (CD)				
Glucocorticoid-remediable aldosteronism (GRA)	AD	Hyperaldosteronism; low renin; hypertension; mild hypokalaemia; risk of haemorrhagic stroke	*CYP11B1-CYP11B2* chimera	steroids: dexamethasone/ hydrocortisone/prednisolone spironolactone/eplerenone
Distal renal tubular acidosis (dRTA) Type 1	AD (AR)	Hyperchloraemia; mild hypokalaemia; mild acidosis; late onset nephrolithiasis; nephrocalcinosis; mineral bone loss (asymptomatic)	*SLC4A1*: anion exchanger 1	Correction of acidosis and hypokalaemia Alkali therapy: Na^+ & K^+ bicarbonate/citrate; Potassium citrate if hypokalaemia/calcium stones Vit. D/Ca^{2+} supplementation *ADV7103 – alkali therapy at clinical trial phase*
Distal renal tubular acidosis (dRTA) Type 1 with Deafness	AR	Hyperchloraemia; hypokalaemia; severe acidosis; growth failure; vomiting/dehydration; progressive sensorineural hearing loss; rickets; nephrolithiasis	*ATP6V0A4*: V-ATPase subunit A4 *ATP6V1B1*: V-ATPase subunit B1	Correction of acidosis and hypokalaemia Alkali therapy: Na^+ & K^+ bicarbonate/citrate; Potassium citrate if hypokalaemia/calcium stones Vit. D/Ca^{2+} supplementation MDT approach Audiologist input
SeSAME syndrome (EAST syndrome)	AR	Seizures, Sensorineural deafness, Ataxia, Mental disability, Electrolyte imbalance (SeSAME); metabolic alkalosis; hypomagnesaemia; hypokalaemia Epilepsy, Ataxia, Sensorineural deafness, Tubulopathy (EAST)	*KCNJ10*: K^+channel	Antiepileptic medication Electrolyte replacement Physical, educational and speech therapy, audiologist input
Liddle syndrome	AD	Pseudoaldosteronism, low renin, hypertension, hypokalaemia, metabolic alkalosis, arrhythmia; constipation	*SCNN1B*: ENaC-β *SCNN1G*: ENaC-γ *(gain-of-function)*	Reduce BP; normalise K^+: Low Na+ diet K^+-sparing diuretics conventional antihypertensives ineffective
Pseudohypo-aldosteronism Type 1a	AD	Pseudohypoaldosteronism type 1, ↓Na^+, ↑K^+, ↑aldosterone, ↑renin Neonatal vomiting and dehydration	*MLR1*: mineralo-corticoid receptor 1	Fluid balance Na^+ supplementation K^+ binding resins Improves with age
Pseudohypo-aldosteronism Type 1b	AR	Pseudohypoaldosteronism type 1, ↓Na^+, ↑K^+, ↑aldosterone, ↑renin Severe neonatal vomiting and dehydration Respiratory distress	*SCNN1A*: ENaC-α *SCNN1B*: ENaC-β *SCNN1G*: ENaC-γ *(loss of function)*	Manage fluid balance; high Na^+ /low K^+ diet; K+ binding resins; Prostaglandin inhibitors; Alkalizing agents; Thiazide diuretics
Pseudohypo-aldosteronism Type 2 (PHA2; Gordon syndrome)	AD	Pseudohypoaldosteronism, low renin; ↑K+; ↑Cl–;; metabolic acidosis; hypertension low/high aldosterone	*WNK1*: serine/ threonine-protein kinase WNK1 *WNK4*:	Dietary Na^+ restriction; K^+ binding resins; Prostaglandin inhibitors; Alkalizing agents; Thiazide diuretics

(continued)

Table 15.15 (continued)

			serine/ threonine-protein kinase WNK4	
Nephrogenic diabetes insipidus	XD, AR	Polyuria; polydipsia; hypernatraemia	*AVPR2*: AVP2 receptor *AQP2*: aquaporin-2	replace urinary H_2O losses; thiazide diuretics; amiloride; low Na^+ diet
Secondary Tubulopathy				
Lowe syndrome	XR	Fanconi type tubular dysfunction, Aminoaciduria, RTA, CKD, vit. D-resistant rickets Congenital Cataract, , hypotonia, motor developmental delay, intellectual disability,	*OLRL1, PIB5PA*	Alkali therapy: Na^+ & K^+ bicarbonate/citrate; K^+ & Ca^{2+} supplementation; oral carnitine; oral PO_4 & calcitriol; KRT: kidney transplant; seizure control
Cystinosis[‡‡‡]	AR	Early Fanconi syndrome; progressive CKD; ESKD <12yrs; Eye involvement: (photophobia, retinal depigmentation, visual impairment; hypothyroidism, portal hypertension, hepato-splenomegaly, T_2DM, muscle weakness, low testosterone; incomplete pubertal development; encephalopathy; pyramidal signs; cranial nerve palsies may occur	*CTNS:* lysosomal membrane protein	See table 18
Maternally-inherited diabetes and deafness (MIDD)	Mt	Proteinuria, progressive CKD (FSGS, TIN); Sensorineural hearing loss; diabetes mellitus in adults (seek maternal inheritance); pigmentary retinopathy; ptosis; cardiomyopathy; myopathy; neuropsychiatric symptoms	*MT-TL1; MT-TK; MT-TE*	Early treatment advocated to avoid kidney complications/ MELAS syndrome Symptomatic management; oral antidiabetic agents +/- insulin for T2DM; hearing aids/cochlear implants; Co-enzyme Q10 supplementation proposed to treat mitochondrial defect

Abbreviations: AD Autosomal dominant, *AR* Autosomal recessive, *FSGS* Focal segmental glomerulosclerosis, *Glu* Glucose, *GS* Gitelman syndrome, H_2O Water, K^+ Potassium, *LMW* Low molecular weight, Mg^{2+} Magnesium, *MOI* Mode of inheritance, *Mt* Mitochondrial inheritance, Na^+ Sodium, $NaHCO_3$ Sodium bicarbonate, *NaCl* Sodium chloride, PO_4 Phosphate, *PTH* Parathyroid hormone, *TIN* Tubulo-interstitial nephritis, *TmG* Tubular maximum rate for glucose transport, T_2DM Type 2 diabetes mellitus, *Vit. D* Vitamin D, *XD* X-linked dominant, *XR* X-linked recessive

[a] See Table 15.16

[b] See Table 15.17

[c] See Table 15.18

Table 15.16 Diagnosis & Management of X-linked hypophosphataemia (XLH)[±] [18]

X-Linked Hypophosphataemia (XLH) [18]	
Clinical Presentation	• X-linked dominant disorder caused by mutations in *PHEX*, encoding fibroblast growth factor 23 (FGF23), a cell-surface-bound protein-cleavage enzyme expressed in osteoblasts, osteocytes and teeth • Commonest cause of inherited phosphate wasting • Presentation with signs of rickets (children)/osteomalacia (adults) in association with hypophosphataemia and renal PO_4 wasting in absence of Vit. D/Ca^{2+} deficiency • Diagnosis confirmed by measuring fibroblast growth factor 23 (FGF23) levels
Genetic Diagnosis	• Confirmation of genetic mutation in *PHEX*
Management	**General principles** • Reduce osteomalacia, and improve oral health • Monitor serum Ca^{2+} • Conventional treatment: treat symptomatic adults with: • active vitamin D (calcitriol), • oral phosphorus (phosphate salts) • Burosumab: recombinant human mAb against FGF23 approved to treat XLH • if available - should be considered in adult XLH patients with: • persistent bone and/or joint pain • osteomalacia that limits daily activities • pseudo-fractures • osteomalacia-related fractures • an insufficient response or refractory to conventional therapy • should be discontinued if fasting serum PO_4 level > upper limit of normal [18] • must not be given alongside conventional treatment when PO_4 levels normal pre-treatment • must not be given in presence of advanced CKD [18]

Abbreviations: Ca^{2+} Calcium, *CKD* Chronic kidney disease, *mAb* Monoclonal antibody, *PO_4* Phosphate, *Vit. D* Vitamin D;
[±]refers to where XLH is referenced in other tables in the chapter

secondary kidney tubulopathies the genetic defect does not directly affect a tubular transport or transport signalling protein, but rather non-specifically leads to damage of kidney tubular cells, and thereby to kidney tubular dysfunction. Gene identification has rendered this heterogeneous disease group of tubulopathies more accessible to unequivocal diagnostics, and thereby to the promise of more refined management strategies [3].

Table 15.17 Diagnosis & Management of Gitelman Syndrome (GS)±± [19]

Gitelman syndrome (GS)		
Clinical Presentation	**Criteria for suspecting GS** • Usually detected during adolescence or adulthood. • Electrolytes: Chronic hypokalemia (<3.5 mmol/l) with inappropriate renal potassium wasting (spot potassium:creatinine ratio >2.0 mmol/mmol [>18 mmol/g]) • Metabolic alkalosis • Hypomagnesaemia (<0.7 mmol/L [<1.70 mg/dL]) with inappropriate renal magnesium wasting (fractional excretion of magnesium >4%) • High plasma renin • Urine: Hypocalciuria (spot calcium-creatinine ratio < 0.2 mmol/mmol [<0.07 mg/mg]) in adults • Fractional excretion of chloride >0.5% • BP: Low/low-normal Ultrasound: Normal kidneys	**Features against a diagnosis of GS** • Use of thiazide diuretics/laxatives • AD family history of kidney disease • Electrolytes: Hypokalemia absent (except in CKD/ESKD) • Inconsistent hypokalemia in absence of substitutive therapy • Metabolic alkalosis absent (unless coexisting bicarbonate loss/acid gain) • Low plasma renin • Urine: Low urinary potassium excretion (spot potassium-creatinine ratio < 2.0 mmol/mmol [<18 mmol/g]); Hypercalciuria • BP: Hypertension/clinically increased extracellular fluid volume • Ultrasound: nephrocalcinosis, nephrolithiasis, unilateral/cystic kidneys • Prenatal history of polyhydramnios, hyperechogenic kidneys • Presentation before age 3 years
Genetic Diagnosis	**Criteria for establishing a diagnosis of GS** • Identification of biallelic inactivating mutations in *SLC12A3*, encoding thiazide-sensitive sodium-chloride cotransporter (NCC) • Hydrochlorothiazide testing no longer recommended as a diagnostic tool in GS: when used diagnostically to differentiate from Bartter syndrome, there is a risk of acute volume depletion in subjects with loop of Henle defect • Unless specific manifestations (e.g., significant proteinuria) are encountered, kidney biopsy is not necessary for the diagnosis of GS [19] • NGS–based gene panel to include differentials for GS: *SLC12A3; CLCNKB; HNF1B* • If only a single variant identified by NGS panel sequencing, analysis should be complemented with a test for a deletion on the other allele [19]	

Table 15.17 (continued)

Gitelman syndrome (GS)	
Management	**Individualised lifelong oral NaCl, K & Mg supplementation:** • GS is caused by a primary defect in a NaCl cotransporter, and is broadly managed by a liberal NaCl intake together with oral Mg and K supplements: • In hypomagnesaemia, Mg supplementation should occur first: Mg repletion facilitates K repletion, reducing risk of tetany/other complications • Cornerstone of preventing chondrocalcinosis is Mg supplementation • No evidence correlating severity of blood levels with symptom intensity
	Monitoring for side effects of supplementation • Target K level around 3.0 mmol/L • Target Mg level 0.6 mmol/L (1.46 mg/dL) • Achieving target electrolyte levels sometimes challenging • Supplementation with large doses may result in serious side effects: gastric ulcers, vomiting, diarrhoea with worsening electrolyte levels • An individual balance between improvement in blood values and side effects should be established • Realistic target values may be lower for some patients and may also change with time
	Drugs to be avoided/used with caution: • The following drug groups to be avoided/used with caution in GS: • Drugs slowing sinus rhythm/affecting QT interval (e.g. negative chronotropic drugs) • Drugs potentially exacerbating hypomagnesaemia (e.g. PPIs, gentamicin, antiviral drugs), acetazolamide
	Intravenous potassium chloride (KCl) • May be necessary when patient cannot take oral drugs/when the K deficit is very severe, causing cardiac arrhythmia/quadriplegia/respiratory failure/rhabdomyolysis
	Intravenous Magnesium Chloride (MgCl2) • Intravenous Mg infusion should be reserved for patients presenting with acute, severe complications of hypomagnesemia (e.g., tetany, cardiac arrhythmias), or in cases of digestive intolerance to oral supplements
	Potassium-sparing diuretics – Amiloride, spironolactone, potassium canrenoate, and eplerenone can increase serum potassium levels resistant to supplements and treat magnesium depletion that is worsened by elevated aldosterone levels – Use of spironolactône complicated by antiandrogenic effects, which are difficult in adolescents and young adults – Eplerenone is a selective aldosterone antagonist, with fewer antiandrogenic side-effects K-sparing diuretics compound renal salt wasting, so should be started cautiously to avoid hypotension, and concomitant salt supplementation should be considered
	RAAS blockade • The use of RAAS blockade has been occasionally reported in the treatment of GS: they may also aggravate renal sodium wasting and increase risk of symptomatic hypovolemia. RAAS inhibitors (ACEi/ARBs) should be stopped in cases of acute, salt-losing complications, e.g. vomiting/diarrhoea
	NSAIDs **Prostaglandin synthase inhibitors** • Prostaglandin synthase inhibitors such as indomethacin are rarely used in GS, because urinary prostaglandin E2 levels in GS are usually normal • Refractory hypokalemia has also been treated with the specific COX-2 inhibitor rofecoxib, but the use of this drug is limited by its long-term cardiovascular effects
	Analgesia for chondrocalcinosis • Both oral NSAIDs and low-dose oral colchicine are effective systemic treatments for acute chondrocalcinosis • NSAIDs must be used with caution in GS due to risk of AKI; • Colchicine treatment can increase the laxative effect of oral magnesium supplementation • Intra-articular corticosteroids may be considered in patients in whom other drugs are contraindicated
	Genetic Counselling • Genetic counselling should be offered to any patient with GS and to parents with a young child suffering from the disease • Could discuss testing of parents, siblings and partner • Prenatal diagnosis and preimplantation genetic diagnosis are technically feasible when 2 pathogenic *SLC12A3* mutations have been identified, although the prognosis is good for most GS patients: In very severe cases of GS, the possible use of these predictive tests can be discussed
	Considerations in Pregnancy • Aggravation of hypokalaemia and hypomagnesaemia during pregnancy necessitates early institution of a joint management plan and adaptations in Na/Mg/K supplementation • ACEi/ARB must be stopped during pregnancy due to significant foetal risk • Monitoring of plasma electrolyte levels advised during labour • After delivery, the treatment of the mother may return to baseline supplementation and follow-up

Abbreviations: ACEi Angiotensin converting enzyme inhibitor, *AD* Autosomal dominant, *AR* Autosomal recessive, *ARB* Angiotensin receptor blocker, *BP* Blood pressure, *CKD* Chronic kidney disease, *ESKD* End stage kidney disease, *K* Potassium, *Mg* Magnesium. *NaCl* Sodium chloride, *NGS* Next generation sequencing, *PPIs* Proton pump inhibitors
±±is shorthand for where Gitelman Syndrome (GS) is referenced in other tables in the chapter

Table 15.18 Diagnosis & Management of Cystinosis[±±±] [20]

Cystinosis [20]	
Clinical Presentation	• Cystinosis is an autosomal recessive lysosomal storage disease caused by mutations in the *CTNS* gene, leading to intralysosomal accumulation of cystine crystals, which damages several organs, including the kidneys • Nephropathic infantile cystinosis is commonest and most severe variant • Symptoms of multiorgan involvement may be mild to severe, depending on patient's age at diagnosis, the age when treatment was instituted, and genetic factors: Patients usually present during the first year of life with polyuria, polydipsia, dehydration, metabolic acidosis (normal anion gap hyperchloremic acidosis), hypophosphatemic rickets, failure to thrive, and laboratory findings consistent with Fanconi syndrome. If untreated, ESKD develops by age 7–10 years • Late-onset (intermediate) nephropathic cystinosis is more indolent: age at manifestation is most commonly in early adolescence. Symptoms usually restricted to kidneys: (less severe form of Fanconi syndrome, proteinuria) and eyes (photophobia). Disease progression is slower: ESKD occurs after age 15 years
Genetic Diagnosis	• Intracellular cystine concentrations (in white blood cells [WBC] or selected WBC types) are used clinically as the only available biomarker for diagnosis, and for gauging therapeutic success at the reduction in intracellular cystine accumulation. Monitoring therapeutic response in this manner is associated with better long-term outcomes, despite inconsistencies between laboratories [20] • Bi-allelic mutations in the *CTNS* gene confirms the genetic diagnosis
Management	**General principles** • Early oral administration of cysteamine, which reverses cystine accumulation via a newly described PQLC2 heptahelical protein substantially delays onset of ESKD, and the development of other complications [20] • Despite substantial improvement in prognosis due to cystine-depleting therapy with cysteamine, no cure of the disease is currently available [1] • A pre-emptive kidney transplant remains the best choice of KRT: widely accepted that there is no risk of recurrence, since the genetic defect is not transferred with the allograft • Cysteamine treatment is usually withdrawn for kidney transplantation, but the delay in resuming treatment should be limited to a few days: it is strongly recommended that there be a continuation of cysteamine treatment in patients treated by dialysis or transplantation [20]
	Primary Hypogonadism in male patients • Testosterone-replacement therapy allows pubertal development, but doesn't prevent infertility
	Pubertal delay in female patients • Female patients with cystinosis are fertile. • Protective effect on gonads from early cysteamine treatment has been shown. • Successful pregnancies have been described • Pre-conception counselling should be offered to all women contemplating pregnancy • Cysteamine therapy should be stopped during pregnancy: the optimal time for stopping cysteamine should be part of the preconception counselling
	Cystinosis Myopathy • Continue cystine reduction therapy • Muscle testing, electromyogram, and changes in pulmonary function should be used as endpoints for therapeutic intervention studies • Physiotherapy and exercise may be useful adjunctive therapies

[±±±]is shorthand for where Cystinosis is referred to elsewhere in other tables in the chapter

Nephrolithiasis

Genetic causes of kidney stones (nephrolithiasis) are described in Table 15.19, the general management of nephrolithiasis in Table 15.20; and the diagnosis and management of Cystinuria in Table 15.21, and that of Primary Hyperoxaluria Type 1 in Table 15.22.

Table 15.19 Nephrolithiasis [3]

Genetic Disorder	MOI	Characteristic signs and features	Gene symbol(s): Gene product(s)	Management
Cystinuria^	AR	Aminoaciduria, cystine calculi, recurrent UTI, haematuria, dysuria Mixed AB genotype rarely develop stones	*SLC3A1*: amino acid transporter 1 **(Type A)** *SLC7A9*: CSNU3 **(Type B)**	See table 15.21
Dent's disease	XR	Fanconi syndrome with CKD (men); Hypercalciuria; Radiopaque Ca^{2+} stones; rickets	*CLCN5*: renal Cl-Channel	Increased fluid intake, diuretics, high citrate diet, refer for bone studies
Primary hyperoxaluria type 1(PH1)^^	AR	Oxalate nephrolithiasis; metabolic acidosis; failure to thrive; nephrocalcinosis; ESKD; hypothyroidism; cardiac failure; myopathy	*AGXT*: Ala-glyoxylate aminotransferase	See table 15.22
Primary hyperoxaluria type 2 (PH2)	AR	Oxalate nephrolithiasis metabolic acidosis; failure to thrive; nephrocalcinosis; ESKD; hypothyroidism; cardiac failure; myopathy	*GRHPR*: glyoxylate reductase	High fluid intake Urinary alkalinization NO rationale for pyridoxine (Type 2); KRT
Primary hyperoxaluria type 3 (PH3)	AR	Oxalate nephrolithiasis metabolic acidosis; failure to thrive; nephrocalcinosis; ESKD; hypothyroidism; cardiac failure; myopathy	*HOGA1*: 4-hydroxy-2-oxoglutarate aldolase 1	High fluid intake Urinary alkalinization vegetarian diet (Type 3) KRT
Adenine-phosphoribosyl-transferase deficiency	AR	Urate nephrolithiasis; radiolucent stones; DHA nephropathy	*APRT*: adenine phosphoribosyl transferase	Allopurinol High fluid intake Low purine diet Monitor crystalluria
Xanthinuria	AR	xanthine calculi; failure to thrive; gross/microscopic haematuria; pyuria; renal colic; UTI; arthropathy; myopathy; low serum urate	*XDH*: xanthine dehydrogenase	High fluid intake Low purine diet Surgical care for xanthine stones - ESWL
Medullary Sponge Kidney (MSK)	(AD)	Haematuria; medullary nephrocalcinosis; nephrolithiasis; urolithiasis; UTI; metabolic acidosis	*GDNF*: Glial-derived neurotrophic factor	High fluid intake Diet modification Thiazide diuretics (Ca^{2+} stones), allopurinol (urate stones), Ca^{2+} citrate (oxalate stones) Antibiotic therapy

(continued)

Table 15.19 (continued)

				Stone management – ESWL Surveillance for Wilms Tumour in children
Familial Hypercalciuria	AD	Ca^{2+} nephrolithiasis, nephrocalcinosis, osteoporosis	*ADCY10*: Adenylate cyclase 10	High fluid intake Diet modification Allopurinol Thiazide diuretics
Calcium Oxalate kidney stones	AR	Oxalate nephrolithiasis kidney colic; UTIs	*SLC26A1*: Sulphate anion transporter 1	High fluid intake Diet modification – reduce oxalate rich foods, reduce Na+ Surgical management – ESWL

Abbreviations: ESWL Extracorporeal shock wave lithotripsy, *UTI* Urinary tract infection

^See Table 15.21

^^See Table 15.22

Table 15.20 General diagnosis & management of nephrolithiasis [21, 22]

Management of Nephrolithiasis[19,20]		
Initial Investigations	Integrating American Urological Association (AUA) and European Urological Association (EUA guidelines: • Clinicians should perform additional metabolic testing in high-risk or interested first-time stone formers and recurrent stone formers • Metabolic testing should consist of one or two 24-hour urine collections obtained on a random diet and analysed at minimum for total volume, pH, calcium, oxalate, uric acid, citrate, sodium, potassium and creatinine	
High risk stone-formers	**Table High Risk Stone formers**[20]	
	General Factors	Early onset of urolithiasis Familial stone formation Brushite-containing stones Uric acid and urate-containing stones Infection stones Solitary kidney
	Diseases associated with stone formation	Hyperparathyroidism Metabolic syndrome Nephrocalcinosis Gastrointestinal diseases (i.e. Crohn's, Malabsorptive conditions, ileal resection) Sarcoidosis
	Genetically determined stone formation	Cystinuria Primary hyperoxaluria Renal tubular acidosis (RTA) type I 2,8-Dihydroxyadeninuria Xanthinuria Lesch-Nyhan syndrome Cystic fibrosis
	Anatomical abnormalities associated with stone formation	Medullary sponge kidney (tubular ectasia) Ureteropelvic junction (UPJ) obstruction Calyceal diverticulum, calyceal cyst Ureteral stricture Vesico-uretero-renal reflux Horseshoe kidney Ureterocele
Stone types	• Stone type is the deciding factor for further diagnostic tests - Different stone types include[20]: • calcium oxalate; • calcium phosphate; • uric acid; • ammonium urate; • struvite (and infection stones); • cystine; • xanthine; • 2,8-dihydroxyadenine; • drug stones; • unknown composition	

(continued)

Table 15.20 (continued)

Management	**General Principles** • Recommend to all stone formers to achieve a fluid intake that will achieve a urine volume of at least 2.5 litres/day • Counsel patients with calcium stones and relatively high urinary calcium to limit sodium intake and consume 1,000 - 1,200 mg per day of dietary calcium Table adapted from European Urological Association (EUA) Urolithiasis Guidelines[20]

Agent	Rationale	Specifics and Side effects	Stone type
Alkaline citrates	Alkalinisation Hypocitraturia Inhibition of calcium oxalate crystallisation	Daily dose for alkalinisation depends on urine pH	Calcium oxalate Uric acid Cystine
Allopurinol	Hyperuricosuria Hyperuricaemia	Renal insufficiency demands dose correction	Calcium oxalate Uric acid Ammonium urate 2,8-Dihydroxyadenine
Captopril	Cystinuria Active decrease of urinary cystine levels	Second-line option due to significant side effects	Cystine
Febuxostat	Hyperuricosuria Hyperuricaemia	Acute gout contraindicated, pregnancy, xanthine stone formation	Calcium oxalate Uric acid
Sodium bicarbonate	Alkalinisation Hypocitraturia		Calcium oxalate Uric acid, Cystine
Pyridoxine	Primary hyperoxaluria	Polyneuropathia	Calcium oxalate
Thiazide (Hydrochloro-thiazide)	Hypercalciuria	Risk for agent-induced hypotonic blood pressure, diabetes, hyperuricaemia, hypokalaemia, followed by intracellular acidosis and hypocitraturia	Calcium oxalate Calcium phosphate
Tiopronin	Cystinuria Active decrease of urinary cystine levels	Risk for tachyphylaxis and proteinuria.	Cystine

Table 15.21 Diagnosis & Management of Cystinuria^ [23]

Cystinuria [23]	
Clinical Presentation	• AR condition: high urinary cystine and dibasic amino acid excretion leads to formation of cystine stones due to low solubility of cystine at normal urinary pH • Detection of hyperechoic colon during routine ultrasound before 36 weeks' gestation may suggest diagnosis of cystinuria, with a high PPV • In most patients, first stone detection occurs during childhood or adolescence • Diagnosis of cystinuria can be made by kidney stone analysis, observation of cystine crystals in urinary sediment, or detection of an abnormal excretion of cystine and dibasic amino acids in urine in adults and children [23]
Genetic Diagnosis	• Type A: *SLC3A1*: amino acid transporter 1 • Type B: *SLC7A9*: CSNU3 amino acid transporter • Genetic analysis should be performed in patients with cystinuria, allowing diagnostic confirmation, disease classification, and counselling of other family members, (although no strong genotype-phenotype correlations yet demonstrated)
Management	**General principles** • Patients with cystinuria are at higher risk of CKD and early onset hypertension • Conservative treatment is based on a stepwise strategy, addressing hydration, diet, and urinary alkalinization as basic measures, specific treatment of kidney tract stones, and thiol derivatives in refractory cases **Specific measures** • **Hydration:** Increased Fluid intake to guarantee a urine output large enough to maintain a cystine concentration of <250 mg/L • **Diet:** Dietary restriction of methionine and sodium • **Urinary alkalization:** oral potassium citrate – monitor urinary pH • **Managing kidney tract stones:** • Patients with cystinuria and ureteral stones who are well, with no infection or kidney impairment can be observed for up to 4 weeks for stone passage • Ongoing pain, kidney impairment, and low chance of spontaneous passage are indications for prompt treatment of stones • An NSAID should be the first drug of choice in the absence of contraindications. • Decompression (stent/nephrostomy) should be undertaken in patients with infected or obstructed kidneys • Due to recurrent nature of cystine stones, complete stone clearance should be achieved whenever possible • **Thiol derivatives**: (alpha-mercaptopropionylglycine (Tiopronin) and D-penicillamine) effective in reducing free urine cystine levels: monitor complete blood cell count and urinary protein excretion regularly

Abbreviations: CKD Chronic kidney disease, *NSAIDs* Non-steroidal anti-inflammatory drugs, *PPV* Positive predictive value

Table 15.22 Diagnosis & Management of Primary Hyperoxaluria Type 1^^ [24]

Primary Hyperoxaluria Type 1 [24]	
Clinical Presentation	• Rare autosomal recessive inborn error of glyoxylate metabolism, caused by deficiency of the liver-specific enzyme alanine:glyoxylate aminotransferase • Results in overproduction and excessive urinary excretion of oxalate, causing recurrent urolithiasis and nephrocalcinosis
Genetic Diagnosis	• Genetic tests for mutations in *AGXT* recommended in subjects with phenotypic characteristics of PH1 • Mutation analysis should be extended to siblings and parents, offering prenatal diagnosis using mutation analysis to parents of an affected child [24]
Management	**General principles** • Early initiation of conservative treatment • High Fluid intake (at least 3 L/m^2 per 24 h) • Vitamin B6 (pyroxidine) in patients with proven PH1 aiming to decrease urine oxalate excretion • Calcium oxalate crystallization inhibition by use of alkalization with oral potassium citrate aims at maintaining renal function [24] • Conservative measures should be initiated as soon as investigations are completed and while renal function is maintained. • Once ESKD established, pyridoxine is the only specific treatment that should be pursued. These measures apply to all types of PH, with the exception of pyridoxine, which is specific to PH1 [24]. • Endoscopic removal is recommended as preferential strategy to manage urolithiasis in patients who require intervention. • Avoiding any form of dialysis unless absolutely necessary is recommended and to consider pre-emptive transplantation in PH1 patients with progressive CKD • Where pre-emptive transplantation is not possible high efficacy dialysis is recommended as conventional dialysis is unable to remove sufficient quantities of oxalate proportionate to the continuous daily production; avoid loop diuretics post transplantation; dialyse pre-emptively immediately post transplantation to help clear residual oxalate load [24] • In ESKD due to PH1, simultaneous liver-kidney transplantation should be considered

^^is shorthand referring to where PH1 is referred to back in tables earlier in the chapter

Congenital Abnormalities of Kidney and Urinary Tract (CAKUT)

CAKUT are a group of disorders of characterised by anatomical abnormalities the kidneys, ureter, urine bladder and urethra present from birth (Table 15.23).

Hereditary Systemic Amyloidosis

Genetic causes of Hereditary Systemic Amyloidosis are described in Table 15.24.

Table 15.23 Congenital abnormalities of the kidney and urinary tract CAKUT [3]

Genetic Disorder	MOI	Characteristic Signs and Features	Gene symbol(s): Gene product(s)	Management
CAKUT	AD	CAKUT iridogoniodysgenesis	*FOXC1*: forkhead box C1, *DSTYK*: Dual serine/ threonine and tyrosine protein kinase	Manage hypertension KRT
Renal agenesis (RA)	AD	Kidney agenesis/dysplasia; VUR; Allelic with *MEN2A;* Facial defects, Males more commonly affected	*RET*: Ret protooncogen; *UPK3A*: uroplakin 3A	Prognosis for patients with unilateral kidney agenesis is excellent, with normal survival rate compared with controls; some data suggest increased risk of CKD, proteinuria, and hypertension, and a high risk for KRT
Renal tubular dysgenesis	AR	Kidney tubular dysgenesis; foetal anuria; oligohydramnios; hypotension; respiratory failure; pulmonary hypoplasia; Potter sequence; skull ossification defects; high mortality	*ACE:* Angiotensin I Converting Enzyme *AGT:* *Angiotensinogen* *AGTR1:* Angiotensinogen receptor 1 *REN:* Renin	CKD Management
Renal hypodysplasia (RHD)	AD	RHD; neonatal feeding issues; metabolic acidosis; pneumothorax; failure to thrive; polyuria; polydipsia; FSGS; CKD	*BMP4*: bone morpho-genetic protein 4; *SIX2*: sine oculis 2	Patients with **unilateral** hypodysplasia: follow-up US to monitor growth of contralateral kidney; Patients with **bilateral** hypodysplasia need supportive management, including maintaining fluid and electrolyte balance, and growth promotion Anti-HTN therapy – ACEi/ARBs CKD due partly to FSGS; ESKD: KRT, Kidney transplantation
Cystic Renal dysplasia	AD	Cystic kidney dysplasia, PUJO	*CDC5L*: cell division cycle; *USF2*: upstream uranscription factor 2	Monitor kidney function; urological intervention if required
Vesicoureteral reflux	AD	VUR Subtle facial and limb defects	*ROBO2*: roundabout 2; *SLIT2:* Slit Guidance Ligand 2 *SOX17:*	Treatment based on VUR grading, UTI and if bladder/bowel dysfunction present; Antibiotic prophylaxis for children <1 yr; continued in some circumstances;

(continued)

Table 15.23 (continued)

			SRY-Box Transcription Factor 17; *TNXB*: tenascin XB	Urinalysis for proteinuria & bacteriuria annually, including urine mcs if urinalysis suggests infection; Ultrasonography and voiding cystography; Surgical treatment
Branchio-oto-renal syndrome (BOR)	AD	CAKUT, RHD, VUR Deafness, ear malformation, branchial cysts, Unilateral/bilateral agenesis/dysplasia, hypoplasia, collecting system anomalies	*EYA1*: (eyes absent 1); *MYOG*: (myogenin); *SIX1*: (sine oculis 1); *SIX5*: (sine oculis 5)	Surgical treatment for Branchial cleft KRT: Kidney Transplantation
Fraser syndrome	AR	kidney agenesis/ hypo/dysplasia; cryptophthalmos; syndactyly; ambiguous genitalia; laryngeal stenosis/atresia	*FRAS1*: ECM protein; *FREM2*: Fras1-related ECM protein, *GRIP1*	Patients who survive may have unilateral kidney agenesis and/or kidney cystic dysplasia. Corrective surgery Treat CKD
HDR syndrome	AD	CAKUT, dysplasia, VUR Hypoparathyroidism, deafne ss, renal defects (HDR), hypocalcaemia	*GATA3*: GATA binding protein 3	Treatment of hypocalcaemia Symptomatic management CKD management Prognosis depends on severity of renal disease
Kallman syndrome	XR AD AR	Kidney agenesis; anosmia, hypogonadotrophic hypogonadism; cleft lip; heart defects	*KAL1*: anosmin, *FGFR1*: fibroblast growth factor receptor 1	Hormone replacement therapy Treatment for decreased bone mass Management of ESKD
Renal coloboma syndrome	AD	kidney hypoplasia, VUR, oligomeganephronia optic nerve coloboma	*PAX2*: paired box gene 2	kidney function testing, kidney US, urinalysis (proteinuria), BP monitoring; evaluation for VUR, KRT, kidney transplantation
Renal cysts and diabetes (RCAD) syndrome	AD	Kidney cysts/malformation (90%); diabetes mellitus (45%); hypomagnesaemia (40%); genital tract abnormalities (20%); hyperuricaemia (20%); elevated liver enzymes (15%) FHx: 50% de novo mutations	*HNF1B (TCF2)*: hepatocyte nuclear factor-β (transcription factor 2)	Electrolyte correction Diabetes treatment ESKD – KRT, kidney transplant Monitor for renal cell carcinoma
Split-hand/split-foot malformatio n (SHFM)	AD AR XR	Urethral malformation, kidney hypoplasia, oligodactyly, syndactyly, aniridia	*BMP7:* Bone morphogenetic protein 7; *DLX5/DLX6:* distal-less homeobox 5/6 *TP63*: tumour protein P63	Reconstructive surgery
Townes-Brocks syndrome	AD	Kidney agenesis, RHD, VUR, horseshoe kidney; Limb, ear, anal abnormalities; cardiac anomalies	*SALL1*: Spalt Like Transcription Factor 1	Surgery for malformations Surgery for congenital heart defects Hearing assessment ESKD: KRT, kidney transplant

Table 15.23 (continued)

Alagille Syndrome	AD	Kidney dysplasia (most common), distal renal tubular acidosis (dRTA), kidney cysts, urinary tract obstruction, kidney agenesis, tubulointerstitial nephritis and vesicoureteral reflux, Glomerular changes, (mesangiolipidosis/FSGS) also described; arterial hypertension secondary to RAS/other vascular involvement, cholestasis, jaundice, failure to thrive, congenital heart defect, posterior embryotoxon	*NOTCH2*: Notch Receptor 2 *JAGGED1:* jagged 1	Treatment for arterial hypertension; KRT; kidney transplant; Liver transplant
16p11.2 microdeletion syndrome	AD	CAKUT; developmental delay; intellectual disability; seizures	*TBX6*: *T-Box Transcription Factor 6*	Supportive management
Apert syndrome	AD	Hydronephrosis; craniosynostosis; acrocephaly; hydrocephalus; hypertelorism; maxillary hypoplasia; syndactyly; developmental delay	*FGFR2*: fibroblast growth factor receptor-2	MDT approach Symptomatic and supportive management
Beckwith-Wiedermann syndrome (BWS)	AD	Kidney medullary dysplasia, nephromegaly, nephrocalcinosis; high risk embryonal tumour development; overgrowth; neonatal hypoglycaemia; abdominal wall defects;	Dysregulation of imprinting in chromosome 11p15.5	MDT approach Regular abdominal and kidney imaging; measurement of serum AFP enables early detection & treatment of associated malignancies (e.g. Wilms tumor, hepatoblastoma).
Campomelic dysplasia	AD	Kidney dysplasia, hydronephrosis; cleft palate; skeletal anomalies; respiratory distress; genital anomalies	*SOX9*: SRY-box 9	Mechanical or physical breathing assistance Surgery for bone deformities Sexual re-assignment Guarded prognosis
Cenani-Lenz syndrome	AR	Kidney agenesis/ hypodysplasia; PUJO; syndactyly; distal limb defects	*LRP4*: LDL Receptor Related Protein 4	Surgical treatment and reconstruction
DiGeorge Syndrome	AD	Kidney agenesis/hypoplasia/ dysplasia; cardiac malformations; hypoparathyroidism; immune deficiency; developmental delay	22q11.2 deletion	Management of hypocalcaemia Immunological management: monitor T cells. HCT, Thymic transplant Monitor hearing, speech, growth Mental health issues in adolescents and adults
Ulnar-Mammary syndrome (UMS)	AD	Cystic kidney dysplasia; upper limb defects; underdevelopment of mammary & apocrine glands; genital abnormalities; poor temp regulation	*TBX3*: T-box transcription factor 3	Corrective or reconstructive surgery

(continued)

Table 15.23 (continued)

Duane-radial ray syndrome (DRRS)	AD	Unilateral kidney agenesis, hypoplasia, horseshoe kidney, VUR; malrotation; cross-fused ectopia; ocular manifestations; Duane anomaly; bilateral deafness; radial malformation;	*SALL4*: spalt-like transcription factor 4	Treatment of amblyopia or surgery To improve head turn and eye misalignment
Pallister-Hall syndrome (PHS)	AD	Kidney agenesis, hypodysplasia, hydronephrosis; hypothalamic harmartoma; central and postaxial polydactyly; bifid epiglottis; imperforate anus	*GLI3*: GLI Family Zinc Finger 3	Hormone replacement therapy due to hypopituitarism, Assess for cortisol deficiency Urgent visualisation and evaluation of epiglottis Anti-seizure medications Periodic Cranial MRI
Rubinstein-Taybi syndrome (RSTS)	AD	Kidney agenesis, hypoplasia, hydronephrosis; broad thumbs; short stature; distinctive facial features; intellectual disability; eye abnormalities; congenital cardiac defects	*CREBBP*: CREB Binding Protein	Monitoring of growth and feeding Symptomatic treatment MDT approach
Simpson- Golabi Behmel syndrome (SGBS)	XR	Medullary kidney dysplasia; nephromegaly; may develop Wilms tumour; pre and postnatal overgrowth; craniofacial anomalies; organomegaly; increased risk of tumours	*GPC3*: glypican 3 *GPC4*: glypican 4	Regular screening for tumours Glucose monitoring in neonatal period Monitor kidney function MDT approach
Zellweger syndrome	AR	Kidney cystic dysplasia; Neurological deficits; hypotonia; hearing loss; vision problems; liver dysfunction; seizures; adrenal insufficiency	12 genes involved in peroxisome function *PEX1*: peroxisomal bio-genesis factor 1 (70% of cases)	Cholic acid Supportive management MDT approach
Smith-Lemli-Opitz syndrome (SLOS)	AR	Kidney hypoplasia, cysts, aplasia; growth delay, microcephaly; polydactyly; fused second and third toes; cleft palate; underdeveloped male external genitalia; developmental delay	*DHCR7*: 7-dehydro-cholesterol reductase	Severely affected individuals may require surgery to correct cleft palate, heart defects and genital anomalies; Cholesterol supplementation, in combination with bile acids, improves growth and reduces photosensitivity with no harmful side effects

Abbreviations: ACEi Angiotensing converting enzyme inhibitor, *AD* Autosomal dominant, *AFP* Alpha-fetoprotein levels, *AR* Autosomal recessive, *ARB* Angiotensin receptor blocker, *BOR* Branchio-oto-renal syndrome, *CKD* Chronic kidney disease, *ESKD* End stage kidney disease, *FSGS* Focal and segmental glomerulosclerosis, *MOI* Mode of inheritance, *PUJO* Pelvi-ureteric junction obstruction, *RAS* Renal artery stenosis, *US* Ultrasound, *VUR* Vesico-ureteric reflux

Table 15.24 Hereditary Systemic Amyloidosis

Genetic Disorder	MOI	Characteristic signs and features	Gene symbol(s): Gene product(s)	Management
Apolipoprotein AI amyloidosis	AD	Hypertension, proteinuria, haematuria and oedema due to CKD; ESKD. Hepatosplenomegaly; progressive cardiomyopathy; skin, testes and adrenal involvement (hypergonadotropic hypogonadism)	*APOA1*: apolipoprotein A1	KRT; Kidney transplant; Combined liver and kidney transplant
Apolipoprotein AII amyloidosis	AD	Primary kidney deposition CKD; oedema, ESKD; cardiomyopathy and deposition in spleen, liver, adrenal glands, pancreas	*APOA2*: apolipoprotein A2	KRT; Kidney Transplant
Fibrinogen Aα amyloidosis	AD	Neurological, cardiac, visceral, kidney and vascular amyloid deposition: Hypertension, uraemia, nephrotic syndrome, ESKD	*FGA*: fibrinogen α-chain	Control Hypertension; Diuretics; KRT; Kidney Transplant; Combined liver and kidney transplant
Lysozyme amyloidosis	AD	Primary kidney deposition; also GI tract; heart; liver; spleen; slow disease progression; Symptoms: nausea & vomiting; dyspepsia; gastritis; GI haemorrhage; abdominal pain; hepatic rupture; sicca syndrome; purpura & petechiae; lymphadenopathy; CKD	*LYZ*: lysozyme	Supportive and symptomatic therapy; Liver or kidney transplant
Hereditary transthyretin-mediated (hATTR) amyloidosis	AD	Adult onset; proteinuria; peripheral neuropathy; congestive cardiac failure; Glaucoma; orthostatic hypotension; diarrhoea/constipation;	*TTR*: transthyretin	Liver transplantation; Supportive treatment of involved organs; Heart transplant/KRT RNAi therapy reduces transcription of mutant transthyretin protein: Patisiran/Inotersen (polyneuropathy); Tafamidis (cardiomyopathy)
Hereditary gelsolin (AGel) amyloidosis	AD	cranial (facial nerve/bulbar) & sensory peripheral neuropathy; corneal lattice dystrophy; cutis laxa; CKD	*GSN*: gelsolin	Symptomatic treatment; Ophthalmology input

Conclusions

Returning to the patient from the beginning of the chapter, who presents with cystic kidney disease, and an autosomal dominant inheritance pattern of 'CKD': It would be invaluable to supplement the rather scant phenotypic information available from the history with a precise cause of CKD in his father and paternal grandmother, as well as the presence or absence of other discriminating features: these might include the size of his cystic kidneys, presence or absence of cysts in other organs, characteristic skin rashes, epilepsy, learning difficulties, or a history of type 2 diabetes mellitus, ESKD, stroke or sudden death in the family. Without significant further information, it would seem reasonable to counsel him appropriately about the benefits and risks (including of not getting a definitive diagnosis) - of undertaking a genetic sequencing panel, focused on candidate genes associated with cystic kidney disease (Table 15.5).

Despite considerable advances in understanding the molecular cause of many genetic kidney diseases, the aetiologies for most remain unsolved. That said, even where the genetic cause is well-defined, such as in Alport and Bartter syndromes, genetic testing is not commonplace – influenced by the associated high costs, long turnaround times, a preconception that the genetic diagnosis will not alter clinical management, insufficient genetic knowledge amongst clinicians, and differences in access to genetic testing, amongst other factors [1].

As the boundaries of our knowledge of genetic kidney disease move inexorably forward, we appreciate ever more fascinating peculiarities—each with important clinical applications: a number of genetic kidney diseases previously considered part of a single disorders have been shown to be genetically heterogeneous, with mutations in different genes along the same biological pathways, giving rise to similar clinical, biochemical, and histopathological features, which simultaneously reinforces - and develops - our understanding of these pathways [1]. Additionally, we recognise that an individual's carrier status for certain genetic kidney disorders may prove important beyond genetic counselling: with potentially important clinical implications for carriers themselves: where heterozygous carriers of X-linked recessive disorders are usually asymptomatic or mildly affected, in some heterozygotes, a more severe disease outcome is noted, notably in Alport syndrome and Fabry disease. As such, carrier status for certain conditions may yet have important implications, for example in selecting living-related kidney transplant donors [1].

There are many exciting opportunities offered by NGS: lowering costs and the lead-time for results from high-throughput sequencing; alongside the carefully designed, internationally collaborative bioinformatic platforms, such as the European Rare Kidney Disease Network (ERKNet). Other drives such as the Human Phenotype Ontology website, and the Online Mendelian Inheritance in Man "OMIM" catalogue of Human Genes and Genetic Disorders help to continuously refine genomic datasets in clarifying molecular pathways associated with particular phenotypes, and hence driving the identification of novel therapeutic targets for rare kidney diseases. We must acknowledge the reverse argument too – that certain iterations of NGS applied in an individual can generate an enormous amount of incidental data, the therapeutic, moral and ethical implications of interpreting this data are yet to be explored [1].

Taking the global perspective, genetic testing is not equally available in all countries equitably to screen for genetic kidney diseases - indeed there may be unequal access to genetic testing between different areas within the same country. Designing pathways for genetic testing that facilitate timely genetic testing for patients with suspected genetic kidney disease, that is equally affordable and accessible in less well-resourced regions and countries alike, is arguably as important as the continuing drive to develop novel therapies for these diseases.

Questions

1. An 18 year old gentleman of mixed heritage is been found to have isolated microscopic haematuria on dipstick, with a normal ultrasound scan. His serum creatinine is 60 μmol/L, (eGFR >90 mL/min/1.73 m^2). His mother – who was born in China, also has dipstick haematuria, as does his maternal grandmother. His father, from India, does not. There is no family history of deafness, visual disturbance or ESKD requiring KRT.

Genetic testing has identified that he is heterozygous for a *COL4A3* mutation. What should the patient be advised?

A. The diagnosis is consistent with Alport disease
B. The diagnosis is consistent with IgA nephropathy (IgAN)
C. The diagnosis is consistent with thin basement nephropathy (TBMN)
D. He is likely to progress to ESKD
E. He is likely to develop deafness

Answer: C—The patient has been shown to be heterozygous for a *COL4A3* mutation. This is consistent with TBMN, with an AD inheritance pattern of a phenotype demonstrating isolated haematuria. To confirm this, genetic testing should be undertaken on both parents. As a carrier of a gene associated with AR Alport syndrome, there is a risk of his offspring developing Alport syndrome, dependent on any prospective partner's carrier status, and the patient should be signposted toward genetic counselling when the time is appropriate.

2. A 29-year-old male banker is found to have dipstick haematuria, but no significant proteinuria on his routine medical examination. A subsequent ultrasound scan reveals multiple cysts on both kidneys. His blood tests reveal his serum creatinine is 70 μmol/L (eGFR >90 mL/min/1.73 m^2). He has no history of diabetes mellitus, no skin rashes, and no other medical problems of note.

His father and paternal grandmother were both said to have had chronic kidney disease, with 'lots of cysts' on their kidneys, but there is no history in the family of progression to ESKD.

Which of the following is least likely to be included on the list of differential diagnoses?

A. Autosomal dominant polycystic kidney disease (ADPKD)
B. Tuberous sclerosis complex (TSC)
C. Autosomal dominant tubulointerstitial kidney disease (ADTKD)
D. Renal cysts and diabetes (RCAD) syndrome
E. Alport syndrome

Answer: E—Whilst each of the diseases listed can display an AD inheritance pattern, as illustrated in the patient's family history, Alport syndrome is more typically X-linked recessive, and not characterised by cystic kidney disease, but rather by microscopic haematuria, progressive proteinuria, and an association with hearing loss.

3. A 22-year-old female medical student has found to have multiple cysts on both kidneys on a screening ultrasound scan. She had been advised to do so by her father, a doctor, who has recently been diagnosed with autosomal dominant polycystic kidney disease, and has had to start haemodialysis. He has been found to have a pathogenic *PKD1* mutation. To her knowledge, her paternal grandmother had a kidney transplant some years ago, but she doesn't know the cause of her kidney disease.

On examination, her blood pressure is 120/70 mmHg, and her pulse 56 beats/minute. Her cardiac, chest, abdominal and neurological examinations are all unremarkable. Her blood tests reveal a serum creatinine of 56 μmol/L (eGFR >90 mL/min/1.73 m^2). There is no history of diabetes mellitus, no skin rashes, and no other medical problems of note.

What is the next most appropriate step in her management?

A. Drink 1–1.5 L of fluid per day
B. Gene sequencing panel for cystic kidney disease
C. Cross-sectional imaging (CT/MRI)
D. Commence Tolvaptan immediately
E. Counsel her about obtaining a pre-implantation genetic diagnosis

Answer: C—She is highly likely to have inherited the pathogenic *PKD1* mutation from her father, and she is also highly likely to progress to ESKD, as have her father and paternal grandmother. Obtaining baseline cross-sectional imaging to establish her baseline total kidney volume (TKV) can serve to provide a marker to facilitate prognostication, as well as a baseline to evaluate the response to prospective Tolvaptan (or other) therapy. She should be advised to increase her water intake (likely to much more than 2 L per day), alongside close monitoring of her blood pressure. Confirming her genetic diagnosis by sequencing *PKD1* to confirm inheritance of the pathogenic *PKD1* mutation would facilitate discussion about her options with regard to having offspring in future, and should form part of (but not the main focus of) the discussion around genetic testing. Tolvaptan therapy would be indicated where a patient has, or is at risk of rapidly progressing, CKD stages 1–3 in adult ADPKD patients aged <50 years. Whilst she is certainly at risk of progressing, in the clinical context, it would be sensible to obtain baseline cross-sectional imaging first.

4. A 24 year old female airport worker – originally from Ghana - presents to her primary care practitioner with headaches and mild abdominal discomfort, which is affecting her memory and concentration. Her urinalysis revealed dipstick haematuria. A subsequent abdominal ultrasound scan reveals several bilateral solid kidney masses, associated with several cysts. Blood tests reveal a serum creatinine of 80 μmol/L (eGFR >90 mL/min/1.73 m^2).

She experienced a normal childhood in Ghana, and is noted to have a facial rash, which has become more extensive during adolescent years, and painful nodules under the nails of her first and fourth fingers of her right hand. To her knowledge, there is no family history of any similar condition.

What is the most likely diagnosis?

A. Neurofibromatosis Type 1 (NF1)
B. Von Hippel Lindau (VHL) Disease
C. Tuberous sclerosis complex (TSC)
D. Lennox-Gastaut syndrome (LGS)
E. Hereditary leiomyomas and renal cell carcinoma (HLRCC)

Answer: C The patient's physical features are most in keeping with bilateral kidney angiomyolipomas (AMLs) and associated cysts, associated with facial angiofibromas, and subungual fibromas. These would be sufficient to meet the criteria for a definite diagnosis of TSC (Table 11). Whilst her headaches, that may be affecting her memory and concentration may be a non-specific presentation, the clinical context should nevertheless prompt urgent cross-sectional brain imaging to exclude significant mass lesions, such as an obstructing subependymal giant cell astrocytoma (SEGA), causing hydrocephalus, which may necessitate urgent neurosurgical intervention, and subsequent consideration of mTOR inhibitor therapy. There should be further consideration of the possibility of an underlying seizure disorder. The other differentials on the list are associated with skin lesions (NF1), kidney masses (HLRCC, VHL), and Lennox-Gastaut syndrome (LGS) is a rare and severe kind of epilepsy that starts in childhood.

5. A 26-year-old male is referred as an emergency to the kidney service with a plasma creatinine of 1235 μmol/L (eGFR <5 mL/min/1.73m^2). He attended his primary care doctor with a 3-week history of oral thrush, nausea, weight loss, nocturia and pruritus. He does not complain of visual problems, rash or arthralgia and is not taking any medications. His hearing has been impaired since birth, to the point that he has required hearing aids from the age of 11. His mother, maternal grandfather, maternal aunt and uncle, and a brother, are also deaf. His maternal aunt was known to have a moderate kidney impairment. On examination, his blood pressure is 168/97 mmHg, his chest was clear and abdominal examination unremarkable. He is noted to have pre-auricular pits, and a raised skin lesion over his neck. Urinalysis demonstrates proteinuria 4+ and haematuria 3+; urine protein:creatinine ratio is 560 mg/mmol. Blood tests show a haemoglobin of 72 g/L, MCV 90.6 fL, platelets 243 × 109 g/L, potassium 5.9 mmol/L, urea 47.4 mmol/L and creatinine 1235 μmol/L. His serum albumin is 40 g/L, corrected serum calcium 1.97 mmol/L, phosphate 1.96 mmol/L and parathyroid hormone level 64.0 pmol/L. Haematinic levels are normal. His autoimmune screen shows no abnormality. Abdominal ultrasound demonstrates that both kidneys are <8 cm in bipolar length.

What is the most likely diagnosis?

A. Alport syndrome
B. Epstein syndrome
C. Fechtner syndrome
D. Branchio-oto-renal syndrome (BOR)
E. Familial hypo/hyperparathyroidism (HDR)

Answer: D All of the above differentials are characterised by deafness, often associated with kidney dysfunction, and may all present with an AD inheritance pattern. Whilst Alport syndrome would be the commonest cause, the presence of pre-auricular pits and a neck lesion – consistent with a branchial fistula – makes BOR the more likely diagnosis in this context. Genetic testing is warranted to sequence the *EYA*, *SIX1* and *SIX5*, although a panel approach excluding other causes of deafness and kidney dysfunction may be more appropriate.

6. A 24 year old male army recruit presents with complaints of weakness of the right lower limb of two months' duration. Neurological evaluation determines a clinical impression of a compressive myelopathy at cervical vertebral levels C6–7. MRI of the brain and spine reveals a predominantly cystic mass in the left cerebellar hemisphere, with enhancing intramedullary mass lesions, consistent with cerebellar and spinal haemangioblastomas. The patient is further investigated with an abdominal ultrasound, which reveals multiple simple cortical cysts in both kidneys, with some solid components. The liver, pancreas, spleen and adrenals are otherwise normal. There is no history of familial involvement. In view of the imaging findings, a clinical diagnosis of VHL disease is made.

What should be the next investigation?

A. MRI scan of the abdomen
B. CT scan of the chest
C. Genetic sequencing of *VHL*
D. Genetic sequencing of *SDH*, *FH*, *TSC* and *VHL*
E. Brain biopsy

Answer: A Whilst sequencing *VHL* would confirm the genetic diagnosis, it would not immediately alter his management: the first clinical priority should be to obtain cross-sectional imaging of the abdomen to further elucidate the ultrasound findings, in particular the solid elements to the mass lesions on his kidneys, as there is a significant risk of associated malignancy in the kidneys, as well as the pancreas, and phaeochromocytomas, which should be followed with an appropriate multi-disciplinary team discussion about appropriate further treatment.

7. A 45 year old Caucasian man presents with a two year history of burning sensation is his hands and feet, dry skin, palpitations and proteinuria. On examination he is tall, his pulse is 95 beats/min, with a forceful cardiac apex beat and a normal neurological examination. Investigations show a serum creatinine of 87 μmol/L, haemoglobin 122 g/L, normal liver function tests, a fasting glucose of 5.4 mmol/L, and a urine protein:creatinine ratio of 330 mg/mol. His kidney ultrasound and chest X-ray are normal, and his echocardiogram demonstrates left ventricular hypertrophy.

What is the most likely cause of his symptoms and proteinuria?

A. Apolipoprotein deficiency
B. Alpha-galactosidase deficiency
C. Autosomal dominant tubulointerstitial nephritis
D. Amyloidosis
E. Diabetes mellitus

Answer B: His presentation with acroparaesthesia, hypohydrosis, LVH and proteinuria in a 45 year old male are suggestive of Fabry disease (alpha-galactosidase deficiency).

8. A 34 year old female presents with an incidental finding of proteinuria and a raised serum creatinine following living kidney donation 5 years ago. Her mother—the kidney allograft recipient -had been diagnosed with end stage kidney disease of unknown cause, and had presented with minimal proteinuria and a normal blood pressure. Her uncle also received a kidney transplant 5 years ago. On examination her blood pressure is 125/68 mmHg, her pulse 68 beats/min, and examination of all other systems is normal. Urine microscopy shows 50 white cells/high power field, urine protein:creatinine ratio was 105 mg/mol, and her serum creatinine was 150 μmol/L.

What is the most likely genetic defect in the family?

A. Cystinosis
B. Fanconi disease
C. Juvenile nephronophthisis
D. *UMOD* mutation
E. Tuberous sclerosis complex (TSC)

Answer: D With minimal proteinuria, leukocyturia, CKD and a strong family history, a familial form of tubulointerstitial disease is the most likely diagnosis

9. A 54 year old lady presents to the medical intaking service with intermittent nausea, vomiting, muscle cramps and weakness. On examination, her blood pressure is 110/70 mmHg, and her pulse 90 beats per minute. Her chest, abdomen and cardiovascular system examinations are normal; she has proximal muscle weakness, but her remaining neurological exam is normal. Her blood tests at presentation are:

Sodium: 139 mmol/L
Potassium: 2.1 mmol/L
Urea: 5.1 mmol/L
Creatinine: 54 μmol/L
Urine microscopy: normal
Urine dipstick: normal
Urinary potassium: 60 mmol/L

What is the most likely cause of her hypokalaemia?

A. Low potassium diet
B. Lower Gastrointestinal tract loss of potassium
C. Movement of potassium from plasma to cells
D. Renal tubular defect
E. Upper Gastrointestinal loss of potassium

Answer: D With a high urinary potassium, the most likely cause of her hypokalaemia is renal potassium loss

10. A 54 year old lady presents to the medical intaking service with intermittent nausea, vomiting, muscle cramps and weakness. On examination, her blood pressure is 110/70 mmHg, and her pulse 90 beats/min. Her chest, abdomen and cardiovascular system examinations are normal. She has proximal muscle weakness, but her remaining neurological exam is normal. Her blood tests at presentation are:

Sodium: 139 mmol/L
Potassium: 2.1 mmol/L
Urea: 5.1 mmol/L
Creatinine: 54 µmol/L
Urine microscopy: normal
Urine dipstick: normal
Urinary potassium: 60 mmol/L

She recalls that her brother, and a maternal cousin have had 'problems with their potassium'. Which of the following is the most likely cause of her hypokalaemia?

A. Bartter syndrome
B. Gitelman syndrome
C. Liddle syndrome
D. Apparent mineralocorticoid excess
E. Glucocorticoid remediable hypertension

Answer: B In the setting of hypokalaemia, and notably a normal/low blood pressure - alongside proven excessive renal potassium wasting, and without obvious other causes of renal or GI potassium losses such as diuretics or laxatives, as well as a suggestive family history of problems with potassium metabolism, consistent with an AR inheritance pattern, Gitelman syndrome is the most likely of the options.

11. A 20-year old Gujarati woman presented to Renal Outpatients. The referral letter stated that she had recently moved house and wanted a review of her renal condition. It also mentioned that 2–3 years earlier, a renal biopsy at another institution had been reported as showing 'chronic glomerulonephritis'.

The nephrologist noticed that the patient looked at him intently during the consultation, which led to a sense of unease. At the end of the consultation the patient mentioned that for some time her eyesight had been worrying her. Haemoglobin 148 g/L, creatinine 186 µmol/L (we should state mg/dL in brackets too), albumin 40 g/L, urine protein 1.2 g/24 h, Urine: RBC 60/µL, WBC <5/µL, Culture sterile. She was referred to the ophthalmologist for further assessment.

In a chance meeting between the ophthalmologist and nephrologist the following week, the former was triumphant: "I've made both an important ophthalmological diagnosis, and made your diagnosis for you!" What is the most likely diagnosis?

A. Chronic glomerulonephritis
B. Alport syndrome [unspecified]
C. Alport syndrome with anterior lenticonus and hearing defect
D. IgA nephropathy
E. Alport syndrome with hearing defect

Answer: C Alport syndrome with anterior lenticonus and hearing defect.

A. Chronicglomerulonephritis---Incorrect---Answer not sufficiently focused.
B. Alport syndrome [unspecified] --- Incorrect --- Can be more specific.
C. Alport syndrome with anterior lenticonus and hearing defect --- Correct --- Deafness meant that patient had to look carefully at the doctor's mouth when he was speaking. Her recent visual blurring added to her difficulties. The anterior lenticonus of Alport's syndrome typically presents at the age of 20.
D. IgA nephropathy -- Incorrect --- Insufficient information for this option.
E. Alport syndrome with hearing defect --- Incorrect --- Less focused than Option C.

Test your learning and check your understanding of this book's contents: use the "Springer Nature Flashcards" app to access questions using https://sn.pub/cz9Cok. To use the app, please follow the instructions in Chap. 1.

References

1. Devuyst O, et al. Rare inherited kidney diseases: challenges, opportunities, and perspectives. Lancet. 2014;383(9931):1844–59.
2. Groopman EE, Rasouly H, Gharavi AG. Genomic medicine for kidney disease. Nature Rev Nephrol. 2018;14(2):83–104.
3. Hildebrandt F. Genetic kidney diseases. Lancet. 2010;375(9722):1287–95.
4. Pollak MR, Friedman DJ. The genetic architecture of kidney disease. Clin J Am Soc of Nephrol. 2020;15(2):268–75.
5. Aymé S, et al. Common elements in rare kidney diseases: conclusions from a kidney disease: improving global outcomes (KDIGO) controversies conference. Kidney Int. 2017;92(4):796–808.
6. Joly D, Beroud C, Grünfeld JP. Rare inherited disorders with renal involvement—approach to the patient. Kidney Int. 2015;87:901–8.
7. Chapman AB, Eckardt K-U, Gansevoort RT, Harris T, Horie S, Kasiske BL, Odland D, Pei Y, Perron RD. Autosomal-dominant polycystic kidney disease (ADPKD): executive summary from a Kidney Disease: Improving Global Outcomes (KDIGO) Controversies Conference. Int Soc Nephrol. 2015;88(1):17–27.
8. Gansevoort RT, Arici M, Benzing T, Birn H, Capasso G, Covic A, Devuyst O, Drechsler C, Eckardt KU, Emma F, Knebelmann B, Le Meur Y, Massy ZA, Ong AC, Ortiz A, Schaefer F, Torra R, Vanholder R, Więcek A, Zoccali C, Van Biesen W. Recommendations for the use of tolvaptan in autosomal dominant polycystic kidney disease: a position statement on behalf of the ERA-EDTA Working Groups on Inherited Kidney Disorders and European Renal Best Practice. Nephrol Dial Transplant. 2016;31(3):337–48. https://doi.org/10.1093/ndt/gfv456. Epub 2016 Jan 29.
9. Irazabal MV, Rangel LJ, Bergstralh EJ, Osborn SL, Harmon AJ, Sundsbak JL, Bae KT, Chapman AB, Grantham JJ, Mrug M, Hogan MC, El-Zoghby ZM, Harris PC, Erickson BJ, King BF, Torres VE, Investigators CRISP. Imaging classification of autosomal dominant polycystic kidney disease: a simple model for selecting patients for clinical trials. J Am Soc Nephrol. 2015;26(1):160–72. https://doi.org/10.1681/ASN.2013101138. Epub 2014 Jun 5.
10. Guay-Woodford LM, Braun MC, Bockenhauer D, Cadnapaphornchai MA, Dell KM, Kerecuk L, Liebau MC, Alonso-Peclet MH, Shneider B, Emre S, Heller T, Kamath BM, Murray KF, Moise K, Eichenwald EE, Evans J, Keller RL, Wilkins-Haug L, Bergmann C, Gunay-Aygun M, Hooper SR, Hardy KK, Hartung EA, Streisand R, Perrone R, Moxey-Mims M. Consensus expert recommendations for the diagnosis and management of autosomal recessive polycystic kidney disease: report of an international conference. J Paediatr. 2014;165(3):611–7.
11. Kai-Uwe Eckardt SLA, Antignac C, Bleyer AJ, Chauveau D, Dahan K, Deltas C, Hosking A, Kmoch S, Rampoldi L, Wolf MWMT, Devuyst O. Autosomal dominant tubulointerstitial kidney disease: diagnosis, classification, and management—a KDIGO consensus report. Int Soc Nephrol Kidney Int. 2015;88(4):676–83.
12. Binderup MLM, Harbud V, Møller HU, Gimsing S, Friis-Hansen L, van Overeem Hansen T, Bagi P, Knigge U, Kosteljanetz M, Bøgeskov L, Thomsen C, Gerdes A-M, Ousager LB, Sunde L. Von Hippel-Lindau disease (vHL) National clinical guideline for diagnosis and surveillance in Denmark 3rd Edition. Dan Med J. 2013;60(12)
13. Northrup H, Krueger DA. Tuberous sclerosis complex diagnostic criteria update: recommendations of the 2012 International Tuberous Sclerosis Complex Consensus Conference. Pediatr Neurol. 2013;49(4):243–54.
14. Krueger DA, Northrup H. Tuberous sclerosis complex surveillance and management: recommendations of the 2012 International Tuberous Sclerosis Complex Consensus Conference. Pediatr Neurol. 2013;49(4):255–65.
15. Kidney Disease: Improving Global Outcomes (KDIGO) Glomerulonephritis Work Group. KDIGO clinical practice guideline for glomerulonephritis. Kidney Int Suppl. 2012;2:139–274.
16. Goodship TH, Fakhouri F, Fervenza FC, Frémeaux-Bacchi V, Kavanagh D, Nester CM, Noris M, Pickering MC, Rodríguez de Córdoba S, Roumenina LT, Sethi S, Smith RJ. Atypical hemolytic uremic syndrome and C3 glomerulopathy: conclusions from a "Kidney Disease: Improving Global Outcomes" (KDIGO) Controversies Conference. Kidney Int. 2017;91(3):539–51.
17. Schiffmann R, Linthorst GE, Ortiz A, Svarstad E, Warnock DG, West ML, Wanner C. Screening, diagnosis, and management of patients with Fabry disease: conclusions from a "Kidney Disease: Improving

Global Outcomes" (KDIGO) Controversies Conference. Kidney Int. 2017;91(2):284–93.
18. Haffner D, Eastwood DM, Duplan MB, Bacchetta J, Schnabel D, Wicart P, Bockenhauer D, Santos F, Levtchenko E, Harvengt P, Kirchhoff M, Di Rocco F, Chaussain C, Brandi ML, Savendahl L, Briot K, Kamenicky P, Rejnmark L, Linglart A. Clinical practice recommendations for the diagnosis and management of X-linked hypophosphataemia. Nat Rev Nephrol. 2019;15(7):435–55.
19. Blanchard A, et al. Gitelman syndrome: consensus and guidance from a kidney disease: improving global outcomes (KDIGO) controversies conference. Kidney Int. 2017;91(1):24–33.
20. Langman CB, Deschênes G, Emma F, Goodyer P, Lipkin G, Midgley JP, Ottolenghi C, Servais A, Soliman NA, Thoene JG, Levtchenko EN. Controversies and research agenda in nephropathic cystinosis: conclusions from a "Kidney Disease: Improving Global Outcomes" (KDIGO) Controversies Conference. Kidney Int. 2016;89(6):1192–203.
21. Pearle MS, Assimos DG, Curhan G, Denu-Ciocca CJ, Matlaga BR, Monga M, Penniston KL, Preminger GM, Turk TM, White JR. American Urological Assocation. Medical management of kidney stones: AUA guideline. J Urol. 2014;192(2):316–24.
22. Türk C, Knoll T, Petrik A, Sarica K, Skolarikos A, Straub M, Seitz C. Guidelines on urolithiasis. European Association of Urology; 2015.
23. Servais A, Thomas K, Dello Strologo L, Sayer JA, Bekri S, Bertholet-Thomas A, Bultitude M, Capolongo G, Cerkauskiene R, Daudon M, Doizi S, Gillion V, Gràcia-Garcia S, Halbritter J, Heidet L, van den Heijkant M, Lemoine S, Knebelmann B, Emma F, Levtchenko E. Metabolic Nephropathy Workgroup of the European Reference Network for rare kidney diseases (ERKNet) and eUROGEN. Cystinuria: clinical practice recommendation. Kidney Int. 2020;99(1):48–58.
24. Cochat P, Hulton S, Acquaviva C, Danpure CJ, Daudon M, De Marchi M, Fargue S, Groothoff J, Harambat J, Hoppe B, Jamieson NV, Kemper MJ, Mandrile G, Marangella M, Picca S, Rumsby G, Salido E, Straub M, van Woerden CS, OxalEurope. Primary hyperoxaluria Type 1: indications for screening and guidance for diagnosis and treatment. Nephrol Dialysis Transpl. 2012;27(5):1729–36.

Kidney Cancer

16

Rebecca Shone, Anna Walsh, Luke Stroman, Christopher Anderson, and Nicholas M. P. Annear

Clinical Scenario

A 48 year old male with no significant medical history is referred to urology with visible haematuria. A contrast CT reveals bilateral enhancing heterogenous masses; 65 mm in the left upper pole as well as a contralateral 26 mm right upper pole lesion (see CT images below in Fig. 16.1). No other sites of metastases were seen.

What is the most appropriate investigation and management for this patient?

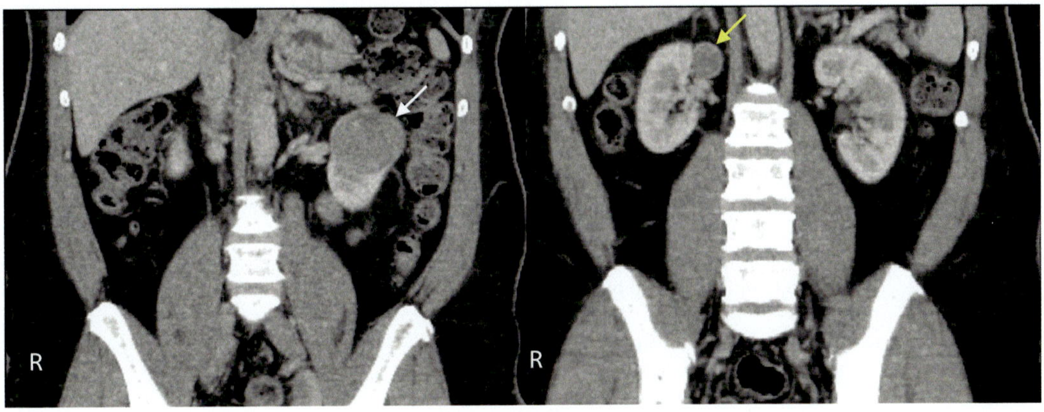

Fig. 16.1 Coronal contrast-enhanced CT scans showing a 65 mm left sided upper pole lesion (white arrow, left) and 23 mm right upper pole lesion (yellow arrow, right)

R. Shone · C. Anderson · N. M. P. Annear (✉)
St George's University Hospitals NHS Foundation Trust, London, UK

St George's University of London, London, UK
e-mail: r.shone@nhs.net; chris.anderson3@nhs.net; nannear@sgul.ac.uk

A. Walsh · L. Stroman
St George's University Hospitals NHS Foundation Trust, London, UK
e-mail: anna.walsh@stgeorges.nhs.uk; luke.stroman@stgeorges.nhs.uk

D. Banerjee et al. (eds.), *Management of Kidney Diseases*,
https://doi.org/10.1007/978-3-031-09131-5_16

Introduction

This chapter will discuss malignancies arising from the renal parenchyma/cortex. These are a heterogenous group of cancers. Renal cell carcinoma (RCC) is the most common solid lesion in the kidney and accounts for the majority of primary renal malignancies (approximately 90%) [1]. It will therefore be our primary focus for the purposes of this chapter (Tables 16.1 and 16.2).

Table 16.1 Principal Subtypes of RCC [1, 2]

	Underlying genetic/histological characteristics	Prognosis
Clear-cell (cc-RCC) *(75% of RCC)*	Loss of chromosome 3p and mutation of the von Hippel-Lindau (*VHL*) gene frequently found.	Worst prognosis of the three subtypes.
Papillary *(15% of RCC)*	Type I—germline mutations of MET Type II—activation of the NRF2-ARE pathway.	Low malignant potential, over 75% can be treated by nephron sparing surgery [1]. Type I has best prognosis.
Chromophobe *(5% of RCC)*	Typical genetic changes include loss of chromosomes Y, 1, 2, 6, 10, 13, 17, 21.	Good prognosis, high 5 and 10 year recurrence free survival [1].

Table 16.2 Other non-RCC renal tumour subtypes [1, 2]

Tumour type	Clinical	Malignant potential	Management
Renal medullary carcinoma	Rare tumour, median age of diagnosis 28 years [1]. Associated with sickle cell disease.	Malignant	Aggressive cancer with most patients presenting with metastatic disease. Radical nephrectomy recommended, even in early disease, along with chemotherapy. Not responsive to targeted anti-angiogenic drugs including tyrosine kinase inhibitors.
Carcinoma associated with ESKD; acquired cystic disease - associated RCC	The lifetime risk of developing RCC is 10 times higher for ESKD patients than the general population [1]. RCCs are generally multifocal and bilateral.	Malignant	RCC associated with ESKD less aggressive than sporadic RCC. Surgical management.
Papillary adenoma	Benign neoplasm arising from renal tubular epithelium. Measure ≤15 mm in diameter. Histologically and genetically indistinguishable from papillary RCC. Estimated prevalence of 20% based on autopsy series [3].	Benign	Surveillance.
Hereditary kidney tumours	5–8% of RCCs are hereditary. Examples of syndromes associated with development of renal tumours include: • Von Hippel-Lindau (VHL) syndrome • Birt-Hogg-Dubé syndrome (BHD) • Hereditary pRCC • Tuberous sclerosis complex (TSC) • Hereditary leiomyomatosis RCC (HLRCC) • Germline succinate dehydrogenase (SDH) mutation	Variable	May require repeated surgeries, nephron sparing approach favoured. • HLRCC and SDH are aggressive and require immediate surgical intervention • Active surveillance for VHL, BHD and HPRCC—monitoring growth, size and location.

Table 16.2 (continued)

Tumour type	Clinical	Malignant potential	Management
Angiomyolipoma (AML)	Benign mesenchymal tumour—occurs sporadically or as part of tuberous sclerosis complex (TSC). Slow growth rate, minimal morbidity. Larger AMLs can cause localised pain and spontaneous bleeding, which can be fatal.	Benign	Active surveillance monitoring risk factors for bleeding—Tumour size, vascularity, and presence of tuberous sclerosis complex [1]. Indications for active treatment include: • Persistent pain • Acute or repeated bleeding • Large size (>4 cm) In patients with tuberous sclerosis complex (TSC), AML size and vascularity may be reduced by mTOR pathway inhibition.
Renal oncocytoma	Benign tumour, representing 18% of solid renal tumours [1]. Slow growing.	Benign	Challenging to diagnose with CT/MRI imaging as similar appearances to RCC. Mainstay of treatment is surveillance; radical/partial nephrectomy is considered if increasing size. Consideration of renal mass biopsy may reduce unnecessary surgical intervention.

Epidemiology and Causes

Kidney cancer is the ninth most commonly occurring cancer in men and the 14th most commonly occurring cancer in women. The age-standardised rate per 100,000 in the US in 2018 was 10.9 per 100,000 [4].

The rate of new kidney cancers has been increasing since the 1990s, though seems to now be plateauing. This rise is thought to be at least partially attributable to the increasing numbers of asymptomatic cancers detected incidentally through CT scanning for other indications.

It is estimated that half of kidney cancers could potentially be prevented by weight loss and tobacco smoking, which are the most potent risk factors [5] (Table 16.3).

Table 16.3 Risk factors associated with kidney cancer

Risk Factor	Comments
Smoking	Risk increases proportional to amount smoked. Kidney cancer risk is 33% higher in current smokers compared with non-smokers [5]
Obesity	There is an increased risk of kidney cancer with increasing BMI. Multiple proposed mechanisms include adipokine secretion from adipose tissue promoting tumour growth
Hypertension	Well established risk factor, proportional to the blood pressure [6]
Workplace exposures	Certain occupation exposures such as asbestos, cadmium, trichloroethylene
Male sex	Twice as common in men as women
Advanced kidney disease	Those with ESKD on dialysis have been shown to have a 2.3 times increased risk of kidney cancer [7] this risk increases further in those with ADPKD [8]
Genetic/ hereditary associations	Von Hippel-Lindau (VHL) syndrome, Hereditary papillary renal cell carcinoma (HPRCC), Hereditary leiomyoma-renal cell carcinoma (HLRCC), Birt-Hogg Dube (BHD) syndrome, Familial renal cancer, Cowden syndrome, Tuberous sclerosis complex (TSC)

Genetic Basis of Kidney Cancer

Kidney cancers are heterogenous and there are many associated genetic mutations. These have an important clinical relevance in that they are the basis of the targeted and immunomodulatory therapies which are key to treating advanced kidney cancer. This will be explored later in the chapter.

The *VHL* tumour suppressor gene is the most frequently mutated gene in sporadic RCC, and it is often the first mutation to occur. In normal cells, the VHL-containing complex targets the alpha subunit of hypoxia inducible factor (HIF-a) for degradation. The mutation of *VHL* and subsequent inactivation of VHL leads to accumulation of HIF-a, leading to uncontrolled activation of HIF target genes, including vascular endothelial growth factor (VEGF), which control angiogenesis and cellular proliferation.

The mutation in *VHL* is one of multiple potential genetic mutations which may occur in the development of RCC. Other genetic mutations frequently associated with RCC include *PBRM1, SETD2, BAP1* which, like *VHL*, are all located on the short arm of chromosome 3 (Fig. 16.2).

Other RCCs are characterised by mutations in mammalian target of rapamycin (*mTOR*), a protein kinase involved in the regulation of cell growth and proliferation which has been implicated in the development of kidney cancer.

In recent years, there has been much interest in the immunological factors that allow tumour cells to proliferate. One such focus is the programmed cell death protein 1 (PD-1) receptor and its ligand (PD-L1). PD-1 is a cell surface receptor which regulates T cell activation, promoting apoptosis in antigen specific T cells. PD-1, PD-L1 and PD-L2 have been found to be abnormally expressed by tumour cells and lymphocytes in the tumour microenvironment, where their inhibitory action assists the cancer cells' evasion of the immune response.

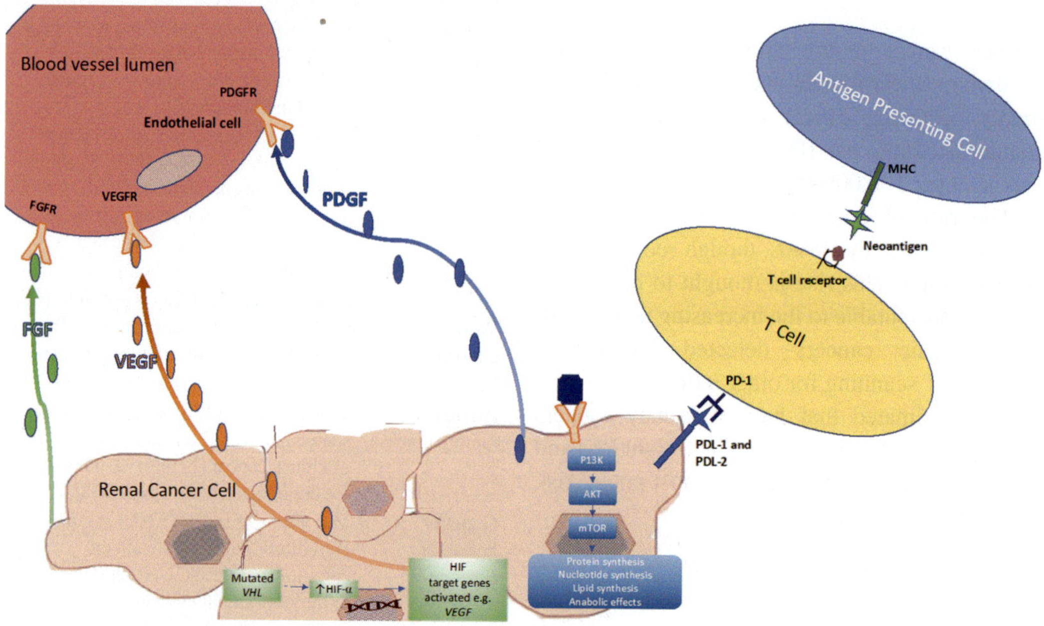

Fig. 16.2 Pathophysiological mechanisms involved in the development of renal cell carcinoma (*Adapted from Choueiri TK, Motzer RJ. Systemic Therapy for Metastatic Renal-Cell Carcinoma. N Engl J Med. 2017 Jan 26;376* (4)*:354–366* [9])
Hypoxia-inducible factor (HIF), VEGF (vascular endothelial growth factor) FGF (fibroblast growth factor), FGFR (FGF receptor), PDGF (platelet-derived growth factor), PDGFR (PDGF receptor) and VEGFR (VEGF receptor), mechanistic target of rapamycin (mTOR), MHC (major histocompatibility complex), PD-1 (programmed cell death protein) PD-L1 (PD-1 ligand, and PI3K (phosphatidylinositol 3-kinase)

Clinical Presentation

More than 50% of RCCs are diagnosed incidentally. The classic presenting triad includes **haematuria, flank pain and a palpable abdominal mass**. Less than 10% of patients present with these symptoms however, and those who do are likely to have locally advanced disease [1] (Fig. 16.3 and Table 16.4).

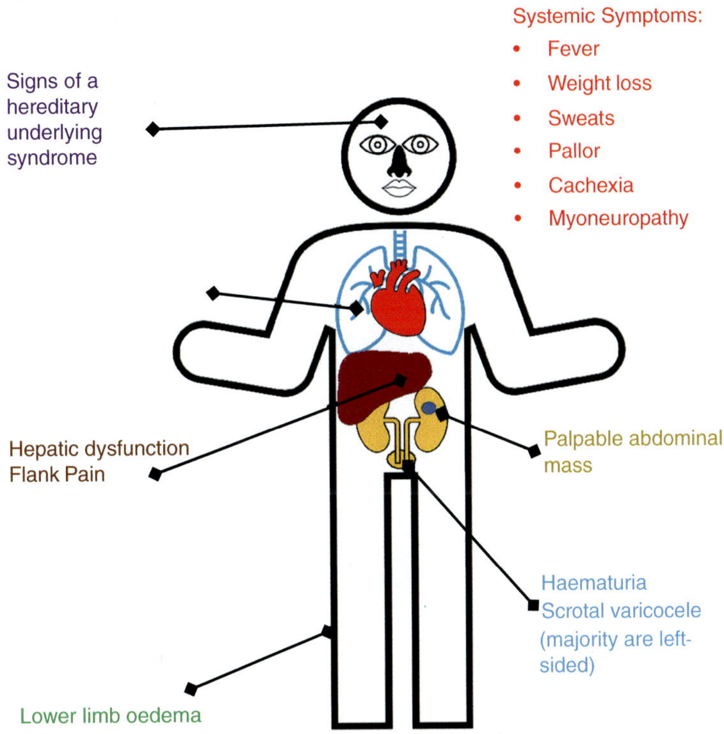

Fig. 16.3 Clinical Presentation of RCC [1]

Table 16.4 Paraneoplastic Syndromes associated with RCC [1]

Paraneoplastic phenomena	Cause(s)	Clinical manifestation
Fever	Cytokine production by the tumour cells, particularly IL-1, IL-6 and TNF-β	Fever, night sweats
Anaemia	Inflammation/chronic disease	Fatigue, breathlessness
Erythrocytosis	Excess erythropoietin (EPO)	Occurs in 1–5% of patients with advanced RCC
Hypercalcaemia	Over production of PTH-r protein. Lytic bone lesions.	Clinical signs of hypercalcaemia—Constipation, confusion Bone pain
Hypercortisolism	Excess ACTH	Cushing's syndrome
Hepatic dysfunction	Liver metastases. Stauffer syndrome refers to hepatic dysfunction in the absence of liver metastases	Jaundice, itch, right upper quadrant pain May be asymptomatic
Secondary (AA) amyloidosis	Deposition of fibril proteins.	Clinical presentation depends on organ affected

Given the paraneoplastic presentations of RCC, patients can present with a myriad of symptoms related to this, including:

- Systemic symptoms of fever, weight loss, sweats, pallor, cachexia, myoneuropathy
- Signs of hepatic dysfunction
- Lower limb oedema—may represent inferior vena cava involvement
- Scrotal varicocele
- Signs of an underlying hereditary syndrome

Investigations

Practice point 1
Imaging is key to diagnosis: Most renal masses can be diagnosed accurately by imaging alone

The most important criterion for differentiating malignant lesions is the presence of enhancement, with contrast enhanced CT and MRI being the modalities of choice. For the diagnosis of complex renal cysts, MRI may be preferable: it has higher sensitivity and specificity for small cystic renal masses and tumour thrombi. Contrast enhanced ultrasound also has a high sensitivity and specificity.

The Bosniak Classification is used to stratify cysts by their radiological features on cross-sectional imaging and thus determine a suitable work up and follow up plan (Table 16.5).

Table 16.5 Bosniak Classification of Renal Cysts [1]

Bosniak Category	Features	Clinical implications
I	• Simple cyst • Hairline-thin wall without septa, calcification or solid components • Non-enhancing	Benign, no follow up needed
II	• Minimally complex • May contain a few hairline-thin septa • Fine calcification in wall or septa • Non-enhancing, high attenuation • <3 cm in size	Benign, no follow up needed
IIF	• Minimally complex • May contain more hairline-thin septa with non-measurable enhancement • May contain calcification, nodular or thick	Some are malignant, require US / CT / MRI follow up over 5 years at 6 monthly intervals
III	• Indeterminate cystic mass • Thickened, irregular walls or septa with enhancement	Over 50% are malignant[1] Need active surveillance or surgery
IV	• Clearly malignant • Solid mass with large cystic or a necrotic component	100% malignant Surgical intervention required.

Renal Tumour Biopsy

The vast majority of kidney cancer diagnoses are made on the basis of the radiological findings. In certain situations however, tumour biopsy is indicated (Table 16.6).

Biopsy should be avoided in comorbid and frail patients who, regardless of histology, would not be considered for active management [1].

Percutaneous sampling can be performed with local anaesthesia under US or CT guidance with needle core biopsy. Given concerns regarding tumour seeding along the needle tract, a co-axial technique is recommended. When performed by experienced operators, core biopsy carries a high diagnostic yield, with a metanalysis reporting sensitivity of 99.1% and specificity of 99.7% for the diagnosis of malignancy [10]. In cases where there is a suspicion of malignancy but the biopsy result is non-diagnostic, a repeat biopsy or surgical exploration should be considered [1] (Fig. 16.4).

> A larger gauge needle or cannula is advanced into the mass; once adequately positioned a smaller needle is placed through it in order to obtain tissue. This allows for multiple needle biopsies via only 1 point of access, thereby reducing risk of tumour seeding.

Table 16.6 Indications for renal tumour biopsy [1]

Indications for renal tumour biopsy [1]
• Further assessment of radiologically indeterminate masses or in the presence of another primary malignancy
• Prior to ablative treatments (cryotherapy/radiofrequency ablation)
• Where active surveillance is being considered
• To select most suitable treatment strategy in metastatic disease

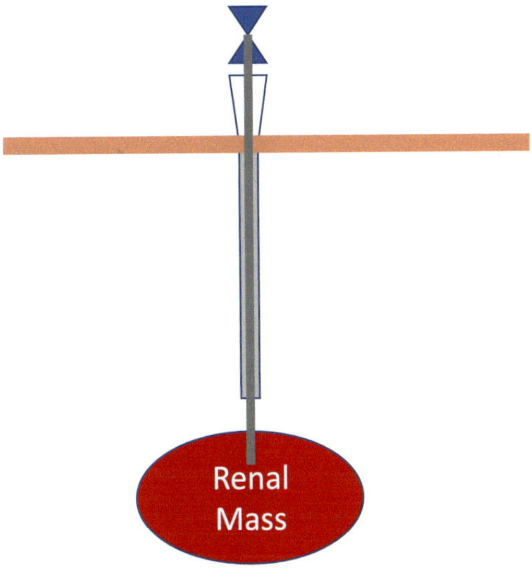

Fig. 16.4 Co-axial technique for biopsy of a kidney mass

Diagnosis and Classification

The approach to classifying renal cell carcinoma involves consideration of both the **stage** (how locally advanced the tumour is) and **grade** (the resemblance of the tumour cells to healthy cells). The TNM classification is universally recognised as the staging tool of choice (Tables 16.7, 16.8, 16.9 and Fig. 16.5).

Table 16.7 TNM Classification [1]

T – Primary Tumour	N – Regional Lymph Nodes	M – Distant metastases
T1 – Tumour ≤ 7 cmin greatest dimension, limited to kidney o **T1a** – Tumour ≤ 4 cm o **T1b** – Tumour >4 cm but ≤ 7cm	**N0** – No regional lymph node metastases	**M0** – No distant metastasis
T2 – Tumour >7 cm in greatest dimension but limited to kidney o **T2a** - Tumour >7 cm but ≤ 10cm o **T2b** – Tumour >10 cm but limited to the kidney	**N1** – Metastasis in regional lymph nodes.	**M1** – Distant metastasis
T3 – Tumour extends into major veins or perinephric tissues but not into ipsilateral adrenal gland and not beyond Gerota's fascia o **T3a** - Tumour extends into renal vein or invades perirenal fat but not beyond Gerota fascia o **T3b** – Tumour extends into vena cava below diaphragm o **T3c** – Tumour extends into vena cava above the diaphragm	**NX** – Regional lymph nodes cannot be assessed	
T4 – Tumour invades beyond Gerota's fascia		

Table 16.8 TNM Stage Grouping [1]

The TNM staging is summarised as RCC Stage 1-4:

Stage 1	T1	N0	M0
Stage 2	T2	N0	M0
Stage 3	T3 T1, T2, T3	N0 N1	M0 M0
Stage 4	T4 Any T	Any N Any N	M0 M1

Table 16.9 World Health Organisation (WHO)/ International Society of Urologic Pathology (ISUP) Tumour Grading [1]

Grade 1	Nucleoli absent or inconspicuous and basophilic at 400 x magnification
Grade 2	Nucleoli clearly visible and eosinophilic at 400 x magnification
Grade 3	Nucleoli conspicuous and eosinophilic at 100 x magnification
Grade 4	Extreme nuclear pleomorphism, multinucleate cells, rhabdoid or sarcomatoid differentiation.

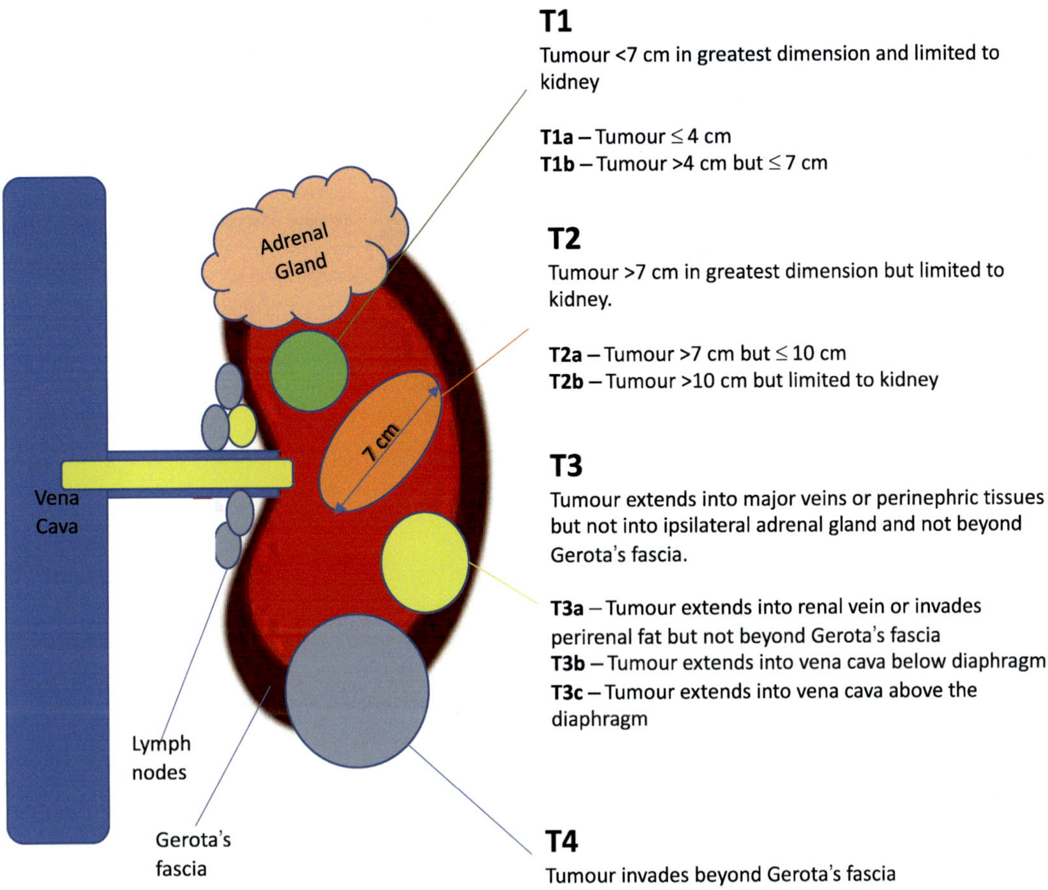

Fig. 16.5 Staging of kidney cancer [1]

Management

Surgery

When patients present with localised disease, the mainstay of treatment is surgery, which can be curative. It is therefore the preferred first line treatment for the majority of patients with stage I, II or III disease.

> **Practice Point 2**
> Surgery is the first line treatment for localised disease

Surgery can include both partial nephrectomy (PN), also known as "nephron sparing" surgery (NSS) or radical nephrectomy (RN), which involves excision of the entire kidney and Gerota's fascia. Excision of the ureter along with the kidney is a nephroureterectomy and performed for urothelial cell malignancy of the upper tract. Imperative indications for PN include a solitary kidney, bilateral renal tumours or patients with syndromes pre-disposing to renal malignancy.

Patients with advanced or metastatic disease with a favourable prognosis who have a resectable primary tumour may also benefit from surgical resection where this is technically feasible

Table 16.10 Comparison between partial and radical nephrectomy [1]

Partial nephrectomy (PN) "Nephron sparing"	Radical nephrectomy (RN)
Preferred option for all T1a and some T1b/T2 tumours.	Option for larger tumours or more locally invasive disease where PN not possible
• A Cochrane review found that for localised disease, PN was associated with reduced time to death of all-cause mortality. Serious adverse events, CSS and time to recurrence were similar between groups[10] • Several retrospective analyses have suggested a decreased cardiovascular specific mortality with PN versus RN[1] • PN should be surgery of choice, even if it necessitates an open procedure where RN could be minimally invasive • Absolute indications for PN include: o a solitary kidney o bilateral renal tumours o patients with syndromes pre-disposing to renal malignancy • PN is preferred option for patients with pre-existing CKD to limit progression of ESKD requiring kidney replacement therapy (KRT)	• Minimally invasive vs open approach – no RCT has addressed oncological outcomes with either approach though minimally invasive associated with lower morbidity • Less likely to have positive surgical margins with RN vs PN[11]

(Table 16.10). For most patients with metastatic disease further systemic treatment is then warranted which will be discussed in more detail below. When surgical resection is performed in the presence of metastatic disease this is termed a cytoreductive nephrectomy (CN).

Adrenalectomy

Ipsilateral adrenalectomy during PN or RN has not been found to have a survival advantage unless there is clinical evidence of gland invasion (T4 disease) [1].

Lymph Node Dissection (LND)

The only randomised trial to date has not shown a survival advantage of LND in localised disease [13]. Retrospective studies have shown a survival benefit with visible LN disease [14].

> **Practice Point 3**
> Despite attempted curative treatment with nephrectomy (either partial or radical), approximately 30% of patients with ccRCC with localised disease will go onto develop metastases [15]

Alternatives to Surgery

Alternatives to surgery include:

- Watchful waiting
- Active Surveillance
- Cryoablation
- Radiofrequency Ablation

Watchful Waiting & Active Surveillance

The increasing incidental detection of small renal masses (SRMs), especially in a predominantly elderly population, has led to the development of active surveillance protocols. In carefully selected patients, this may be an appropriate initial strategy to monitor their renal mass, which could then be treated at a later date if it is seen to progress. Studies suggest that up to 20% of small renal masses are benign, with only 20% having an aggressive phenotype [16].

Active surveillance differs from watchful waiting, which is reserved for those patients who would not be candidates for active treatment, and who therefore do not usually require follow up imaging (Fig. 16.6).

Other less-invasive treatments are also available for those who may not be fit for surgery,

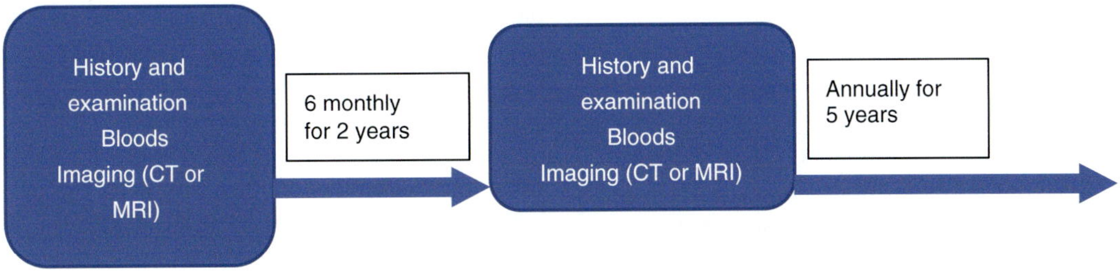

Fig. 16.6 Follow up of patients under active surveillance [1]

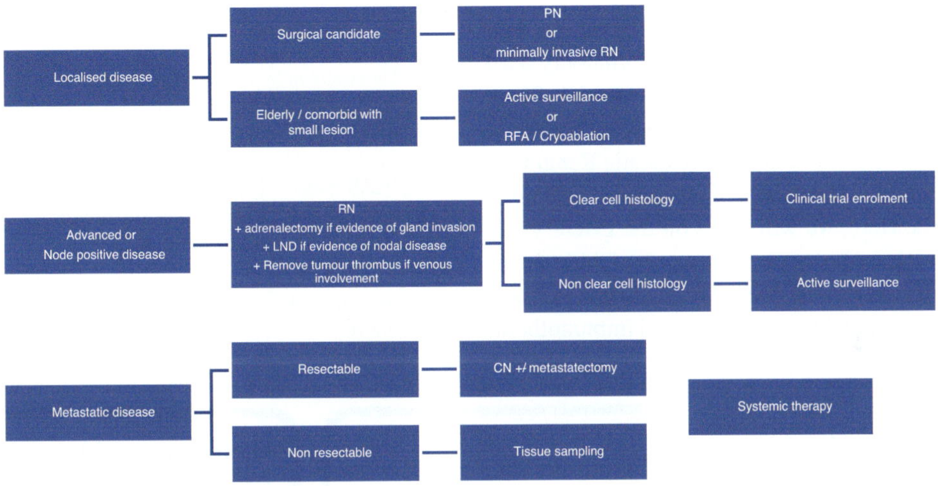

Fig. 16.7 Management of Kidney Cancer [1]
PN Partial nephrectomy, *RN* Radical nephrectomy, *RFA* Radiofrequency ablation, *CN* Cytoreductive nephrectomy, *LND* Lymph node dissection

have small (<4 cm tumours) or those who have multiple and/ or bilateral tumours. These treatments include **cryotherapy** and **radiofrequency ablation**. There are currently no data demonstrating any oncological benefit of these treatments over PN, although benefit has been shown in reduction in loss of kidney function. Increased local recurrence has been seen when compared to partial nephrectomy but cancer specific survival is similar [17].

Cryoablation

Cryoablation can be performed by either the percutaneous or laparoscopic route, with no significant difference in complication between the two routes. Under ultrasound or CT guidance, a probe is inserted into the tumour through which an argon coolant is delivered at subfreezing temperatures. This forms an 'ice ball' around the probe tip, destroying the tumour tissue. Helium is then passed through the probe to induce a slow thaw. In most cases, two freeze-thaw cycles are performed.

Radiofrequency Ablation (RFA)

Percutaneous RFA can be carried out under local anaesthesia and sedation or general anaesthetic. One or more radiofrequency electrodes are inserted percutaneously into the tumour under imaging guidance. Radiofrequency energy is then delivered via the electrode to create high temperatures and destroy the tumour tissue.

Figure 16.7 summarises the approach to management of kidney cancer.

Systemic Therapy

> **Practice Point 4**
>
> **Small molecule inhibitors, targeted therapies and immune checkpoint-based immunotherapy** form the treatment pathway for advanced or metastatic kidney cancer.
>
> **There is no role for chemotherapy** [1]

Treatment options are selected based on risk scoring and histology. The most commonly used risk scoring models are the Memorial Sloan Kettering Cancer Center (MSKCC) Prognostic Model or the International Metastatic Renal Cell Carcinoma Database Consortium (IMDC) Criteria. Here, we will focus on the IMDC criteria which is most commonly used (Table 16.11 and Fig. 16.8). The MSKCC calculator is based on the older and no longer utilised immunotherapies, IL2/IFN-α. The mechanism of action of systemic therapies are shown in Table 16.12 and Fig. 16.9.

Table 16.11 International Metastatic RCC Database Consortium (IMDC) criteria for predicting survival in patients with metastatic RCC [1]

IMDC criteria: Factors predicting poorer outcome include
• Less than one year from time of diagnosis to systemic therapy • Performance status <80% (Karnofsky performance status (KPS) scale) • Haemoglobin less than lower limit of normal • Calcium greater than upper limit of normal • Neutrophils greater than upper limit of normal • Platelets greater than upper limit of normal
Favourable risk: No prognostic factors **Intermediate risk: 1–2 prognostic factors** **Poor risk: 3 or more prognostic factors**

Table adapted from https://www.mdcalc.com/imdc-international-metastatic-rcc-database-consortium-risk-score-rcc

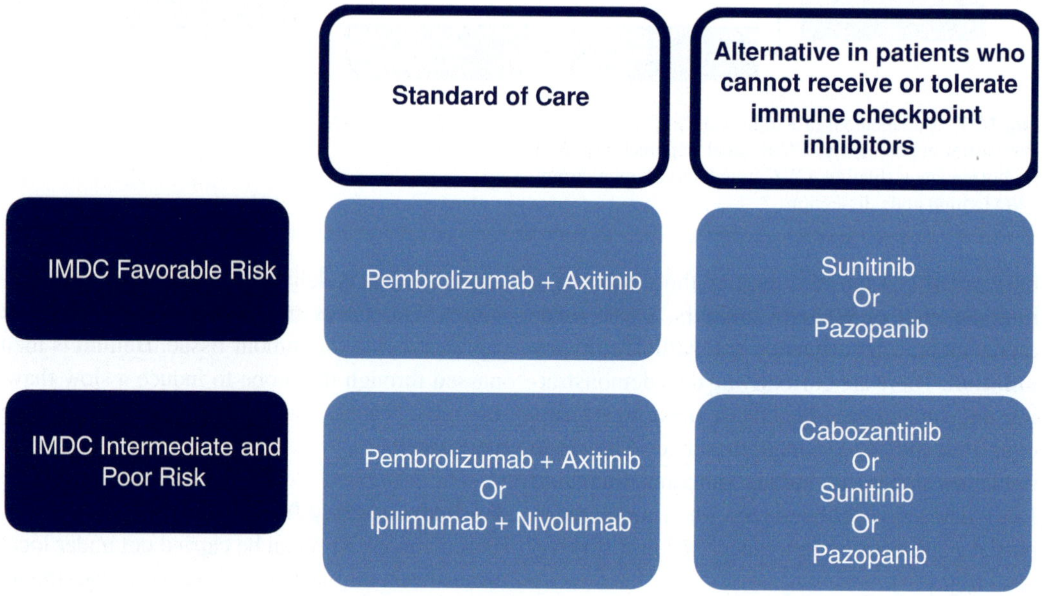

Fig. 16.8 Selection of therapy in metastatic kidney cancer (Adapted from EAU Guidelines [1])

Table 16.12 Systemic therapies used in the treatment of advanced kidney cancer

	Mechanism of Action	Agents
Targeted Therapies	Tyrosine kinase inhibitors	Sorafenib, sunitinib, pazopanib, axitinib, Lenvatinib, cavozantinib
	Monoclonal antibody against circulating VEGF	Bevacizumab
	mTOR inhibitors	Temsirolimus, everolimus
Immunotherapy	PD-1 inhibitors	Pembrolizumab, nivolumab
	PDL-1 inhibitors	Avelumab
	CTLA-4 inhibitors	Ipilimumab

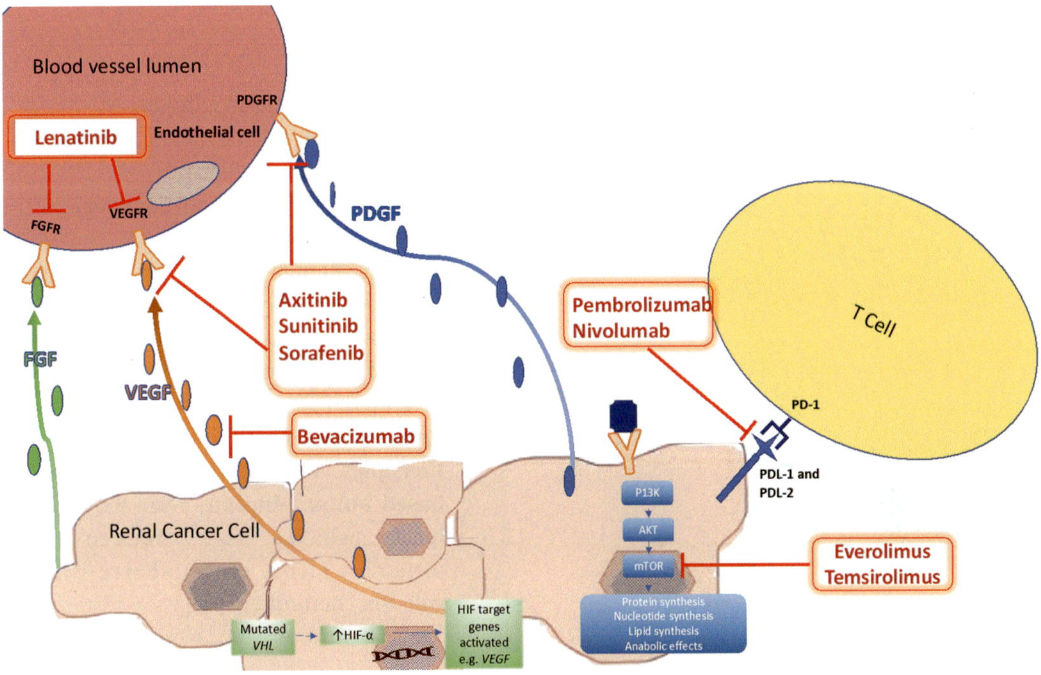

Fig. 16.9 Mechanism of action of targeted and immunological therapies
(*Adapted from Choueiri TK, Motzer RJ. Systemic Therapy for Metastatic Renal-Cell Carcinoma. N Engl J Med. 2017 Jan 26;376* (4)*:354–366* [9])
Hypoxia-inducible factor (HIF), VEGF (vascular endothelial growth factor) FGF (fibroblast growth factor), FGFR (FGF receptor), PDGF (platelet-derived growth factor), PDGFR (PDGF receptor) and VEGFR (VEGF receptor), mechanistic target of rapamycin (mTOR), MHC (major histocompatibility complex), PD-1 (programmed cell death protein) PD-L1 (PD-1 ligand, and PI3K (phosphatidylinositol 3-kinase)

Prognosis

The prognosis depends on stage of the kidney cancer as shown in Fig. 16.10

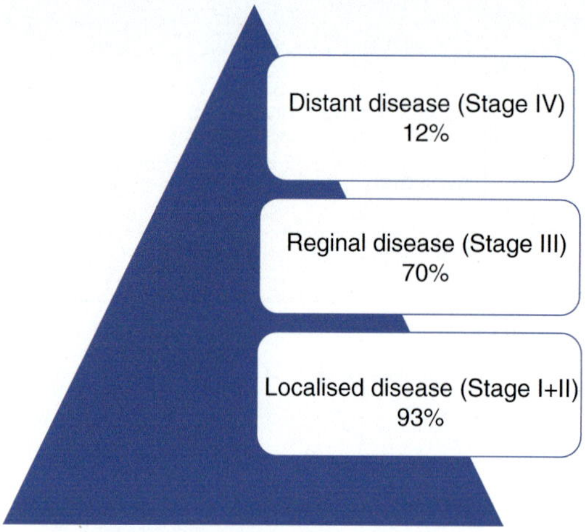

Fig. 16.10 Renal Cell Cancer 5 year percentage survival by stage [18]

Follow up

Surveillance following treatment aims to detect local recurrence or metastatic disease while the patient is still curable. Controversy exists regarding the optimal duration/intervals for follow up of patients who have completed treatment for RCC, and there is no existing evidence base to guide clinicians. The surveillance modality is guided by the individual patient's risk profile. Factors increasing risk include larger tumours (>7 cm), or when there is a positive surgical margin. Follow up following cryoablation or RFA may be more intensive due to the higher recurrence rate (Table 16.13).

Practice Points

1. **Imaging is key to diagnosis:** most renal masses can be diagnosed accurately by imaging alone
2. Surgery is the first line treatment for localised disease
3. Despite attempted curative treatment with nephrectomy (either partial or radical), approximately 30% of patients with ccRCC with localised disease will go onto develop metastases [15]
4. **Small molecule inhibitors, targeted therapies and immune checkpoint-based immunotherapy** form the treatment pathway for advanced or metastatic kidney cancer; **There is no role for chemotherapy** [1]

Table 16.13 Proposed Surveillance Schedule (Adapted from EAU Guidelines [1])

Risk Profile	Surveillance interval							
	3 mo	6 mo	12 mo	18 mo	24 mo	30 mo	36 mo	>3 year
Low	-	CT	-	CT	-	CT	-	CT every 2 years
Intermediate	-	CT	CT	-	CT		CT	CT yearly
High	CT	CT	CT	CT	CT	-	CT	CT yearly

(CT should be contrasted if possible, or appropriate imaging schedule agreed with radiologists)

Conclusions

The treatment of kidney cancer has evolved rapidly over the preceding two decades with the advent of targeted and immunotherapies. In future, these treatment modalities are likely to become more individualised with the use of genetic sequencing and biomarkers.

As we reflect on the 48-year-old gentleman with haematuria and two solid kidney lesions identified on CT imaging, whom we met at the start of this chapter, his case was discussed in a urological multidisciplinary meeting. On review of his imaging, the lesions were thought to be radiologically indeterminate: a needle core biopsy was performed on the left, which revealed an ISUP Grade 2 Papillary RCC. A left-sided laparoscopic radical nephrectomy was performed. Histology confirmed papillary RCC, stage T1a. Follow-up using a CT scan was planned 6 months post-operatively for surveillance of the contralateral mass. A fast rate of growth would prompt a biopsy and subsequent partial nephrectomy if this contralateral lesion was also found to be malignant.

Appendix 1

Table 16.14 Karnofsky Performance Status Score *(adapted from mdcalc.com/karnofsky-performance-status-scale)* [19]

Description	Points Assigned	Description
Normal no complaints; no evidence of disease	100	Able to carry on normal activity and to work; no special care needed
Able to carry on normal activity; minor signs or symptoms of disease	90	
Normal activity with effort; some signs or symptoms of disease	80	
Cares for self; unable to carry on normal activity or to do active work	70	Unable to work; able to live at home and care for most personal needs; varying amount of assistance needed.
Requires occasional assistance, but is able to care for most personal needs	60	
Required considerable assistance and frequent medical care	50	
Disabled; required special care and assistance	40	Unable to care for self; requires equivalent of institutional or hospital care; disease may be progressing rapidly.
Severely disabled; hospital admission is indicated although death not imminent	30	
Very sick; hospital admission necessary; active supportive treatment necessary	20	
Moribund; fatal processes progressing rapidly	10	
Dead	0	n/a

Adapted from: Karnofsky DA Burchenal JH. (1949). 'The Clinical Evaluation of Chemotherapeutic Agents in Cancer.' In: MacLeod CM (Ed), Evaluation of Chemotherapeutic Agents. Columbia Univ Press. Page 196

Questions

1. Which of the following is <u>not</u> a recognised risk factor for the development of kidney cancer?
   A. Smoking
   B. Obesity
   C. Asbestos exposure
   D. Alcohol
   E. Male sex

Answer: D

   A. **Incorrect**—Smoking is a well-established risk factor for kidney cancer.
   B. **Incorrect**—The risk of developing kidney cancer increases with BMI.
   C. **Incorrect**—Asbestos, along with other occupational exposures such as trichloroethylene, increase the risk of kidney cancer
   D. **Correct**—In fact, alcohol has been found to have a protective effect, whereby those who drink up 2 alcoholic drinks per day have a reduced risk of kidney cancer compared with non-drinkers. Alcohol intake is however associated with an increased risk of other diseases and cancers in other solid organs.
   E. **Incorrect**—Kidney cancer is twice as common in men compared to women.

2. As far as the presenting features of kidney cancer are concerned, which of the following statements is true?
   A. Haematuria, flank pain and a palpable abdominal mass is the recognised presenting triad for the majority of patients.
   B. More than half of patients present with a manifestation of a paraneoplastic syndrome rather than symptoms of the RCC itself.
   C. The majority of kidney cancers are diagnosed incidentally
   D. Varicoceles are a common presenting symptom in men.
   E. Absence of haematuria confers a more favourable prognosis**Answer: C**

   A. **Incorrect**—the classical triad of haematuria, flank pain and a palpable abdominal mass is seen in <10% of patients.
   B. **Incorrect**—Most patients are asymptomatic and diagnosed incidentally.
   C. **Correct**—Most kidney cancers are diagnosed incidentally through imaging for other reasons.
   D. **Incorrect**—Scrotal varicoceles are a rare sign of kidney cancer.
   E. **Incorrect**—Absence of haematuria alone does not necessarily confer a more favourable prognosis. However, where patients do present with the classical triad of haematuria, flank pain and a palpable abdominal mass, they are more likely to have locally advanced disease.

3. An 84 year old lady presents to the emergency department with abdominal pain and confusion. She has a known 3 cm lesion on the lower pole of the left kidney (Bosniak IIF) which is under active surveillance by her urologist. On admission her blood tests demonstrate the following: adjusted calcium 3.1 mmol/L, PTH 15 pmol/L, vitamin D 30 nmol/L, creatinine 80 μmol/L (eGFR 64 ml/min/1.73 m [2]). Her other blood tests are unremarkable. What is the most likely cause of her hypercalcaemia?
   A. Production of PTH related peptide
   B. Primary hyperparathyroidism
   C. Metastatic bone disease
   D. Vitamin D deficiency
   E. Secondary hyperparathyroidism.

Answer: B

   A. **Incorrect**—production of PTH related peptide would lead to hypercalcaemia which in turn would cause the PTH to be suppressed, rather than elevated which it is in this case. There is a specific laboratory test for PTHrP. Levels of PTHrP do not cause elevation in native PTH detection.
   B. **Correct**—This patient has primary hyperparathyroidism as evidenced by hypercalcaemia in the setting of a raised

PTH. Given the degree of hypercalcaemia the PTH should be low.
C. **Incorrect**—If the hypercalcaemia was a result of bone metastases, PTH would be suppressed rather than elevated.
D. **Incorrect**—Though the vitamin D is low, this is not responsible for the hypercalcaemia. Low vitamin D is more likely to cause hypocalcaemia.
E. **Incorrect**—Secondary hyperparathyroidism occurs in response to hypocalcaemia where the parathyroid glands hypertrophy and produce excess PTH, commonly seen in chronic kidney disease stage 3 and above.

4. An active 64 year old man with a background of hypertension undergoes a CT scan of the abdomen in his local emergency department after presenting with abdominal pain. He is found to have an 8 cm solid lesion in the upper pole of the right kidney which is staged as T2a N0 M0. Which of the following treatments would be most likely to be recommended?
A. Active surveillance
B. Radical nephrectomy with ipsilateral adrenalectomy
C. Partial nephrectomy
D. Radical nephrectomy
E. Radiofrequency ablation

Answer: C

A. **Incorrect**—Given this man's age and lack of significant co-morbidities, a definitive management strategy by way of partial nephrectomy would be recommended.
B. **Incorrect**—Firstly, partial nephrectomy is preferred over radical nephrectomy, secondly, adrenalectomy in only indicated where there is evidence of gland invasion.
C. **Correct**—Surgery is the management of choice for localised kidney cancer and partial nephrectomy is preferred where possible
D. **Incorrect**—Partial nephrectomy is the preferred option for localised tumours where surgically feasible .
E. **Incorrect**—Surgery would be the management of choice given the size of his tumour and the lack of contraindications to surgery.

5. A 94 year old lady with a background of CKD stage G4, ischaemic heart disease, previous stroke, heart failure with reduced ejection fraction and newly diagnosed Alzheimer's dementia is incidentally found to have an indeterminate 4 cm cystic mass in the right kidney (Bosniak III) Which of the following management options is most appropriate?
A. Renal tumour biopsy
B. Active surveillance
C. Radiofrequency ablation
D. Partial nephrectomy
E. Watchful waiting**Answer: E**

A. **Incorrect**—though the cystic mass is indeterminate, which is an indication for biopsy, the guidelines are clear that renal tumour biopsy should only be undertaken where it is likely to change management. Given this patient's age and co-morbidities she is unlikely to be a candidate for surgical treatment, regardless of the biopsy findings.
B. **Incorrect**—Active surveillance would involve 6 monthly assessment and imaging for 2 years and annual follow up thereafter. Even if the kidney lesion was found to have grown in size, this lady would not be candidate for treatment.
C. **Incorrect**—Given her co-morbidities and age she is not fit for RFA.
D. **Incorrect**—Given her co-morbidities and age she is not fit for surgery.
E. **Correct**—Watchful waiting differs from active surveillance in that no routine re-imaging or regular assessment is requirement. Given this patient's extensive co-morbidities this would be the most appropriate option.

6. A 64 year old male is found to have an isolated enhancing 3 cm solid kidney mass on CT imaging with no evidence of lymph node involvement or metastatic spread. You are

referring to the urology registrar on the telephone, who wants to know what stage his cancer appears to be.

A. T1a; N0; M0
B. T2b; N1; M0
C. T3; N0; M1
D. T4; N1; M1
E. T1b; N0; M0

Answer: A

A. **Correct**—the isolated enhancing solid kidney mass is <4 cm diameter and is limited to the kidney
B. **Incorrect**—the isolated enhancing solid kidney mass is <4 cm diameter and is limited to the kidney
C. **Incorrect**—the isolated enhancing solid kidney mass is <4 cm diameter and is limited to the kidney
D. **Incorrect**—the isolated enhancing solid kidney mass is <4 cm diameter and is limited to the kidney
E. **Incorrect**—the isolated enhancing solid kidney mass is <4 cm diameter and is limited to the kidney

7. A 48 year old female of normal intellect and no other comorbidity is found to have a cystic lesion on her right kidney—of around 3 cm in diameter. What is the most appropriate next investigation?

A. Contrast enhanced CT
B. Contrast enhanced MRI
C. Non-contrast CT
D. Biopsy of the renal lesion
E. MAG-3 scan

Answer: B

A. **Incorrect**—a contrast-enhanced CT or MRI is advocated, with a preference for MRI in cystic lesions, where MRI has a higher sensitivity and specificity for small cystic renal masses and tumour thrombi.
B. **Correct**—a contrast-enhanced CT or MRI is advocated, with a preference for MRI in cystic lesions, where MRI has a higher sensitivity and specificity for small cystic renal masses and tumour thrombi.
C. **Incorrect**—a contrast-enhanced CT or MRI is advocated, with a preference for MRI in cystic lesions, where MRI has a higher sensitivity and specificity for small cystic renal masses and tumour thrombi. The most important criterion for differentiating malignant lesions is the presence of enhancement so the use of contrast is essential.
D. **Incorrect**—a contrast-enhanced CT or MRI is advocated, with a preference for MRI in cystic lesions, where MRI has a higher sensitivity and specificity for small cystic renal masses and tumour thrombi. Most lesions can be diagnosed on the basis of imaging alone, avoiding the need for an unnecessary invasive procedure.
E. **Incorrect**—a contrast-enhanced CT or MRI is advocated, with a preference for MRI in cystic lesions, where MRI has a higher sensitivity and specificity for small cystic renal masses and tumour thrombi. MAG-3 will give functional information about both kidneys only.

8. A fit, independent 72 year old gentleman has a successful laparoscopic partial left nephrectomy for stage T1a N0 M0 renal cell cancer, with clear tumour margins on resection. His serum creatinine at one month post-procedure is 94 μmol/L (1.06 mg/dL). How should he be followed up?

A. Discharge from follow-up
B. Non-contrast CT at 1 year
C. Non-contrast MRI at 3 months
D. Ultrasound at 6 months
E. Contrasted CT at 6 months

Answer: E

A. **Incorrect**—Whilst this gentleman's 5 year survival with localised stage I disease is around 93%, there is still a significant risk of developing recurrence or metastases of up to 30%
B. **Incorrect**—Non-contrast CT is not appropriate to follow up this patient with normal renal function.
C. **Incorrect**—Non-contrast MRI is not optimal to follow up this patient with

normal renal function. Furthermore, imaging within 3 months is only indicated for patients with a high recurrence risk. The history does not suggest that he falls into this category so repeat imaging within 6 months would be sufficient.
D. **Incorrect**—Ultrasound is of insufficient sensitivity to detect metastatic spread.
E. **Correct**—Contrasted CT of the chest and abdomen is the recommended follow up modality for low-risk localised disease post partial nephrectomy with curative intent

9. A 58 year old female with CKD stage G4 secondary to diabetes mellitus, with concomitant ischaemic heart disease is found to have an incidental 2 cm solid kidney lesion on ultrasound, which is confirmed on CT imaging, with no nodal involvement or metastases. She had a non-ST elevation myocardial infarction 3 months ago. What is the most appropriate management for her?
   A. Immediate partial nephrectomy
   B. Urgent radical nephrectomy
   C. Watchful waiting
   D. Active Surveillance
   E. Start Pembrolizumab and Axitinib

Answer: D

A. **Incorrect**—This lady's recent myocardial event makes immediate surgery risky. Given her localised disease and comorbidity, active surveillance would be more appropriate to allow her medical condition to stabilise, with consideration of definitive surgical therapy in the form of partial nephrectomy or ablative therapy—if appropriate—at a later stage.
B. **Incorrect**—This lady's recent myocardial event makes immediate surgery risky. Given her localised disease and comorbidity, active surveillance would be more appropriate to allow her medical condition to stabilise, with consideration of definitive surgical therapy in the form of partial nephrectomy or ablative therapy—if appropriate—at a later stage.
C. **Incorrect**—Watchful waiting is reserved for patients who are not candidates for active treatment and who therefore do not require follow up imaging. In this case, active surveillance with regular imaging is more appropriate as this patient would be a surgical candidate if her lesion was found to have grown rapidly in size or metastasised.
D. **Correct**—This lady's recent myocardial event makes immediate surgery risky. Given her localised disease and comorbidity, active surveillance is the most appropriate option to allow her medical condition to stabilise, with consideration of definitive surgical therapy in the form of partial nephrectomy or ablative therapy—if appropriate—at a later stage.
E. **Incorrect**—This lady's recent myocardial event makes immediate surgery risky. Given her localised disease and comorbidity, active surveillance would be more appropriate to allow her medical condition to stabilise, with consideration of definitive surgical therapy in the form of partial nephrectomy or ablative therapy—if appropriate—at a later stage. There is no evidence of metastatic spread to warrant systemic therapy.

10. A 45 year old female primary school teacher has been found to have T2aN1M1 renal cell cancer on a delayed follow-up scan, having elected for active surveillance 18 months ago. She has CKD stage G3a (serum creatinine 148 μmol/L (1.67 mg/dL)—eGFR 50 ml/min/1.73 m [2]). All full blood count parameters remain in the normal range, as does her serum calcium level. She otherwise remains well, having prospectively arranged cover for her class to attend the renal clinic with you to follow up her scan results. You rightly refer for her case for consideration urgently in the Uro-Oncology MDT meeting. What is the most likely management for her current disease?

A. Urgent partial nephrectomy
B. Urgent radical nephrectomy and metastasectomy
C. Watchful waiting
D. Active Surveillance
E. Consideration for cytoreductive nephrectomy, metastasectomy and consideration of first line systemic therapy with Pembrolizumab and Axitinib

Answer: E

A. **Incorrect**—This lady has new metastatic renal cell cancer, which warrants cytoreductive nephrectomy, metastasectomy and consideration of first line systemic therapy with Pembrolizumab and Axitinib, since partial nephrectomy alone will not be sufficient to fully treat her disease
B. **Incorrect**—This lady has new metastatic renal cell cancer, which warrants cytoreductive nephrectomy, metastasectomy and consideration of first line systemic therapy with Pembrolizumab and Axitinib, since radical nephrectomy and metastasectomy alone are unlikely to fully treat her disease
C. **Incorrect**—This lady has new metastatic renal cell cancer, which warrants cytoreductive nephrectomy, metastasectomy and consideration of first line systemic therapy with Pembrolizumab and Axitinib – watchful waiting would inevitably lead to further disease spread, and would not be the most appropriate line of management for a young, fit patient.
D. **Incorrect**—This lady has new metastatic renal cell cancer, following delayed re-imaging on active surveillance. Her current disease warrants consideration for cytoreductive nephrectomy, metastasectomy and first line systemic therapy with Pembrolizumab and Axitinib
E. **Correct**—This lady has new metastatic renal cell cancer, which warrants consideration of cytoreductive nephrectomy, metastasectomy and first line systemic therapy with Pembrolizumab and Axitinib

Test your learning and check your understanding of this book's contents: use the "Springer Nature Flashcards" app to access questions using https://sn.pub/cz9Cok. To use the app, please follow the instructions in Chap. 1.

References

1. European Association of Urology. Guidelines on Renal Cell Carcinoma. [Online] EAU Guidelines Office, Arnhem, The Netherlands; 2021. https://uroweb.org/guideline/renal-cell-carcinoma/. Accessed 5 July 2021.
2. Cancer Research UK. Kidney cancer: types and grades; 2020. https://www.cancerresearchuk.org/about-cancer/kidney-cancer/stages-types-grades/types-grades. Accessed 30 Nov 2020.
3. Caliò A, Warfel KA, Eble JN. Papillary adenomas and other small epithelial tumors in the kidney: an autopsy study. Am J Surg Pathol. 2019;43(2):277–87.
4. World Cancer Research Fund. Kidney cancer statistics; n.d. https://www.wcrf.org/dietandcancer/kidney-cancer-statistics/. Accessed 30 Nov 2020].
5. Cumberbatch MG, Rota M, Catto JW, et al. The role of tobacco smoke in bladder and kidney carcinogenesis: a comparison of exposures and meta-analysis of incidence and mortality risks. Eur Urol. 2016;70(3):458–66.
6. Hidayat K, Du X, Zou S, et al. Blood pressure and kidney cancer risk. J Hypertens. 2017;35(7):1333–44.
7. Wong G, Staplin N, Emberson J, et al. Chronic kidney disease and the risk of cancer: an individual patient data meta-analysis of 32,057 participants from six prospective studies. BMC Cancer 2016; 16(1).
8. Hajj P, Ferlicot S, Massoud W, Awad A, Hammoudi Y, Charpentier B, Durrbach A, Droupy S, Benoît G. Prevalence of renal cell carcinoma in patients with autosomal dominant polycystic kidney disease and chronic renal failure. Urology. 2009;74(3):631–4.
9. Choueiri TK, Motzer RJ. Systemic therapy for metastatic renal-cell carcinoma. N Engl J Med. 2017;376(4):354–66.
10. Marconi L, Dabestani S, Lam TB, Hofmann F, Stewart F, Norrie J, Bex A, Bensalah K, Canfield SE, Hora M, Kuczyk MA, Merseburger AS, Mulders PFA, Powles T, Staehler M, Ljungberg B, Volpe A. Systematic review and meta-analysis of diagnostic accuracy of percutaneous renal tumour biopsy. Eur Urol. 2016;69(4):660–73.
11. Kunath F, Schmidt S, Krabbe LM, Miernik A, Dahm P, Cleves A, Walther M, Kroeger N. Partial nephrectomy versus radical nephrectomy for clinical localised renal masses. Cochrane Database Syst Rev. 2017;5(5):CD012045.

12. Van Poppel H, Da Pozzo L, Albrecht W, Matveev V, Bono A, Borkowski A, Colombel M, Klotz L, Skinner E, Keane T, Marreaud S, Collette S, Sylvester R. A prospective, randomised EORTC intergroup phase 3 study comparing the oncologic outcome of elective nephron-sparing surgery and radical nephrectomy for low-stage renal cell carcinoma. Eur Urol. 2011;59(4):543–52.
13. Blom JH, van Poppel H, Marechal JM, Jacqmin D, Sylvester R, Schröder FH, de Prijck L. Radical nephrectomy with and without lymph node dissection: preliminary results of the EORTC randomized phase III protocol 30881. EORTC Genitourinary Group. Eur Urol. 1999;36(6):570–5.
14. Whitson JM, Harris CR, Reese AC, Meng MV. Lymphadenectomy improves survival of patients with renal cell carcinoma and nodal metastases. J Urol. 2011;185(5):1615–20.
15. Hsieh JJ, Purdue MP, Signoretti S, Swanton C, Albiges L, Schmidinger M, Heng DY, Larkin J, Ficarra V. Renal cell carcinoma. Nat Rev Dis Primers. 2017;3:17009.
16. Akdogan B, Gudeloglu A, Inci K, Gunay LM, Koni A, Ozen H. Prevalence and predictors of benign lesions in renal masses smaller than 7 cm presumed to be renal cell carcinoma. Clin Genitourin Cancer. 2012;10(2):121–5. https://doi.org/10.1016/j.clgc.2012.01.005. Epub 2012 Mar 7.
17. Pan XW, Cui XM, Huang H, Huang Y, Li L, Wang ZJ, Qu FJ, Gao Y, Cui XG, Xu DF. Radiofrequency ablation versus partial nephrectomy for treatment of renal masses: a systematic review and meta-analysis. Kaohsiung J Med Sci. 2015;31(12):649–58.
18. American Cancer Society. Survival Rates for Kidney Cancer; 2021. Available from: https://www.cancer.org/cancer/kidney-cancer/detection-diagnosis-staging/survival-rates.html. Accessed 2 June 2021.
19. Karnofsky DA. Burchenal JH. 'The Clinical evaluation of chemotherapeutic agents in cancer.' In: macLeod CM (Ed), Evaluation of chemotherapeutic agents. Columbia Univ Press. 1949. p. 196.

Hemodialysis in Clinical Practice

17

Mohamed Elewa and Sandip Mitra

Clinical Scenario

A 64 year old lady with end stage kidney disease secondary to polycystic kidney disease, is now anuric, and has been on treatment with **high flux hemodialysis** for 6 years using a dialysis catheter. She is on **conventional HD** 3.5 h three times week, achieving a **blood flow of 275 mL/min.** Hemodialysis treatment has been complicated by **predialysis hyperkalemia, frequent alarms of high venous pressures, streaky washbacks, high interdialytic weight gains and dialysis cramps.** She has an Arteriovenous (AV) fistula which has a **very short segment,** insufficient for cannulation with two needles. There have been unplanned **hospital admissions** with fluid overload, and an elective decompression procedure for **carpal tunnel syndrome**.

What factors need addressing to optimize this lady's dialysis prescription, and what other practical changes might help improve the quality of haemodialysis treatment that she receives?

M. Elewa
Manchester University Hospitals NHS Foundation Trust, Manchester, UK

Ain Shams University, Cairo, Egypt
e-mail: mohamed.elewa@mft.nhs.uk

S. Mitra (✉)
Manchester University Hospitals NHS Foundation Trust, Manchester, UK

Manchester Academy of Health Sciences Centre, University of Manchester, Manchester, UK
e-mail: sandip.mitra@mft.nhs.uk

Introduction

'Dialysis' is defined as *"The separation of particles in a liquid on the basis of differences in their ability to pass through a membrane"*. Clinically, the movement of substances between the blood and dialysis fluid compartment across an artificial semipermeable membrane for blood purification is hemodialysis. Thomas Graham, often dubbed the "Father of Dialysis", described the diffusion of liquids in 1854. His study of colloids and osmotic forces resulted in the ability to separate colloids and crystalloids, by a process termed "dialysis", which remains the basis for all long-term dialysis technology. That said, it wasn't until 1945, when Dr. Willem Kolff, from the University of Groningen successfully developed an artificial kidney to provide hemodialysis. Using restricted resources during the war, he developed a rotating drum kidney to treat a patient with Acute Kidney Failure. The patient recovered, and lived for another 6 years, ushering in an era of dialysis for sustaining lives despite kidney failure. Major technological and industrial advances over decades have ensured success of the therapy long term and established hemodialysis as a dominant treatment modality for patients with kidney failure across the globe.

D. Banerjee et al. (eds.), *Management of Kidney Diseases*,
https://doi.org/10.1007/978-3-031-09131-5_17

Basic Principles of Dialysis

Diffusion

...is the net movement of solutes from a region of higher concentration to a region of lower concentration driven by a gradient in concentration, on dialysis, across a semi-permeable membrane

This molecular movement is influenced by the size of the molecules of the solute (mass) relative to the size of the pores of the membrane. Depending on the shape or electrical charge of the membrane and the molecules, the rate of this movement across the membrane will be affected. Diffusive clearance of a dialyzer is measured by its K_oA or coefficient of mass transfer for urea. K_oA of a dialysis membrane depends on pore density, pore size distribution, and resistance to solute passage. Higher values indicate more efficient dialyzers [1].

Ultrafiltration

...is a type of membrane filtration in which forces, like hydrostatic pressure or concentration gradients (osmotic force) lead to solvent (e.g. water) moving across a semipermeable membrane

Suspended solutes of high molecular weight are retained in the so-called retentate, while the solvent and low molecular weight solutes can pass through the membrane in the permeate (filtrate). Transmembrane pressure (TMP) is the hydrostatic pressure gradient across the membrane. This is the driving force that causes ultrafiltration (UF), called hydrostatic UF. Alternatively, if ultrafiltration is induced by an osmotic force, created by a substance such as glucose or polymers, it is called osmotic UF.

Convection

"...is described as solvent drag: if a pressure gradient exists between the two sides of a semi-permeable (porous) membrane, when the molecular dimensions of a solute are such that passage through the membrane is possible, the solute is swept ("dragged") across the membrane dissolved in ultra-filtered plasma water"

The Convection is necessary to transfer middle and large molecular solutes that do not transport readily by diffusion such as middle and larger solutes in uremia. The convective clearance is facilitated by permeable membranes and pore size distribution of the membrane. Convective properties of a dialyzer are indicated by its K_{UF} (coefficient of ultrafiltration). K_{UF} refers to the permeability of the membrane to water or 'leakiness' of a membrane. A dialyzer and with K_{UF} >20 mL/h/mmHg is known as high flux dialyzer. Sieving coefficient of a solute indicates the ease with which it can be removed by convection [2].

Clearance

Solute removal is measured in terms of clearance. Dialyzer clearance is "the volume of plasma, from which a given substance has been removed completely in a given time period". Urea is considered a surrogate marker for uremic toxins, and has been used for measurement of dialysis efficiency. Urea transport is flow limited, both within the body and in the extracorporeal system. Within the body, urea easily crosses the cell membrane (between the erythrocyte component and the water component of blood), and with high-efficiency dialyzers, with high mass transfer area coefficient K_0A such that extracorporeal clearance is essentially limited by extracorporeal blood (Qb) and dialysate flow rates (Qd). Thus, the major determinants affecting in vivo urea clearance in hemodialysis are Blood flow rate (Qb), dialysate flow rate (Qd) and dialyser membrane characteristics [3].

Components of the Haemodialysis Machine and Extracorporeal Blood Circuit

Extracorporeal Blood Circuit (ECC)

A closed extracorporeal system starts from the vascular access, and ensures that the blood is delivered to the dialyzer and safely back to the

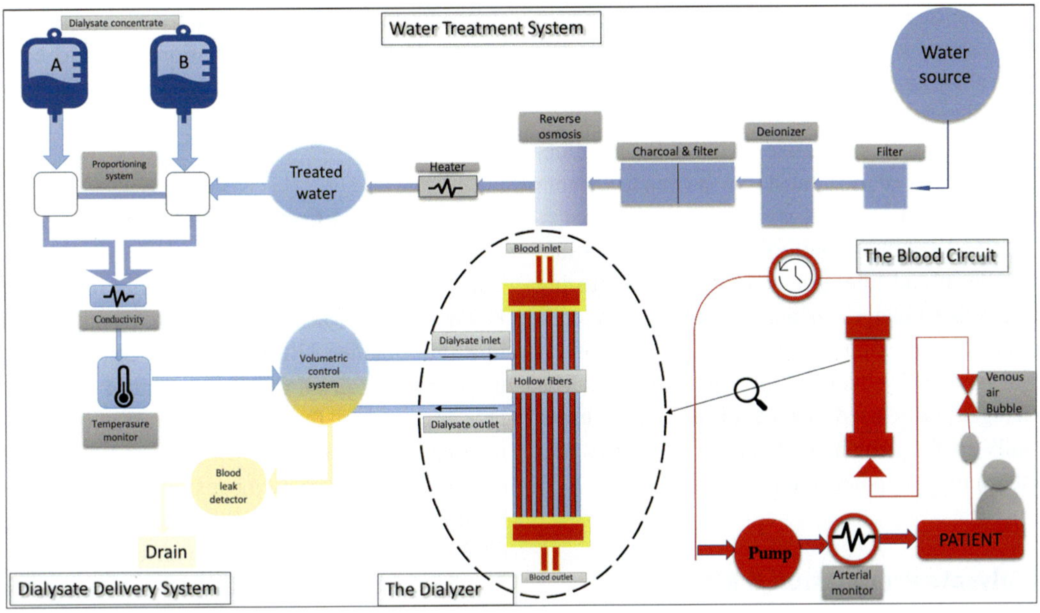

Fig. 17.1 Key Components of Hemodialysis Treatment. Diagram illustrating four key components of haemodialysis treatment: the blood circuit, the dialyser and dialysate delivery system, and the water treatment system

patient. ECC is comprised of a pre-dialyzer limb (arterial) and a post-dialyzer limb (venous). These are manufactured from inert, biocompatible and sterilized materials. A blood pump propels the blood through the tubing system using negative pressure. The commonest blood pump design is the roller design; rotator rollers compress the blood in the tubing system and sweep the blood towards the dialyzer. The pump speed is displayed on the machine as Qb (mL/min), and this can be adjusted, with ranges of up to 500 mL/min. This is automatically calculated from the number of pump revolutions per minute, and the volume of the blood in the tubing system within the pump. It is important to note that the calculated Qb could be higher than the actual blood flow rate. This is due to a negative pressure exerted by the pump on the tubing system to propel the blood. A more accurate measurement is the Effective Blood Flow Rate (EBFR), or corrected Qb for the measured "arterial pressure". After the blood passes through the dialyzer, the blood then moves towards the "venous side" of the circuit, eventually returning back to the patient via the AV access. The tubing design which has integrated blood chambers and drips, ensures monitoring and safety. These chambers are fitted in the dialysis machine so that pressure changes, or air can be detected, and when detected the blood pump would stop, a clamp secures the venous line to prevent blood return, and the alarm sound is activated [4] (Fig. 17.1).

Pressures in the tubing of the ECC is detected by transducer devices inside the machine which convert the pressure changes into electronic signals. Transducer protector act as barrier between the blood in tube and transducer in the machine. If these protector filters are wet, they prevent airflow and need to be changed immediately after inspection. The ECC pressures are dependent of the blood flow rate and resistance to flow across the tubing and at the access sites. Pressure changes will trigger an alarm when it exceeds the set limits of tolerance in the machine.

The arterial pump effect is measured as the "arterial pressure", which is a negative value. At pressures −150 mmHg or lower, EBFR deviates significantly from calculated Qb and can lead to loss of treatment efficiency. Excessive negative pressures may indicate poor arterial inflow, likely due to problematic vascular access. This must be addressed to ensure adequate blood flow. High Venous pressures (VP) are caused by an obstruction distal to the point, kinks in lines or access stenosis. Low VP caused by poor arterial flow, or wet venous isolator. A dislodged venous needle may not trigger a venous alarm, hence vigilance and adherence to taping policy with a risk mitigation strategy is imperative to avoid exsanguination. Venous alarms must not be reset without visual inspection of access site.

Blood volume monitors are sensors built into specific blood lines for noninvasive monitoring of relative changes in plasma volumes by continuously tracking changes in hematocrit or plasma density induced by ultrafiltration. The changes can be used to guide ultrafiltration, especially in frequent hemodynamic instability and intradialytic hypotension [4].

Dialysate Preparation & Monitoring

The purpose of the dialysis circuit or the fluid pathway within the machine is to prepare the dialysate by adding acid concentrate and alkaline buffer to treated water, and deliver it to the dialyzer at a predetermined rate. It is also designed to ensure the dialysate has the appropriate composition, temperature, and pH through a series of monitors and detectors along the dialysate delivery system. Finally, the discarded dialysate is drained along with the excess fluid removed from the patient through ultrafiltration.

The treated water is initially delivered to the dialysis machine, deaerated and warmed, and moved to the proportioning system. The dialysate is prepared here by combining water with specific portions of acid concentrate (comprising of acetate or citrate with chloride salts of sodium, potassium, calcium, magnesium and glucose) and bicarbonate buffer solution or powder to produce a physiological solution (final dialysate) which is fed into the dialyser inlet to come in contact with blood across the semipermeable membrane. The table below describes the essential safety checks that are carried out in the prepared dialysate after proportioning and mixing and prior to it being fed into the dialyser at commencement of HD. The final concentration of electrolytes is generated by a process known as proportioning. Dialysate concentrate can be tailored to each patient's needs. The various combinations of fluid concentrations may be limited by local guidelines and availability (Table 17.1).

Ultrafiltration Control Systems

The goal of ultrafiltration apparatus inside the HD machine is to ensure precise removal of fluid in a safe manner. Ultrafiltration is controlled by the means of an ultrafiltration control unit, that gets input from the information provided pretreatment about desired UF volumes. The unit controls the UF rate by means of an UF pump. A balancing chamber within the machine (***Volumetric Device***) adjusts to ensure that dialysate flow to and from the dialyzer is balanced for accuracy. A ***Flow Control Device*** is an alternative method based on flow sensors on the inlet and outlet of the dialyser to achieve accuracy and balance. The advances in these systems have enabled large fluid volume shifts across high permeable dialysers with relative ease and accuracy.

Water Treatment Systems

For 4 h, thrice weekly standard hemodialysis sessions, an individual patient's blood comes in contact with at approximately 18,000 L of water per annum at a dialysate flow rate of 500 mL/min. This underpins the importance of high-quality standards, adequate water treatment systems, and its effective monitoring in order to ensure patient safety. The water purification systems in use are Reverse Osmosis (R/O) or Deionizer (D/I) systems. The water is "pre-treated" by passing through a series of filters: sediment filter, softener, a carbon filter, and micro-filters. Each of these acts to remove contaminants, sediments, and minerals. Local guidelines set recommended specification of water treatment systems and quality, along with the recommended frequency of monitoring of dialysis water. Ultrapure water is defined as water with a bacterial count below 0.1 colony-forming unit

Table 17.1 Safety measures in the Dialysate circuit

Safety Measure	Description	Effect
Dialysate temperature:	- The dialysis water is warmed inside the machine with the temperature control set by the user in units typically operating between 35.5-37°C.	- Lower dialysate temperature has been associated with lower risk of intradialytic hypotension. - The use of dialysate at lower temperatures (35.5-36°C) during dialysis proven to improve BP stability should be balanced against against patient tolerability. - High temperatures > 42° C can cause hemolysis, protein degeneration and instability.
Dialysate conductivity:	- Conductive potential of the fluid determined by positively charged ions of Na, Ca, K, Mg. The conductivity measures the rate of flow of an electric current to verify the concentration of salts in the solution. Maintained between 12-16 mS/cm.	- Fluid ionic composition changes will trigger alarm. - An empty concentrate jug towards end of dialysis a common cause of low conductivity. - Unsafe dialysate will be automatically discarded. - After necessary corrections the alarm would reset itself.
Dialysate pH:	- Dialysate pH recommended 6.8-7.6 and checked prior to entry to a dialyser inlet	- Extremes pH lead to oxidative stress and hemolysis
Blood leak in dialysate detector	- Photoelectric sensor located downstream of the dialyzer outlet, can detect presence of red cells and trigger an alarm	- Persistent blood leak alarm requires cessation of treatment, discard lines and dialyser without washback

(CFU)/mL and endotoxin below 0.03 endotoxin unit (EU)/mL and is recommended for use in hemodiafiltration. This is made feasible by additional highly reliable endotoxin adsorption filters in the dialysate fluid pathway within the machine.

Dialyser Membranes and its Performance

The blood is propelled from the "arterial" side of the circuit towards the hemodialyzer, where the dialysis process, an exchange of molecules occurs across the dialyser semipermeable membrane, can take place. Most dialyzers available today are designed as rigid cylinders, packed with membrane material configured in the form of capillary fibres (Hollow Fibre design).

Membranes are either synthetic or non-synthetic. Non-synthetic membranes are derived from natural materials, they are less biocompatible. Biocompatibility can be improved by substituting hydroxyl groups, which reduces the ability of cellulose membranes to activate complement and cause leukopenia. Synthetic membranes are more biocompatible and have higher permeability. Some examples of membrane materials commonly in clinical use include polysulfone, polyethersulfone, cellulose triacetate, polyacrylonitrile, polycarbonate, and polymethylmethacrylate.

The primary mode of removal of small solutes is diffusion. The rate of diffusion of a solute is dependent on thickness of the membrane, pore sizes and shape, and diffusivity of the solute. This is expressed as K_0A, and is an *in-vitro* measurement provided in specification by manufacturers. High-efficiency dialyzers can achieve greater urea clearances than low flux dialysers at comparable blood flow rates.

The main mode of removal of large solutes, on the other hand, is convection. The ability of a larger solute to pass through the pores of a membrane is expressed as the sieving coefficient of the membrane for a given solute. Dialyzer manufacturers provide sieving coefficients of albumin, B12, beta-2 microglobulin and others, as a measure of convective performance.

The ultrafiltration coefficient (K_{UF}) is a measure of the water permeability of a membrane, and values above 20 mL/h/mmHg indicate high flux dialyzers which can readily move large volumes of fluid at low transmembrane pressure gradients. A dialyzer with higher K_{UF} will typically have higher diffusive and sieving coefficient values.

Majority of international guidelines recommend the use of high flux, high efficiency dialyzers and Information about membrane properties is provided by manufacturers. For intensive care units, small surface area dialyzers may be preferred in acute kidney injury with severe uremia to prevent dialysis disequilibrium syndrome, whilst large surface area dialyzers are indicated in the treatment of poisoning, drug overdose and toxicity [1].

Hemodialysis Techniques

Three principle hemodialysis techniques are used in clinical practice (Table 17.2).

Hemodiafiltration may be considered as a treatment for intra-dialytic hypotension refractory to other measures, and for dialysis patients with favorable prognosis who are unable or unlikely to be transplanted. There has been a growth in the use of HDF as a treatment modality and is recommended for consideration for Incentre and satellite hemodialysis by NICE, UK (2019). Further evidence generating studies in HDF are ongoing [5].

Table 17.2 Hemodialysis Techniques *(Mitra & Elewa 2021)*

Haemodialysis Technique	Description
Conventional Hemodialysis (Low Flux or High Flux Membrane)	• The setup allows blood flow into a dialyser compartment, and the dialysate flow in the other compartment, in opposing direction to maximize solute movement using a low or high flux dialyser acting as the interface membrane. High flux hemodialysis, predominantly a diffusive treatment combined with limited volumes of convective clearances.
Hemodiafiltration (with an additional HDF pump and reinfusion)	• Hemodiafiltration (HDF), combines both diffusive and high dose convective therapy. • Newer technology has enabled ultrapure replacement solution to be generated and delivered by the device (on-line HDF), allowing higher convective volumes and easier delivery of this therapy to patients. • A large convective volume creates a solute drag for middle and large middle molecules, the convective volume replaced by reinfusion of online generated substitution fluid or using packaged solutions by a separate HDF pump for reinfusion. • The volume control is achieved by balancing the rate of fluid replacement using precise volumetric devices with in the machine.
Expanded Hemodialysis (Using a dedicated membrane)	• Expanded HD (HDX) define a treatment where diffusion and convection are technically integrated inside a hollow-fiber dialyzer equipped with a medium cut-off membrane (MCO) without the need for substitution fluid. • The MCO Dialyzer, through its innovative design, combines the functional features of enhanced permeability, increased selectivity, controlled retention, and improved internal filtration into a single dialyzer, enabling removal of small, conventional middle molecules and large middle molecular uremic toxins without the need for additional pump or reinfusion fluid.

Prescribing Hemodialysis

Standard Prescription

Practice Point 1

The standard hemodialysis prescription should include:

- Dialyzer (material, surface area, flux)
- Modality (e.g., HFD, HDF predilution, HDF post dilution)
- Dialysate concentrate composition.
- Dialysate flow rate
- Dialysate temperature, Conductivity, Bicarbonate
- Blood flow rate
- Ultrafiltration volume and rate
- Treatment Time
- Access Connection: Needle gauze, Connection (SNHD, reverse) Catheter Locks
- Anticoagulation (anticoagulant, coagulopathy, monitoring)
- Medications to be administered.
- Specific blood tests or monitoring required.
- Special Instruction for Nurses (Access issues, Post HD instructions)
- Any limitations to be considered e.g., timing, logistical constraints, preferences

The prescription of dialysis should take into account patient characteristics such as predialysis clinical observations such as blood pressure, temperature and oxygen saturation, new onset symptoms, glycemic and electrolyte status. Particular attention to predictable rapid changes in weight as a result of illnesses or recent hospitalization would improve accuracy of the ultrafiltration prescription. All these factors enable the clinical staff to individualize the treatment to changes in patient health status.

Anticoagulation in Haemodialysis

As the blood moves through the extracorporeal circuit, it is exposed to surfaces of varying thrombogenicity. Anticoagulation is therefore essential to prevent the formation of microthrombi, or blood coagulation which can result in circuit loss. The formation of microthrombi in the dialyzer causes partial clotting of the membrane pores, reducing the effective membrane surface area, reducing dialysis efficacy.

Clinical practice guidelines on anticoagulation in hemodialysis published by professional societies are provides the best practice guidance. Practice should be defined by Unit Protocol along with instructions for reversing anticoagulation as required. The use of either unfractionated heparin, or low molecular weight heparin is the mainstay in HD. Regional citrate recommended in situations with high bleeding requires expertise and is rarely practiced in chronic HD. Use of high blood flow rates with frequent saline flushes could reduce anticoagulation requirement significantly particularly for shorter duration sessions. In patients with HIT (heparin induced thrombocytopenia) danaparoid, direct thrombin inhibitors or regional citrate are recommended [6]. Systemic anticoagulation should be avoided in the presence of active bleeding. Minimal anticoagulation protocols must be applied in specific settings.

Practice Point 2

Signs of clotting in the extracorporeal circuit include:

- Raised venous pressure
- Reduced arterial pressure
- Raised trans membrane pressure (TMP)
- Visible signs of clotting, streaky dialyser

Acute Heparin Free/Minimal Anticoagulant Dialysis

In patients with acute trauma, clotting disorders, active bleeding, or in the immediate pre- or post-

Home Hemodialysis

Maintenance dialysis patients who receive in-center dialysis thrice weekly have to endure an extended 72-hr interdialytic gap during the weekend, which has been strongly linked with higher hospitalizations and increased risk of mortality. Avoidance of a long gap through an alternate day dialysis schedule or extended dialysis regimen of more frequent dialysis, or intensive HD, can most feasibly be delivered in the Home setting. The avoidance of regular trips to hospital for dialysis may also be advantageous for convenience and lifestyle reasons. The adaptive dialysis regimen at home often allows patients more liberty with dietary and fluid restrictions positively impacting on quality of life.

Poor prognosis outcome indicators such as high interdialytic fluid gains, refractory hypertension, hemodynamic instability and severe hyperphosphatemia can be more effectively managed through extended dialysis in the home setting. Home HD also alleviates strain on available capacity and workforce benefitting the provider and the health system overall. It is therefore a key recommendation with a call to action to offer the choice of Home HD to Incentre Dialysis patients.

The key barriers to a successful home HD transition are available space at home, needle phobia, lack of support at home and treatment burden. Barriers can be overcome with specific clinical strategies e.g., use of blunt needles for Button-Hole cannulation to overcome needle phobia where clinically appropriate.

A successful Home program is driven by a dedicated patient training program, a robust home support system and clinical leadership from the multidisciplinary team members.

Several HD modalities (Table 17.3) may be offered in the home setting to fit in with patient preferences and lifestyle but each will require adjustments to prescription accordingly. For example, in comparison to a Incentre session, a Nocturnal dialysis session with longer hours, will require lower blood flow rates, more anticoagulation to avoid circuit loss, dialysate settings suitable for longer hours, and specific interventions such as appropriate supplementation of water-soluble vitamins and where necessary, dialysate phosphate supplementation for hypophosphatemia [11].

Buttonhole Cannulation

Practice Point 4

The advantages and disadvantages of buttonhole cannulation

Advantages:

- Helpful in needle-phobic patients
- Reduce cannulation attempts
- Reduce aneurysms & aneurysm size
- May be less painful
- Helpful when a narrow segment available to needle
- Fewer hematomas

Disadvantages:

- Association with higher infection rate
- May require re-siting

Haemodialysis Governance and Quality Assurance

Treatment safety in HD is a broad concept and entails not only preventing clinical and mechanical complications during treatment, but also ensuring patient and staff safety, robust infection control measures, and continued quality assurance. This requires a multidisciplinary team in order to cover the various aspects of dialysis care. Errors in HD can cause harm and fatality. Although an in-center dialysis facility is a health care provider; management of dialysis unit encompasses a lot more than just dialysis provision.

The Medical Director is primarily responsible for the quality assessment and performance improvement programs within the facility. An administrator is responsible for fiscal management, staff training and coverage. Physicians, Nurse in charge, Nursing staff, Support workers, Technicians, Dietitian, and Social worker comprise a multidisciplinary team within a facility, working together to improve system process and clinical outcomes through quality assurance. Attention should also be paid to the physical

Table 17.3 Different Modalities for Home HD [12]

Modality	Prescription parameters	Key Points
Short Daily HD (SDHD)	2-3 hours, 5-7x/week Bicarbonate mmol/l 32-36 Qb ml/min 350-400 Qd ml/min 300-600	• RCT evidence of benefit (FHN Study) • Can be accommodated in the day for patients who work. • Effective in high fluid gains and heart failure • Fluid gain between treatments is less; however, with shorter treatment times, UF rate per hour may be too high • Greater use of consumables & storage requirements
Nocturnal HD (NHD)	6-8 hours, 4-6x/week including alternate nights. Bicarbonate mmol/l 28-35 Qb ml/min 200-300 Qd ml/min 300-400	• Keeps patients free during the day, allows for more liberal diet • Enhanced phosphate and middle molecule removal • Phosphate supplementation may be required in 20 % • Can disrupt sleep and patients may fear needle dislodgement. • Greater loss of water -soluble vitamins. Routine replacement of vitamins C, B and folic acid recommended.
Alternate daytime HD (ADHD)	4-6 hours, alternate days Bicarbonate mmol/l 28-35 Qb ml/min 300-400 Qd ml/min 300-600	• Avoid long interdialytic gap, allows dialysis free days in the week • Most popular regimen with HHD patients • Minimal increase in consumables • Lack of published research in this modality
Conventional HD	4-5 hours, 3/week Bicarbonate mmol/l 32-36 Qb ml/min 300-400 Qd ml/min 500-800	• Often used in those who do not wish to consider more frequent schedules • Compared with in-centre HD may have an added benefit associated with patients performing their own treatment at home • More flexibility with timings compared in-centre HD, saved travel time • Excellent initial regimen for units new to home HD while experience is gained
Hemodiafiltration at Home	Conv, SDHD, ADHD, NHD Prescription Identical to	• Can be performed with ultrapure water • Enhanced larger middle molecule clearance. • High convective volumes associated with clinical outcome benefits may be more readily achieved
Low Flow Dialysate HD systems (20-60 L dialysate per treatment)	SDHD or NHD or Alt day Lactate mmol/l 40-45 Qb ml/min 300-500 Qd ml/min 90-300 (NHD) 80-160 (SDHD)	• No comparative study between high and low flow dialysate HD systems • Can achieve similar Kt/V with extended time and frequency. • Not suitable for thrice weekly schedule • Portability options-an advantage for some patients

environment such as equipment standards, fire safety, patient care settings, water quality, and infection control measures. Several standard and quality metrics are being used to report quality and performance improvement. These are either Process metrics (such as targets for dialysis adequacy, vascular access, hemoglobin, infection rates, immunizations) or Outcome measures (mortality, hospitalization, transplant rates, quality adjusted life years and patient experience). An embedded facility culture of incident reporting of adverse events and "near misses" supported by Root Cause Analysis (RCA) is essential to good governance and safety for staff and patients [13, 14] (Fig. 17.2).

Practice Point 5

Common, potentially avoidable adverse events in HD facility [15]

- Needle dislodgements and catheter disconnection
- Hygiene lapses
- Access related blood stream infections
- Access infiltrations
- Medication errors
- Errors at Care transitions
- Patient falls
- Adverse clinical incidents with disasters (water failures, outage)

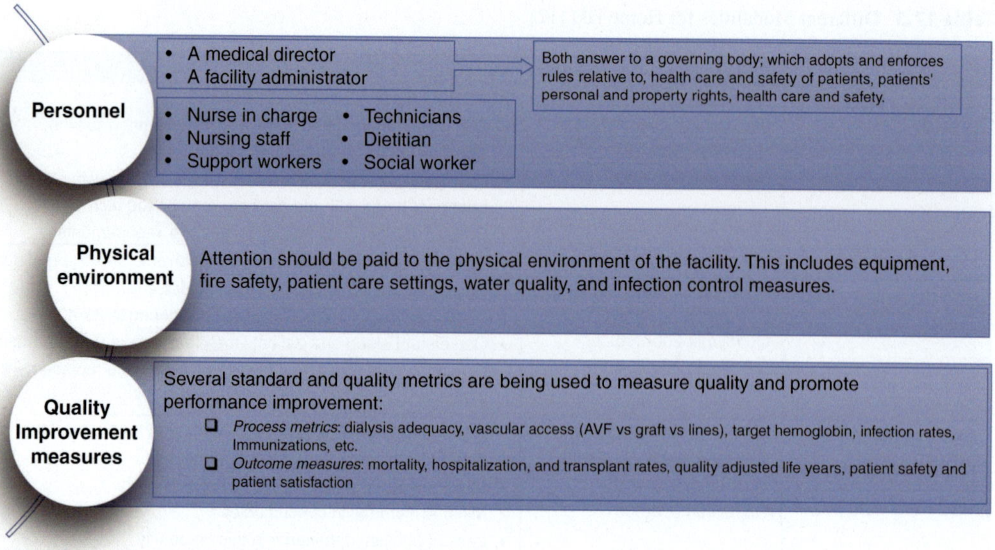

Fig. 17.2 Managing a Dialysis Facility. Diagram illustrates the elements recommended to manage a dialysis facility; divided into three domains: personnel, physical environment and quality improvement measures

Personalized Dialysis: Future and Emerging Opportunities

Research and innovation in biomaterials, sensors and engineering, provides the opportunity to potentially disrupt and advance technology in dialysis. There has been an intense focus on enhancing dialysis by creating miniaturized, portable, wearable and implantable devices to potentially improve both blood purification and patient experience. In modern devices, predictive algorithms allow adaptation in real time to allow biofeedback of ultrafiltration rate in response to changing blood volume parameters to improve hemodynamic and volume management. Applications of Artificial Intelligence (AI) in dialysis can further improve treatment safety, troubleshoot dialysis delivery, preemptive management and personalized treatment to promote good health in dialysis. AI algorithms may also address real time monitoring of vascular access and its patency.

Advanced technology must include assessments of care, enhanced monitoring, and enabling independence, efficiency and safety but also aim to reduce burden for staff and patients. Big data analytics can be applied both at an individual level and in programs to standardize and improve efficiency. Ultimately, precision dialysis therapy, will become more feasible as we better understand biological, behavioral and social determinants of good health in dialysis [16].

Conclusions

The 65 year old HD patient discussed at the beginning of the chapter highlights the importance of good dialysis practice and high quality blood purification. She is anuric and perhaps not receiving adequate blood purification for both small and middle molecules (e.g predialysis hyperkalemia and carpal tunnel syndrome). The dialytic clearance can be augmented by strict adherence to the dialysis prescription and HD prescription changes as discussed in this chapter. Prescription considerations should include higher blood flows, improved anticoagulation regimen and enhancing convective clearances, through increasing dialysis time or adding haemodiafiltration mode or expanded hemodialysis, if available. Reducing interdialytic weight gain and limiting the rate of ultrafiltration will improve fluid related complications. Button hole cannulation may be considered to allow use of short segment AVF, to achieve higher blood flows and mitigate against future catheter related complications. Extended dialysis, ideally in the home settting, could improve adherence, resolve many of the restrictions of incentre HD, and potentially improve cardiovascular outcomes.

Since its inception nearly six decades ago, Hemodialysis therapy for clinical use, has undergone a massive technological progress led by unprecedented engineering advances and entrepreneurship. Fundamentally, the current dialysis machine is not dissimilar to the early models set up by the forefathers of modern dialysis, and constitutes, a blood circuit, a dialyzer and the dialysate pathway with precise control systems to ensure safety. Further advances have led to increased safety, tolerability, and greater efficacy and flexibility of treatment. The efficacy of the treatment, however, is still critically reliant on a reliable access to the bloodstream and an effective anticoagulation regimen to maintain extracorporeal patency and blood flow.

Hemodialysis therapy remains one of the greatest technological inventions in modern medicine and the cornerstone therapy for sustaining human lives afflicted by kidney failure. The improvements in HD safety and technology have seen an unprecedented uptake and increase in HD prevalence. Further innovation is necessary to improve patient experience, outcomes and quality of life on dialysis.

Questions

1. The single most effective means of increasing diffusive clearance of small solutes during HD such as in Predialysis Hyperkalemia is:
   A. Increasing Dialysate flow rate
   B. Increase Dialyser Size
   C. Administer Insulin dextrose
   D. Increasing haemodialysis machine blood flow rate
   E. Increasing Time on dialysis

Correct answer (D)

2. The signs that indicate excessive clotting in circuit during treatment are:
   A. Raised venous pressure
   B. Reduced arterial pressure
   C. Raised trans membrane pressure (TMP)
   D. Visible signs of clotting, streaky dialyser
   E. Low dialysate conductivity

Correct answer (A, B, C, D)

3. Indicate which of these factors will not trigger alarms for High venous pressures
   A. Blood Circuit connection error
   B. AVF stenosis
   C. Kink in the blood tubing, returning limb
   D. Kink in blood tubing pre dialyser
   E. Occluded venous limb of dialysis catheter

Correct answer (A, D)

4. Disconnection haemorrhage from a catheter can be prevented by
   A. Keeping access site visible at all time during a treatment
   B. Adherence to a Safe Taping policy
   C. Optimum securement of the lines
   D. A robust HD governance structure
   E. Specific modules incorporated in staff competency training and assessment

Correct answer (A, B, C, D, E)

5. Which of these constitute good practice in Ultrafiltration?
   A. Limit Interdialytic weight gain to 3% body weight
   B. UF rate should vary between 10–20 mL/kg/h
   C. Empower patients with knowledge on fluid balance
   D. Reassess target weight on a monthly basis
   E. Use relative blood volume monitoring for unstable patients
   F. Use Iso UF regularly for fluid overload

Correct answer (A, C, D, E)

6. The following are some clinical features of middle molecule toxicity (Residual syndrome)
   A. Macroglossia
   B. Arthropathy
   C. Haemochromatosis

   D. Carpal Tunnel syndrome
   E. Neuropathy

Correct answer (A, B, D, E)

7. Convective clearances can be augmented in Haemodiafiltration by the following
   A. Switch from 15 g to 16 g needles for cannulation
   B. Use of higher surface area dialysers
   C. Adequate Anticoagulation
   D. Higher blood pump speeds
   E. Increased treatment time

Correct answer (B, C, D, E)

8. Expanded HD therapy delivers improved dialytic toxin clearances on middle and large middle molecules through the use of:
   A. Large surface area dialysers
   B. High pore density dialyser
   C. Homogenous dialyser pore size distribution
   D. Substitution fluid and additional pump
   E. HD machine special design and adaptation

Correct answer (B, C)

9. Advantages of Button-hole cannulation strategy for AVF include
   A. needling short AVF segments
   B. lower risk of infections
   C. addressing needle phobia
   D. requires skilled expertise and resiting
   E. use of sharp needles in a preformed track to alleviate pain

Correct answer (A, C)

10. The key clinical indications for recommending extended HD at Home are
   A. Persistent fluid overload and hypertension
   B. High interdialytic weight gain and ultrafiltration rate
   C. Dialysis via Catheter
   D. Uncontrolled anemia
   E. Severe LVH (increased LV mass)

Correct answer (A, B, E)

Test your learning and check your understanding of this book's contents: use the "Springer Nature Flashcards" app to access questions using https://sn.pub/cz9Cok. To use the app, please follow the instructions in Chap. 1.

References

1. Haroon S, Davenport A. Choosing a dialyzer: what clinicians need to know. Hemodial Int. 2018;22(S2):S65–74.
2. Khan MA, Hussain A. Hemodialysis membranes: a review. J Membr Sci Technol. 2019;9:199.
3. Eloot S, Schneditz D, Vanholder R. What can the dialysis physician learn from kinetic modelling beyond kt/v urea? Nephrol Dialysis Transpl. 2012;27(11):4021–9.
4. Mitra S, Mitsides N. Technical aspects of hemodialysis. Core concepts in dialysis and continuous therapies; 2016, pp. 15–26.
5. Canaud B, Busink E, Apel C, Bowry SK. Is there not sufficient evidence to show that haemodiafiltration is superior to conventional haemodialysis in treating end-stage kidney disease patients? Blood Purif. 2018;46(1):7–11.
6. Cronin RE, Reilly RF. Unfractionated heparin for hemodialysis: still the best option. In: Seminars in dialysis, vol. 23. Oxford: Blackwell Publishing Ltd.; 2010. p. 510–5, No. 5.
7. Assimon MM, Flythe JE. Rapid ultrafiltration rates and outcomes among hemodialysis patients: re-examining the evidence base. Curr Opin Nephrol Hypertens. 2015;24(6):525–30.
8. Vanholder R. Single needle hemodialysis: is the past the future? J Nephrol. 2020;33(1):49–58.
9. Upadhyay A. Dialyzer reuse: is it safe and worth it? Brazil J Nephrol. 2019;41(3):312–4.
10. Lowrie EG, Li Z, Ofsthun N, Lazarus JM. Reprocessing dialysers for multiple uses: recent analysis of death risks for patients. Nephrology Dialysis Transplantation. 2004;19(11):2823–30.
11. Young BA, Chan C, Blagg C, Lockridge R, Golper T, Finkelstein F, et al. How to overcome barriers and establish a successful home HD program. Clin J Am Soc Nephrol. 2012;7(12):2023–32.
12. Mitra S, Kharbanda K. Home haemodialysis and haemodiafiltration. IntechOpen; 2016.
13. Himmelfarb J, Kliger AS. End-stage renal disease measures of quality. Annu Rev Med. 2007;58:387–99.
14. Blankschaen SM, Saha S, Wish JB. Management of the hemodialysis unit: core curriculum 2016. Am J Kidney Dis. 2016;68(2):316–27.
15. Garrick R, Kliger A, Stefanchik B. Patient and facility safety in hemodialysis: opportunities and strategies to develop a culture of safety. Clin J Am Soc Nephrol. 2012;7(4):680–8.
16. Burlacu A, Iftene A, Jugrin D, Popa IV, Lupu PM, Vlad C, Covic A. Using artificial intelligence resources in dialysis and kidney transplant patients: a literature review. BioMed Res Int. 2020, 2020;

Complications of Haemodialysis

18

Oluwatoyin I. Ameh, Udeme E. Ekrikpo, Aminu K. Bello, and Ikechi G. Okpechi

Clinical Scenario

You are called to assess an unwell 67-year-old male with End Stage Kidney Disease (ESKD) secondary to hypertensive nephropathy on the haemodialysis unit. On initial assessment, he is dialysing via a native left brachiocephalic arteriovenous fistula: he is conscious, with a GCS of 15/15, but is pale, clammy and cool to touch. He has a blood pressure of 80/60 mmHg and a pulse of 115 beats per minute. His oxygen saturations are 98% on air. His blood glucose is 7 mmol/L; he has no concurrent chest pain, and his ECG shows a sinus tachycardia, with voltage criteria for left ventricular hypertrophy.

How would you manage this patient acutely, and what further information would help establish the cause of his presentation?

Introduction

Worldwide, haemodialysis (HD) is the commonest form of kidney replacement therapy (KRT), and can be associated with various complications related to uremia, vascular access, fluid and electrolyte management, as well as increased potential for bleeding due to use of anticoagulation. Progressive loss of kidney function leads to a uraemic state, associated with accumulation of fluid, acid-base disorders, multi-organ dysfunction, and retention of various solutes. Haemodialysis can be used to correct several of these abnormalities, but can cause problems related to technique, frequency or other pathophysiological processes occurring. For instance, repeated needling of a fistula can lead to aneurysmal dilatation, rupture and severe bleeding requiring transfusion, hospitalisation or death. Similarly, anaemia may be worsened by repeated blood loss due to clotting of the dialysis line. Although most HD complications occur acutely (e.g. seizures, febrile episodes, etc), others are insidious and take to develop and diagnose (e.g. dialysis-related dementia). In this chapter, we present an overview of common complications associated with HD with available treatment

O. I. Ameh
Division of Nephrology, Zenith Medical & Kidney Centre, Gudu, Abuja, Nigeria

U. E. Ekrikpo
Renal Unit, Department of Internal Medicine, University of Uyo, Uyo, Nigeria

A. K. Bello
Division of Nephrology and Immunology, Faculty of Medicine and Dentistry, University of Alberta, Edmonton, AB, Canada
e-mail: aminu1@ualberta.ca

I. G. Okpechi (✉)
Division of Nephrology and Immunology, Faculty of Medicine and Dentistry, University of Alberta, Edmonton, AB, Canada

Division of Nephrology and Hypertension, Kidney and Hypertension Research Unit, University of Cape Town, Cape Town, South Africa
e-mail: ikechi.okpechi@uct.ac.za

D. Banerjee et al. (eds.), *Management of Kidney Diseases*,
https://doi.org/10.1007/978-3-031-09131-5_18

options. Complications of continuous ambulatory peritoneal dialysis (CAPD) are discussed in a separate chapter.

Cardiovascular Complications of Haemodialysis

Intradialytic Hypotension

Definition of intradialytic Hypotension [1, 2]:

Intradialytic hypotension was defined by KDOQI in 2005 as a reduction in systolic blood pressure (SBP) ≥20 mmHg or a reduction in mean arterial pressure (MAP) by 10 mmHg with associated symptoms of cardiovascular (CV) compromise such as dizziness, nausea, vomiting, deep sighing or yawning [1]. More recently, KDIGO proposed in 2020 this be amended to "*Any symptomatic decrease in SBP or a nadir intradialytic BP <90 mmHg should prompt reassessment of BP and volume management* [2]"

Intradialytic hypotension is prevalent in between 15 and 50% of dialysis sessions, depending on the case definition criteria employed [2, 3]. Pathophysiologically, it is a maladaptive response to the acute and apparently fixed fluid (water) shifts that occur during a dialysis session i.e. a target ultrafiltration volume that has to be removed within a time constraint of usually 4 h. Normally in the setting of volume loss, cardiovascular and neurohormonal mechanisms are activated, including: increased heart rate and myocardial contractility, increased peripheral resistance and activation of the sympathetic nervous system and the renin angiotensin aldosterone system. These all promote plasma refilling, and thereby maintain intravascular volume and BP. With intradialytic hypotension however, certain procedure-related and/or patient-related factors lead to ineffectual responses with resulting hypotension (Fig. 18.1). Dialysis-related factors usually include dialysate composition (low sodium, low calcium), use of warm dialysate, acetate dialysate buffer, aggressive ultrafiltration, and low plasma osmolality. Large interdialytic weight gain, pre-dialysis use of antihypertensive medications, ingestion of meals during dialysis sessions (leading to significant splanchnic bed pooling of blood volume), hypoalbuminemia, pre-existing comorbidities (e.g. pericardial effusion, peripheral vascular disease, autonomic dysfunction in diabetic patients) are all examples of patient-related factors that are associated with intradialytic hypotension.

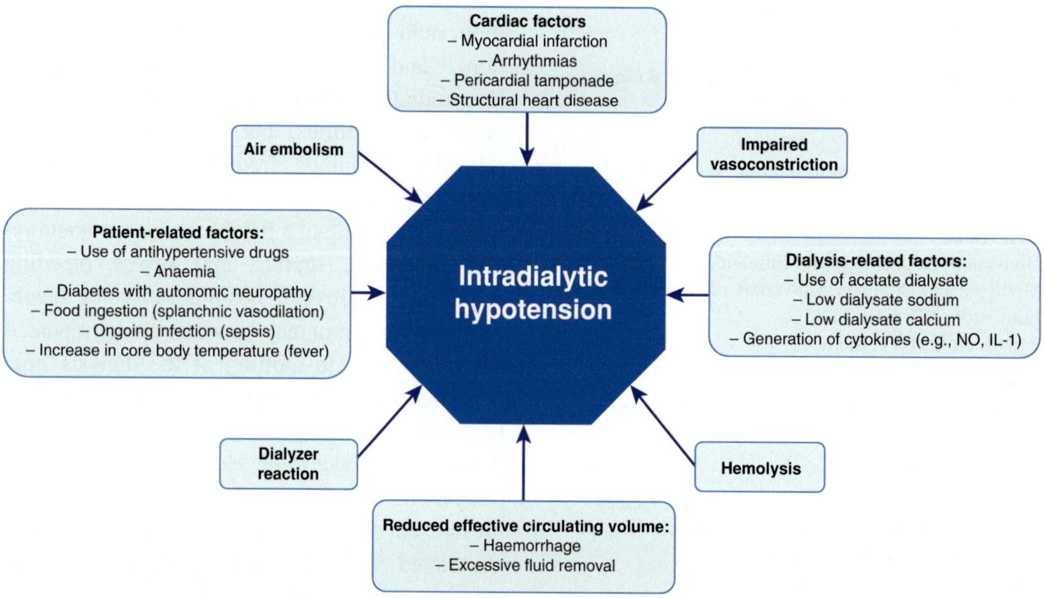

Fig. 18.1 Factors contributing to intradialytic hypotension. *NO* Nitric oxide, *IL-1* Interleukin-1

The acute management of symptomatic intradialytic hypotension episodes is dictated by the severity of each episode and can entail postural adjustments to improve venous return (e.g. the Trendelenburg position), stopping ultrafiltration—with or without terminating the dialysis session altogether, and the administration of intravenous fluid and oxygen.

There are long term sequelae to repeated intradialytic hypotension. Hence, this should be minimised in HD patients, as it portends adverse morbidity and mortality outcomes. The consequences of repeated intradialytic hypotension includes repeated myocardial stunning with resultant myocardial fibrosis and cardiac hypertrophy [4, 5], endotoxin translocation due to gut ischaemia associated with chronic systemic inflammation [6, 7], and loss of residual kidney function due to repeated kidney parenchymal ischaemia (Fig. 18.2).

Given the serious consequences, preventive strategies must be implemented in the HD patient who suffers repeated episodes of intradialytic hypotension: First line preventive measures, as outlined by the European best practices guidelines [8], include dietary sodium restriction, bicarbonate buffer use, a clinical reappraisal of patient's dry weight, adjusting dialysate temperature to 36.5 °C, avoiding meals during dialysis, and adjusting the doses and timing of administration of antihypertensive medication. In more refractory cases, Midodrine—a selective alpha-1 adrenoceptor agonist—may be used, and L-carnitine supplementation is also advocated. If all measures are unsuccessful, the patient may benefit from a change in dialysis modality.

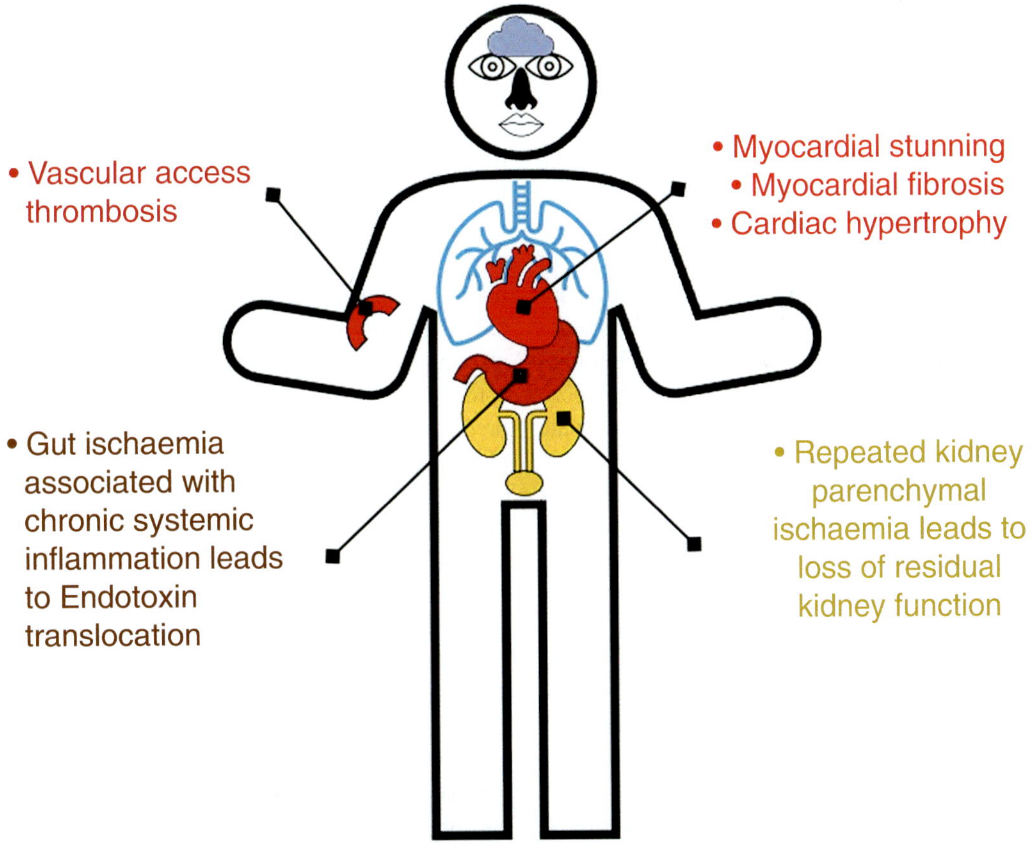

Fig. 18.2 **Consequences of Intradialytic Hypotension**

Intradialytic Hypertension

Definition of intradialytic Hypertension [2]:
Intradialytic hypertension has not hitherto been defined in international consensus guidelines, although KDIGO recently proposed in 2020 a definition of: "*An SBP rise >10 mmHg from pre- to post-dialysis in the hypertensive range in at least 4 of 6 consecutive dialysis treatments should prompt a more extensive evaluation of BP and volume management, including home and/or ABPM* [2]".

Whilst haemodialysis is physiologically more likely to lead to a fall in BP, in a subgroup of patients, a paradoxical increase in BP is recurrently observed during most treatment sessions. Intradialytic Hypertension has hitherto variously been classified as an increase in mean arterial pressure (MAP) of >15 mmHg during a treatment session or shortly after a session, or as hypertension occurring in the second or third hour of dialysis treatment following substantial ultrafiltration, and as a pre- to post-dialysis increase in SBP of 5–10 mmHg [9]. KDIGO's has recently issued a statement defining it as an SBP rise >10 mmHg from pre- to post-dialysis in the hypertensive range in at least 4 of 6 consecutive dialysis treatments should prompt a more extensive evaluation of BP and volume management, including home and/or ABPM [10]. Intradialytic hypertension occurs in 5–15% of HD patients [11] and is associated with poor short- and long-term cardiovascular outcomes [12–14]. Patients prone to developing intradialytic hypertension are characterized by non-modifiable factors such as increased age, male gender, and Caucasian race [15]. In addition, modality-related factors such as short dialysis duration, short dialysis vintage, and smaller interdialytic weight gain and hence low ultrafiltration volumes per treatment have also been noted to typify HD patients who develop recurrent intradialytic hypertension [15]. These patients' metabolic profile is characterized by lower Hb, creatinine, albumin, calcium and phosphate levels, and a lower total iron binding capacity [15].

The pathophysiologic mechanisms underlying intradialytic hypertension have not been fully elucidated, but a few associations have been identified and include a chronically expanded extracellular volume, osmolality shifts and endothelial cell dysfunction. Chronic extracellular volume overload has consistently been demonstrated in patients with intradialytic hypertension. Paradoxically, these patients weigh relatively less, have smaller interdialytic weight gains and have relatively lower pre-dialysis BP readings [12]. They however, have a higher post-dialysis extracellular water-to-total body water ratio (ECW/TBW) despite adequate ultrafiltration volumes. Ultrafiltration goals in HD are usually dictated by the acute ECW gain in the inter-dialytic period and not the overall ECW gain over time and as such, in intradialytic hypertension there is a persistence of extracellular space overload. This is the rationale for ultrafiltration probing as a management strategy in intradialytic hypertension (see below).

As previously discussed under intradialytic hypotension, serum osmolality changes due to solute shifts during dialysis usually cause a BP decline. However, in patients with recurrent intradialytic hypertension, the gradient of solute shift is not significant enough to cause BP reductions. This is because these patients tend to have lower pre-dialysis serum levels of osmotically active solutes such as creatinine, blood urea nitrogen, phosphate, albumin and a lower interdialytic weight gain relative to other HD patients [12]. The dialysate-to-plasma sodium gradient is also an important contributor to intradialytic osmolar shifts and intradialytic hypertension in predisposed patients. A higher dialysate-to-plasma sodium gradient results in less effective extracellular fluid (ECF) removal as a higher gradient favors both ECF and intracellular fluid removal rather than ECF removal alone [16, 17]. The absence of active therapeutic intradialysis BP control with antihypertensives occurring either as a result of withholding all BP lowering agents prior dialysis sessions, or their loss into the dialysate during dialysis sessions has additionally been identified as a contributing factor to the occurrence of recurrent intradialytic hypertension [18].

Intradialysis BP levels may become severely elevated necessitating the use of immediate release or short acting BP lowering agents to lower the BP. The long-term management of intradialytic hypertension involves a downward review of dry weight over time i.e. dry-weight probing, reducing dialysate sodium to reduce the dialysate-plasma gradient, and the use of antihypertensives prior to commencing dialysis sessions. Dry weight probing addresses the chronic ECW excess state in these patients while a less steep or flat dialysate-plasma sodium gradient ensures that ultrafiltration effectively addresses the ECV compartment alone. Withholding antihypertensives prior to dialysis sessions should not be a broad approach applied to all dialysis patients. In patients with recurrent intradialytic hypertension, non-dialyzable antihypertensives (e.g. Amlodipine) can be administered [19]. While the choice of antihypertensives is driven by factors such as comorbid states and underlying CV risk factors, ACEis/ARBs and β-blockers are particularly beneficial.

Cardiac Arrhythmias, Sudden Cardiac Arrest, and Sudden Cardiac Death

Cardiovascular disease remains an important cause of mortality in kidney failure patients with sudden cardiac death (SCD) accounting for 78% of CV causes of death [20]. SCD has been defined as "an unexpected death due to cardiac causes in a person with known or unknown cardiac disease, within 1 h of symptom onset (witnessed SCD) or within 24 h of the last proof of life (unwitnessed SCD) [20, 21]". Included in this definition is a distinct subgroup of patients in whom sudden cardiac arrest (SCA) in dialysis is the cause of SCD. The risk for arrhythmias and SCA is higher among HD patients relative to CAPD patients in the first 2 years of dialysis initiation but this risk equalizes thereafter [16]. Forty percent of deaths among dialysis patients are attributable to arrhythmias and SCA with the reported event rates of occurrence ranging between 4.5–7.0 per 100,000 HD sessions [22–24]. Prognosis following intradialysis SCA is dismal with 7.8% dying intradialysis following unsuccessful resuscitative attempts while only 40% remain alive 2 days post event [23].

SCA represents an interplay between a triggering event for a fatal arrhythmia and a predisposing/underlying CV disease. CKD and kidney failure are associated with myocardial structural changes, such as left ventricular hypertrophy (LVH), coronary vascular calcification, and myocardial fibrosis, which in turn disrupt the architecture of cardiac electrical pathways resulting in arrhythmogenic zones and conduction delays in fibrotic areas [25]. Fluxes in electrolyte levels especially with regards to dialysate potassium and calcium (low levels of both predispose to prolonged QT interval and QT dispersion on ECG), intracorporeal fluid compartment volume fluctuations, and myocardial stunning, constitute identified triggers [26, 27]. A relationship exists between dialysis timing and the occurrence of SCD. HD patients are most at risk after a long interdialytic interval (>2 days), with the risk being highest in the last 12 h of the interdialytic period, during or after the first dialysis session of the week and within 6 h after a dialysis session [28–31]. Both tachy- and bradyarrhythmias are known to occur in the dialysis population. While tachyarrhythmias have been widely held to be the commoner cause of SCA, more recent data suggests that bradyarrhythmias account more for fatal intradialysis arrests. Tachyarrhythmias include atrial fibrillation, supraventricular tachycardia, and non-sustained ventricular tachycardia [32].

Management strategies are directed towards the prevention of arrhythmias and encompass avoiding rapid electrolyte shifts during dialysis sessions, more frequent dialysis session scheduling to avoid long interdialytic intervals, the use of cardioprotective agents such as ACEi/ARB which are known to have a beneficial effect on modifying myocardial hypertrophy and fibrosis, and β-blockers with pleiotropic benefits beyond BP control including inhibitory effect on the sympathetic system, promoting of heart rate variability, and improving baroreceptor sensitivity. The use of cardiac devices such as implantable defibrillators has also been advocated. Other causes of SCD in dialysis patients other than fatal arrhythmias identified from autopsy series include acute myocardial infarction and dissecting aortic aneurysms [33].

Dialysis Pericarditis

Dialysis pericarditis refers to pericarditis occurring 8 weeks after the initiation of dialysis [34]. The exact incidence and prevalence of dialysis pericarditis is unknown as most data usually do not make the distinction between uremic and dialysis pericarditis. While uremic and dialysis-related pericarditis share a similar etiologic factor of the accumulation of uremic toxins, dialysis-related pericarditis is perpetuated by inefficient solute clearance during dialysis (not achieving kt/V), infrequent scheduling, and suboptimal dialysis flow rates [34, 35]. It must be borne in mind that pericarditis from other etiologies such as Dressler's syndrome, connective tissue disorders like systemic lupus erythematosus, infections or malignancies can also account for pericarditis in the dialysis patient. For diagnostic purposes, atypical electrocardiographic (ECG) findings are more commonly observed [36]. An associated infection should be suspected in the patient with dialysis pericarditis who has the representative ECG tracings of widespread ST elevation or PR segment depression seen in pericarditis unrelated to kidney failure. Inflammatory markers and white cell counts are also elevated [37, 38].

The characteristic chest pain of pericarditis is infrequently observed in these patients. More frequently, intradialysis hypotension and clinical features of heart failure from complicating pericardial effusion are the clinical manifestations in this patient group [34–36]. Non-specific constitutional symptoms of malaise, chills and fever, cough, and dyspnea have also been observed. Treatment approaches involve improving solute clearance by augmenting dialysis parameters—improving blood flow, increasing dialysis duration, and/or increasing frequency. Trial data [39, 40] demonstrates no benefit of non-steroidal anti-inflammatory drug (NSAID) use while data is poor for the efficacy of steroids or colchicine. Surgical treatment—needle pericardiocentesis, pericardiotomy with continuous drainage, partial or complete pericardiectomy—may be necessary in dialysis pericarditis with recurrent pericardial effusions [38].

Dialysis Access Ischemia Steal Syndrome

Dialysis access ischemic steal syndrome (DAISS) is an access-related complication seen in 1–8% of HD patients with arteriovenous (AV) dialysis accesses [41]. While most AV access demonstrates evidence of distal arterial steal, not all patients will develop the ischemic symptoms that typify this complication. It occurs as a result of decreased distal arterial blood flow beyond the point of an AV anastomosis; blood diversion through the anastomosis accounts for the distal "steal" of blood supply while resultant distal hypoperfusion and ischemia rather than the steal alone accounts for symptoms. Risk factors for DAISS include a proximally placed AV access i.e. brachial artery access points, diabetes mellitus, peripheral vascular disease, age > 60 years, and female gender [41]. Clinical manifestations include cold hands, pain in the hands during dialysis (could also occur off dialysis), tingling and numbness in the hands, sensory and motor deficits, and skin changes such as ischemic fingertip ulcers and dry gangrene of the digits in chronic cases [42]. In addition to typical history and examination findings, a doppler ultrasonography to assess access flow and establish improved digital pressures with compression at the AV anastomotic site strongly suggest the presence of significant steal [42]. An arteriography is critical to making a diagnosis of steal and associated distal hypoperfusion and helps to guide the best treatment approach. The available treatment modalities are varied depending on the severity of symptoms and the pathophysiologic vascular hemodynamic processes at play and range from observation of symptoms to ligation of the AV access in extreme situations [42, 43].

Practice Point 1: Cardiovascular Complications of Haemodialysis

Complication	Causes	Management
Intradialytic hypotension	See Fig. 18.1	Acutely: – rendelenburg, stop ultrafiltration, fluid bolus. – Consider underlying cause (see Fig. 18.1) – Dietary sodium restriction – Bicarbonate buffer – Review patient's dry weight – Adjust dialysate temperature to 36.5 – Avoid meals during dialysis, adjust timing of anti-hypertensives. – Consider midodrine or L-carnitine supplementation
Intradialytic hypertension	– Chronically expanded extracellular volume – Lower pre-dialysis levels of osmotically active solutes – Lower intra-dialytic weight gain – Inadequate BP control prior to dialysis – Loss of anti-hypertensives into dialysate	– Review dry weight – Consider reduction in dialysate sodium – Review and optimise medications – Consider use of non-dialyzable antihypertensives, e.g. amlodipine.
Cardiac arrhythmias	Both tachy- and bradyarrhythmias – Underlying cardiovascular disease with resultant myocardial structural abnormalities – Fluxes in electrolyte levels – Intracorporeal fluid compartment volume fluctuations	Prevention is key – Avoidance of rapid electrolyte shifts – Avoiding long interdialytic intervals – Use and up-titration of cardioprotective drugs
Dialysis pericarditis	Overlap between uraemic/dialysis-related pericarditis – inefficient solute clearance – suboptimal dialysis flow rates Consider other aetiologies for instance connective tissue disease	– Improvement of solute clearance – Augmentation of dialysis parameters – Consider steroids, colchicine (though a paucity of evidence)
Dialysis ischaemia steal syndrome (DAISS)	Risk factors include: – Proximally placed AV access – Diabetes, peripheral vascular disease, age >60 years, females.	Severe ischaemia warrants invasive treatment. Options depend on individual anatomy and pathology but include: – Angioplasty to inflow arterial stenosis – Precision banding – Ligation

Neurological Complications of Haemodialysis

Seizures

Hemodialysis-related seizure (HRS) is a common complication frequently observed in the younger age dialysis population. It has been reported in 7–50% of children with kidney failure [44, 45]. Young age, a medical history of seizures, dyselectrolytemias such as hypocalcemia and hypomagnesemia, as well as metabolic factors (e.g. hypoglycemia) and sustained acid-base abnormalities are known risk factors (Fig. 18.3). Rapid clearance of anti-convulsant drugs during dialysis (in patients known with epilepsy), or use

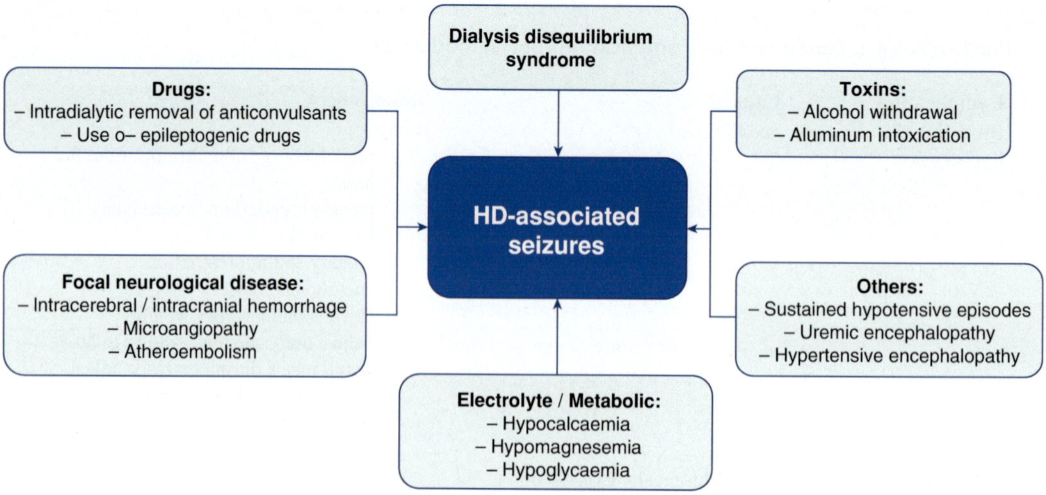

Fig. 18.3 Factors implicated in haemodialysis-associated seizures

of epileptogenic drugs (e.g. theophylline) can be triggers of a seizure disorder during dialysis. In addition, HD-related processes such as a relatively rapid clearance of solutes such as urea can lead to an osmotic gradient between the brain and the plasma, leading to dialysis disequilibrium syndrome (DDS): brain edema that manifests as neurological symptoms such as headache, nausea, vomiting, muscle cramps, tremors, disturbed consciousness, and convulsions. Other HD-related processes including the use of acetate buffer, heparinization-related intracerebral hemorrhage, and erythropoietin administration have also been associated with HRS [45, 46]. Generalized tonic-clonic seizures are more commonly observed than non-convulsive seizures [45]. There is a dearth of clinical trial efficacy data regarding the efficacy of antiepileptic drugs in the prevention and management of HRS. Diazepam, a benzodiazepine that is non-dialyzable has been reported to prevent the recurrence of HRS [44].

Headache

Dialysis-related headache (DRH) is a common neurologic complication of HD and is described by the International Headache society as a secondary form of headache occurring during, and as a result of HD, with no particular pathognomonic characteristics, and which spontaneously resolves within 72 h of the termination of the dialysis session [47]. Diagnostic criteria help to distinguish DRH from other headache phenomena that may be observed in HD patients [47]:

Diagnostic criteria for dialysis-related headaches (DRH) [47]

1. Patient is on HD
2. Two of the following to demonstrate HD causality:
   (a) Headache occurring during an HD session
   (b) Each headache episode worsening during the dialysis session and/or each headache episode resolving within 72 hours of HD completion,
3. Three headache episodes meeting the specifics above
4. Headaches no longer occurring after renal transplantation and cessation of HD altogether

A previous diagnosis of primary headache appears to be a risk factor for DRH. Pathophysiologic mechanisms have been attributed to changes in levels of solutes such as sodium, magnesium, and urea as well as intradialytic changes in blood pressure and volume status [48, 49]. No clinical trial data is available to guide prophylactic and therapeutic approaches to DRH management. There are case reports [50, 51] describing the prophylactic role of chlorpromazine, ACE-i [51], magnesium oxide and nortriptyline, while paracetamol and the ergot alkaloids (ergotamine, dihydroergotamine) have also been shown to have therapeutic benefits [50]. The risk of AV fistula closure with alkaloid derivatives necessitates caution in its application for the treatment of DRH.

Dialysis Dementia

Dialysis dementia is prevalent in about 4% of the HD population [52], and is associated with an increased risk of dialysis withdrawal and death. With the highly restricted use of aluminum-containing phosphate binders and improved water treatment systems that safeguard against aluminum contamination of dialysates, dialysis dementia in HD patients is now rarely observed [53]. It is a subacute, progressive, and fatal dementia occurring due to aluminum deposition in the cerebral cortex. More recently, risk factors for dialysis-related dementia include the poor clearance of middle-molecules with neurotoxin activity; the preservation of residual renal function in HD patients which ensures to an extent the excretion of middle molecules has been associated with reduced odds of dialysis dementia [52]. The chronic oxidative stress and inflammatory states induced by HD have also been implicated. Risk factors for dementia in the general population (increased age, race, low educational status, comorbidities such as cerebrovascular disease and diabetes) are also observed in patients with dialysis dementia. The management of aluminum-related dementia includes aluminum chelation with deferoxamine, improved water treatment methods, and substituting aluminum-containing phosphate binders with non-aluminum alternatives (calcium- or non-calcium-based binders) [54]. The clinical efficacy of medications for dementia in the general population have not been defined in the dialysis population, but hold promise.

Dialysis-Related Muscle Cramps

Muscle cramps are a frequent muscular complication in HD and typically present, usually towards the end of a dialysis session and may result in the premature termination of a session of dialysis. Cramps have been reported in up to 86% of HD patients [55]. Short-term painful discomfort to the patient and long-term inadequacy of dialysis sessions are consequences of muscle cramps that should be avoided. Muscle cramps usually occur in the lower extremities but can also manifest in the arm, hand, and abdominal muscles. The exact causes of cramps during dialysis are unknown but the temporal occurrence towards the end of a treatment session lend credence to the role of changes in ECV and solute/osmolarity shifts in promoting the abnormal muscular energy utilization and cramp triggering. Muscle cramps are observed in up to 74% of intradialytic hypotensive episodes [56]. It is believed that volume contraction from high ultrafiltration rates account for this. Preventive and treatment approaches thus involve limiting interdialytic weight gain (which limits dialysis sessions UF goals) and sequential/controlled ultrafiltration, respectively. Hyponatremia has also been implicated as a predisposing factor to muscle cramping by its role in influencing serum osmolarity and influencing water shifts across the various human volume compartments. Magnesium plays a critical role in skeletal metabolism influencing neuromuscular excitability. It also plays a regulatory role in sodium, potassium, and calcium ion channels transport. Hypomagnesemia among HD patients contributes to the occurrence of dialysis-related cramps. Magnesium is freely diffusible across the dialysis membrane and increasing dialysate magnesium concentrations cause an increase in serum magnesium thus promoting neuromuscular excitability stability. The use of magnesium-based phosphate binders can also be employed to improve serum magnesium levels in the HD population [57]. Broad non-specific treatment approaches employed include carnitine, and vitamins C and E supplementation [58, 59]. The use of benzodiazepines has also been documented [60].

Practice Point 2: Neurological Complications of Haemodialysis

Complication	Causes	Management
Seizures	See Fig. 18.2	Acutely: – stop dialysis, check glucose and bloods, rule out hypoglycaemia, manage as per local emergency protocols. Identify and treat underlying causes. Consider antiepileptics in conjunction with a neurologist—no specific evidence to guide choice of agent.
Dialysis related headache	Proposed mechanisms include: – changes in solute levels – intradialytic blood pressure and volume changes	– Rule out other potential causes of headache – Analgesia No specific clinical trial data to support prophylactic or therapeutic measures.
Dialysis Dementia	– Chronic oxidative stress and inflammatory state associated with haemodialysis – Metabolic and uremic factors – Underlying cardiovascular risk factors – Aluminium intoxication (now rarely seen)	– Investigate and treat as per non-CKD patients. – Chelators for treatment of aluminium toxicity
Dialysis related muscle cramps	– Changes in extracellular volume – Solute/osmolarity shifts. – Hypomagnesemia	Focussed on prevention: – Avoid excessive interdialytic weight gain – Avoid eating during haemodialysis – Consider increasing dialysate magnesium concentration and/or use of magnesium containing phosphate binders Stretching/warm compresses may help relieve symptoms

Haematologic Complications of Haemodialysis

Intra-Dialytic Haemolysis

This is an uncommon but important complication of HD because of the significant risk of morbidity and mortality [61]. Fig. 18.4 summarizes the possible aetiology of intradialytic haemolysis. Factors that increase mechanical or shear stress on the red blood cells include defective blood lines causing kinking in the lines, dialysis techniques that increase turbulence of flow like using a single needle technique, and when relatively high blood flow rates occur in the presence of small cannula size [10]. Contaminants, including chemicals used for water disinfection like chloramine, formaldehyde, chlorine are common causes of intradialytic haemolysis [62, 63]. Metals including Copper, zinc and aluminium and nitrates have also been implicated [64]. Overheated dialysate (usually above 47 °C). If the patient's osmolality falls below 250 mOsm/kg, either because of error in mixing dialysate (hypo-osmolar dialysate) or use of plasma expanders, intravascular haemolysis may occur [65, 66]. A host of patient factors predispose to intravascular haemolysis—malignant hypertension, autoimmune conditions like Systemic lupus erythematosus and thrombotic thrombocytopenic purpura, sickle cell anaemia, G6PD deficiency and hypersplenism. Medications that may induce haemolysis in dialysis patients include aspirin, sulphonamides, nitrofurantoin, quinidine and hydralazine [61, 67].

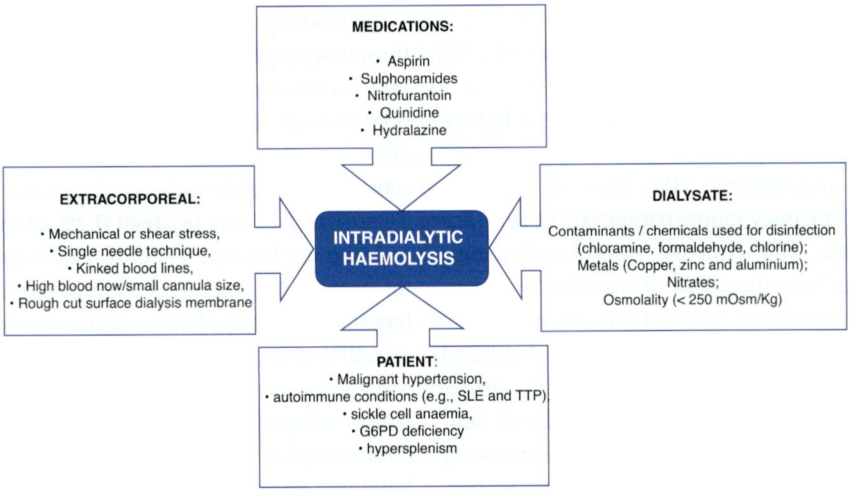

Fig. 18.4 **Proposed aetiological factors for the development of intradialytic haemolysis** *SLE* **Systemic lupus erythematosus,** *TTP* **Thrombotic thrombocytopenic purpura,** *G6PD* **Glucose-6-phosphate dehydrogenase**

The symptoms are non-specific. Chronic intradialysis haemolysis is usually asymptomatic, presenting as chronic anaemia with fatigue or erythropoietin resistance. Acute intradialysis haemolysis presents with nausea, vomiting, abdominal pain, diarrhoea, increasing dyspnoea and hypertension, headache, dark urine and possibly death. Inspection of the extracorporeal circuit may reveal a cherry red (less opaque) colour which may be associated with a pink tinged dialysate fluid if haemolysis is massive. Another indicator is a reduction in both arterial and venous circuits suggesting a kink in the bloodline. Important investigations include haptoglobin, LDH, Coomb's test, blood film, serum free haemoglobin and methaemalbumin.

Once acute haemolysis has been identified, it is important to stop dialysis immediately and not to return the blood in the extracorporeal circulation to prevent fatal arrythmias from hyperkalaemia. Some patients may require ICU care. Serum potassium levels should be monitored closely. Blood products should be given as indicated. The aetiology of the haemolysis should be investigated immediately and identified to prevent repeat episodes [68]. Prevention of this complication requires strict adherence to protocols for dialysis water safety by appropriately trained staff; avoidance of small needle/large flow rates and ensuring correct positioning of tubings in the dialysis machine pumps.

Haemorrhage

The need for extracorporeal anticoagulation during HD has introduced an increased likelihood for bleeding complications especially for individuals who are at increased risk. Major bleeding episodes occur in 1.7% to 3.7% of HD patients [69]. Bleeding can occur at any site—vascular access site [70], gastrointestinal, gall bladder, intracerebral, subdural, retroperitoneum, perinephric or even into the vitreous humor. Factors that increase risk of intradialysis haemorrhage include suboptimal control of BP, pre-existing gastrointestinal lesions, renal cystic disease, diabetic retinopathy, recent surgery or trauma, concomitant use of warfarin or aspirin and acute stroke [71]. The clinical presentation usually depends on the site of bleeding. Prevention or minimization of bleeding may be done by using dialysis modes that do not require use of systemic anticoagulation including using CAPD, heparin-free HD, regional anticoagulation with citrate, prostacyclin or mesilates. Regional heparin anticoagulation may also be employed.

erythropoietin or androgen therapy [85]. Dialysis induced hypoxaemia and acidosis have also been suggested as risk factors. Priapism may resolve spontaneously or require the use of surgical intervention.

Hearing Loss

Hearing impairment affecting low, middle and high frequency sounds is not uncommon among adult HD patients. The stria vascularis and renal tubular cells have similar modes of active transport of fluids and electrolytes and may be responsible for the simultaneous affectations in medications that have ototoxic and nephrotoxic properties [86]. An inhibition of the Na^+-K^+ ATPase in the cochlea has also been implicated as a pathophysiologic pathway for sensorineural hearing loss in HD patients [86]. Some have suggested osmotic disequilibrium in the inner ear initiated or worsened by HD. Patients on HD will benefit from pure tone audiometry for monitoring of hearing function [87].

Acute visual loss following HD is an uncommon complication which could be caused by sudden hypotension or rapid ultrafiltration leading to a non-arteritic anterior ischaemic optic neuropathy [88]. The risk factors for visual loss caused by HD include diabetes mellitus, dyslipidaemia, smoking and hypertension. Immediate post-dialysis reduction in ocular perfusion pressure, choroidal and retinal thickness has been reported [89].

Practice Point 4: Other Complications of Haemodialysis

Complication	Causes	Management
Acute visual loss	• Causes include sudden hypotension or rapid ultrafiltration leading to a ischaemic optic neuropathy • Immediate post-dialysis reduction in ocular perfusion pressure, choroidal and retinal thickness has been reported	
Hearing loss	• Cochlear stria vascularis and renal tubular cells have similar modes of active transport of fluids and electrolytes • Suggested mechanisms include HD-induced: • Osmotic disequilibrium in the inner ear • Inhibition of the the Na^+-K^+ ATPase in the cochlea • Inadequate BP control prior to dialysis • Loss of anti-hypertensives into dialysate	
Priapism	• Rare complication, associated with erythropoietin or androgen therapy. • Dialysis induced hypoxaemia and acidosis suggested as risk factors.	• May resolve spontaneously • Surgical intervention
Post-dialysis fatigue	Associated with: • Rapid changes in BP during dialysis • High ultrafiltration levels • Osmotic disequilibrium Concomitant depression	• Increased frequency of HD • Adjust dialysis prescription • Treat depression • Optimise nutrition and treatment of co-morbidities such as anaemia and heart failure
Dialysis-associated pruritus	Multifactorial—following all implicated • Dialysis inadequacy • Hyperparathyroidism • Hypercalcaemia • Hypermagnesaemia	• Topical—Moisturisers, mild topical steroids, topical tacrolimus, • Oral—antihistamines, pregabalin, nalfurafine.

Conclusions

Returning to our patient: He has been a dialysis patient for several years. His blood pressure at the start of haemodialysis was 130/80 mmHg, which was usual for him after taking his antihypertensive medications each morning. He was afebrile, and had been otherwise well. He noted that he had been passing less urine recently, and that his interdialytic weight gains have over the last few weeks increased to around 4 kg, and he freely admits to having difficulty with fluid and salt restriction. At the point of review, he had completed 3 h of haemodialysis with an ultrafiltration of 3.5 L. You advise his nurse to administer a 250 mL bolus of 0.9% sodium chloride, following which his blood pressure improves to 110/80 mmHg, and he is able to successfully complete 4 h of dialysis without further ultrafiltration.

The likely cause of his intradialytic hypotension is multifactorial: whilst fluid restriction can be difficult, particularly for those new to dialysis, it is also an issue where patients with a significant native urine output become oligo-anuric on haemodialysis. Having excluded other contributory acutely reversible causes, in addition to better adherence to fluid restriction to limit interdialytic weight gains, the patient may be advised to reduce or omit their antihypertensive medication on dialysis days in order to facilitate ultrafiltration to euvolaemia.

Questions

1. A 43-year-old female who has been on maintenance hemodialysis for 11 months presented with unilateral leg swelling and was noticed to have fever, chills, flushing, worsening breathlessness and chest pain following a bolus of IV Unfractionated heparin injection. A doppler ultrasound scan of the limb was suggestive of a deep venous thrombosis. At presentation for the next hemodialysis session, she was noticed to have gangrene of three toes in her left lower limb. CBC was normal except for a platelet count of 81,200/mm^3. His platelet count was 223,400 two months ago. She had no splenomegaly and no abnormal bleeding. What is the best management option for this patient?
   A. Blood culture and commence empirical IV antibiotics
   B. Use low molecular weight heparin for treatment of DVT and continue hemodialysis using standard protocol
   C. Use dabigatran for treatment of DVT and continue hemodialysis using standard protocol
   D. Use warfarin for the treatment of DVT, discontinue all heparin products and use argatroban for hemodialysis.
   E. Give platelet concentrate infusion, IV antibiotics, low molecular weight heparin and continue hemodialysis using standard protocol.

The correct answer is D.

This patient has developed heparin-induced thrombocytopenia (HIT). Paradoxically, they present with thrombotic phenomena instead of bleeding tendencies. Differential diagnoses include drug-induced thrombocytopenia from use of quinine, quinidine, chloroquine and sulfonamides; bacterial sepsis; TTP, ITP, disseminated intravascular coagulopathy and splenomegaly. We do not have any information regarding medication use except heparin. CBC would have shown neutrophilia if there is bacterial sepsis. The patient had no splenomegaly. Use of any heparin preparation will worsen the condition. Platelet concentrate is known to worsen thrombosis. Argatroban, bivalirudin, fondaparinux are non-heparin anticoagulants used in HIT.

2. Which of the following is **not** useful for the treatment of dialysis-associated pruritus?
   A. Naltrexone
   B. Skin moisturizers and low potency topical steroids
   C. Nalfurafine
   D. Propoxyphene
   E. Gabapentin

The correct answer is D.

Propoxyphene is a narcotic pain reliever which is not known to have any effect on pruritus. All others have been shown to have beneficial effect in individuals with pruritus.

3. A 56-year-old woman with end-stage renal disease secondary to diabetic nephropathy uses a cuffed, tunneled, right internal jugular catheter as vascular access for hemodialysis for 5 months. After the first 35 minutes of HD, she develops nausea and rigors and has a temperature of 38.3 °C. Her BP drops from 157/80 to 100/61 mmHg, and her heart rate is 113 beats per minute, regular. She had a similar experience during dialysis 3 days ago, but the temperature was 37.7 °C and she had transient rigors. Examination revealed mild erythema and tenderness of the exit site but no purulent discharge. No other patient having dialysis at the centre has similar occurrence. What is the most correct statement?
   A. Take a swab from the exit site and start empiric antibiotic
   B. The most likely cause of this intradialysis complication is bacterial contamination of dialysis water
   C. Commence IV antibiotic following local resistance pattern for Gram positive and negative bacteria after taking samples from the exit site, one from the catheter lumen (hub), and one from the bloodline.
   D. The most common causative organisms are Gram negative organisms
   E. Catheter removal is not essential if a fungal organism is cultured.

The correct answer is C.

This is most likely a catheter-related blood stream infection.

The identification of the offending organism and sensitivity pattern is critical in the establishment of correct treatment and prevention of metastatic infection and death. Taking a swab sample from the exit site only may not establish the offending organism(s) as catheter and bloodline samples are also important. Bacterial contamination of water would present with chills/rigors within one hour of treatment associated with fever one to two hours after treatment, hypotension and reducing hemoglobin levels. However, the latter will affect multiple dialysis patients in the same centre. Gram positive organisms like *Staph Aureus* are the commonest organisms implicated and having an established fungal catheter-related infection is an indication for removing the catheter.

4. A 60-year-old diabetic female with a current weight of 102 kg has recently commenced hemodialysis. Dry weight estimation by bioelectrical impedance analysis is 93 kg. She has been unable to complete her last 3 scheduled HD sessions due to intra-dialysis MAP drops up to 15 mmHg. The following are cardiovascular and neuroendocrine mechanisms that are expected to have occurred in this patient except
   A. Augmented myocardial contractility
   B. Increased peripheral resistance
   C. Activation of the parasympathetic nervous system
   D. Activation of the Renin-Angiotensin-Aldosterone system
   E. Increased heart rate

The correct answer: C.

Options A, B, D and E are all known compensatory, adaptive mechanisms that occur during hemodialysis to prevent blood pressure drops intradialysis.

5. One of the following can prevent the occurrence of intradialytic hypertension
   A. A steep dialysate-to-plasma sodium gradient favoring intracellular fluid shifts alone
   B. A moderate dialysate-to-plasma sodium gradient favoring net extracellular fluid shifts
   C. A moderate dialysate-to-plasma calcium gradient favoring total body water fluid loss
   D. A steep dialysate-to-plasma sodium gradient favoring total body water fluid loss
   E. A zero dialysate-to-plasma sodium gradient to prevent rebound hypervolemia

Correct answer: B.

As sodium plays a central role in determining serum osmolarity and thus intravascular volume, sodium shifts induced by dialysate-serum sodium gradients induce fluid movement across the various fluid compartments, principally the intracellular and plasma/extracellular fluid compartments. It has been demonstrated by bioimpedance techniques that steeper sodium gradients of the dialysate relative to serum promotes intracellular fluid loss rather than plasma/extracellular fluid loss. With high gradients the extracellular fluid compartment remains expanded. It has thus been suggested that in the management of dialysis patients with intradialytic hypertension less steep dialysate-to-plasma sodium gradients be maintained and thus facilitate extracellular fluid loss.

6. A 54-year-old with end-stage renal disease from lupus nephritis who was transferred 10 weeks ago from peritoneal dialysis to hemodialysis following fungal peritonitis, has come into the HD unit with complaints of low-grade, continuous fever, malaise, and central chest pain. The pain is rather constant and is mildly improved by a change in posture to a seated position. There is no associated cough or dyspnea. A bedside 12-lead ECG done showed features of LVH and non-specific ST segment changes, while an echocardiogram revealed mild pericardial effusion. White blood cell count was 14,000cells/mm^3 while CRP was 62 mg/dL. B-D-Glucan assay was indeterminate. A highly likely diagnosis in this patient is:
   A. Uremic gastritis
   B. Tietze's disease
   C. Fungal pericarditis
   D. Lupus pericarditis
   E. Dialysis pericarditis

The correct answer: E.

Unlike pericarditis in non-uremic, non-dialysis patients, dialysis-related pericarditis usually presents without the classic ECG findings of diffuse PR segment depression and saddle-shaped ST segment elevation. The lack of associated epicardial inflammation in uremic and dialysis patients accounts for the absence of these typical ECG findings. Intensification dialysis schedule is known to improve associated pericardial effusions while anti-inflammatory agents such as steroids and NSAIDs have not been consistently shown to be helpful.

7. A 56-year-old woman with end-stage renal disease secondary to diabetic nephropathy uses a cuffed, tunneled, right internal jugular catheter as vascular access for hemodialysis for 5 months. After the first 35 minutes of HD, she develops nausea and rigors and has a temperature of 38.3 °C. Her BP drops from 157/80 to 100/61 mmHg, and her heart rate is 113 beats per minute, regular. She had a similar experience during dialysis 3 days ago, but the temperature was 37.7 °C and she had transient rigors. Examination revealed mild erythema and tenderness of the exit site but no purulent discharge. No other patient having dialysis at the centre has similar occurrence. What is the most likely cause of clinical scenario?
   A. Gram positive infection
   B. Gram negative infection
   C. Fungal infection
   D. Virus infection
   E. Parasite infection

The correct answer is C.

This is most likely a catheter-related blood stream infection and Gram positive organisms like *Staph Aureus* are the commonest organisms

Test your learning and check your understanding of this book's contents: use the "Springer Nature Flashcards" app to access questions using https://sn.pub/cz9Cok. To use the app, please follow the instructions in Chap. 1.

References

1. K/DOQI clinical practice guidelines on hypertension and antihypertensive agents in chronic kidney disease. Am J Kidney Dis. 2004;43:S1–290.
2. Flythe JE, Chang TI, et al. Blood pressure and volume management in dialysis: conclusions from a kidney disease: improving global outcomes (KDIGO) controversies conference. Kidney Int. 2020;97:861–76.
3. Flythe JE, Xue H, Lynch KE, Curhan GC, Brunelli SM. Association of mortality risk with various definitions of intradialytic hypotension. J Am Soc Nephrol. 2015;26:724–34.

4. Burton JO, Jefferies HJ, Selby NM, McIntyre CW. Hemodialysis-induced cardiac injury: determinants and associated outcomes. Clin J Am Soc Nephrol. 2009;4:914–20.
5. Burton JO, Jefferies HJ, Selby NM, McIntyre CW. Hemodialysis-induced repetitive myocardial injury results in global and segmental reduction in systolic cardiac function. Clin J Am Soc Nephrol. 2009;4:1925–31.
6. McIntyre CW, Harrison LE, Eldehni MT, et al. Circulating endotoxemia: a novel factor in systemic inflammation and cardiovascular disease in chronic kidney disease. Clin J Am Soc Nephrol. 2011;6:133–41.
7. Shafi T, Jaar BG, Plantinga LC, et al. Association of residual urine output with mortality, quality of life, and inflammation in incident hemodialysis patients: the Choices for Healthy Outcomes in Caring for End-Stage Renal Disease (CHOICE) Study. Am J Kidney Dis. 2010;56:348–58.
8. Kooman J, Basci A, Pizzarelli F, et al. EBPG guideline on haemodynamic instability. Nephrol Dialysis Transpl. 2007;22:ii22–44.
9. Van Buren PN. Pathophysiology and implications of intradialytic hypertension. Curr Opin Nephrol Hypertens. 2017;26:303.
10. Polaschegg HD. Red blood cell damage from extracorporeal circulation in hemodialysis. Seminars in dialysis; 2009: Wiley Online Library. p. 524–31.
11. Van Buren PN, Kim C, Toto RD, Inrig JK. The prevalence of persistent intradialytic hypertension in a hemodialysis population with extended follow-up. Int J Artif Organs. 2012;35:1031–8.
12. Park J, Rhee CM, Sim JJ, et al. A comparative effectiveness research study of the change in blood pressure during hemodialysis treatment and survival. Kidney Int. 2013;84:795–802.
13. Assimon MM, Wang L, Flythe JE. Intradialytic hypertension frequency and short-term clinical outcomes among individuals receiving maintenance hemodialysis. Am J Hypertens. 2018;31:329–39.
14. Inrig JK, Patel UD, Toto RD, Szczech LA. Association of blood pressure increases during hemodialysis with 2-year mortality in incident hemodialysis patients: a secondary analysis of the Dialysis Morbidity and Mortality Wave 2 Study. Am J Kidney Dis. 2009;54:881–90.
15. Van Buren PN, Inrig JK. Special situations: Intradialytic hypertension/chronic hypertension and intradialytic hypotension. Seminars in dialysis; 2017: Wiley Online Library. p. 545–52.
16. Sarkar SR, Wystrychowski G, Zhu F, Usvyat LA, Kotanko P, Levin NW. Fluid dynamics during hemodialysis in relationship to sodium gradient between dialysate and plasma. ASAIO J. 2007;53:339–42.
17. Inrig JK, Molina C, D'Silva K, et al. Effect of low versus high dialysate sodium concentration on blood pressure and endothelial-derived vasoregulators during hemodialysis: a randomized crossover study. Am J Kidney Dis. 2015;65:464–73.
18. Krishnan N, Peixoto AJ. We hold antihypertensives prior to dialysis. Seminars in dialysis; 2016: Wiley Online Library. p. 323–5.
19. Santos SF, Peixoto AJ, Perazella MA. How should we manage adverse intradialytic blood pressure changes? Adv Chronic Kidney Dis. 2012;19:158–65.
20. Saran R, Robinson B, Abbott KC, et al. US renal data system 2017 annual data report: epidemiology of kidney disease in the United States. Am J Kidney Dis. 2018;71:A7.
21. Organization WH. Sudden cardiac death: report of a WHO Scientific Group. World Health Organization; 1985.
22. Saran R, Robinson B, Abbott K, Agodoa L, Bhave N, Bragg-Gresham J. US renal data system 2018 annual data report: epidemiology of kidney disease in the United States. Am J Kidney Dis:71.
23. Karnik JA, Young BS, Lew NL, et al. Cardiac arrest and sudden death in dialysis units. Kidney Int. 2001;60:350–7.
24. Pun PH, Lehrich RW, Honeycutt EF, Herzog CA, Middleton JP. Modifiable risk factors associated with sudden cardiac arrest within hemodialysis clinics. Kidney Int. 2011;79:218–27.
25. Whitman IR, Feldman HI, Deo R. CKD and sudden cardiac death: epidemiology, mechanisms, and therapeutic approaches. J Am Soc Nephrol. 2012;23:1929–39.
26. Näppi SE, Virtanen VK, Saha HH, Mustonen JT, Pasternack AI. QTc dispersion increases during hemodialysis with low-calcium dialysate. Kidney Int. 2000;57:2117–22.
27. Genovesi S, Dossi C, Vigano MR, et al. Electrolyte concentration during haemodialysis and QT interval prolongation in uraemic patients. Europace. 2008;10:771–7.
28. Bleyer A, Hartman J, Brannon P, Reeves-Daniel A, Satko S, Russell G. Characteristics of sudden death in hemodialysis patients. Kidney Int. 2006;69:2268–73.
29. Genovesi S, Valsecchi MG, Rossi E, et al. Sudden death and associated factors in a historical cohort of chronic haemodialysis patients. Nephrol Dialysis Transpl. 2009;24:2529–36.
30. Foley RN, Gilbertson DT, Murray T, Collins AJ. Long interdialytic interval and mortality among patients receiving hemodialysis. N Engl J Med. 2011;365:1099–107.
31. Roy-Chaudhury P, Tumlin JA, Koplan BA, et al. Primary outcomes of the monitoring in dialysis study indicate that clinically significant arrhythmias are common in hemodialysis patients and related to dialytic cycle. Kidney Int. 2018;93:941–51.
32. Rogovoy NM, Howell SJ, Lee TL, et al. Hemodialysis procedure–associated autonomic imbalance and cardiac arrhythmias: insights from continuous 14-Day ECG monitoring. J Am Heart Assoc. 2019;8:e013748.

33. Takeda K, Harada A, Okuda S, et al. Sudden death in chronic dialysis patients. Nephrol Dialysis Transpl. 1997;12:952–5.
34. Alpert MA, Ravenscraft MD. Pericardial involvement in end-stage renal disease. Am J Med Sci. 2003;325:228–36.
35. Wood JE, Mahnensmith RL. Pericarditis associated with renal failure: evolution and management. Seminars in dialysis; 2001: Wiley Online Library. p. 61–6.
36. COMTY CM, COHEN SL, SHAPIRO FL. Pericarditis in chronic uremia and its sequels. Ann Intern Med. 1971;75:173–83.
37. Horstkotte D, Follath F, Gutschik E, et al. European Society of Cardiology Guidelines. Guidelines on prevention, diagnosis and treatment of infective endocarditis executive summary. The task force on infective endocarditis of the European society of cardiology. Eur Heart J. 2004;25:267–76.
38. Dad T, Sarnak MJ. Pericarditis and pericardial effusions in end-stage renal disease. Seminars in dialysis; 2016: Wiley Online Library. p. 366–73.
39. Spector D, Alfred H, Siedlecki M, Briefel G. A controlled study of the effect of indomethacin in uremic pericarditis. Kidney Int. 1983;24:663–9.
40. Rutsky EA, Rostand SG. Treatment of uremic pericarditis and pericardial effusion. Am J Kidney Dis. 1987;10:2–8.
41. Tordoir J, Dammers R, Van der Sande F. Upper extremity ischemia and hemodialysis vascular access. Eur J Vasc Endovasc Surg. 2004;27:1–5.
42. Malik J, Tuka V, Kasalova Z, et al. Understanding the dialysis access steal syndrome. A review of the etiologies, diagnosis, prevention and treatment strategies. J Vasc Access. 2008;9:155–66.
43. Asif A, Leon C, Merrill D, et al. Arterial steal syndrome: a modest proposal for an old paradigm. Am J Kidney Dis. 2006;48:88–97.
44. Sönmez F, Mir S, Tütüncüoğlu S. Potential prophylactic use of benzodiazepines for hemodialysis-associated seizures. Pediatr Nephrol. 2000;14:367–9.
45. Glenn CM, Astley SJ, Watkins SL. Dialysis-associated seizures in children and adolescents. Pediatr Nephrol. 1992;6:182–6.
46. Scorza FA, Md A, Arida RM, et al. Seizure occurrence in patients with chronic renal insufficiency in regular hemodialysis program. Arq Neuropsiquiatr. 2005;63:757–60.
47. Arnold M. Headache classification committee of the international headache society (ihs) the international classification of headache disorders. Cephalalgia. 2018;38:1–211.
48. Göksan B, Karaali-Savrun F, Ertan S, Savrun M. Haemodialysis-related headache. Cephalalgia. 2004;24:284–7.
49. Goksel BK, Torun D, Karaca S, et al. Is low blood magnesium level associated with hemodialysis headache? Headache. 2006;46:40–5.
50. Levin M. Resident and fellow section. Headache. 2013;53:181–5.
51. Leinisch-Dahlke E, Schmidt-Wilcke T, Krämer B, May A. Improvement of dialysis headache after treatment with ACE-inhibitors but not angiotensin II receptor blocker: a case report with pathophysiological considerations. Cephalalgia. 2005;25:71–4.
52. Kurella M, Mapes DL, Port FK, Chertow GM. Correlates and outcomes of dementia among dialysis patients: the Dialysis Outcomes and Practice Patterns Study. Nephrol Dialysis Transpl. 2006;21:2543–8.
53. Dunea G. Dialysis dementia: an epidemic that came and went. ASAIO J. 2001;47:192–4.
54. Rob PM, Niederstadt C, Reusche E. Dementia in patients undergoing long-term dialysis. CNS Drugs. 2001;15:691–9.
55. Sena Ulu M, Ahsen A. Muscle cramps during hemodialysis. Eur J Gen Med. 2015;12
56. Caplin B, Kumar S, Davenport A. Patients' perspective of haemodialysis-associated symptoms. Nephrol Dialysis Transpl. 2011;26:2656–63.
57. de Francisco AL, Leidig M, Covic AC, et al. Evaluation of calcium acetate/magnesium carbonate as a phosphate binder compared with sevelamer hydrochloride in haemodialysis patients: a controlled randomized study (CALMAG study) assessing efficacy and tolerability. Nephrol Dialysis Transpl. 2010;25: 3707–17.
58. Canzanello VJ, Burkart JM. Hemodialysis-Associated Muscle Cramps. Seminars in dialysis; 1992: Wiley Online Library. p. 299–304.
59. Khajehdehi P, Mojerlou M, Behzadi S, Rais-Jalali GA. A randomized, double-blind, placebo-controlled trial of supplementary vitamins E, C and their combination for treatment of haemodialysis cramps. Nephrol Dialysis Transpl. 2001;16:1448–51.
60. Holley JL, Bems J, Sheridan AM. Muscle cramps in dialysis patients. Available on the Up To Date website: http://www.uptodate.com/contents/muscle-cramps-in-dialysispatients; 2012.
61. Saha M, Allon M. Diagnosis, treatment, and prevention of hemodialysis emergencies. Clin J Am Soc Nephrol. 2017;12:357–69.
62. de Oliveira RM, de los Santos CA, Antonello I, d'Avila D. Warning: an anemia outbreak due to chloramine exposure in a clean hemodialysis unit—an issue to be revisited. Ren Fail. 2009;31:81–3.
63. Gordon SM, Bland LA, Alexander SR, Newman F, Arduino MJ, Jarvis WR. Hemolysis associated with hydrogen peroxide at a pediatric dialysis center. Am J Nephrol. 1990;10:123–7.
64. Coulliette AD, Arduino MJ. Hemodialysis and water quality. Seminars in dialysis; 2013: Wiley Online Library. p. 427–38.
65. Berkes SL, Kahn SI, Chazan JA, Garella S. Prolonged hemolysis from overheated dialysate. Ann Intern Med. 1975;83:363–4.
66. Jepson R, Alonso E. Overheated dialysate: a case study and review. Nephrol Nurs J. 2009;36:551.
67. Daugirdas JT, Blake PG, Ing TS. Handbook of dialysis. Lippincott Williams & Wilkins; 2007.

68. Tharmaraj D, Kerr PG. Haemolysis in haemodialysis. Nephrology. 2017;22:838–47.
69. Holden RM, Harman GJ, Wang M, Holland D, Day AG. Major bleeding in hemodialysis patients. Clin J Am Soc Nephrol. 2008;3:105–10.
70. Jose MD, Marshall MR, Read G, et al. Fatal dialysis vascular access hemorrhage. Am J Kidney Dis. 2017;70:570–5.
71. Lohr JW, Schwab SJ. Minimizing hemorrhagic complications in dialysis patients. J Am Soc Nephrol. 1991;2:961–75.
72. Daugirdas JT, Bernardo AA. Hemodialysis effect on platelet count and function and hemodialysis-associated thrombocytopenia. Kidney Int. 2012;82:147–57.
73. Knudsen F, Nielsen AH. Polycarbonate versus cuprophan dialyzers: effect on platelet function. Blood Purif. 1984;2:173–80.
74. El Golli-Bennour E, Kouidhi B, Dey M, et al. Cytotoxic effects exerted by polyarylsulfone dialyser membranes depend on different sterilization processes. Int Urol Nephrol. 2011;43:483–90.
75. Gameiro J, Jorge S, Lopes JA. Haemodialysis-related-heparin-induced thrombocytopenia: case series and literature review. Nefrología (English Edition). 2018;38:551–7.
76. Hu X, Sang Y, Yang M, Chen X, Tang W. Prevalence of chronic kidney disease-associated pruritus among adult dialysis patients: a meta-analysis of cross-sectional studies. Medicine. 2018;97
77. Verduzco HA, Shirazian S. CKD-associated pruritus: new insights into diagnosis, pathogenesis, and management. Kidney Int Reports. 2020;5:1387–402.
78. Inui S. Nalfurafine hydrochloride to treat pruritus: a review. Clin Cosmetic Investig Dermatol. 2015;8:249.
79. Sklar AH, Riesenberg LA, Silber AK, Ahmed W, Ali A. Postdialysis fatigue. Am J Kidney Dis. 1996;28:732–6.
80. Sklar A, Newman N, Scott R, Semenyuk L, Schultz J, Fiacco V. Identification of factors responsible for post-dialysis fatigue. Am J Kidney Dis. 1999;34:464–70.
81. Jadoul M, Poignet J-L, Geddes C, et al. The changing epidemiology of hepatitis C virus (HCV) infection in haemodialysis: European multicentre study. Nephrol Dialysis Transpl. 2004;19:904–9.
82. Jadoul M, Bieber BA, Martin P, et al. Prevalence, incidence, and risk factors for hepatitis C virus infection in hemodialysis patients. Kidney Int. 2019;95:939–47.
83. Rahnavardi M, Moghaddam SMH, Alavian SM. Hepatitis C in hemodialysis patients: current global magnitude, natural history, diagnostic difficulties, and preventive measures. Am J Nephrol. 2008;28:628–40.
84. Soi V, Moore CL, Kumbar L, Yee J. Prevention of catheter-related bloodstream infections in patients on hemodialysis: challenges and management strategies. Int J Nephrol Renov Dis. 2016;9:95.
85. Shih WV, Wong C. Priapism and hemodialysis: case report and literature review. Clin Nephrol. 2018;90:64.
86. Gatland D, Tucker B, Chalstrey S, Keene M, Baker L. Hearing loss in chronic renal failure-hearing threshold changes following haemodialysis. J R Soc Med. 1991;84:587.
87. Bazzi C, Venturini C, Pagani C, Arrigo G, D'Amico G. Hearing loss in short-and long-term haemodialysed patients. Nephrol Dialysis Transpl. 1995;10:1865–8.
88. Bansal S, Ansons A, Vishwanath M. Hypotension-induced blindness in haemodialysis patients. Clin Kidney J. 2014;7:387–90.
89. Wang L, Yin G, Yu Z, Chen N, Wang D. Effect of hemodialysis on eye coats, axial length, and ocular perfusion pressure in patients with chronic renal failure. J Ophthalmol. 2018;2018

19 Peritoneal Dialysis

Angela Yee-Moon Wang

Clinical Scenario

A 68-year old woman with long-standing diabetes mellitus and stage 4 chronic kidney disease (CKD), followed up at the renal clinic showed gradual deterioration in kidney function over the last few years. In the past 6 months, her kidney function has deteriorated further. She lives with her husband, and carries out her daily activities independently, and also looks after her family. Clinically, she is asymptomatic. On examination, her blood pressure is 150/95, she has a mild pallor over her palmar creases and conjunctiva. Her chest is clear on auscultation, but there is mild bilateral pedal edema. Her blood tests show a blood haemoglobin of 9 g/dL, her serum sodium 142 mmol/L, and potassium 5.4 mmol/L, urea is 37.8 mmol/L, and creatinine 450 μmol/L, her estimated glomerular filtration rate (eGFR) using CKD-EPI equation is 8.1 mL/min/1.73 m^2, her serum bicarbonate is 19 mmol/L, serum albumin is 35 g/L, and adjusted serum calcium is 2.34 mmol/L, and phosphate is 2.10 mmol/L.

How would you counsel the patient about her options for kidney replacement therapy?

A. Y.-M. Wang (✉)
Department of Medicine, Queen Mary Hospital, the University of Hong Kong, Pokfulam, Hong Kong
e-mail: angela_wang@connect.hku.hk

Introduction

Peritoneal dialysis (PD) is one of the main kidney replacement therapies (KRT) that can be carried out at home for patients with end stage kidney disease (ESKD). To carry out PD, patients need to have a catheter placement into peritoneal cavity. Dialysis fluid is instilled into the peritoneal cavity through the catheter and allowed to dwell for 4–6 h. Uraemic retention solutes are removed through the semi-permeable peritoneal membrane by diffusion. Simultaneously, ultrafiltration takes place through the peritoneal membrane, with the dialysis fluid glucose acting as an osmotic agent. The peritoneal membrane characteristics differ among patients and affect peritoneal membrane transport kinetics of fluid and solutes. Peritoneal membrane characteristics may change over time in individual patients due to uremia, diabetes, dialysis procedure, dialysis fluids, drugs, peritoneal infections or inflammation. This chapter aims to give a practical guidance to clinicians delivering PD therapy. The topics include: assessing and preparing kidney failure patients for PD and contraindications to PD. A brief description of the different PD modalities, solutions, prescription, and key principles in delivering high quality goal-directed PD will be given. The chapter will outline assessments of residual kidney function (RKF), indices of dialysis adequacy, peritoneal membrane transport characteristics as well as quality of PD therapy. A

D. Banerjee et al. (eds.), *Management of Kidney Diseases*,
https://doi.org/10.1007/978-3-031-09131-5_19

clinical approach to low clearance and low drain volume in PD will be discussed.

Assessing and Preparing Kidney Failure Patients for PD

The provision of pre-dialysis education and decision aids increase the likelihood of patients choosing home dialysis therapy such as PD. Home dialysis or PD provides patients more freedom and flexibility with their time and improves their sense of well-being. When being told of the need for dialysis, patients very often have difficulties accepting it and are fearful that dialysis initiation might impact their work, personal life, travel and quality of life. Pre-dialysis education provided by a multidisciplinary team of experienced staff plays an essential role in alleviating fear and anxiety of patients, help patients to better understand kidney failure, face and accept dialysis, make their preferred choice of dialysis modality, prepare and cope with life on dialysis better and maintain a feeling of control with their health condition. Generally, patients should be referred to pre-dialysis education at least 4–6 months before dialysis initiation or when their eGFR falls below 15 mL/min/1.73 m. The multidisciplinary team involved in giving pre-dialysis education should include experienced nephrologist, renal nurse, dietitian, physiotherapist, psychologist, and social worker. The program should be designed according to local settings, culture, staff availability and patient load in individual hospitals. Lack of patient preparedness and an urgent start to dialysis are associated with lower survival and higher morbidity.

In assessing patients planning for PD therapy, a careful history should be taken in relation to their co-morbidities, bowel habits, personal hygiene, and prior abdominal surgeries. Patients' general condition, ability to perform PD, family support and home environment need assessment. Assisted PD may be considered in elderly patients or patients with mental or physical disabilities who choose PD.

PD is contraindicated if the peritoneal cavity is obliterated or the membrane is not functional, for example due to peritoneal adhesions or catheter placement is not possible. Obesity may present a challenge but is not a contraindication to PD. Obese patients receiving PD may be at an increased risk of catheter leak, hernias, exit site infection, and peritonitis compared with non-obese patients. A high body mass index may lead to inadequate solute clearance especially with loss of RKF, thus requiring larger dwell volumes. In morbidly obese patient, an extended catheter with a high abdominal or pre-sternal exit site may be used to avoid placement in a skin fold or the pannus region, but this would require considerable operator experience. A history of previous abdominal surgery does not preclude percutaneous PD catheter placement unless extensive adhesions are present or anticipated. Polycystic kidneys may increase intra-abdominal pressure and increase risk of hernias. However, PD has been successfully performed in these patients. Thus, the decision of modality choice in patients with polycystic kidneys need to be individualized, taking into consideration the enlarged kidneys and/or liver size, patients' body build and sense of abdominal fullness with the enlarged kidneys and/or liver. Patients with chronic constipation, diverticular disease and other causes of abnormal colonic distention may be unsuitable candidates for PD. Patients with cirrhosis and ascites are at an increased risk of spontaneous bacterial peritonitis and protein loss, but PD is not contraindicated. PD has been successfully performed in these patients and the PD catheter allows drainage of ascites.

Choice in PD Modality

The choice of PD modality should be personalized, involving a shared decision-making approach between physicians and patients and is the modality that patient chooses after receiving dialysis education and decision support. Patients and caregivers need to be informed of the challenges, considerations, and trade-offs of the different dialysis modalities so that modality selection can be tailored to their individual health and social circumstances.

PD Catheter Placement

PD catheter can be placed by traditional open surgical techniques, laparoscopic implantation, or percutaneous insertion. Percutaneous insertion is preferred because it can be done under local anaesthesia, is less invasive and less costly. Physicians can be easily trained to perform percutaneous PD catheter insertion and this significantly minimizes delays in arranging catheter insertions. Both laparoscopy and open surgery typically require general anaesthesia, are most costly and usually reserved for cases with previous abdominal surgeries. In placing a PD catheter (double cuffed preferred), the catheter coil must be positioned in the most dependent region of the peritoneal space: the posterior low pelvis. Meticulous attention should be placed to the location of the catheter exit site, creation of an inferiorly angled tunnel through the rectus abdominis muscle, and establish a stable position of catheter coil within the pelvic cul-de-sac. Prophylactic antibiotics should be given prior to catheter operation. After catheter placement, a breathable dressing must completely cover the abdominal incision wound and catheter exit site. Both the wound and exit site dressing should be kept dry and intact. Unless the catheter is used immediately as part of an urgent-start program, a minimum 2-week healing time is needed to ensure tissue ingrowth of the catheter cuffs and prevent fluid leaks prior to starting PD.

Urgent Start PD

Urgent start PD is defined as the situation in which PD needs initiation in less than 48 h after presentation to correct life-threatening complications. Non-urgent start refers to those in which dialysis initiation can be delayed more than 48 h after presentation. A planned approach is one in which the modality has been chosen prior to the need for dialysis and there is an access ready for use at the initiation of dialysis. An unplanned start is dialysis initiation when access is not ready for use or requires hospitalization or when dialysis is initiated with a modality that is not the patient's choice.

PD is possible in both planned or unplanned and urgent or nonurgent start. However, patients with hyperkalemia, volume overload, or marked uremia are not good candidates for urgent-start PD.

The major barriers to an urgent-start PD program are lack of operators who can place a PD catheter within the urgent start time frame and limited capacity of the health care facility to support PD for urgent-start patients and nursing manpower to train patients at short notice (Table 19.1). Where technical expertise in PD catheter placement is lacking, this can be addressed by increasing training of nephrologists. In urgent start, PD patients may have limited time to receive required education for an informed decision making on their initial choice of modality. These patients need to be provided with the required education and support to enable transition to their preferred modality when feasible.

Starting PD exchanges shortly after PD catheter placement instead of waiting for 2 weeks period for the cuff ingrowth and abdominal wound healing requires treatment modifications include doing intermittent PD in hospital in

Table 19.1 Institutional infrastructure setup required for urgent-start PD programs

(i) Ability to place a peritoneal catheter immediately within 48 h;
(ii) Staff education regarding use of catheter immediately after placement;
(iii) Administrative support in inpatient and outpatient settings;
(iv) Identification of appropriate candidates for urgent-start PD;
(v) Utilization of protocols in every step of the urgent-start process from patient selection for PD through appropriate post-discharge follow-up.

recumbent position and reducing instillation volume to prevent leaks.

Initiation of PD Therapy for End-Stage Kidney Disease

For patients who choose PD modality, initiation of therapy should be considered when one or more of the following are present:

(i) symptoms or signs attributable to kidney failure (e.g., neurological signs and symptoms attributable to uremia, pericarditis, anorexia, medically resistant acid-base or electrolyte abnormalities, reduced energy level, weight loss with no other potential explanation, intractable pruritus, or bleeding);

(ii) inability to control volume status or blood pressure;

(iii) progressive deterioration in nutritional status refractory to interventions.

Initiation of PD therapy should not solely be based on numerical values of eGFR.

PD Modalities

PD can be performed manually or via automated system. Continuous ambulatory peritoneal dialysis (CAPD) is done manually. Automated peritoneal dialysis (APD) includes: continuous cyclic peritoneal dialysis (CCPD), intermittent peritoneal dialysis (IPD), tidal peritoneal dialysis (TPD). Details of the different modalities are outlined in Table 19.2.

Table 19.2 A Summary of Different forms of PD modalities prescription

CAPD	Introduced in 1976 by Popovich and Moncrief and later modified by Oreopoulos as a wearable, portable form of dialysis, not requiring any equipment other than the disposable PD solution bags and a tube connecting the bag to patient's PD catheter to instill PD fluids into patient's peritoneal cavity. Prescription can be modified based on clinical status, sense of well-being, nutrition status, volume and blood pressure control, dietary compliance, biochemical parameters and indices of dialysis adequacy, taking into account patient's work and lifestyle pattern. Prescription can be initiated with 1.5% 2 L × 2 or 3 exchanges and one night time exchange of around 8–10 days, taking into consideration patient's body build, amount of RKF, urine volume and dietary intake. CAPD can maintain a relatively steady physiological state, control volume status and blood pressure in most patients.
APD	Automated PD was introduced in the late 1970s with an aim to achieve higher solute and fluid removal than CAPD and to automate PD with a cycler during patient sleep time.
CCPD	Continuous PD performed using a cycler. Typical prescription includes 3–4 night time exchanges each of 2–3 L, depending on body build, clearance needs and residual kidney function (RKF) and a single long day dwell with 1.5–2 L PD fluid. It allows more flexibility in the number and volume of exchanges carried out during night time, and reduces to a single daytime exchange, allowing patients more free time during the day. CCPD also allows larger volumes to be used in the supine position and minimizes the risk of touch contamination.
IPD	Usually consists of frequent, short cycles performed over 12–24 h per session and peritoneal cavity was drained dry between sessions. Nocturnal IPD (NIPD) is performed nightly and is usually reserved for patients with high peritoneal solute transport and low ultrafiltration. The short cycles of NIPD allow better ultrafiltration than longer cycles of CAPD or CCPD in high transporter. The total PD exchange volume per treatment usually ranges between 8 and 12 L.
PD Plus	PD Plus refers to CCPD with an exchange added to the long day dwell hours. Usually 3 or 4 × 2 L PD exchanges are performed during the night for 8–10 h. The long day dwell is then split into two shorter daytime exchanges performed manually or cycler assisted to improve both clearance and ultrafiltration. It limits daytime exchanges to less than 7 h. It is usually used for patients of larger body build, anuric patients or patients who need more solute clearance.

Table 19.2 (continued)

TPD	It consists of an initial fill usually in the range of 2–2.5 L then a variable dwell and partial drain, usually half of the PD volume, leaving a residual volume in the peritoneal cavity. The cavity is refilled and this will repeat until the last exchange when all PD fluids are drained. There is usually a daytime exchange. The principle purpose of TPD is to enhance clearance of small solutes by reducing the normal loss of dialysis time with inflow and outflow of PD fluid. However, TPD has not been shown to be superior to APD in terms of clearance or ultrafiltration. TPD may be useful for patients with inflow or outflow pain, slow drainage or multiple alarms due to drainage problems. It is more costly and complex to implement.
Assisted PD	It is usually adopted in patients of which a caregiver, helper or nursing staff is required to carry out the PD procedure such as in elderly patients, patients with multi-morbidities who are unable to do the procedure themselves or those in aged home. It can be done either manually by CAPD or using a cycler.
Incremental PD	A strategy by which less than standard full dose PD is prescribed in patients starting PD treatment and the combination of RKF and peritoneal clearance achieved remains sufficient to achieve individual clearance goals. It can be adopted in patients with relatively well preserved RKF. It incurs less workload for patients and their caregivers to do PD, thus enabling them more free time for life participation. It also has the advantage of minimizing patients' exposure to glucose solutions. Incremental PD is more cost-saving for emerging countries.

PD Solutions

Constituents of PD Solutions

Commercially available PD solutions contain sodium (132–135 mmol/L), calcium (1.25–1.75 mmol/L), magnesium (0.5 mmol/L), chloride (95–103.5 mmol/L) and lactate (35–40 mmol/L) and varying concentrations of glucose/dextrose ranging from 1.36%/1.5%, 2.27%/2.5% and 3.86%/4.25%. The overall osmolality was 344–347, 395–398, and 483–486 mOsmol/L, respectively and aimed to facilitate ultrafiltration and removal of water-soluble uremic toxins through the peritoneal membrane while maintaining electrolyte and acid-base balance of PD patients.

Standard glucose solutions are acidic in pH (5.0–5.8) to prevent dextrose caramelization during the sterilization procedure. Lactate concentration varies between 35 to 40 mmol/L. Lactate is rapidly metabolized to bicarbonate in a 1:1 ratio in patients with normal liver function and maintains a high dialysate to plasma lactate concentration gradient required for continued absorption without lactate accumulation in the circulation.

With high lactate, high glucose concentration, high osmolality and high levels of glucose degradation products (GDPs) generated, long term use of these solutions are associated with progressive peritoneal membrane injury, neovascularization, peritoneal sclerosis and fibrosis. The low pH, high osmolarity and high glucose content of these solutions also inhibit phagocytic functions of peritoneal leukocytes and impair host immune defense mechanisms. Some patients may complain of inflow pain with these solutions.

Calcium concentration of these solutions varies between 1.25 and 1.75 mM with 1.75 mM being termed standard calcium and 1.25 mM being termed 'low calcium' but 1.25 mM is the more physiological calcium concentration. Use of 1.75 mM calcium dialysate is associated with more progression in coronary artery calcium score over 24 months than 1.25 mM calcium dialysate in hemodialysis, especially with poor phosphorus control. Furthermore, use of 1.25 mM calcium dialysate showed a significantly lower prevalence of histologically diagnosed low bone turnover than 1.75 mM calcium dialysate group. Although similar study is not available in PD patients, Kidney Disease Improving Global outcomes (KDIGO) 2017 CKD-mineral bone disease (MBD) guideline and International Society of Peritoneal Dialysis (ISPD) Adult Cardiovascular and Metabolic guideline 2015 suggested the use of 1.25 mM calcium-containing PD solution to avoid positive calcium balance or hypercalcemia.

Types of PD Solutions

Glucose-Based Solutions

The ultrafiltration rate across the peritoneum is directly proportional to the initial glucose osmotic gradient (Table 19.3)

Adverse Effects of Glucose-Based PD Solution

Cumulative glucose absorption through the peritoneum incurs negative effects to the peritoneum and systemically including worsening of insulin resistance, hyperglycemia, accumulation of atherogenic visceral fat, weight gain, dyslipidemia and worsening glycemic control in PD patients with diabetes.

The standard heat sterilization of glucose-based solutions accelerates the generation of GDPs. Glycated local proteins form advanced glycation end-products (AGEs). Both GDPs and AGEs are directly cytotoxic to the peritoneal mesothelial cells and contribute to the long-term bio-incompatibility of glucose-based solutions (Fig. 19.1). They cause mesothelial cell loss, inflammation, submesothelial fibrosis and thick-

Table 19.3 Ultrafiltration volume with different glucose concentrations

Glucose solution concentration	Average ultrafiltration volume (mL)
1.36%/1.5%	100–200
2.27%/2.5%	200–400
3.86%/4.25%	>400

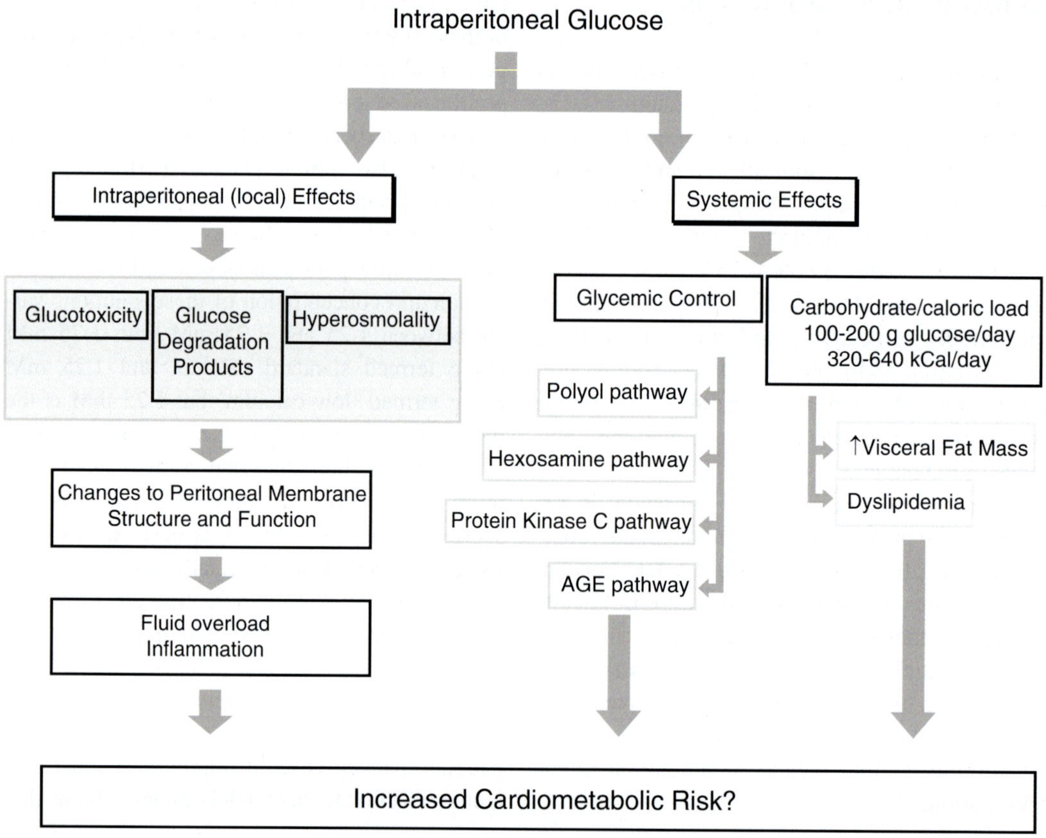

Fig. 19.1 Negative local and systemic impact of peritoneal glucose

ening, calcification, vasculopathy and diabetiform neoangiogenesis, resulting in changes to the peritoneal membrane structure and increased peritoneal solute transport (PSTR) with time on dialysis, requiring use of higher glucose concentration solutions for ultrafiltration. This would eventually lead to peritoneal membrane failure (PMF) over time and increase risk of volume overload. A high PSTR is associated with worse patient survival and a trend towards worse PD technique survival. Thus, a glucose sparing or glucose minimization PD regimen should be adopted in all PD patients as clinical condition and financial situation permit.

Almost two thirds of the PD fluid glucose are absorbed during a 4-h dwell and over 85% in an 8-h dwell with an average PSTR. This translates to an obligatory absorption of 43 g and 73 g of glucose with an 8-h dwell of 2.5% and 4.25% solutions, respectively. Exposure to glucose-based PD solution is associated with more weight gain, truncal fat mass and visceral adiposity increase than use of non-glucose-based PD solutions. Increased abdominal adiposity also contributes to a higher cardiovascular risk in PD patients. High glucose solutions may also add satiety and reduce appetite.

Glucose Polymer Solution or Icodextrin

Icodextrin is a starch-derived, branched, water soluble glucose polymer with an average molecular weight between 13,000 and 19,000 Daltons. Commercially available 7.5% icodextrin solution has a sodium concentration of 133 mmol/L and a lactate concentration of 40 mmol/L and is iso-osmotic (284 mOsmol/L). Icodextrin is not significantly metabolized in the peritoneum and is slowly absorbed into the bloodstream via the lymph vessels, with around 40% being absorbed after a 12 h period and is metabolized into oligosaccharides and maltose by circulating α-amylase (Fig. 19.2). Maltose cannot be metabolized in the circulation of humans as maltase is not in the circulation but is present in the kidney and intracellularly in the body. As icodextrin does not get reabsorbed, it is a superior osmotic agent and has superior ultrafiltration capacity than glucose solution, especially when dwell for long hours.

Icodextrin is a useful salvage therapy in PD patients with refractory fluid overload or ultrafiltration failure and may prolong PD technique survival (Table 19.4). PD patients using icodextrin achieved significantly better daily peritoneal ultrafiltration and had lower incidence of uncon-

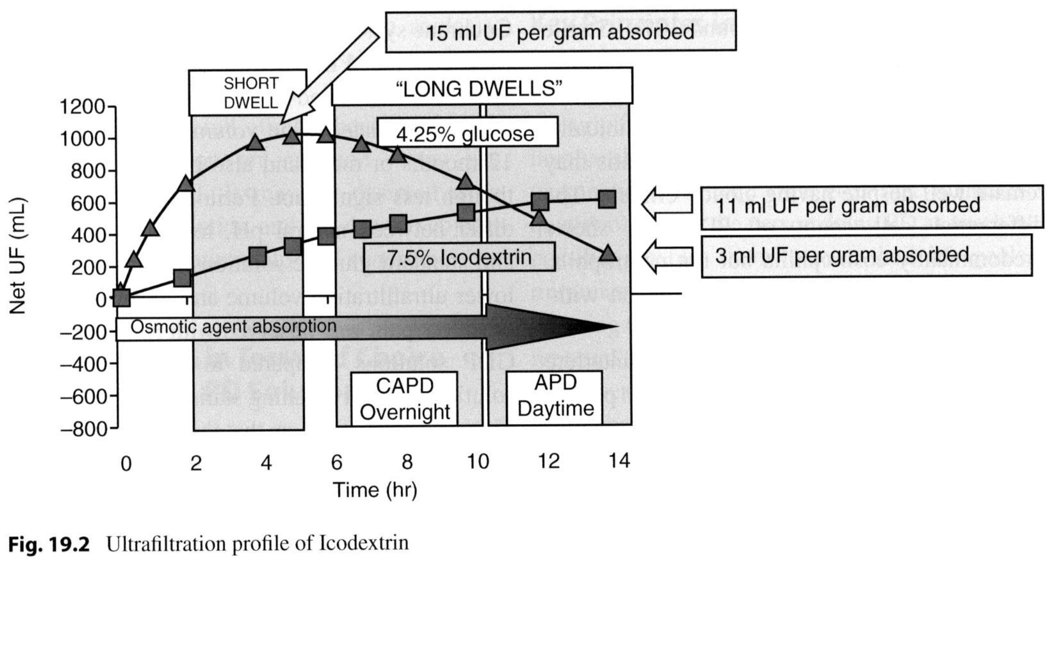

Fig. 19.2 Ultrafiltration profile of Icodextrin

PD prescription they receive. Patients doing PD should be educated about their condition and be informed about their prognosis and be given the opportunity to define their goals of care. PD can be prescribed in a variety of ways and should take into account local resources, person's wishes regarding lifestyle and the family's/caregivers' wishes if they are providing assistance (Fig. 19.3). PD infection, cardiovascular disease, mortality, PD failure and life participation were ranked the top core outcome domains in the Standardized Outcomes in Nephrology (SONG) initiative by all stakeholders (Table 19.7).

The following assessments should be included to ensure high-quality PD care.

(a) Patient reported outcome measures assess how a person doing PD is experiencing life and his/her feeling of well-being. It should take into consideration the person's symptoms, impact of the PD regimen on the person's life, mental health and social circumstances.

According to the ISPD 2020 guideline, patient's perception of their health-related quality of life (HRQOL) should be assessed routinely. This should take into account assessment of patient's symptoms, experience, patient reported outcome measures (PROMS), impact of the dialysis treatment regimen, and the psychosocial status of the patient. Treatment should be adjusted and modified based on patients' HRQOL, including symptom management, adjustments in dialysis treatment regimens, and clearly defining the goals of care.

Table 19.7 Domains to be addressed in patients receiving PD

Cognitive dysfunction	Uremic pruritus
Family and marital discord	Anorexia, nausea
Depression	Restless legs
Anxiety	Satisfaction with dialysis treatment regimen
Fatigue	Impact of the treatment regimen on their life
Lethargy	Satisfaction with care provided
Physical functioning	Caregiver burden
Sexual dysfunction	Abdominal discomfort, anorexia appetite, nausea, vomiting
Symptoms of neuropathy	Additional physical symptoms
Sleep disturbances	

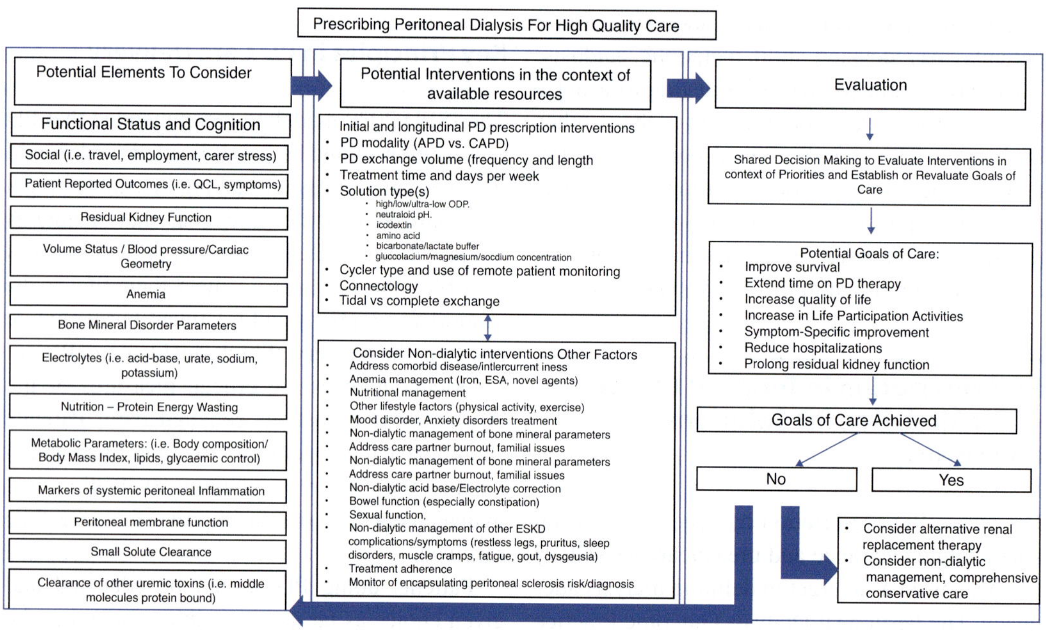

Fig. 19.3 Prescribing high quality PD

(b) Volume status is an important part of PD delivery. Urine output and fluid removed by PD both contribute to euvolemia. Regular assessment of volume status, including blood pressure and clinical examination, should be part of routine PD care.

(c) Nutrition status should be assessed regularly through evaluation of the patient's appetite, clinical examination, body weight measurements and blood tests (potassium, bicarbonate, phosphate, albumin). Dietary intake of potassium, phosphate, sodium, protein, carbohydrate and fat may need to be assessed and adjusted as well.

Various nutritional indices including body weight changes, appetite, subjective global assessment (SGA), serum albumin, handgrip strength may be used.

Hypokalemia is associated with poor nutritional status and adverse outcomes including peritonitis. Hypoalbuminemia is more common in PD than hemodialysis and is associated with PEW and peritoneal protein losses (Table 19.8). Hyperphosphatemia is multifactorial and associated with adverse outcomes in PD. Factors to consider include patients' dietary intake, compliance to phosphate binders, RKF and PD prescription.

Table 19.8 International Society of Renal Nutrition and Metabolism Consensus Criteria to diagnose protein-energy wasting (PEW)

Dietary intake
Unintentional low dietary energy intake <25 kcal/kg/day for at least 2 months
Unintentional low dietary protein intake <0.8 g/kg/day for at least 2 months
Body mass
Body mass index <23 kg/m^2
Unintentional weight loss over time: 5% over 3 month or 10% over 6 month
Total body fat <10%
Muscle mass
Muscle wasting: Reduced muscle mass 5% over 3 m or 10% over 6 month
Reduced mid-arm muscle circumfrence area >10% in relation to 50th percentile of reference population
Creatinine appearance
Serum biochemical parameters
Serum albumen <38 g/L (bromcresol green method)
Serum prealbumin (transthyretin) <300 mg/L
Serum cholesterol <100 mg/L

The diagnosis of PEW is made based on the presence of three out of the four characteristics listed in the table above. Unintentional weight loss should lead one to consider the presence of PEW. Loss of 5% of non-edematous weight within 3 months or an unintentional loss of 10% of non-edematous weight over the past 6 months is an indicator of PEW, independent of weight-for-height measures. Loss of body fat and muscle mass are considered as important criteria for diagnosing PEW. Inflammatory markers such as C-reactive protein are usually elevated in the setting of PEW.

(d) Removal of uremic solutes may be estimated using Kt/Vurea and/or creatinine clearance. Both are measures of small solute clearance.

Residual Kidney Function

RKF is an important parameter in predicting clinical outcomes of PD patients and its contribution is stronger than PD clearance. Having a better preserved RKF is associated with better small solutes and middle molecule uremic retention solutes clearance, better extracellular volume control, less inflammation, better control of CKD-bone mineral disease, better nutrition status and less resting hypercatabolism, thus contributing to overall better survival and cardiovascular outcomes and better quality of life (Fig. 19.4). PD patients with faster decline in RKF or urine volume were associated with worse patient survival and technique survival. It is therefore imperative to measure urine volume or RKF regularly in PD patients (Table 19.9).

Preserving Residual Kidney Function in PD Patients

It is generally recognized that avoid overdehydration and hypotensive episodes as well as avoid nephrotoxins and iodinated contrast use may be important. Diuretics increases urine volume and sodium excretion and minimizes use of hypertonic PD glucose solutions but did not preserve RKF.

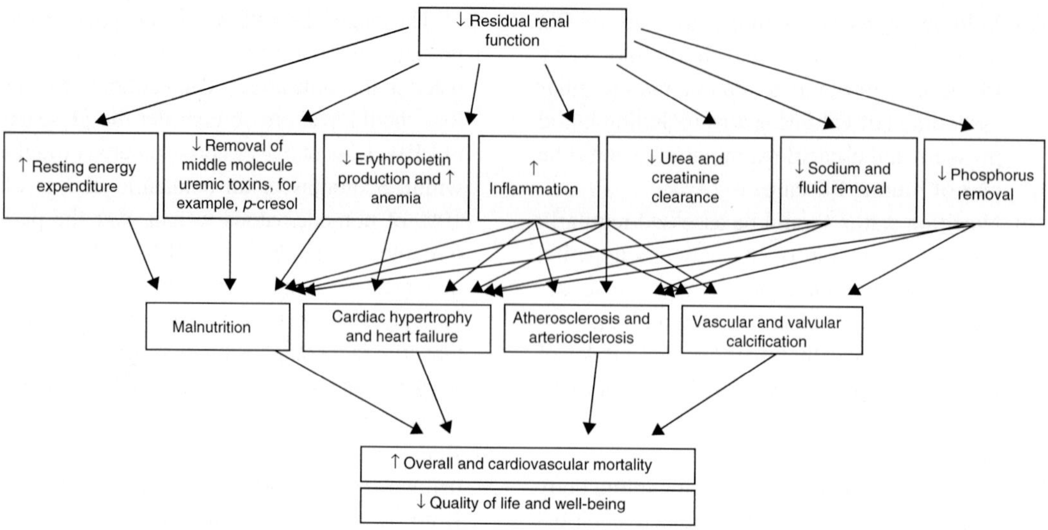

Fig. 19.4 Importance of RKF

Table 19.9 Recommendations on RKF

• RKF should be monitored at least once every 6 months in PD patients with urine output
• Management should focus on preserving RKF as long as possible in PD patients.

Neutral pH, low GDP biocompatible PD solution was associated with better preserved RKF and greater urine volumes for use greater than 12 months. The ISPD Adult Cardiovascular and Metabolic Guidelines recommended that neutral pH, low GDP solutions should be considered for better preservation of RKF if used for 12 months or more (2B). On the other hand, glucose polymer or icodextrin solution has no significant effect on RKF in PD patients (Fig. 19.5).

Two very small trials suggested better preservation of RKF with angiotensin converting enzyme inhibitors or angiotensin receptor blockers. A small trial suggested benefit of ketoacid supplemented low protein diet in preserving RKF in PD patients. Two small single-arm pilot studies suggested that oral N-acetylcysteine 1200 mg twice daily for 2–4 weeks may be useful in increasing urine volume and residual GFR. These preliminary findings need further confirmation in adequately powered RCTs. There is no conclusive evidence to suggest the modality of PD, namely APD versus continuous form of PD may influence the rate of decline in RKF differentially.

Assessment of RKF

Residual glomerular filtration rate (GFR) is estimated by averaging 24-hour urine urea and creatinine clearance and is normalized to body surface area. Unmodified urine creatinine clearance substantially overestimates the true GFR due to tubular secretion of creatinine while renal urea clearance underestimates GFR. At a minimum, urine volume should be measured and tracked regularly.

Assessment of Indices of Dialysis Adequacy

'Dialysis adequacy' is used to denote small solute clearance, namely urea clearance normalized to total body water (Kt/V) and creatinine clearance, normalized to body surface area (CrCl) (150) in PD patients. Both are comprised of two components, namely clearance from RKF and clearance from PD. Kt/V and CrCl are estimated from the urea and creatinine output from the

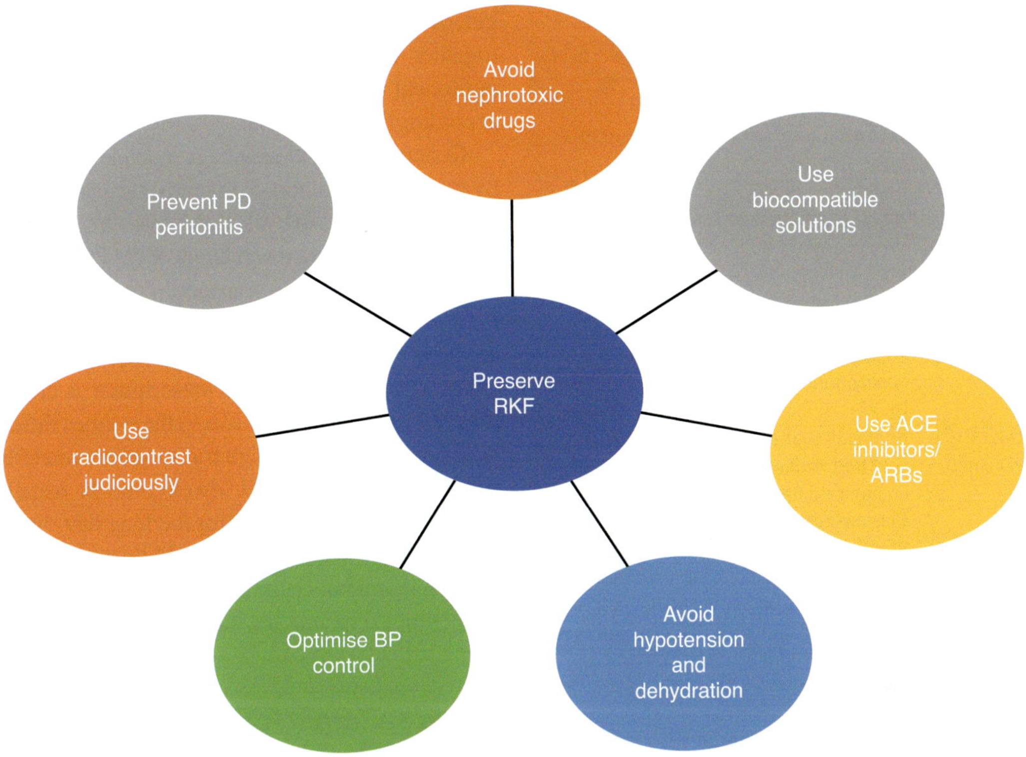

Fig. 19.5 Potential therapeutic strategies that may preserve RKF

drained effluent and urine collected during a simultaneous 24 h period together with a blood sample collected for serum urea and creatinine. Both Kt/V and CrCl values are conventionally expressed as weekly. In APD, the effluent volumes involved may be larger. APD patients are usually trained to record or measure total effluent volumes at home using the machine reading and bring back a representative aliquot of the dialysate to clinic for measurement of urea and creatinine concentrations.

In CAPD, serum urea and creatinine may not fluctuate much during the day and the timing of blood sampling for urea and creatinine may not be as critical. In APD, however, serum urea and creatinine may vary 10% or more from a trough value after stopping PD in the morning to peak levels before patient resumes PD in the evening. Thus, in patients receiving APD with no day dwell, serum samples should be collected approximately half way between the hours with no day dwell.

Estimation of Normalized Protein Nitrogen Appearance (nPNA)

nPNA, a surrogate of dietary protein intake can be estimated using the Randerson formula. However, the equation assumes that the patient is metabolically stable and urea generation, excretion and other nitrogen losses are proportional and in equilibrium to the amount of protein intake. These formulas are derived using the same variables as Kt/V (Table 19.10).

Kidney Disease Outcome Quality Initiative (KDOQI) 2020 recommended a dietary protein intake of 1.0–1.2 g /kg body weight for metabolically stable PD patients to maintain a stable nutritional status. A daily energy intake of 25–35 kcal/kg ideal body weight per day (including energy derived from peritoneal glucose absorption) based on age, gender, level of physical activity, body composition, weight status goals, CKD stage, and concurrent illness or presence of inflammation to maintain normal nutritional sta-

Table 19.10 Summary of various equations

nPNA by Randerson	10.76[a](UNA/1.44 + 1.46) and UNA is in g/day
Residual GFR	Average of (24 h urine urea clearance + creatinine clearance in mL/min)
Total Kt/V	Summation of PD Kt/V and renal Kt/V
PD KT/V	[(24 h PD volume in L)[a](24 h PD fluid urea concentration in mmol/L)/Plasma urea concentration in mmol/L] and normalized by V
Renal Kt/V	[(24 h urine volume in L)[a](24 h urine urea concentration in mmol/L)/Plasma urea concentration in mmol/L] and normalized by V
Total CrCl	Summation of PD CrCl and renal CrCl
PD CrCl	[(24 h PD volume in L)[a](24 h PD fluid creatinine concentration in umol/L)/Plasma creatinine concentration in umol/L] and normalized by BSA
Renal CrCl	[(24 h urine volume in L)[a](average of 24 h urine urea and creatinine concentration in umol/L)/Plasma creatinine concentration in umol/L] and normalized by BSA
V	2.447 + (0.3362 × BW in kg) + (0.1074 × BH in cm) − (0.09516 × age in years) for male −2.097 + (0.2466 × BW in kg) + (0.1069 × BH in cm) for female
BSA	$0.007184 \times \text{BW in kg}^{0.425} \times \text{BH in cm}^{0.725}$

UNA Urea nitrogen appearance, *V* Total body water estimated by Watson method, *BSA* Body surface area, *BW* Body weight, *BH* Body height

[a]These equations assumed a steady state, where urea nitrogen output equals to urea generation. The Randerson equation assumed the average daily dialysate protein loss is 7.3 g per day. In PD patients with substantial protein losses in dialysate or urine, these losses must be added to the equation in calculating nPNA

tus is recommended for metabolically stable PD patients.

Peritoneal Equilibration Test (PET)

It is a simple bedside test that assesses the diffusive transport capacity of urea, creatinine and other solutes and ultrafiltration across the semi-permeable membrane. It involves doing a 4 h dwell with a 2 L bag of 2.5% PD solution during which the ratio of dialysate to plasma creatinine concentration at 4 hour and the ratio of dialysate glucose concentration at 4 h to 0 h are estimated together with ultrafiltration volume at 4 h. The peritoneal transport characteristics are defined accordingly (Fig. 19.6).

Generally, urea clearance is much less affected by peritoneal transport characteristics than CrCl in CAPD as over 90% of Kt/V and equilibration occurs with the long dwell hours of CAPD, regardless of peritoneal transport characteristics. Peritoneal membrane transport characteristics is an important consideration in PD modality (APD versus CAPD) and regimen prescription as creatinine clearance may show two to three times difference between low and high transporters even after a 4–6 h dwell. In APD, dwell time is usually shorter than CAPD except for the long day dwell. In anuric PD patients, there could be problems in achieving optimal clearance targets, depending on the peritoneal membrane transport characteristics.

Is There a Target for Small Solute Clearance?

Two large prospective RCTs did not observe any significant benefit on overall survival of PD patients by increasing peritoneal small solute clearance. In the Adequacy of PD in MEXico (ADEMEX) study, increasing weekly Kt/V from 1.62 to 2.13 (or weekly CrCl from 46.1 to 56.9 L/wk. per 1.73 m^2) had no significant effect on mortality risk in PD patients. In the randomized trial from Hong Kong of which PD patients were randomized to Kt/V targets of 1.7–2.0 and >2.0. no significant difference was observed in the overall survival between the group reaching Kt/V target of 1.7–2.0 and the group reaching Kt/V >2.0. There is no data to support benefit of further increasing total weekly Kt/V beyond 2.0 or total CrCl of over 60 L/week per 1.73 m^2.

The 2 trials raised important questions about previous focus on achieving small solute clearance targets in PD care delivery. In the 2020 ISPD guideline, high quality goal-directed PD should aim to achieve and maintain clinical euvolemia and blood pressure while taking RKF and its preservation into consideration, as well maintain good

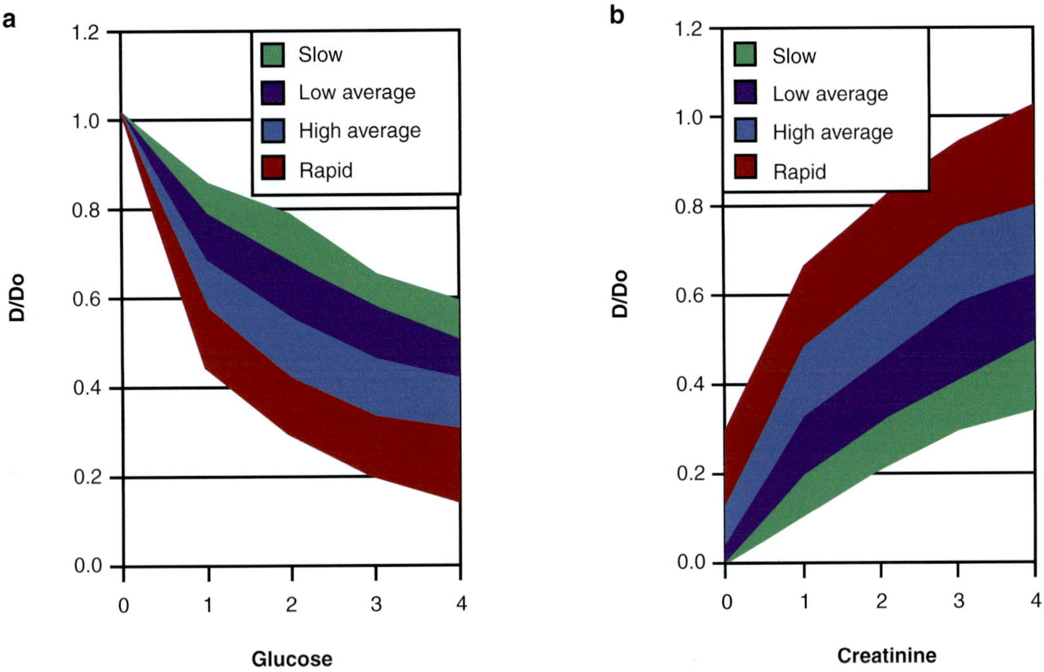

Fig. 19.6 Peritoneal equilibration test

Fig. 19.7 Factors to be reviewed in patients who remain symptomatic despite achieving a Kt/V >1.7

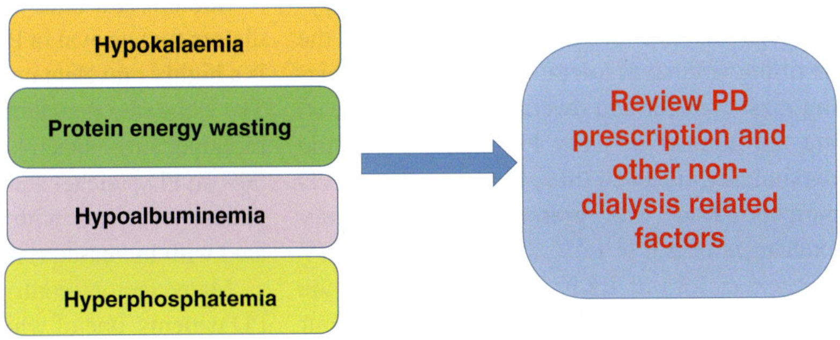

nutrition status, perceived well-being and quality of life of PD patients so for their life participation and not for the role purpose of reaching an arbitrary numerical clearance target.

Patients who remain symptomatic despite a Kt/V >1.7 should have other dialysis and non-dialysis related factors reviewed as possible contributing factors. In emerging countries, every effort should be made to conform to the same principles in PD prescription, taking into account resources limitation (Fig. 19.7).

There was weak evidence to suggest that anuric PD patients should have a weekly Kt/V of at least 1.7. In the NECOSAD (Netherlands Cooperative Study on the Adequacy of Dialysis) observational Study, peritoneal Kt/V <1.5 and CrCl <40 L/week per 1.73 m^2 were associated with higher mortality (175).

In elderly patients who are frail or have a poor prognosis, there may be a quality of life benefit from a modified dialysis prescription to minimize treatment burden (Table 19.11).

Table 19.11 Evaluations in PD patients with a low Kt/V or CrCl result

1. Are there incomplete or missed collection of 24 h urine and dialysate?
2. Any non-adherence to the dialysis prescription or missed cycles?
3. Any clinical and other biochemical evidence of inadequate dialysis?
4. Are the dialysis prescription, namely the number of cycles and the concentration of PD solutions optimal for the patient?
5. Are actual dwell times differ from that prescribed?
6. Any recent loss in residual urine volume and RKF?
7. Any incomplete drain
8. Any hypercatabolic conditions?

Evaluation of Patients with Low Delivered Urea/Creatinine Clearance Values

General Principles in Adjusting PD Prescription

If dialysis dose is confirmed inadequate, dialysis dose may be increased by increasing the instilling volume as tolerated, thereby maximizing mass transfer and dwell time or by increasing the number of daily PD exchanges while maximizing the dwell time. For example, for PD patients who are prescribed three daily exchanges of 2 L × 1.5% and have a low Kt/V because of loss of RKF, one may increase the dialysis dose by either increasing to four exchanges daily of 2 L × 1.5% or by increasing the volume per exchange to 2.3–2.5 L × 1.5% as required and as tolerated. If there is a need to increase ultrafiltration volume as well, then one may consider replacing 1.5% with 2.5% solution.

Ultrafiltration and Volume Control as a Treatment Target

Generally, a net ultrafiltration >200 mL from a standard 4-hour dwell of 2.27%/2.5% glucose/dextrose or > 400 ml from a standard 4-h dwell of 3.86%/4.25% glucose/dextrose solution is regarded as sufficient ultrafiltration. Values below this indicate relative ultrafiltration failure (UFF). Symptoms of UFF may not manifest overtly until RKF has declined significantly or completely lost.

Ultrafiltration is an important parameter for assessing adequacy of dialysis, and ultrafiltration has been shown to be associated with survival in anuric APD patients; low ultrafiltration volume below 750 ml per day was associated with a higher mortality (176). However, a numerical target for daily ultrafiltration volume was not recommended as the overall volume status depends also on the residual urine volume as well as salt and fluid intake of patients and there may be substantial intra-individual variation.

The ISPD guideline 2020 as well as the ISPD Cardiovascular and Metabolic guidelines 2015 emphasized the importance of maintaining euvolemia as one of the key treatment goals in PD. Attention should be paid to both urine volumes and PD ultrafiltration volumes.

Sodium and fluid removal are important predictors for survival in PD patients. Fluid overload is a highly prevalent complication in PD patients. The estimated prevalence of fluid overload using bioimpedance spectroscopy, was at least over 50% in PD patients and was even higher in anuric patients. Patients with fluid overload is associated with increased risk of mortality.

Many factors contribute to fluid overload in PD patients, one of which is low drain volume or ultrafiltration (Table 19.12). It is essential to take a thorough history and physical examination (Fig. 19.8 and Table 19.13).

High Transporters

Patients who are high transporters equilibrate very quickly and have excellent diffusive transport capacity. However, a major clinical problem encountered by high transporters is suboptimal ultrafiltration, low drain volume and inadequate solute clearance as the osmotic gradient for glucose dissipates relatively quickly. High transporters would be more suited to do short dwell times as in APD or NIPD using standard glucose solution and then a long day dwell using icodextrin.

Some patients may start as high transporters but some may gradually become high transporters over time on PD. A high peritoneal transport status is associated with an increased mortality. Proposed mechanisms for increased mortality observed in high transporters include fluid overload, chronic inflammation, increased peritoneal protein loss and increased risk of PEW.

Table 19.12 Factors contributing to fluid overload in PD patients

Patient related factors
- Adherence to dietary salt and fluid intake
- Compliance to PD regimen
- Loss of residual kidney function
- Blood glucose control
- Health literacy
- Heart disease and heart failure
- Inflammation
- Protein-energy wasting syndrome

Dialysis related factors
- Mechanical factors eg. catheter function, leaks, hernias, fibrin
- Low ultrafiltration due to
  - high peritoneal solute transport
  - peritoneal membrane failure
  - constipation
  - encapsulating peritoneal sclerosis

Low Transporters

Low transporters ultrafiltrate well but equilibrate slowly. Low transporters may do best with longer day dwells such as CAPD with a single overnight exchange or CCPD with fewer overnight exchanges.

Acute Peritoneal Membrane Dysfunction

Patients with acute peritonitis may develop acute reduction in drain volume and increased peritoneal solute transport. as a result of an increased effective surface are and an increased vascular

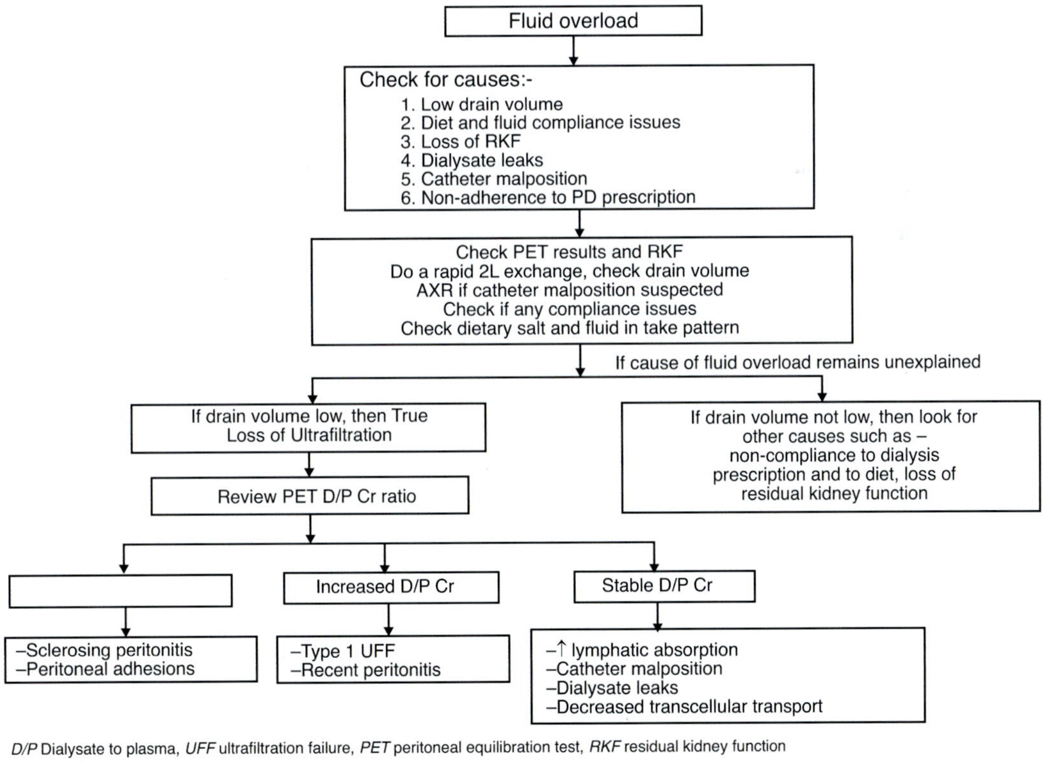

Fig. 19.8 Approach to patients with fluid overload

Table 19.13 Clinical evaluation in patient with low drain volume

If drain volume is low, review:
(i) any mechanical issues that may explain low drain volume
(ii) any constipation
(iii) is outflow position related
(iv) catheter position
(v) Any fibrin clots that may obstruct outflow
(vi) Any omental wrap
(vii) Peritoneal membrane transport characteristics
(viii) Any features to suggest peritoneal adhesions or encapsulating peritoneal sclerosis

permeability. Short term adjustment of PD prescription may be needed to improve ultrafiltration.

Ultrafiltration Failure (UFF)

Conventionally, UFF is defined as having a net ultrafiltration volume below 400mls with a standard 2 L 3.86% glucose solution during a 4 h exchange.

There are 3 types of UFF. Type I UFF is the commonest and is partly attributed to long-standing glucose exposure of the peritoneal membrane. Peritoneal membrane showed submesothelial fibrosis, vasculopathic changes and neovascularization. The neovascularization increases the effective peritoneal surface area, leading to more rapid PSTR. The process is thought to be mediated by vascular endothelial growth factor (VEGF) through induction of nitric oxide. Clinically, the osmotic gradient for glucose dissipates rapidly before adequate ultrafiltration has occurred due to very high PSTR. It usually has a more gradual onset and increases with time on PD. In some cases, temporary cessation of PD or resting the peritoneal membrane may allow re-mesothelialization and may transiently improve ultrafiltration capacity (216). However, in some cases, encapsulating peritoneal sclerosis (EPS) may develop after switching to hemodialysis.

The cumulative incidence of UFF was estimated to be 2.6% after 1 year on PD, rising to 9.5% after 2 years and to 30.9% after 6 years. Peritonitis may partly influence the time course of small solute and solute-free water transport. Patients with previous peritonitis showed an earlier and more pronounced increase in the mass transfer area coefficient for creatinine and glucose and a decrease in solute-free water transport and ultrafiltration rate compared to patients with no peritonitis. In long-term peritonitis-free PD patients, small solute transport decreased, while ultrafiltration increased.

Type II UFF occurs as a result of loss of peritoneal surface area, resulting in decrease in peritoneal transport of small solutes and water. This is less common and usually occurs in the context of peritoneal adhesions secondary to severe peritonitis or after surgical complications that substantially reduces peritoneal surface area and transport capacity for both solutes and water. Type II UFF may be a manifestation of encapsulating EPS although in early stages of EPS, a high rather than a low peritoneal transport is usually seen. EPS can be diagnosed by contrast CT abdomen.

Type III UFF occurs when lymphatic reabsorption of fluid from the peritoneal cavity is large enough to reduce ultrafiltration. It is a diagnosis by exclusion since peritoneal lymphatic flow is not measured in most PD centers (Table 19.14).

To evaluate UFF, a modified PET using 3.86% glucose solution is preferred over 2.5% dextrose solution to maximize osmotic drive (227). During the PET, the D/P sodium curve typically shows an initial fall due to high ultrafiltration rate. Ultrafiltration is low in sodium concentration initially due to sodium sieving. Dialysate sodium concentration reduces, resulting in a fall in the D/P sodium ratio. With the cessation of ultrafiltration later in the dwell, dialysate sodium gradually equilibrates with that of plasma, and D/P sodium ratio gradually returns back to baseline. Absence of the initial fall in D/P sodium ratio is a

Table 19.14 Summary of Characteristics in the 3 types of UFF

Types	Characteristics
I	Patients classically on PD for years, presented with a low drain volume, PET showed a high D/P creatinine ratio. Attributed to long exposure of peritoneal membrane to glucose solutions, leading to submesothelial fibrosis, vasculopathic changes and neovascularization of the peritoneum and an increase in the effective peritoneal surface area.
II	Patients classically presented with a low drain volume and PET showed a low D/P creatinine ratio. Decrease in peritoneal transport of small solutes and water due to loss of peritoneal surface area. Characterized by a decrease in the osmotic conductance to glucose and an attenuation of sodium sieving. Usually occurs in the context of peritoneal adhesions secondary to severe peritonitis, encapsulating peritonitis or after surgical complications.
III	Occurs when there is high lymphatic reabsorption of fluid from the peritoneal cavity that reduces ultrafiltration.

feature of UFF and typically seen in the early phase of EPS.

Current treatment for UFF is lacking. For Type 1 UFF, a period of peritoneal rest may transiently improve ultrafiltration capacity. For type II and III, permanent switch to hemodialysis is required.

Practice Points

- Pre-dialysis education involving a multidisciplinary team help patients to better understand kidney failure, accept dialysis, make their preferred choice of dialysis modality and maintain a feeling of control with their health condition. Pre-dialysis education has also been shown to facilitate patients choosing home peritoneal dialysis as the modality.
- In assessing patients suitability for PD therapy, it is important to assess patients' medical history, comorbidities, bowel habits, personal hygiene and prior abdominal surgeries as well as general condition, ability to perform PD, family support and home environment.
- PD is contraindicated if the peritoneal cavity is obliterated or membrane not functional due to peritoneal adhesions.
- Choice of PD modality should be personalized involving a shared decision-making approach between physicians and patients after patients are educated on the different modalities.
- PD is possible in both planned and unplanned and urgent or nonurgent start. In urgent start PD, patients have limited time to receive education for an informed decision making, these patients need to be provided the required education and support to enable transition to their preferred modality where feasible.
- For patients who chose PD modality, Initiation of therapy should be considered in the presence of symptoms or signs attributable to kidney failure, inability to control volume status or blood pressure and progressive deterioration in nutrition status due to uremic symptoms.
- In prescribing PD solutions, icodextrin is recommended to improve ultrafiltration independent of the dialysate to plasma creatinine ratio by the 2020 International Society of Peritoneal Dialysis (ISPD) Guideline.
- Neutral pH, low glucose degradation products solutions is recommended for better preservation of residual kidney function if used for 12 months or more according to the ISPD 2020 and 2015 guidelines.

- PD prescription should be 'goal-directed' and should involve shared decision-making in establishing a personalized realistic care goal that maintains quality of life for the person doing PD as much as possible, enables them to meet their life goals, minimize symptoms and treatment burden while ensuring the delivery of high quality care.
- In order to ensure high quality PD care, the following assessments should be included: (1) Patient reported outcome measures, (2) volume status, (3) nutrition status, (4) uremic solutes removal.
- Preserving residual kidney function (RKF) is an important treatment strategy in PD patients as having better preserved RKF is predictive of better clinical outcomes. RKF should be monitored at least once every 6 months in PD patients with urine output. Management should focus on preserving it as long as possible.
- Patients who remain symptomatic despite a Kt/V > 1.7 should have other dialysis and non-dialysis related factors reviewed as possible contributing factors. This include hypokalemia, protein energy wasting, hypoalbuminemia and hyperphosphatemia.
- Maintaining euvolemia is one of the key treatment goals in PD patients and attention should be paid to both urine volumes, PD ultrafiltration volumes as well as salt and fluid intake pattern of patients.
- Patients with low drain volume should evaluate any mechanical issues, constipation, whether drain is position-related, catheter position, any fibrin clots that may obstruct outflow, any omental wrap, peritoneal membrane function and any features to suggest peritoneal adhesions or encapsulating peritoneal sclerosis.

Conclusions

For the 68 year old lady discussed in the clinical case, peritoneal dialysis offers the advantages of being able to undergo kidney replacement therapy at home, while enjoying her family life, maintaining her residual kidney function, fewer dietary restrictions, a more gradual correction of her metabolic acidosis, whilst avoiding the complications, inconvenience and costs associated with in-centre haemodialysis. She will nevertheless require close monitoring of her peritoneal dialysis adequacy and ultrafiltration, and preparation for transplantation.

Questions

1. A 36-year-old man with end stage kidney failure due focal segmental glomerulosclerosis, on peritoneal dialysis for six years presented with shortness of breath and leg swelling. He used 15 L of glucose based peritoneal dialysis fluid with an osmolality of 395 mosmol/L for nighttime daily dialysis for the last few months. His ultrafiltration was 300 mL per day. He produced very little urine. On examination his blood pressure was 160/80 mmHg pulse 90 beats per min respiratory rate 20 breaths per minute, with leg oedema. His respiratory system exam revealed bibasilar crackles.

   What is most likely cause of his fluid retention?

   A. Increased plasma hydrostatic pressure
   B. Decreased plasma hydrostatic pressure
   C. Heart failure with preserved ejection fraction
   D. Low plasma osmotic pressure
   E. Lack of osmosis across the peritoneal membrane

Answer E Increased glucose concentration is associated with damage and fibrosis of the peritoneal membrane

2. A 55-year-old end stage kidney failure patient on peritoneal dialysis presented with recurrent abdominal pain fever and cloudy peritoneal effluent. She was treated for staphylococcal peritonitis a month before. On exam she had blood pressure of 130/84 mmHg, pulse 84 beats per minute, temperature 36 degrees Celsius. Her abdomen was soft and non-tender. Her peritoneal fluid showed 600 white cells per ml and culture grew Candida albicans.

   What is the next best step management?
   A. Start intraperitoneal vancomycin and intravenous gentamicin
   B. Start oral fluconazole
   C. Start intravenous amphotericin
   D. Start oral fluconazole and remove peritoneal dialysis catheter
   E. Start intravenous cefuroxime

Answer D Fungal infection is an indication for catheter removal, difficult to eradicate

3. A 56-year-old woman with known liver cirrhosis and ascites due to autoimmune hepatitis and ESKD due to IgA nephropathy was referred to advanced CKD clinic. Her eGFR was 15 ml/min. Physical examination showed ascites. She opted to have peritoneal dialysis for her ESKD.

   What is true about peritoneal dialysis in patients with liver cirrhosis?
   A. Associated with increased risk of peritonitis
   B. Associated with increased risk of peritoneal leak
   C. Increased risk of encapsulating peritonitis
   D. Does not help the drainage of ascites
   E. Peritoneal dialysis as a therapy for ESKD is contraindicated

Answer A PD in Cirrhosis patients can be done, helps drain the ascites but increases risk of infection

4. A 55 year-old man with IgA nephropathy presented in the advanced CKD clinic with an eGFR of 10 mL/min/1.73 m2, haemoglobin 102 g/L and leg oedema. He was slim and without any history of diabetes, hypertension or heart disease. He was prepared for a peritoneal catheter placement as PD was his modality of choice. What measures help and uncomplicated start of dialysis.
   A. Erythropoietin therapy before catheter placement
   B. Iron therapy before catheter placement
   C. Prophylactic antibiotic at catheter placement
   D. A surgical catheter placement as opposed to medical catheter placement
   E. Prophylactic anticoagulation

Answer C Prophylactic antibiotic is beneficial to prevent infections

5. A 56-year-old female with polycystic presented with tiredness and eGFR of 10 mL/min/1.73 m^2. She opted for peritoneal dialysis.

   What is not an indication to start dialysis?
   A. An eGFR of 10 mL/min/1.73 m^2
   B. Symptoms of nausea, vomiting and anorexia
   C. Fluid overload not responding to diuretic therapy
   D. Recurrent hyperkalaemia
   E. Weight loss and poor nutritional status

Answer A all but an absolute eGFR are indications for starting dialysis

Test your learning and check your understanding of this book's contents: use the "Springer Nature Flashcards" app to access questions using https://sn.pub/cz9Cok. To use the app, please follow the instructions in Chap. 1.

Further Reading

Brown EA, Blake PG, Boudville N, Davies S, de Arteaga J, Dong J, Finkelstein F, Foo M, Hurst H, Johnson DW, Johnson M, Liew A, Moraes T, Perl J, Shroff R, Teitelbaum I, Wang AY, Warady B. International Society for Peritoneal Dialysis practice recommendations: prescribing high-quality goal-directed peritoneal dialysis. Perit Dial Int. 2020;40(3):244–53. https://doi.org/10.1177/0896860819895364. Epub 2020 Jan 21.

Morelle J, Stachowska-Pietka J, Öberg C, Gadola L, La Milia V, Yu Z, Lambie M, Mehrotra R, de Arteaga J, Davies S. ISPD recommendations for the evaluation of peritoneal membrane dysfunction in adults: classification, measurement, interpretation and rationale for intervention. Perit Dial Int. 2021;41(4):352–72. https://doi.org/10.1177/0896860820982218. Epub 2021 Feb 10.

Boudville N, de Moraes TP. 2005 Guidelines on targets for solute and fluid removal in adults being treated with chronic peritoneal dialysis: 2019 update of the literature and revision of recommendations. Perit Dial Int. 2020;40(3):254–60. https://doi.org/10.1177/0896860819898307. Epub 2020 Jan 14.

Crabtree JH, Shrestha BM, Chow KM, Figueiredo AE, Povlsen JV, Wilkie M, Abdel-Aal A, Cullis B, Goh BL, Briggs VR, Brown EA, Dor FJMF. Creating and maintaining optimal peritoneal dialysis access in the adult patient: 2019 update. Perit Dial Int. 2019;39(5):414–36. https://doi.org/10.3747/pdi.2018.00232. Epub 2019 Apr 26.

Complications of Peritoneal Dialysis: Prevention and Management

20

Brett Cullis and Robert Freercks

Clinical Scenario

A 35 year old male PD patient presents with a 24 h history of nausea, vomiting and generalised abdominal pains. He has end stage kidney disease (ESKD) due to diabetes mellitus, and started dialysing via automated peritoneal dialysis (APD) six months ago. He has not noted any problems with drainage; he says that his bags have remained clear, and he continues to manage ultrafiltration of around 1 L per day, alongside a native urine output of 1 L per day. His most recent PET test, undertaken earlier this month, showed him to be a high average transporter. His PD catheter exit site is clean, and there is no purulent discharge emanating from this. He is currently apyrexial, is able to lie flat, and has no peripheral pitting oedema. His blood pressure was 124/84, and his pulse 64 beats per minute.

B. Cullis (✉)
Hilton Life Renal Unit, Hilton, South Africa

Department of Nephrology and Child Health, University of Cape Town, Cape Town, South Africa

R. Freercks
Department of Nephtrology, Livingstone Hospital, Port Elizabeth, South Africa

Department of Nephrology and hypertension, University of Cape Town, Cape Town, South Africa

Introduction

Peritoneal dialysis (PD) is a vital form of kidney replacement therapy, that—once patients (and their carers), are trained and comfortable with the rigorous hygiene involved in catheter care techniques—enables patients to dialyse safely and independently at home, often with very limited specialist support, for many years. Conversely, PD complications are not uncommon, and can lead to significant morbidity and mortality—particularly in lower middle income countries (LMIC), where the provision of alternative forms of kidney replacement therapy (KRT) is not guaranteed. PD complications can be simply divided into infective (75%) and non-infective causes (25%). Clinicians need to be well-versed in prevention, investigation and management of PD complications. In this chapter, we shall discuss in detail the complications of PD, and their appropriate management pathways and strategies for prevention.

Infective Complications

Apart from catheter malfunction, infections pose the biggest threat to the continuity of PD in an individual, and represent an important barrier to the uptake of PD. Where there may be no alternative forms of KRT in LMIC, this can lead to significant morbidity and mortality [1]. Clinicians must therefore be well-versed in the effective prevention and

D. Banerjee et al. (eds.), *Management of Kidney Diseases*,
https://doi.org/10.1007/978-3-031-09131-5_20

management of infection in PD, and should develop clear protocols in their own units for use by all staff.

Much progress has been made over the last few decades in addressing the prevention and treatment of infections in PD, and in providing sound recommendations for clinical practice. To this end, the International Society for Peritoneal Dialysis (ISPD) has published graded and pragmatic guidelines for clinical use which were recently updated in 2016 (peritonitis) and 2017 (catheter-related infection) [2, 3]. We will focus on many of these recommendation in this chapter, but it is important to note that the local context will determine which problems are prevalent in any specific area and recommendations will need to be adapted accordingly. Patients on PD are also at increased risk for systemic infections such as tuberculosis (TB), and other severe bacterial and viral illnesses, but this chapter will focus on those specific to PD.

It is recommended that each PD unit monitors the incidence of peritonitis as a quality control indicator. While the overall peritonitis rate should be less than 0.5 episodes per year at risk, the rate achieved will depend on local factors, including whether patients have been given a choice in terms of dialysis modality, clinic attendance, and possibly sociodemographic factors and comorbidities such as HIV and diabetes. Lower socioeconomic status has not been consistently shown to associate with peritonitis risk [4, 5].

Prevention of Infection

The key emphasis needs to be placed on adequate training of the patient by experienced staff in terms of hand hygiene, exit site care and exchange technique. Further specific measures have also been shown to be effective:

1. The administration of prophylactic antibiotics (with gram positive cover such as cefazolin or vancomycin) prior to catheter insertion.
2. Daily topical application of mupirocin or gentamicin preparations to the catheter exit site.
3. Adequate catheter immobilisation during daily care.
4. Modern connectology: The use of disconnect systems that utilize a "flush before fill" design and avoidance of manual spike systems.
5. The use of anti-fungal prophylaxis during antibiotic treatment for peritonitis (with nystatin or fluconazole, depending on local resistance and drug interaction concerns).
6. Soaking of the transfer set adapter in 10% povidone iodine solution at transfer set change [6].

Observational data has shown that automated peritoneal dialysis (APD) may be associated with a lower risk of peritonitis, but definitive data is lacking. Other measures that appear to be helpful but lack randomised data include the use of prophylactic antibiotics for touch contamination or accidental disconnection (gram positive cover) and prior to most endoscopic/dental procedures (gram positive and negative cover) and the avoidance of hypokalaemia and constipation to reduce bacterial translocation. Loss of patient motivation and depression are also risk factors for infection and should be actively enquired after during patient interactions.

The ideal exit site should be situated away from the belt line and skin folds and be downward and lateral facing to allow for good drainage. Showering is permissible, as is swimming in the sea or private pools, however baths and communal pools should be avoided, and are associated with pseudomonal infections. Many recommend covering the exit site during swimming with an occlusive dressing such as an stoma bag. Patients should keep their nails trimmed and inspect and clean the exit site at least twice weekly or after every shower, following hand hygiene in a clean environment free of wind and pets. The exit site can be cleansed with soap and water or 2% chlorhexidine or similar antiseptic. After rinsing and drying the exit site well, a small amount of antibacterial ointment can be applied with a cotton bud or gauze and then dressed with gauze and secured with tape. In warm climates, leaving the exit site open has also been shown to be a safe option. Avoidance of excessive movement at the exit site is very important and taping the catheter to the skin about 2 cm away from the exit site should be done. Securing the catheter extension set in a purpose-made fabric belt has proven very useful in assisting immobilisation. There are currently no firm data to recommend one dressing or cleaning solution over any other.

Diagnosis of Infection

Effective treatment involves the rapid recognition of infection in order to preserve PD as a technique. Patients should be taught how to recognise infection at home to facilitate early presentation for assessment. Infections in PD can present as either, or a combination of both catheter-related infection and/or peritonitis:

Catheter-Related Infections

Exit site infections are often associated with poor catheter care and subsequent peritonitis and catheter loss. Scoring systems can be used to assist with the evaluation of the exit site (see Table 20.2). Tunnel infection usually occurs in association with an exit site infection. Signs of inflammation are present along the catheter tunnel tract, although this may be occult, in which case fluid can be demonstrated ultrasonographically around the catheter tract [7]. This distinction is important, due to the higher risk of refractory infection or progression to peritonitis, especially in the presence of *Staphylococcus aureus* infection. Any discharge present should be cultured.

Table 20.1 Presentations of PD infections

Presentations of PD infections
1. Catheter-related infection
(a) Exit site infection—purulent discharge at catheter exit site with or without erythema; confirmed on culture of exit site specimen.
Tunnel infection—clinical inflammation or ultrasonographic evidence of fluid collection along the subcutaneous catheter tract.
2. Peritonitis
(a) Diagnosed in the presence of *two of the following three*:
• Generalised abdominal pain with or without other symptoms.
• Cloudy dialysis effluent with a white cell count $>100/\mu L$ ($0.1 \times 10^9/L$) and >50% polymorphonuclear (after minimum 2 h dwell).
• A positive dialysis effluent culture.
(b) For patients on APD, a percentage neutrophils >50% should be considered indicative of peritonitis even if the WCC is <100, due to the short dwell times. Alternatively, a 1 L manual 2 h dwell can be performed in the unit in order to obtain sample for culture.
(c) Note the differential diagnosis of cloudy effluent also includes: Chemical peritonitis due to batch contamination or dihydropyridine calcium channel blockers, eosinophilic peritonitis, hemoperitoneum, chylous effluent, pancreatitis, malignancy and specimen after a prolonged period when PD has been interrupted.
(d) The presence of a lymphocytic pleocytosis should also prompt investigation for TB peritonitis which is not rare in endemic areas, although it is often initially neutrophilic.

Table 20.2 Exit site scoring system[a]

Parameter	0	1	2
Swelling	No	Exit only (<0.5 cm)	>0.5 cm and/or tunnel
Crust	No	<0.5 cm	>0.5 cm
Redness	No	<0.5 cm	>0.5 cm
Pain	No	Slight	Severe
Drainage	No	Serous	Purulent[b]

Infection should be assumed with a score of 4 or higher

[a]Modified from Schaefer F et al.

[b]Purulent drainage, even by itself, is sufficient to indicate infection. A score of less than 4 may or may not represent infection

Peritonitis

Peritonitis can be catheter-related through touch contamination or through extension of exit site/tunnel infection into the peritoneal space. It can also be secondary to translocation of bacteria from the gut or though transient bacteraemia, either spontaneously, after invasive procedures or following a bowel perforation. Peritonitis should be suspected in the presence of abdominal pain or a cloudy dialysis effluent and should be promptly investigated (Table 20.3). While cloudy dialysate is usually associated with infection, other non-infectious causes should be considered, especially in the absence of abdominal pain (see above). Localised abdominal pain or polymicrobial infection should raise the suspicion for surgical causes such as appendicitis and may warrant specific imaging, surgical assessment and the addition of anaerobic cover.

Table 20.3 Steps in Investigating for PD peritonitis

Steps in investigating for PD peritonitis
• Dialysate fluid should be drained and inspected then sent for an urgent cell count, gram stain and culture prior to initiation of antibiotics. • Culture yields should be >85%, and are increased by placing 5–10 mL directly into aerobic and anaerobic blood culture bottles and through re-suspended sediment culture after centrifuge of a 50 mL aliquot. • It is important to liaise with the local microbiology lab in order to increase diagnostic yields. • The exit site and tunnel should be carefully evaluated for signs of infection and any purulent discharge cultured. • The Gram stain is only predictive of the final organism, or if fungal elements are present. • The presence of gram-negative rods indicates the need for pseudomonal cover if not already in place.

Treatment of Infections

Catheter-Related Infection

Clinical judgement is required to distinguish bacterial colonisation (positive culture without evidence of inflammation) from true infection in order to avoid unnecessary antibiotic prescription and the promotion of antimicrobial resistance. Apart from culturing any exit site discharge, peritonitis should also be ruled out through fluid assessment and culture. Mild exit site infection in the absence of tunnel involvement or peritonitis can initially be managed with intensified local care. The presence of *S. Aureus* or *Pseudomonas* on initial cultures, or a failure to respond to this regimen within 1 week would indicate the need for systemic antibiotics, even if initially mild. Chronic exit site inflammation can lead to the formation of a pyogenic granuloma, which can further become infected. Topical application of silver nitrate is often successful in this context and any associated infection should also be treated.

Concomitant peritonitis or abdominal wall abscess implies deep cuff involvement and mandates catheter removal as well as the use of intraperitoneal antibiotics until catheter removal. In this instance and depending on residual renal function, temporary haemodialysis may be required.

More severe exit site and/or superficial tunnel infection and any febrile patient should be treated with systemic antibiotics along with intensified daily exit site care and careful clinical follow up. The initial empirical antibiotic choice should cover *S. Aureus,* according to local or known sensitivity patterns but cover for *Pseudomonas* should be added where the patient has a history of such an infection. The prescription should be adapted according to culture results as soon as available. Common appropriate initial empiric choices are cloxacillin/flucloxacillin or Clindamycin/Linezolid, depending on local sensitivities. The duration of treatment should be a minimum of 2 weeks and until the exit site looks normal, but 3 weeks for associated tunnel infection or pseudomonas. Where pseudomonas is cultured and is susceptible, an effective treatment consists of combined oral ciprofloxacin with topical ciprofloxacin drops and gauze soaks 4 times per day. The gauze is soaked in a solution made up of 125 ml of vinegar (acetic acid) mixed with 125 ml of sterile (or cooled boiled) water and 1 teaspoon of salt. Resolution of any tunnel infection should be confirmed by the absence of fluid around the catheter on follow-up sonography—persistent fluid around the catheter would indicate refractory infection.

For refractory/relapsing exit site or tunnel infections in the absence of peritonitis, simultaneous catheter removal and replacement under antibiotic cover is recommended [8, 9]. In this instance, low volume PD (or supine APD) can be used initially to avoid the need for temporary HD. However, catheter salvage therapy has been successfully performed by shaving off the external cuff and re-tunnelling the catheter through a new exit site under ongoing antibiotic cover. This technique may be preferable, particularly in resource-constrained areas, and allows continued PD immediately.

Peritonitis

Initial Management of Suspected Peritonitis

Send appropriate cultures and cell count, examine the exit site and tunnel carefully and culture any purulent discharge present. Initiate empiric broad-spectrum antibiotics (see Table 20.4) while awaiting culture and it is an option to add heparin 500u/L to the first few exchanges to prevent fibrinous catheter occlusion. Approximately 70%

Table 20.4 Commonly used antibiotics and their dosing (adapted from ISPD 2016 update [2])

DRUG	ONCE DAILY DOSING[a] (per exchange, once dly)	EACH BAG EQUIVALENT (mg/L, unless indicated otherwise)
Vancomycin	20–30 mg/kg every 5–7 days or if level <15	LD 30 mg/kg, MD 1.5 mg/kg/bag
Teicoplanin	15 mg/kg every 5 days	LD400 mg/bag/MD 20 mg/bag
Cefazolin	15–20 mg/kg	LD 500/MD 125
Cloxacillin	ND	LD 500/MD 125
Clindamycin	ND	MD 600 mg/bag
Ampicillin	2 g BD	MD 125
Ceftazidime	3 g stat, then 1–1.5 g/day	LD 500/MD 125
Ceftriaxone	2 g stat, then 1 g/day	ND
Cefipime	1 g	LD 500/MD 125
Ciprofloxacin	ND (can use orally)	MD 50
Gentamycin	0.6 mg/kg	LD 8/MD 4
Tobramycin	0.6 mg/kg	LD 3 mg/kg/MD 0.3 mg/kg
Amikacin	2 mg/kg	LD 25/MD 12
Cotrimoxazole	960 mg orally BD	
Fluconazole	200 mg	ND
Meropenem	1 g	LD250/MD125
Imipenem/Cilastatin	1 g BD	LD250/MD50

Note: Most antibiotics are stable for at least 5 days when mixed in the bag and stored at room temperature. The exception to this is ampicillin (12 h) where intermittent mixing/dosing required. (At room temperature: Vancomycin is stable 28 days, Gentamycin 14 days, cefazolin 8 days; Ceftazidime 4 days, but 7 days if refrigerated). First line agents are all stable in icodextrin if refrigerated

[a]Once daily dosing requires a dwell of at least 6 h

LD = loading dose per litre in first bag, MD = maintanence dose per litre in each bag, ND = No data

of infections are related to gram positive organisms, with the balance being gram negative or other (such as fungal or mycobacterial). Consider whether a surgical cause for peritonitis may be present and manage appropriately. Patients who have systemic sepsis should be admitted and considered for IV antibiotics, although most patients will be able to be treated as outpatients, provided they have ready access to transport back, and their pain is not severe. Ancilliary use of antifungal prophylaxis (nystatin orally or fluconazole 200 mg po alternate days) should be given. Note that a temporary increase in dialysate glucose concentration or use of icodextrin may also be necessary since an increase in membrane transport due to inflammation is common in peritonitis, and may result in fluid overload.

Basic principles of Antibiotic Therapy for Peritonitis:

- Broad spectrum antibiotics to cover both gram positive and gram negative organisms are initiated empirically but narrowed down after positive culture is obtained. The combination of a glycopeptide and ceftazidime has been shown to be superior to other regimens [10]. Glycopeptides cover many inherently penicillin-resistant gram positive organisms and ceftazidime affords pseudomonal in addition to other gram negatives. There are many rational combinations and the choice should be tailored according to local susceptibility data and ecology (Table 20.4).
- Intraperitoneal (IP) antibiotics are superior in efficacy compared to IV, with the exception being in the presence of systemic sepsis. They should be added to the dialysate in a sterile fashion (after 5 min of disinfection of the injection port) by trained personnel.
- Once-daily IP treatment of most antibiotics is possible and has equivalent efficacy to intermittent dosing, provided the dwell is at least 6 h.
- Antibiotics can be added to the same bag but should not be mixed in the same syringe.
- Antibiotics can be mixed in the unit and provided to patients to take home with them. They can be mixed at home, but given the stability of the agents, in-unit mixing is preferable.
- Serum vancomycin levels can be checked after 3–5 days, and a trough concentration of >15 μg/ml should be maintained, although there is no good evidence to support this prac-

tice. Dosing is usually required every 7 days, but every 3–5 days in those with good residual kidney function.

- Aminoglycosides appear largely safe when necessary and do not impact residual kidney function or cause ototoxicity when dosed correctly, daily and for ≤1 week. However, where an alternative non-toxic therapy is unavailable, safe use has been reported over up to 3 weeks.
- Data concerning APD are scant, but strategies for dosing include dosing per bag as for CAPD (preferred strategy), reprogramming the cycler to allow a daily 6-hour dwell, switching to CAPD for the duration of treatment, and intermittent instillation of a 6-hour dwell for glycopeptide dosing [11].

Further Assessment of the Patient Should Occur Within 2–3 Days:

- Most patients improve rapidly within 2–3 days and failure to do so demands re-consideration of the diagnosis, possible further imaging (Chest radiograph/CT Abdomen/ultrasonography of the tunnel), repeat cell count/cultures including TB/fungal cultures and a possible switch in therapy to broaden cover. Failure to respond by day 5 necessitates prompt catheter removal to protect the membrane. A high index of suspicion for TB should also be maintained in endemic areas.
- Dialysate cell count >1090 cells/μL (1.09×10^9/L) on day 3 strongly predicts treatment failure [12].
- For patients that have responded well clinically, antibiotic therapy should be narrowed according to culture results.
- For those patients with a rapid clinical response but negative culture, it is usually safe to continue only gram positive cover provided the cell count has dropped markedly by day 3, since most culture negative episodes are gram positive in origin. An alternative is to continue an oral quinolone antibiotic for 10 days.
- The presence of fungal elements on initial gram stain or subsequent culture demands immediate removal of the catheter and a switch to include antifungal treatment (Table 20.5). Cure rates for fungal peritonitis are less than 10%.
- Early catheter removal is mandatory for all organisms if there is concomitant tunnel infection (or where an exit site organism is the same as peritoneal fluid), with the exception for coagulase negative staphylococcal (CNS) and streptococcal infection that is rapidly responding (Table 20.5).

Specific Organisms and Their Treatment

In general, the narrowest spectrum antibiotic available should be used to limit the development of resistance. Some specific recommendations can be made regarding certain organisms (Table 20.6):

Final Assessment of the Patient:

- The duration of therapy should be 3 weeks, but 2 weeks in CNS/streptococcal infection with a rapid response.
- After catheter removal, treatment should continue for 10–14 days.
- Each peritonitis episode should be interrogated and patients should be re-trained regarding hygiene and aseptic technique plus touch contamination protocols.
- The transfer set should be changed once fluid clears.

Table 20.5 Indications for PD catheter removal

Catheter removal is considered necessary for:
1. Refractory peritonitis (failure to resolve by day 5).
2. Fungal peritonitis
3. Relapsing peritonitis (peritonitis with same organism ≤4 weeks after successful treatment)
4. Refractory exit site or tunnel infection.

Note: For relapsing peritonitis due to non-virulent organisms or in the presence of persistent exit site/tunnel infection with resolved peritonitis, simultaneous removal and replacement of the catheter can be safely performed after 2–3 week's treatment, sometimes avoiding HD. However, for refractory peritonitis, a new catheter should only be placed a minimum of two weeks after full resolution of peritonitis. Successful return to peritoneal dialysis after catheter removal for infection is successful in a large number of patients, but should be carefully considered in those with repeated infections (peritonitis with a different organism ≥4 weeks after successful treatment) or after fungal peritonitis

Table 20.6 Specific recommendations for management of PD peritonitis due to isolated organisms

Organism	Management
Coagulase negative Staphylococci (CNS)	• Where methicillin sensitive, continuous instead of daily treatment with first generation cephalosporins is preferred.
Staphylococcus aureus	• High risk for catheter removal. • Where methicillin sensitive, first generation cephalosporins are preferred. • A nasal swab for *S. aureus* should be performed, and where positive, eradication measures should be attempted.
Pseudomonas	• High risk for catheter removal. • Two antibiotics with different mechanisms of action should be used (also for *Stenotrophomonas*): *Oral ciprofloxacin can be combined successfully, but must be dosed apart from phosphate binders, as these can bind ciprofloxacin in the gut, and markedly reduce its absorption.* • Consider extending treatment to 28 days in some cases.
Enterococcus species	• Vancomycin is the preferred agent where sensitive.
Other *enterobacteriaceae*	• Due regard should be given to increasing antibiotic resistance and the use of two agents should be considered for those organisms with inducible beta lactamase inhibition. • Consultation with microbiologists is recommended where possible.
Tuberculosis	• There is a neutrophilic effluent in 75% of cases. Standard anti-TB therapy is used, and catheter removal is often not necessary. • Some patients may develop a protein-losing state via their dialysate, which may necessitate a transfer to HD.

Prognosis

Most patients recover rapidly, but the risk of requiring catheter removal is approximately 20%. The overall mortality rate is approximately 5% but is highest for those with fungal, gram negative, *S. aureus* or TB infections. While the reasons are poorly understood, a recent episode of peritonitis is also associated with an increased odds of all-cause death for the next few months, but especially in the first 30 days. Other possible consequences of peritonitis include the formation of infected intra-abdominal collections, fibrous adhesions and encapsulating peritoneal sclerosis.

Non-Infective Complications

Approximately 25% of cases of technique failure in PD occurs as a result of some form of mechanical complication. These can involve the catheter itself with poor drainage or alternatively the boundaries of the peritoneal space leading to hernias or leaks. The vast majority of these complications can be dealt with and patients can return to PD shortly thereafter. This section will address these issues and how to prevent and manage them.

PD Catheter Obstruction

There are several possible causes of PD catheter flow complications, as listed in Table 20.7.

Table 20.7 Causes of PD catheter obstruction & Specific treatments

Cause of PD catheter obstruction	Treatment
Catheter obstruction due to fibrin	Intraluminal tissue plasminogen activator (tPA)
Catheter migration out of the pelvis	Guidewire manipulation of PD catheter
Catheter entrapment in the omentum	Laparoscopic replacement and omentopexy
Severe constipation	Oral bowel preparation solution

As the PD fluid drains into the true pelvis in the upright position, a catheter sited there is much more likely to drain effectively and to near completion. If the catheter has moved out of the pelvis it often (but not universally) leads to poor drainage. The migration of the catheter may be because of significant constipation with the loaded sigmoid colon moving the catheter into the upper abdomen and this is by far the most common cause. It is easily diagnosed with a plain abdominal x-ray which shows both the catheter migration as well as the faecal loading. The catheter may also migrate when the omentum wraps around the catheter and with traction pulls it out of the pelvis. Omental wrapping cannot be distinguished from other causes of migration without the use of laparoscopy. Catheters may also become blocked with fibrin. This usually leads to problems with both drainage into and out of the abdomen, but occasionally a ball valve effect may be seen and only inflow drainage occurs. In this situation, the abdominal x-ray usually shows the catheter in the correct position. Some rarer causes of obstruction are reported in the literature, such as obstruction due to fallopian tubes, appendices and other mobile structures in the abdomen. It is also relatively common for patients with significant peritonitis or following surgery to develop adhesions, and these can obliterate the pelvis or create pockets where fluid collects and drains slowly. All of the above need to be diagnosed at laparoscopy or laparotomy.

Prevention of PD Catheter Obstruction

In recently published ISPD access guidelines, practical methods to ensure optimal PD access and reduced complications are discussed (Table 20.8) [13]. These guidelines analyse methods of insertion of catheters, as well as some techniques to prevent complications. Although there is no evidence of superiority of different methods of insertion of PD catheters in the hands of a skilled operator, if the laparoscopic route is chosen, then advanced laparoscopic techniques such as musculofascial tunnelling, omentectomy, omentopexy and tip suturing have been shown in a large meta-analysis to lead to better long term outcomes, with fewer mechanical complications.

As constipation is by far the most common reason for catheter migration, maintenance of a regular bowel habit through the regular use of laxatives in PD patients is recommended to prevent catheter migration.

Table 20.8 Advanced laparoscopic techniques to prevent PD catheter blockage

Laparoscopic technique	Description
Musculofascial tunnelling	• Involves the formation of a tunnel along the posterior rectus sheath in a caudal direction prior to the catheter entering the peritoneal space. • Keeps the catheter directed into the pelvis, and if migration occurs will allow it to return to its original position through its elastic memory.
Omentectomy	• Was used historically, and can be performed via either laparotomy or laparoscopic approaches. • Removal of a large proportion of the omentum prevents it reaching into the pelvis and entrapping the catheter: Unfortunately, the omentum is a highly vascular structure, and extreme care needs to be taken to ensure haemostasis as post-operative bleeding results in both fibrin occlusion of the catheter, as well as formation of adhesions.
Omentopexy	• Is preferred over omentectomy. • Involves suturing the end of the omentum to either the mesocolon or a point on the anterior abdominal wall in one of the upper quadrants. Only needs to be performed when the omentum is long enough to reach the level of the pelvic brim, and can be confirmed at the time of surgery.

Table 20.8 (continued)

Laparoscopic technique	Description
Tip suturing	• Is a controversial technique, as it can be argued that having a foreign object may be a nidus for infection, and if the catheter is immobilised too tightly it may result in rectal or vaginal pain. • Significantly reduces the incidence of catheter migration. • Various techniques have been described from a propylene loop of suture protruding from the lower third of the anterior abdominal wall into the abdominal cavity through which the catheter travels, to a loop on the dome of the bladder, directing the catheter into the retrovesical space: Both of these techniques allow easy removal of the catheter if necessary, since the catheter slides through the loop unimpeded. Alternatively, the catheter can be fixed using sutures to the pelvic sidewall.

Note: These techniques cannot be performed if the catheter is inserted percutaneously, however it should be noted that although these methods reduce mechanical complications, many studies show percutaneously inserted catheters have patency in excess of 80% at one year despite this, and therefore if using this approach the above laparoscopic techniques can be performed later if a catheter does become problematic

Obstruction of the catheter due to fibrin can be prevented by the addition of heparin 500-1000iu/l to the PD solution when PD fluid is bloodstained or has significant amounts of fibrin present.

Management of PD Catheter Obstruction

Catheter migration with constipation: This is diagnosed by plain abdominal x-ray showing faecal loading with or without migration of the catheter. In the vast majority of cases, this can be remedied with a single dose of a solution used for bowel preparation for colonoscopy (e.g. sodium picosulphate or macrogol). The patient takes the preparation and waits until the bowel has emptied significantly before performing the next dialysis exchange.

Catheter migration without constipation: Occasionally the catheter will not move into the pelvis of its own accord. This could be due to omental wrapping in which case it is unlikely to move without surgical intervention, however it may simply be that it is in the incorrect position and a much less invasive method may be used to manipulate the catheter to get it into position. This involves fluoroscopy, and use of a flexible guidewire. There are numerous published techniques, ranging from a stiff wire bent into a 270° arc, to various guidewires and angiography catheters, which are advanced under fluoroscopic guidance in order to manipulate the tip of the catheter back into the pelvis. The most commonly used method uses a relatively stiff angiography guidewire with a flexible or j-shaped tip, which is advanced through the catheter and beyond. As the wire is advanced through the tip, it presses against the abdominal side wall and the catheter is pushed downward into the pelvis. Results from most of the published studies show a technique success rate of approximately 80%, however publication bias may overestimate the success rate achieved in clinical practice. It is a very low risk, minimally invasive procedure though, and if facilities exist, may prevent the need for surgery and should be considered [14, 15].

It is imperative that the technique is performed in a sterile manner, and a dose of intraperitoneal antibiotic is administered as per the unit protocol for catheter contamination episodes, in order to prevent PD peritonitis.

Should the above not prove successful, then repositioning of the catheter should be performed surgically. It is preferable to reposition using laparoscopy, as it allows for the above advanced techniques to prevent further complications, but also allows direct visualisation of the catheter, division of adhesions, and placement of the catheter back in the pelvis under direct vision. Finally, the smaller incisions associated with laparoscopy than for open laparotomy may facilitate a return to PD immediately, provided that the laparoscopic port sites are sutured internally.

Laparoscopy is not available in many centres due to a lack of expertise, and expensive consumable devices. In this situation, the catheter can be replaced by performing a mini-laparotomy, or alternatively, the catheter can be replaced at the bedside. This latter technique involves dissection and freeing of the deep cuff under local anaesthesia. The catheter is slowly withdrawn until the first side hole is visualised. Using a peel-away sheath PD catheter insertion kit, the guidewire is fed through the side-hole into the abdomen. The catheter can then be completely withdrawn, leaving the guidewire with the distal tip in the peritoneal cavity. The catheter can be freed of any fibrin, and then is replaced in the abdomen using the peel-away sheath percutaneous technique, over the guidewire.

Catheter obstruction secondary to fibrin deposition: It is common for fibrin to be found in the PD effluent, and this can cause occlusion of the lumen and side-holes. This can cause both uni- and bi-directional flow obstruction. Under sterile conditions, the catheter can be flushed vigorously with saline or PD solution, using a 20 ml syringe. Avoid aspirating rapidly, as it is possible to entrap mobile structures, such as omental folds in the tip of the catheter. Gentle aspiration may alternatively result in removal of the responsible fibrin plug, and restore PD fluid flow. If this is unsuccessful, then the catheter may be locked with a thrombolytic solution. The most commonly recommended is tissue plasminogen Activator (tPA), which is made up to a 1 mg/mL solution and 8 mls (in an adult Tenckhoff catheter) is slowly injected and left for 1 h, then aspirated. This will usually result in restoration of flow if fibrin is the cause of the obstruction.

Hernia and Leak

Hernias and leaks occur in approximately 15% of patients on PD, and appear to be more prevalent than the general population due to the increased abdominal pressure associated with PD solutions, which makes defects in the abdominal wall more apparent. Other factors such as malnutrition, polycystic kidney disease and surgery for catheter placement also increase the risk. They may become apparent initially, with initiation of dialysis or after many years. Hernias are defects in the abdominal with an intact peritoneum, whereas a leak is a defect where the peritoneal membrane has been disrupted. The latter can commonly occur after an episode of peritonitis or surgery, and with rest may resolve, however hernias almost always need to be repaired.

Hernias

The most common sites for hernias in PD patients are inguinal, umbilical and paraumbilical. Other hernias occurring less commonly are femoral, diaphragmatic and Spigelian, along with recto/vaginocoeles. The usual presentation is a sudden swelling over the affected area, however there are reports of patients presenting with recurrent peritonitis associated with intermittent subacute obstruction of bowel.

If it is uncertain as to whether there is a hernia or not, then further imaging may be helpful. The simplest is CT peritoneography (Fig. 20.1). Magnetic resonance imaging (MRI) may also be used, with the PD solution acting as the contrast media (Gadolinium is usually avoided due to the risk of nephrogenic systemic fibrosis and possible peritoneal fibrosis). This technique may be more helpful for diagnosing a leak as discussed later [16].

Hernia Prevention and Management

Prior to insertion of a PD catheter, all patients should have all potential hernia sites inspected; if a hernia is present, this needs to be repaired at the time of surgery to place the PD catheter.

If a hernia is diagnosed at a later point, it is usually advisable for the hernia to be repaired, but occasionally if it is small, not increasing in size, and has a wide neck, it can be left in patients who have a limited life expectancy. In other patients, due to the likelihood of significant worsening, it should be repaired. Inguinal hernias can often be repaired using an extraperitoneal approach which will allow early reinstatement of

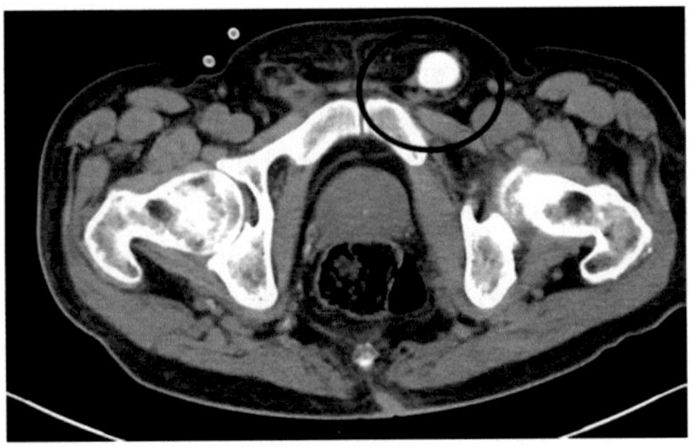

Fig. 20.1 CT Peritoneogram demonstrating an inguinal hernia in a patient who presented with recurrent peritonitis of unknown cause. *Notes: 2 mL/kg of intravenous contrast is injected into a 2 L dialysate bag and instilled into the abdomen. The patient is asked to perform manoeuvres, which increase the intra-abdominal pressure, such as coughing, bending and squatting. 30 min after installation, a standard CT scan of the abdomen is performed, then the fluid is drained out*

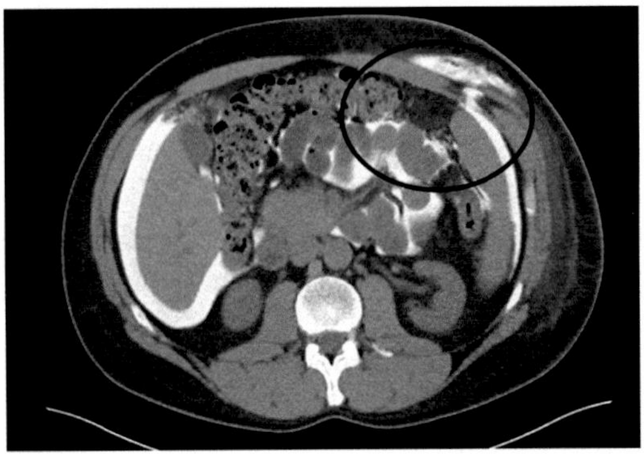

Fig. 20.2 CT peritoneogram demonstrating an extraperitoneal leak into the subcutaneous tissues of the left anterior abdominal wall

PD (see below), however umbilical and paraumbilical hernias usually require a procedure which breaches the peritoneum, and requires a period of rest from PD.

Repair of hernias almost always require the use of a synthetic mesh to prevent recurrence. There is debate as to whether this should be placed intra- or extra-peritoneally. Intraperitoneal mesh has the risk of being infected if the patient develops peritonitis in the 2–4 weeks following repair, however there is little evidence of this occurring in the literature. Until further evidence comes to light, if there is the surgical expertise available, the extraperitoneal approach should be considered.

Although there is little evidence as to the optimal timing for reinitiating PD, if the patient can delay dialysis then 4 weeks is recommended, however if the peritoneum is not breached then 10 days is the minimum before resumption of ambulatory PD. If the patient is on automated PD (APD), a low volume fill program (1–1.5 L) may be used, with a dry abdomen when ambulating, in order to allow an immediate return to PD, without the need for bridging HD.

A patent processus vaginalis is where there is a potential connection between the abdominal cavity and the scrotum. This often presents as a unilateral or bilateral scrotal swelling, and must be distinguished from a leak as discussed below. When this is noted unilaterally, there is a significant risk of a contralateral leak, such that a bilateral repair should be performed.

Leaks

Leaks may occur at any point where there is a defect in the peritoneal membrane, with the most common sites being along the PD catheter tunnel and trans-diaphragmatic, however numerous other potential sites may occur, including pericardial, transvaginal and retroperitoneal. Figure 20.2 shows a leak in the left flank, which would occur after heavy exercise. Identification of a leak may be more difficult than a hernia, as it may be subtle. Features which should alert one to a leak is poor ultrafiltration in the early phase after starting PD, abdominal wall oedema, with a peau d'orange appearance, genital oedema, and in the case of a transdiaphragmatic leak, shortness of breath. Hydrothorax and transdiaphragmatic leaks will be discussed separately.

If there is poor ultrafiltration due to leakage into the soft tissues, this can be identified by performing a peritoneal equilibration test (PET) which should be discordant with the clinical picture. If a patient has ultrafiltration failure (<200 mL with a 2.5% glucose solution) but is a low, low average or even high average transporter, one should consider a leak and proceed to imaging. There are 3 modalities which are helpful: the first is nuclear scintigraphy, where 2 mCi of Technetium radionuclide is added to a 2 L PD bag. This may identify a leak, but does not give good definition. CT or MR peritoneography, as discussed earlier, may offer better definition and demonstration of the site of the leak, and where a repair is needed (Fig. 20.2).

Most leaks may resolve if PD is withheld for a period of 2 weeks, allowing the peritoneum to seal itself. If following this rest period, the leak recurs, then it will usually require surgical repair.

Hydrothorax

Hydrothorax occurs due to leakage through a defect in the peritoneum and diaphragm. This may be a congenital defect, or alternatively a rupture of a pleural bleb. The usual presentation is an asymptomatic pleural effusion on chest radiograph (CXR), however it may cause shortness of breath and in extremely rare cases, tension hydrothorax. As with other PD leaks, there is frequently associated poor ultrafiltration, and the patient may present with oedema and signs of fluid overload. It may therefore be difficult to distinguish between a pleural effusion secondary to a leak and one due to fluid overload, or right ventricular failure on clinical grounds. A confident diagnosis may be made by measuring the glucose in the fluid aspirated from the pleural space is >40 mmol/L or >3 mmol/L above that of the serum. CT/MR Peritoneography or scintigraphy may also be helpful in diagnosing a leak, and the former may even demonstrate the exact position which can be sutured thoracoscopically.

Management of Hydrothorax

This is determined by whether the leak occurred following an episode of peritonitis or not. If so, then following a period of 2 weeks' rest, the healed mesothelium may prevent further leakage. If it occurs at the start of PD, it is unlikely to resolve spontaneously. The options are then to perform a thoracoscopic surgical repair, or more commonly pleurodesis. This will usually result in a good functional outcome, and very seldom recurs.

Encapsulating Peritoneal Sclerosis (EPS)

Encapsulating peritoneal sclerosis is a condition that occurs in 1–2.5% of patients on PD, can have dire consequences for the patient, and requires early identification. Significant thickening of the peritoneal membrane results in adhesion of bowel loops, and cocooning of the bowel, resulting in bowel obstruction (Table 20.9). There is often associated ascites associated with this, especially in patients who have transferred to haemodialysis or had a kidney transplant.

The most common clinical features are vomiting and abdominal pain, with rarer symptoms being ascites, blood stained dialysate and an abdominal mass.

The cause remains uncertain, with numerous theories under investigation. One prevalent theory is that there is a predisposition to membrane thickening such as increased time on PD, or an as yet unidentified genetic cause, following which a second insult leads to excessive peritoneal membrane fibrosis: this could be an environmental toxin, or infection. Underlying this theory is a strong association with time on dialysis, with more than 90% of cases presenting after 3 years on PD. Although it was initially considered important, there is no clear link between number of peritonitis episodes and the development of EPS. Many studies have demonstrated a disconnect between ultrafiltration failure (UFF) and peritoneal transporter status: normally, patients with UFF are high transporters, whereas this is not necessarily the case in EPS, presumably due to the fibrotic thickening disrupting the usual performance of the membrane in the PET test. This is important, as many studies have shown that patients continuing PD for 3 years or more after the development of ultrafiltration failure are at exceptionally high risk of EPS.

Table 20.9 Clinical and Radiological features of Encapsulating Peritoneal Sclerosis (EPS)

Clinical presentation	Radiological findings on CT
• Typically after >3 years on PD • Vomiting • Abdominal pain • Ascites • Blood stained dialysate • Abdominal mass	• Thickened bowel loops and peritoneum • Diffuse peritoneal membrane calcification • Loculated ascites

The diagnosis of EPS is usually made with radiological imaging, on the background of the appropriate clinical picture. The gold standard diagnostic test is CT imaging, demonstrating features of thickened bowel loops and peritoneum, diffuse calcification of the membrane, and loculated ascites. None of these features is diagnostic. Normally in the supine patient, bowel loops tend to "float" on the ascites, and are in contact with the anterior abdominal wall. In patients with EPS, the bowel loops are often posterior to the ascites which collects anterior to them. Ultrasound can be used to look for bowel wall thickening, but is very operator dependant, and therefore less reliable for making the diagnosis.

The optimal therapy for EPS remains uncertain. If patients are young, with a reasonable prognosis, then a transfer to haemodialysis is recommended. Small case series have suggested some benefit with the use of tamoxifen, corticosteroids and other immunosuppressants. No randomised controlled trials have been done to determine the best treatment, and publication bias makes it difficult to determine the best option. Also, as EPS has different phases from early inflammatory phase to late fibrotic phase, it may be important to target different therapies at different stages. Once the patient has developed symptoms of bowel obstruction, surgical intervention may be necessary. It is recommended that this be undertaken in a centre experienced with performing peritonectomy, where a multidisciplinary approach to parenteral nutrition, and a combination of peritonectomy and plication of the intestine can be performed. EPS has a high mortality, and malnutrition is thought to play a key role in this, hence the need for aggressively treating this prior to surgery.

Conclusions

Returning to our 35 year old PD patient, who presented in the initial clinical scenario with nausea, vomiting and generalised abdominal pain: with good drainage of his PD fluid, preserved ultrafiltration, and physical signs consistent with euvolaemia, we may consider catheter obstruction, a hernia or fluid leak all less likely causes of his presentation. Further, the fact that he is a relatively new starter on APD makes EPS improbable. The absence of a purulent discharge from around his catheter is only part reassuring—from the perspective of helping to exclude an exit site infection. However, as in 75% of cases, the most likely cause of his presentation remains PD-associated infection, and we must therefore pay careful attention to excluding PD peritonitis, for which shorter dwell times associated with APD may explain his clear bags: sending an urgent PD fluid cell count, gram stain and culture prior to initiation of antibiotics is essential, as per the local PD peritonitis protocol, ensuring at least a 6 h dwell time, and with a view to revising antibiotics according to the results of the gram stain and culture.

In conclusion, infectious and non-infectious complications of PD are common: Through rigorous patient training and ensuring familiarity amongst clinicians of local protocols, we can facilitate timely and pro-active investigation and management of PD complications, and in the majority of cases, allow patients to return to PD for long term dialysis.

Questions

1. Which of the following are most important in a patient presenting with cloudy effluent?
   A. Peritoneal fluid culture and cell count
   B. Exit site inspection and pus swab if inflamed
   C. Start on intraperitoneal antibiotics with both gram positive and gram negative cover
   D. Discussion on the possible causes for peritonitis and consider retraining the patient
   E. All of the above

Answer: E.

PD peritonitis is usually simply a coagulase negative staphylococcal infection which is easily treated, however if appropriate investigation of the cause and rapid initiation of antibiotics to cover gram negative organisms is not performed then there is a higher chance of catheter loss in those with other causes.

2. The ISPD guidelines recommend a culture negative rate of <20% for peritonitis. Which methods can be used to increase this yield?
   A. Centrifuge 50mls of fluid, resuspend the pellet and culture
   B. Inoculate blood culture bottles with 10mls of PD fluid
   C. Ensure fluid samples are collected before antibiotics are added to the bag
   D. Discuss with local microbiology lab the importance of the primary samples
   E. All of the above

Answer: E.

Discsussion with local microbiologists can be extremely helpful as peritoneal fluid specimens are often not regarded as particularly important in the lab and may not be given appropriate consideration. Understanding of the value of centrifugation and use of blood culture bottles to increase yield and peritonitis outcomes are essential.

3. Exit site infections should be managed with:
   A. Warm compresses with a towel soaked in boiling water
   B. Increased exit site care if mild
   C. Shaving of the cuff and retunneling
   D. Antibiotics appropriate to cultures for 2 weeks
   E. B and D

Answer E.

Exit site infections may be very mild and immobilisation of the catheter and increased exit site care can resolve it. If there is a purulent discharge or pain though then appropriate antibiotics are necessary and should be continued for 2 weeks

4. Which of the following is incorrect?
   A. Peritonitis which does not resolve by day 5 is called refractory peritonitis
   B. If PD effluent has not cleared by day 5 the catheter should be removed to preserve the membrane for future use
   C. Fungal peritonitis can be safely treated with fluconazole but if not cleared by day 5 then the catheter should be removed
   D. A PD effluent cell count >1000 on day 3 is predictive of failure to clear by day 5
   E. In relapsing (same organism within 4 weeks) peritonitis simultaneous removal and replacement of the PD catheter after 2 weeks antbiotics is feasible

Answer: C.

Fungal peritonitis carries a very high treatment failure rate and a 25% mortality. Although there are case reports of successful treatment with antifungals but this is not recommended.

5. A patient presents with a case of PD peritonitis secondary to pseudomonas aeriginosa, the following are the most appropriate treatment options:
   A. Remove the PD catheter immediately
   B. Continue ceftazidime/gentamicin for 2 weeks
   C. Treat with 2 anti-pseudomonal antibiotics for 3 weeks
   D. Shave the cuff on the catheter as it is the most likely source.

Answer: C.

Gram negative peritonitis requires 2 agents to improve treatment success. Although an exit site infection and peritonitis with pseudomonas with likely require tube removal it is not necessary unless refractory peritonitis or recurrent peritonitis occur.

6. A patient who has poor ultrafiltration, with a PET test result showing slow average transporter status should be considered to have a mechanical complication until proven otherwise.
   A. True
   B. False

Answer: A.

Patients with poor ultrafiltration especially early in the course of PD and not associated with hyperglycaemia are likely to have a mechanical complication, most especially a leak and CT peritoneography should be considered.

7. A patient presents with a right sided pleural effusion. Which of the following are not likely to assist in the diagnosis of a leak:
   A. Pleural aspiration showing a fluid:serum gradient >3 mmol/L

B. Echocardiogram to exclude right heart failure
C. Pleural biopsy
D. Nuclear scintigraphy
E. MRI of the thorax

Answer: C.

All of the investigations are helpful in distinguishing between a pleural effusion due to fluid overload and a leak except c. A pleural biopsy may be necessary in the case of an exudative effusion but hydrothorax is always a transudate.

8. Encapsulating peritoneal sclerosis (EPS) is a rare complication of PD associated with thickening and cocooning of the peritoneal membrane. The following are options for therapy except:
   A. Tamoxifen
   B. Peritonectomy
   C. Prednisone
   D. Intraperitoneal antibiotics
   E. Sirolimus

Answer: D.

Although all of the above are treatment options, there is no consensus on the optimal treatment regimen and randomised trials are needed, however given the paucity of cases it is unlikely this will be achievable.

9. Rapid of inflow of fluid and poor drainage thereof is likely to be secondary to:
   A. Catheter migration out of the pelvis
   B. Constipation and faecal loading
   C. Omental wrapping of the catheter
   D. Fibrin
   E. All of the above

Answer: E.

Poor drainage may be due to any of these causes however the most common and easily treatable is faecal loading and should be aggressively treated.

10. Polycystic kidney disease patients should not be treated with PD due to the high risk of hernia and lack of space in the abdomen?
   A. True
   B. False

Answer: B.

PKD patients often do well on PD and although those with massively enlarged kidneys may find large fill volumes uncomfortable, it is not a contraindication to therapy. Hernias are more common in these patients, and should be sought and repaired pro-actively, before or at the time of PD catheter placement.

Test your learning and check your understanding of this book's contents: use the "Springer Nature Flashcards" app to access questions using https://sn.pub/cz9Cok. To use the app, please follow the instructions in Chap. 1.

References

1. Boudville N, et al. Recent peritonitis associates with mortality among patients treated with peritoneal dialysis. J Am Soc Nephrol. 2012;23(8):1398–405.
2. Li PK-T, et al. ISPD peritonitis recommendations: 2016 update on prevention and treatment. Perit Dial Int. 2016;36(5):481–508.
3. Szeto C-C, et al. ISPD catheter-related infection recommendations: 2017 update. Perit Dial Int. 2017;37(2):141–54.
4. Davidson B, et al. Outcomes and challenges of a PD-first program, a south-African perspective. Perit Dial Int. 2018;38(3):179–86.
5. Htay H, et al. Center effects and peritoneal dialysis peritonitis outcomes: analysis of a national registry. Am J Kidney Dis. 2018;71(6):814–21.
6. Firanek C, et al. Comparison of disinfection procedures on the catheter adapter-transfer set junction. Peritoneal Dialysis Int. 2016;36(2):225–7.
7. Kwan TH, et al. Ultrasonography in the management of exit site infections in peritoneal dialysis patients. Nephrology. 2004;9(6):348–52.
8. Kirmizis D, et al. Exit-site relocation: a novel, straightforward technique for exit-site infections. Perit Dial Int. 2019;39(4):350–5.
9. Wong FS. Use of cleansing agents at the peritoneal catheter exit site. Perit Dial Int. 2003;23(2_suppl):148–52.
10. Morimoto K, et al. The impact of intraperitoneal antibiotic administration in patients with peritoneal dialysis-related peritonitis: systematic review and meta-analysis. Renal Replacement Ther. 2020;6:1–6.
11. Schaefer F, et al. Intermittent versus continuous intraperitoneal glycopeptide/ceftazidime treatment in children with peritoneal dialysis-associated peritonitis. J Am Soc Nephrol. 1999;10(1):136–45.

12. Chow KM, et al. Predictive value of dialysate cell counts in peritonitis complicating peritoneal dialysis. Clin J Am Soc Nephrol. 2006;1(4):768–73.
13. Crabtree JH, et al. Creating and maintaining optimal peritoneal dialysis access in the adult patient: 2019 update. Perit Dial Int. 2019;39(5):414–36.
14. Jones B, et al. Tenckhoff catheter salvage by closed stiff-wire manipulation without fluoroscopic control. Perit Dial Int. 1998;18(4):415–8.
15. Hevia C, et al. Alpha replacement method for displaced peritoneal catheter: a simple and effective maneuver. Adv Perit Dial. 2001;17:138–41.
16. Prischl FC, et al. Magnetic resonance imaging of the peritoneal cavity among peritoneal dialysis patients, using the dialysate as "contrast medium". J Am Soc Nephrol. 2002;13(1):197–203.

Kidney Transplantation: The Pre-Transplantation Recipient & Donor Work-Up

21

Pankaj Jawa, Prabir Roy-Chaudhury, and Roberto Ceratti Manfro

Clinical Scenario
A 55-year-old woman with diabetic nephropathy and sarcoidosis and declining kidney function, eGFR 20 mL/min/1.73 m^2 was referred for pre-emptive kidney transplantation. Her body mass index was 35 kg/m^2 and blood pressure 130/75 mmHg. What investigations would she need as part of her kidney transplant work up?

Introduction

Recipient Evaluation

Patients with End-Stage Renal Disease (ESRD) have a few treatment options. Renal transplantation is undoubtedly the one that provides more prolonged survival and better quality of life and must be offered for suitable patients with CKD stage 5 progressing to ESRD or patients already on dialysis. The transplant evaluation is a screening process to exclude patients for whom transplant will be detrimental [1, 2] (Table 21.1).

Referral for Kidney Transplantation

The education for kidney transplant should start once the eGFR <30 mL/min/1.73 m^2 [2]. At this time, necessary vaccinations and cancer screening are performed (Table 21.2). Patients could be referred for preemptive transplantation when the eGFR is <20 mL/min/1.73 m^2. If a living donor is available, the time that it takes by the transplant program to evaluate the donors should be considered. Efforts should be made for a preemptive kidney transplant, especially in countries where preemptive deceased donor transplantation is not allowed, to put patients on the waiting list early to minimize their time on dialysis.

Recipient Evaluation Team

The journey from transplant evaluation to surgery can be very tiring for patients requiring multiple visits with providers from various disciplines. The evaluation time will depend on their comorbidities. The transplant team involves health professionals from different fields who have experience and understand the complexity

P. Jawa
University of North Carolina, Chapel Hill, USA

P. Roy-Chaudhury (✉)
University of North Carolina, Chapel Hill, USA

WG (Bill) Hefner, Salisbury VA Medical Center, Salisbury, NC, USA
e-mail: prabir_roy-chaudhury@med.unc.edu

R. C. Manfro
Federal University of Rio Grande do Sul, Porto Alegre, Brazil

D. Banerjee et al. (eds.), *Management of Kidney Diseases*,
https://doi.org/10.1007/978-3-031-09131-5_21

Table 21.1 Contraindications for a kidney transplant

Absolute contraindications for a kidney transplant, but are not limited to:
1. Active infections such as tuberculosis.
2. Active substance abuse
3. Severe cardiac, vascular, pulmonary, or other comorbid conditions that create an unacceptable risk for transplant surgery or immunosuppression
4. Factors limiting the candidate's ability to adhere to medical care post-transplant, such as living situation, active mental illness, or psychosocial condition.
5. Malignancy with prognosis suggesting an anticipated survival of <5 years
Relative contraindications for a kidney transplant, but are not limited to:
1. Active infection (HIV, HCV, HBV, tuberculosis)
2. Active systemic diseases such as Good pasture's Syndrome with the persistent presence of anti-GBM antibodies, Systemic lupus erythematosus, or Antineutrophil cytoplasmic antibodies.
3. BMI >40%
4. Inadequate social support system
5. Malnutrition
6. Frailty

Table 21.2 Vaccinations and Cancer screening

Pre-transplant vaccinations:
– Tetanus/diphtheria (Td)
– Pertussis (Tdap)
– Influenza vaccine (yearly)
– MMR
– Pneumococcal vaccine (recommended with a booster every 3–5 years)
– Neisseria meningitides (MCV4. For patients at high epidemiological risk)
– Hepatitis A, hepatitis B
– Varicella vaccine—Varivax (seronegative patients)
– Polio (inactivated/live-activated)
– HPV (Females 9–45 years and males 9–26 years and MSM > 26)
Do not administer to post-transplant patients.
– Varicella-Zoster
– Influenza (live-attenuated)
– MMR
– Polio (live-attenuated)
– Tdap (Td was >5 years ago)
Cancer screening:
– Pap smear (Women >21 years)
– Mammogram (Women >40 years)
– Colonoscopy (> 50 years)
– PSA (Men >50 years)
– CT chest (for patients >30 pack-years of smoking)
– Renal ultrasound (long dialysis vintage, cystic disease, or strong family history)
– Cystoscopy (long history of tobacco or use of cyclophosphamide)
– Ultrasound liver (history of cirrhosis of liver)

Table 21.3 The transplant team

Transplant team
• Transplant surgeon—to evaluate for any surgical issues.
• Nephrologist—to evaluate for any medical issues
• Transplant co-ordinator—primary contact for the patient to help navigate through the transplant process
• Social worker—to assess socio-economic condition.
• Financial co-ordinator (optional)—to get medical insurance clearance.
• Pharmacist (optional)—to educate the patient about medications post-transplant.
• Psychologist (optional)—to evaluate for mental disorders
• Dietician (optional)—overweight and underweight patients

of transplants. The role of a recipient evaluation team is to provide constant support and encouragement to the patient and help them understand and navigate the evaluation process (Table 21.3). The team must frequently meet to address patient needs and clear them medically and surgically for transplant. It is also necessary to evaluate if the patient has adequate social support and means to support visits and medications post-transplant.

Transplant Recipient Testing

The necessary cardiac screening and work-up for infectious diseases follow a thorough medical history and physical examination. Additionally, transplant centers can determine their required and optional testing based on the local environment and demographics of the population they serve (Tables 21.4 and 21.5).

Comorbid Conditions in Renal Transplant Recipient

Cardiovascular Disease

In many developed and developing countries, CVD is the most common cause of death at all points post-transplant. The risk factors are older age, pre-existing CVD, time on dialysis, and diabetes mellitus. Most of the deaths occur

Table 21.4 Pre-transplant evaluation required testing

Transplant recipient required testing
– ABO compatibility
– HLA typing and anti-HLA antibody screening
– Complete blood count—TLC with differential, Hemoglobin, Hematocrit, Platelets.
– Complete chemistry panel—sodium, potassium, bicarbonate, urea or blood urea nitrogen, creatinine, calcium, PTH
– Liver function tests—AST, ALT, Total bilirubin, Direct Bilirubin, Total protein, Albumin.
– Serum/Urine toxicology screen.
– HbA1C or 2-h glucose tolerance test
– Hepatitis A IgG, Hepatitis B surface antigen, b core antibody, Hepatitis C antibody, HIV antibody.
– Type and screen for blood
– VDRL, CMV IgG,
– Coagulation panel (PT, INR, PTT)
– PPD (TB skin test) or interferon-gamma release assay (IGRA)
– Beta HCG (women of childbearing age)
– Chest X-ray
– Electrocardiogram
– Abdominal ultrasound or computed tomography

Table 21.5 Pre-transplant evaluation complementary optional testing

Optional testing
– Alkaline phosphate, uric acid, fasting lipids, glucose, magnesium, phosphorus.
– EBV, HSV, HTLV, Varicella, Toxoplasmosis, Rubella, Strongyloides, T. Cruzi, West Nile, Chagas disease.
– Cardiac ECHO or Stress test (depending on age and comorbidities)
– 24-h blood pressure monitoring
– Hypercoagulable work up (history of bleeding, thrombosis, miscarriages)
– Cardiology clearance (patients with a history of CAD, arrhythmia, abnormal cardiac imaging tests).
– Transplant psychologist (history of mental disorder, e.g., depression or anxiety)
– Nutrition assessment (uncontrolled diabetes, BMI >40%, frailty, weight loss, undernourished)
– Cystoscopy (cyclophosphamide exposure)
– Pulmonary function tests with pulmonary consult (patients with COPD)
– CT angiography of abdomen and pelvis and lower limbs (vasculature evaluation)

within 30 days post-transplant. In the pre-transplant evaluation, it is needed to identify moderate to high-risk patients and work on their risk factor management, such as treatment of hypertension, hyperlipidemia and stop cigarette smoking.

CAD is very prevalent in CKD and ESKD patients compared to the general population. CKD patients undergoing transplant evaluation should undergo a comprehensive screening with either non-invasive or invasive testing. There are no uniform guidelines from various medical societies (Table 21.6). The assessment will depend mainly on the history of diabetes and cardiovascular disease. In patients without diabetes or other risk factors, the cardiovascular review could be limited to history, physical examination, and electrocardiogram. However, the presence of risk factors determines further assessment by echocardiogram and stress test (treadmill or dobutamine) or nuclear imaging. A long history of diabetes and the presence of cardiovascular risk factors may require an evaluation by a cardiologist and possible cardiac angiography [2, 3].

Recipients with heart failure due to left ventricular systolic or diastolic dysfunction should undergo evaluation by history, physical examination, chest X-ray, electrocardiogram, and echocardiogram. Like CAD, there is a need to determine the etiology of cardiac dysfunction and work on the risk factors. It also includes looking at dialysis adequacy and volume control. The presence of LVH and higher LA volume are independent predictors of death in patients who are wait-listed for renal transplantation. AST and Canadian guidelines do not recommend listing for kidney transplantation alone in patients with severe irreversible (non-uremic) cardiac dysfunction. [see Chap. 11 for more information].

Cerebrovascular Disease

The rate of patients hospitalized with stroke is markedly higher for dialysis patients compared to the general population even after adjustment for age, gender, and race [4]. The risk continues to be increased close to 8% even after renal transplant. The main predictors are age, peripheral vascular disease, and diabetic nephropathy. Similar to cardiovascular evaluation, there is a need for the identification of patients at a high risk of cerebrovascular disease and work on risk modifications such as the use of statin therapy. The patients' evaluation should include an electrocardiogram, carotid Doppler +/− CT of the head, or MRI. Carotid endarterectomy indica-

Table 21.6 Guidelines from transplant societies for cardiovascular evaluation

Canadian guidelines:
1. All patients should be assessed for the presence of ischemic heart disease with an ECG and a chest radiograph
2. Further testing for IHD depends on the pretest probability of coronary artery disease (CAD). The following patients should have further non-invasive testing:
• Symptomatic patients or patients with a prior history of CAD, including:
– Previous history of myocardial infarction (Grade A)
– Symptoms of angina (Grade A)
– Signs or symptoms of congestive heart failure (Grade A)
• Asymptomatic patients with:
– Diabetes (type 1 or type 2) (Grade B)
– Multiple risk factors for CAD (3 or more) (Grade B):
Age >50 years
Prolonged duration of chronic kidney disease
Family history of CAD (first-degree relative)
Significant smoking history
Dyslipidemia (high-density lipoprotein level <0.9 mmol/L or total cholesterol >5.2 mmol/L), BMI $\geq$ 30 kg/m^2
History of hypertension
3. A cardiologist should assess all patients with a positive non-invasive test to undergo angiography (Grade B).
4. Very high-risk patients should be considered for angiography even with a negative non-invasive test (Grade C).
KDIGO guidelines:
1. All patients evaluated for kidney transplantation should undergo assessment for the presence and severity of cardiac disease with history, physical examination, and electrocardiogram (ECG).
2. Patients with signs or symptoms of active cardiac disease (e.g., angina, arrhythmia, heart failure, symptomatic valvular heart disease) should undergo an assessment by a cardiologist and be managed according to current local cardiac guidelines before further consideration for a kidney transplant.
3. Asymptomatic KTCs at high risk for coronary artery disease (CAD) or reduced functional capacity undergo non-invasive CAD screening.
4. Asymptomatic KTCs with known CAD not be revascularized exclusively to reduce perioperative cardiac events.
5. Exclude candidates with advanced triple vessel coronary disease from kidney transplantation. However, the risk of a post-transplant major cardiac event should be a significant consideration and discussed with the candidate

tions are similar to the general population. As per Canadian guidelines, kidney transplantation should be deferred in patients with a history of stroke or transient ischemic events for six months following the event.

Patients with autosomal dominant polycystic kidney (ADPK) disease have 4 to 5 times higher prevalence of intracranial aneurysm. The guidelines suggest screening patients with ADPK disease and a family history of an intracranial aneurysm, history of headaches, or those who have an at-risk activity. Evaluation by MRA or CT angiogram is indicated for high-risk patients, and neurosurgery should be consulted for further assessment and management. The intervention is recommended if the size of the aneurysm is >7 mm.

Peripheral Vascular Disease

Peripheral vascular occlusive disease after renal transplantation has been associated with lower 10-year patient and graft survival [5]. The risk factors are age, preoperative peripheral vascular disease, diabetes, and smoking. There is a higher incidence of peripheral arterial disease and death in patients waiting for a kidney transplant. At the time of transplantation, abnormal toe brachial index and history of diabetes are the most significant risk factors for proximal foot amputation. The vasculature should be evaluated by Doppler's or computed tomography of the abdomen, pelvis and lower limbs for all high-risk patients such as diabetics or with a history of claudication.

Malignancy

Patients with ESKD and on dialysis have a higher risk of cancer than patients not on dialysis, especially kidney and bladder cancer. The mortality among transplant recipients with a history of cancer is 30% higher compared to other patients. Therefore, transplant candidates should be screened for cancer, depending on their age and risk factors.

Patients with a malignancy history have a waiting time from 2–5 years after their curative treatment, depending on the type and stage of cancer; some malignancies do not require a wait time prior to transplantation (Table 21.7). The

Table 21.7 Malignancy with no waiting time

Malignancies with no waiting time (KDIGO guidelines)
• Non-melanoma skin cancers (surgically or otherwise treated) • Small renal cell cancer (<3 cm) • Prostate cancer (Gleason score ≤6) • Carcinoma in situ • Thyroid cancer (follicular/papillary <2 cm of low-grade histology) • Superficial bladder cancer

Table 21.8 Malignancy and its recurrence risk

Cancer	Recurrence risk
Incidental renal cancer	1%
Uterus (body)	4%
Testicular cancer (including seminomas, teratomas, embryomas, choriocarcinomas, mixed cell, and unclassified tumors)	5%
Cervix of uterus	6%
Thyroid and other endocrine tumors	7%
Colon Cancer	21%
Prostate cancer	18%
Lymphoma (Hodgkin's and Non-Hodgkin's)	11%
Malignant Melanoma	21%
Wilm's tumor	13%
Breast Cancer	23%
Clinically apparent or symptomatic renal cancer	27%
Bladder cancer	29%
Kaposi's and other sarcomas	29%
Multiple myeloma	67%
Non-melanoma skin cancer	48%

waiting time for cancers after treatment is two years for malignancy with low recurrence rates (1–7%) and 2–5 years for cancers with intermediate (11–21%) and high recurrence risk (>23%). Cancers such as leukemia have minimal data to propose waiting time, and for patients treated for liver cancer, there is a high rate of recurrence, so renal transplantation is not recommended (Table 21.8 illustrates common malignancies and their recurrence risk).

Obesity

KDIGO recommends using BMI or waist to hip circumference ratio to evaluate for obesity. In terms of BMI, obesity is defined as BMI >30 kg/m^2 and super obese as >35 kg/m^2. For candidates of Asian ethnicity, obesity is defined as a BMI >27.5 kg/m^2. As per WHO, waist to hip ratio of >0.85 for women or >0.9 for men is considered obese. Obese patients have a similar graft survival compared to non-obese patients; however, the risk of DGF is higher. Most of the transplant centers do recommend weight loss before transplantation; however, the threshold for a kidney transplant is dependent on the transplant center and its policies. Most centers decline patients with BMI >40 kg/m^2 and recommend some intervention for weight loss.

Age

At all ages, renal transplantation offers a substantial survival advantage over dialysis. In patients older than 60, the 5-year survival is 90% compared to 27% for patients on dialysis. However, one-year survival is almost similar between the two groups. Therefore, elderly patients should be considered for transplant if their life expectancy is >2 years. Currently, as per SRTR (Scientific Registry of Transplant Recipients) data, 23.8% of wait-listed patients are 65-year-old or older.

Age alone can be misleading in transplant recipient evaluations. Elderly patients should undergo a frailty assessment by Hopkins frailty phenotype scoring. Frail alone increases the risk of death by two-fold. In the Hopkins phenotype frailty measure, the definition of frailty, as a clinical syndrome, relies on having three or more following five criteria: unintentional weight loss, self-reported exhaustion, weakness, slow walking speed, and low physical activity.

The cognitive function should also be evaluated in detail, as the ten-year dementia risk is 17% for patients 75 years and older.

Infections—HIV, Hepatitis B, Hepatitis C, Tuberculosis

HIV

These patients are currently considered for a kidney transplant if they are compliant with their medical treatment, have an undetectable viral load for more than six months, CD4 count is >200/μL, and no opportunistic infections.

The 5-year graft survival in well-controlled HIV infected patients is similar to non-HIV patients. The antiretroviral regimen should be adjusted and modified before the transplant. Patients must be adherent and tolerant to HIV medications, and ideally, no significant interaction among antiretroviral and immunosuppressive drugs should exist. The risk of DGF and acute rejection is higher, and the risk of de novo malignancy and infections is acceptable in HIV renal transplant recipients.

Hepatitis B

The serological status of recipients should be determined before transplantation. The presence of HBV DNA or hepatitis B antigen pre-transplant has been associated with an increased probability of death from liver disease post-transplant. Immunosuppressive therapy may also enhance viral replication in both HbsAg positive and negative patients. Patients with chronic HBV should be evaluated further with HBV DNA levels and ultrasound for cirrhosis. Patients with compensated cirrhosis can be considered for kidney transplantation alone. In recipients with high risk or HBV reactivation, treatment with entecavir or tenofovir should be initiated.

Hepatitis C

Patients on chronic hemodialysis with positive anti-HCV antibodies have an increased incidence of liver cirrhosis and hepatocellular carcinoma leading to increased mortality. Renal transplant recipients with hepatitis C have an increased risk of death and graft loss. Therefore, every patient is screened for hepatitis C before transplant. HCV-positive patients should undergo investigation for liver cirrhosis. Patients should be treated for Hepatitis C before transplant if they present with decompensated cirrhosis or extrahepatic manifestations of hepatitis C. In the absence of such conditions, patients may accept a kidney from HCV positive or negative donors balancing the risks and benefits of shortening the waiting time. Irrespective of the timing, all patients should be treated with the direct antiviral drug.

Tuberculosis

There is a risk of reactivation of tuberculosis post-transplant, especially for those who have the latent disease and live in endemic areas. Therefore, all kidney transplant recipients are screened for tuberculosis with either PPD or IGRA. If available, the more sensitive IGRA should be used for the diagnosis of latent tuberculosis. As per European guidelines, patients considered to have latent TB infection are defined by:

- A 5 mm (renal transplant recipients) or a 10 mm (dialysis patients) induration after tuberculin skin testing
- Chest X-ray images suggestive of past TB infection
- History of prior TB infection that was not treated adequately; and
- Close contact with infectious patients.

Patients with latent tuberculosis isoniazid (for nine months) or rifampin (for four months) is recommended before transplant for treatment. Patients with active tuberculosis should not be considered for kidney transplantation until they undergo successful treatment.

Pulmonary Disorder

Currently, the guidelines recommend screening for transplant recipients, similar to the general population. However, Canadian guidelines have defined criteria for candidates who have pulmonary disease and are not candidates. However, all guidelines (AST, European, and Canadian) recommend stopping smoking, as patients who are current smokers are at a higher risk for perioperative complications (Table 21.9).

Hematologic Disorders

Hypercoagulable states undiagnosed before transplant have been associated with acute vascular rejections, venous thrombosis, and transplant failure. However, routine hematological screening is not recommended for every transplant recipient. The testing should be limited to patients with a history of recurrent venous thrombosis

Table 21.9 Canadian guidelines for patients with pulmonary disorders

Canadian guidelines for pulmonary disorders

1. Patients with the following respiratory conditions and severity are not candidates for kidney transplantation:
   - A requirement for home oxygen therapy
   - Uncontrolled asthma
   - Severe cor pulmonale
   - Severe chronic obstructive pulmonary disease (COPD)–pulmonary fibrosis or restrictive disease with any of the following parameters: best forced expiratory volume in 1 s (FEV1) <25% predicted value, PO_2 room air <60 mmHg with exercise desaturation, SaO_2 < 90% > 4 lower respiratory infections in the last 12 months, a moderate disease with evidence of progression
2. Patients with moderate COPD–pulmonary fibrosis or restrictive disease with any of the following parameters have a relative contraindication for kidney transplantation (Grade C):
   - Best FEV1 25–50% of the predicted value
   - PO2 room air <60–70 mmHg
   - Restrictive disease with exercise desaturation, SaO_2 90%

(dialysis access or thrombosis of the portal, hepatic, mesenteric veins), arterial thrombosis, family history of thrombosis, and recurrent miscarriage. Perioperative anticoagulation can decrease the risk of allograft thrombosis.

Living Donor Evaluation

Living donor kidney transplantation, more frequently than deceased donor kidney transplantation, provides excellent graft function and, depending on HLA compatibility, longer graft longevity. As per the Global Observatory on Donation and Transplant, 36% of 90.306 kidney transplants performed worldwide in 2017 were from living donors. The number of living donor transplants were more in Africa, the Eastern Mediterranean, and Southeast Asia compared to the Americas and European region. In the United States, the number of living donors increased in 2018 and 2019 after being stable for most of the decade. In the United States, according to the Organ Procurement and Transplantation Network data, 38% of the kidney transplants performed in 2019 were from living donors. In Europe, 28% of total kidney transplants were from living donors (Table 21.10).

Kidney Donation Evaluation

Ideally, living donor candidates should be evaluated by a team, preferably separate from the kidney recipient team. The kidney donation team should include a nephrologist and transplant surgeon (both not involved in the recipient's care), co-ordinator, social worker, and other optional members, including dietitians, psychologists, and psychiatrists. The advocate for the living donor helps a well-informed decision for donation providing independent information and assuring the absence of coercion. Every living donor should have informed consent, which details their rights, consent for donation, risks involved not limited to the medical or surgical, and the psychosocial risk related to donation. Kidney donors undergo a thorough evaluation to identify medical, surgical, or psychosocial conditions that may put them at a high risk of chronic kidney disease in the future [6, 7]. Every center can modify the testing based on the endemic disease in their patient population, but necessary work-up should be standard for any donor (Tables 21.11 and 21.12). There are a few absolute and relative contraindications for donors to donate (Table 21.13).

Donor History

A detailed history helps us to understand better as well as inform donors of their risk of chronic kidney disease in the future. During history taking and laboratory review, if the risk of immediate kidney disease is considerable, one should not proceed with the donation.

Donor Medical history: It should focus on their past medical history and their future risk of developing the disease, especially diabetes,

Table 21.10 Kidney transplants by world region in 2018. Data from the Global Observatory on Donation and Transplantation (GODT)

Region	All kidney transplants in 2018	LD kidney transplants	DD Kidney transplants
Americas	36,541	11,021	25,308
South East Asia	7963	6772	1164
Europe	27,879	7820	20,059
Western pacific	16,315	3823	12,492
Africa	268	268	–
Eastern Mediterranean	1858	1685	173

Data from the Global Observatory on Donation and Transplantation (GODT). LD, living donor; DD, deceased donor

Table 21.11 Required evaluations, testing, and donor follow-up

Complete medical history and physical examination: (including a family history of kidney disease, kidney stones, gout, lifestyle, habits. Measure blood pressure on at least two occasions)

Testing:

- ABO blood typing
- Human Leucocyte antigens (HLA) class I and II typing
- Pre donation kidney function (glomerular filtration rate):
  - Estimate GFR using serum creatinine-based estimating equations
  - Confirm with one or more of the following: measured GFR using an exogenous filtration marker (Iothalamate, iohexol, radionuclides), measured creatinine clearance, eGFR from the combination of serum creatinine and cystatin C,
  - If none available: repeat eGFR with serum creatinine
- Predonation albuminuria:
  - Assess albuminuria using albumin-to-creatinine ratio in a spot urine specimen
  - Confirm albuminuria with albumin excretion rate in a timed urine specimen or by repeating albumin-to-creatinine ratio if albumin excretion rate is not possible
- Urine: urinalysis, urine culture, toxicology screen
- Blood: complete blood count—TLC with differential, Hemoglobin, Hematocrit, Platelets.Complete chemistry panel: sodium, potassium, bicarbonate, urea or blood urea nitrogen, creatinine, calcium, fasting blood glucose or glycated hemoglobin (hemoglobin A1c) or 2-h glucose tolerance testing, fasting lipid profile, including total cholesterol, LDL-cholesterol, HDL-cholesterol, and triglycerides.
- Infection transmission: HIV, Hepatitis B virus, Hepatitis C virus, Cytomegalovirus, Epstein–Barr virus, Treponema pallidum (syphilis), and other potential infections as per geography and environmental exposures. PPD or IGRA
- Coagulation (PT, INR, PTT)
- Beta HCG: immediately before donation, women of childbearing age
- Image: chest x-ray, an image of the kidneys and urinary tract
- ECG
- Cancer Screening (as per local guidelines, including):
  - Pap smear (women over 21 yo)
  - Mammogram (women over 40 yo, should be current within 12 months)
  - Colonoscopy (patients over 50)
- Psychosocial evaluation
- Ethical, legal, and policy considerations (respect donor autonomy) at all phases
- Nephrology evaluation for medical clearance.
- Transplant surgeon evaluation for surgical clearance

Post donation follow-up (yearly intervals):

- Blood pressure measurement, body mass index measurement,
- Serum creatinine measurement with GFR estimation and albuminuria measurement
- Promotion of healthy lifestyle (exercise, diet, and abstinence from tobacco
- Promote psychologic health and well-being
- Urine protein quantification

Table 21.12 Optional testing for Donors according to individual characteristics and environmental exposures

Optional testing:
– Alkaline phosphatase, total protein, albumin, total bilirubin, uric acid, AST, ALT, fasting lipids, glucose, magnesium, phosphorus.
– Varicella, Toxoplasmosis, Rubella, Strongyloidosis, T. Cruzi, West Nile, Chagas disease and hypercoagulable work up in donors with a history of bleeding or thrombosis.
– Nuclear medicine kidney scan for evaluation of split GFR (DTPA, MAG 3)
– Donors older than 50 years: echo and stress testing (treadmill test for men, Adenosine Sesti for women)
– CT-angiogram (CTA)
– 24 h Blood pressure monitoring if needed
– Nutrition assessment (Hypertension, BMI >30%, unexplained weight loss)
– Psychosocial evaluation with transplant social worker or transplant psychologist.

Table 21.13 Absolute and Relative Contraindications for Donation

Absolute Contraindications for kidney donation:
– GFR <60 mL/min per 1.73 m^2
– Solitary kidney
– Albuminuria >100 mg/d
– History of overt proteinuria or hematuria of glomerular origin (except thin basement membrane)
– Age <18 years-old
– Type 1 Diabetes and Type 2 diabetes, not well controlled.
– Active cancer
– Active drug abuse (including alcohol)
– Uncontrolled psychiatric disorder
Relative Contraindications for kidney donation:
– GFR 60–90 mL/min per 1.73 m^2
– Type 2 diabetes
– History of malignancy
– Chronic illness
– Obesity with a BMI >35
– History of nephrolithiasis
– History of hypertension on more than two drugs or with organ damage
– Impaired glucose tolerance

hypertension, coronary heart disease, obesity, nephrolithiasis. Medical history of cancer is vital along with their medication history (nephrotoxic medications such as but not limited to non-steroidal anti-inflammatory drugs). History of infections is significant, especially for donors from endemic areas to avoid transmission of disease to recipients.

Surgical history: Should focus on previous abdominal surgeries, which could cause unexpected problems during kidney retrieval—also, any surgery, which was complicated by kidney, ureter, or bladder injury.

Social history: a history of smoking (both active and passive is essential), excessive alcohol intake, intravenous or illicit drug use may have caused some other organ damage which may need further evaluation.

Family history: the focus should be to identify any genetic kidney disease (such as polycystic kidney disease) which may manifest in the donor later. Detailed family history may help guide future risk of illness in the living donor.

Risk of Donation

Surgical Risk

Living donor surgery is considered safe. Surgical mortality is 3.1 per 10,000 donors. The risk of complications has been evaluated in various studies to date. As per the European association guidelines (based on the US transplant registry), 16.8% of donors experienced a perioperative complication, most commonly gastrointestinal (4.4%), bleeding (3.0%), respiratory (2.5%), surgical/anesthesia-related injuries (2.4%). After adjustment of the demographics, African-American are at higher risk of complications. The perioperative complication rate at Canadian transplant centers was also close to 13%. The re-hospitalization rate following donor nephrectomy is higher among donors who are older and have more comorbid conditions.

Medical Risk

The risk of ESRD is slightly high compared to non-donors. In one report, the relative risk increased between 3.5 and 5.3 for 15-year kidney failure, according to sex and race. An online tool (http://www.transplantmodels.com/esrdrisk/)

may be used to estimate the projected lifetime risk of ESRD in the absence of donation according to baseline demographic and clinical characteristics. The projected pre-donation risk can be multiplied by the estimated donation attributable risk to calculate the projected post-donation risk. However, the absolute risk is generally low. Moreover, it seems to be no increased risk for chronic diseases such as hypertension, diabetes or cardiovascular disease, or any adverse psychosocial outcomes. In living donors, eGFR at six months may be an independent predictor for ESRD. The incidence of ESRD 15 years post-donation with eGFR <50 mL/mim/1.73 m^2 at 6 months mark is 33 per 10,000 donors compared to 11.7 donors per 10,000 with eGFR >70 mL/min/1.73 m^2.

Pre-Eclampsia

The risk of pre-eclampsia and HTN is double in female living kidney donors. However, there is no significant risk of preterm birth or low birth weight.

Special Considerations in Kidney Donors

Glomerular Filtration Rate

Ideally, donors should have a GFR of 90 mL/min per 1.73 m^2 or greater. When the GFR is between 60 and 89 mL/min per 1.73 m^2, the decision for donation must take into account the demographic and health profile of the donor in relation to what the transplant program considers an acceptable risk. Donor candidates with GFR less than 60 mL/min per 1.73 m^2 should not donate. When GFR is asymmetric or in the presence of parenchymal, vascular abnormalities, or urological abnormalities that do not preclude donation, the affected kidney should be used for donation.

Albuminuria

Patients with albuminuria <30 mg/d can be considered for kidney donation. If albuminuria ranges between 30 and 100 mg/day, the donation should be on a case by case basis taking into account other risk factors. Candidates with albuminuria >100 mg/d should not donate.

Hematuria

Donors with microscopic hematuria should be considered as kidney donors after they have been evaluated in detail. In the concomitance of albuminuria (> 30 mg/d), genetic risk, abnormal urologic or urinary stone evaluation donation should not proceed. In some cases, the evaluation may include a cystoscopy or a kidney biopsy.

Prediabetes

Living donors with impaired glucose tolerance may be able to donate without any significant comorbidity. KDIGO guidelines recommend considering patients with prediabetes if their risk of developing diabetes is low and with no other comorbidities.

BMI >35

There is an increased risk of ESRD in obese patients. For an increase in BMI >27 kg/m^2, there is a 7% increase in ESRD risk [8]. It is similar for all donors irrespective of gender, race or baseline eGFR spectrum. Therefore, most transplant centers are hesitant in considering donors with high BMI, especially with a higher prevalence of metabolic syndrome.

Hypertension

Ideally, donors should have normal blood pressure, as defined for the general population. According to the KDIGO guideline, donor candidates without evidence of organ damage and hypertension controlled to systolic blood pressure less than 140 mmHg and diastolic blood pressure less than 90 mmHg using one or two antihypertensive agents may be acceptable for donation.

Gout

Kidney donation is associated with an increase in serum uric acid concentration, which may increase the risk of gout. In non-donor populations, hyperuricemia is associated with a higher risk of CKD. In a large kidney-donor cohort study in the incidence of gout was not increased in donors; however, donors with gout had more frequent diagnoses of acute kidney injury, CKD, and other disorders of the kidney. An increased risk occurred in African Americans, older donors, and men. Therefore, donor candidates should be asked about prior episodes of gout.

Older Donors

For kidney donation, older age is classified as older than 60 years of age. Kidney donation from older donors is a safe surgical procedure. The long-term result from transplantation from an old living donor is similar to deceased donor transplantation from a younger donor. Therefore, it should be considered on a case-by-case basis. For hypertensive older donors with high blood pressure lower than 140/90 mmHg, with no end-organ damage and BMI <30, there is no increased incidence of kidney disease in the short term. However, long-term older hypertensive donors have an increased relative risk of ESRD (HR of 3.04) 15 years post-donation [9]. The absolute risk of ESRD is minimal. There is no increased mortality for older donors.

APOL1 Genetic Testing

There is an increased interest in the transplant community about the risk of the *APOL1* gene in donor candidates with sub-Saharan African ancestors and its likelihood of nephropathy in the future. Some centers are testing for the *APOL1* gene in patients of African descent and ruling them out for donation with two *APOL1* renal risk variants [10]. These kidneys have been associated with shorter graft survival and lower post-donation eGFR. In terms of cost-effectiveness, it is beneficial to prevent the earlier onset of chronic kidney disease in some of the African American donors.

Family History of Polycystic Kidney Disease

Age-dependent imaging criteria have been established for adults with a family history of ADPKD (PKD1 or PKD2). In candidates 40 years old or older, the absence or a limited number of cysts on kidney computed tomography or magnetic resonance imaging may be used to rule out ADPKD. DNA testing can also sometimes help diagnose or exclude the condition. PKD1 and PKD2 mutation screening, with a good technique, may help to elucidate whether or not the donor candidate is acceptable.

Conclusions

It was very important to take a full history and examine the patient to identify any other issues such as asymptomatic atherosclerotic artery disease and active sarcoidosis. She needed a dobutamine stress test with inducible ischaemia in 3/17 myocardial segments. The coronary angiogram showed atherosclerotic disease in the left anterior coronary artery which was managed with a coronary stent. She was started on aspirin and clopidogrel. Her full blood count, calcium, phosphate, liver function tests and chest Xray were normal. She was positive of CMV, EBV but negative for HepB, HepC, HIV. She was listed for kidney deceased donor list 3 months after the coronary angiogram when her clogidogrel was discontinued by cardiologist.

Questions

1. A 44 year old male, an intravenous drug user on haemodialysis with history of incidental renal cell carcinoma removed 10 years ago was referred for kidney transplantation. His BP was 170/80, height 168 cm weight 110 kg. He was on treatment for HIV infection with normal CD4 count.

   What is a contraindication for transplantation in this man?

   A. Active intravenous drug use
   B. High BMI
   C. High blood pressure
   D. HIV infection
   E. Past history of renal cell carcinoma

Answer A

2. A 55 year old man with diabetes, hypertension with advanced CKD and eGFR 15 mL/min/1.73 m^2 was referred for kidney trans-

plantation. What is the best possible test for screening for coronary artery disease?
   A. coronary angiography
   B. CT calcium score
   C. Exercise treadmill test
   D. Dobutamine stress test
   E. MRI of the heart

Answer D

3. Which vaccine should be avoided in the immediate post transplant period?
   A. Hepatitis A
   B. Influenza
   C. MMR
   D. Pneumococcus
   E. Tetanus

Answer MMR vaccine, as it is a live virus

4. Which of the following malignancies requires a long waiting time before kidney transplantation?
   A. Breast Cancer
   B. Carcinoma in situ
   C. Non-melanoma skin cancers (surgically or otherwise treated)
   D. Small renal cell cancer (<3 cm)
   E. Prostate cancer (Gleason score ≤6)

Answer A, the rest of the malignancies do not require any waiting

5. What is not an absolute contraindication for living kidney donation
   A. GFR <60 mL/min per 1.73 m^2
   B. History of nephrolithiasis
   C. Solitary kidney
   D. Type 1 Diabetes and Type 2 diabetes, not well controlled.
   E. Uncontrolled psychiatric disorder

Answer B

6. A 57 year old male was willing to donate a kidney to his wife. His blood group was A+ and his wife was B+.

   What is best option to improve graft survival?
   A. Anti-A/B antibody depletion at the time of transplantation using PP, double-filtration PP/membrane filtration, or selective or unselective immunoadsorption
   B. Continue with kidney transplantation without any measures
   C. Modulation of the recipient's immune system by the use of intravenous immunoglobulins
   D. Organise a paired exchange using the national paired exchange scheme
   E. Reduction of the B lymphocyte pool anti-CD20 antibody rituximab

Answer D, as this is has the best possible outcome

7. A 55 year old man with diabetes, hypertension with advanced CKD and eGFR 15 ml/min/1.73 m^2 was referred for kidney transplantation. A dobutamine stress test showed reversible ischaemia in 4/17 myocardial segments.

   What is the best possible test for management for possible coronary artery disease?
   A. CT coronary angiogram
   B. Coronary angiogram
   C. Exercise treadmill test
   D. MRI without gadolinium
   E. Myocardial perfusion scan

Answer A

8. A 55 year old man with diabetes, hypertension with advanced CKD and eGFR 15 mL/min/1.73 m^2 was referred for kidney transplantation. A dobutamine stress test showed reversible ischaemia in 4/17 myocardial segments. A coronary angiogram showed left anterior descending artery stenosis which was treated with coronary stent.

   What is next best possible step in management?
   A. Offer no antiplatelet therapy
   B. Start aspirin and wait 1 year before kidney transplantation
   C. Start aspirin and clopidogrel and wait 1 year before transplantation
   D. Start aspirin and clopidogrel and wait 3 months, then stop clopidogrel, continue aspirin proceed to transplantation
   E. Start clopidogrel and proceed to transplantation

Answer D

9. A 55 year old man with diabetes, hypertension on dialysis was referred for kidney transplantation. A dobutamine stress test showed reversible ischaemia in 5/17 myocar-

dial segments. A coronary angiogram showed triple vessel disease.

What is next best possible step in management

A. Do nothing as patient is asymptomatic
B. Plan for coronary stent
C. Plan for coronary artery bypass graft
D. Start calcium channel blocker
E. Start isosorbide and hydralazine

Answer C, will be the most common step though the evidence is not clear

10. A 45 year old patient was referred for a live donor kidney transplant from his mother. He has not received his COVID-19 vaccines and has not suffered from COVID-19.

What is the best possible advice for COVID-19 vaccination?

A. Avoid vaccination
B. Receive both doses at least two weeks before transplantation
C. Receive the last dose the day before kidney transplant
D. Receive both doses after transplantation
E. Receive the second dose a day after transplantation

Answer B, as this gives the best chance for immunity

Test your learning and check your understanding of this book's contents: use the "Springer Nature Flashcards" app to access questions using https://sn.pub/cz9Cok. To use the app, please follow the instructions in Chap. 1.

References

1. Contra-indications for transplantation. Nephrol Dialysis Transpl. 2000;15(suppl_7):5–6. https://doi.org/10.1093/ndt/15.suppl_7.5-a.
2. Kidney Disease: Improving Global Outcomes (KDIGO) Kidney Transplant Candidate Work Group. K/DOQI clinical practice guidelines on the evaluation and management of candidates for kidney transplantation. Transplantation. 2010;104:S1–S103. https://doi.org/10.1053/j.ajkd.2005.01.019.
3. Tabriziani H, Baron P, Abudayyeh I, Lipkowitz M. Cardiac risk assessment for end-stage renal disease patients on the renal transplant waiting list. Clin Kidney J. 2019;12(4):576–85. https://doi.org/10.1093/ckj/sfz039.
4. Seliger SL, Gillen DL, Longstreth W, Kestenbaum B, Stehman-Breen CO. Elevated risk of stroke among patients with end-stage renal disease. Kidney Int. 2003;64(2):603–9. https://doi.org/10.1046/j.1523-1755.2003.00101.x.
5. Sung RS, Althoen M, Howell TA, Merion RM. Peripheral vascular occlusive disease in renal transplant recipients: risk factors and impact on kidney allograft survival. Transplantation. 2000;70(7):1049–54. https://doi.org/10.1097/00007890-200010150-00010.
6. Lentine KL, Kasiske BL, Levey AS, Adams PL, Alberú J, et al. KDIGO clinical practice guideline on the evaluation and care of living kidney donors. Transplantation. 2017;101(8S):S1–S109.
7. Garg AX, Levey AS, Kasiske BL, Cheung M, Lentine KL, et al. Application of the 2017 KDIGO guideline for the evaluation and care of living kidney donors to clinical practice. Clin J Am Soc Nephrol 15: 896–905, 2020. doi: https://doi.org/10.2215/CJN.12141019.
8. Locke JE, Reed RD, Massie A, Maclennan PA, Sawinski D, Kumar V, et al. Obesity increases the risk of end-stage renal disease among living kidney donors. Kidney Int. 2017;91(3):699–703. https://doi.org/10.1016/j.kint.2016.10.014.
9. Ammary FA, Luo X, Muzaale AD, Massie AB, Crews DC, Waldram MM, et al. Risk of ESKD in older live kidney donors with hypertension. Clin J Am Soc Nephrol. 2019;14(7):1048–55. https://doi.org/10.2215/cjn.14031118.
10. Mena-Gutierrez, A. M., Reeves-Daniel, A. M., Jay, C. L., & Freedman, B. I. (2020). Practical considerations for APOL1 genotyping in the living kidney donor evaluation. Transplantation, 104(1), 27–32. doi: https://doi.org/10.1097/tp.0000000000002933.

Management of the Patient After Kidney Transplantation

22

Madhu Bhaskaran and Shahrzad Ossareh

Clinical Scenario

A 55-year-old male kidney transplant recipient, 4 years post-transplant, presented to the emergency department with fever, shortness of breath and fresh bleeding from the rectum. He was tender over the transplanted kidney. On examination, he was pale, tired and breathless. His haemoglobin was 54 g/L [previously 100 g/L], creatinine 1024 μmol/L [previously 230 μmol/L], serum potassium 6.5 mmol/L [previously 5.1 mmol/L] and platelets 63×10^9/L [previously 120×10^9/L], tacrolimus 19 ng/L [previously 8 ng/L].

What are next steps in management?

Introduction

Kidney transplantation changes quality of life and improves survival. Careful management in the immediate post-transplant period prevents graft loss due to rejection and infection. Longer term management maintains quality of life, prevents rejection, atypical infection and malignancy. This chapter will discuss recipient- and donor-related factors that influence post-transplant care, possible peri-operative events, hospital discharge and patient education, post-operative care, post-transplant clinic visits, common clinical and laboratory abnormalities and triage, post-transplant medications, post-transplant infections, indications for allograft biopsy and necessary allograft imaging studies. It will also discuss management of the failing renal allograft and kidney replacement therapy, long term care for patients, and other special considerations in follow-up care.

M. Bhaskaran (✉)
Northwell Healthcare, New York, USA
e-mail: MBhaskar@northwell.edu

S. Ossareh
Iran University of Medical Sciences, Tehran, Iran

Pre Transplant Evaluation and Factors that Influence Post-Transplant Care

There are several important factors that need to be considered during the short and longer term after kidney transplantation. The consequences and management of such factors are discussed as follows:

Aetiology of Kidney Disease

- Availability of native kidney biopsy: it is important to understand the nature of the native kidney disease leading to ESKD, that may have implications for the post-transplant course.
- Alport syndrome: this will increase the risk of anti-GBM disease, recurrence of which in a

D. Banerjee et al. (eds.), *Management of Kidney Diseases*,
https://doi.org/10.1007/978-3-031-09131-5_22

kidney allograft, can lead to rapid allograft loss

- SLE: previously thought to have low risk of recurrence, however transplant needs to be delayed until disease is quiescent; There is increasing awareness of recurrence in the transplant kidney
- Paraproteinemia: unrecognized pre-transplant can lead to recurrence and allograft loss early post-transplant
- Oxalosis: in many instances will require a simultaneous liver-kidney transplant to avoid recurrence in the transplanted kidney

> **Practice Point 1**
> - Obtain as much information about native kidney disease, including prior transplant course, any biopsies, recurrent disease
> - Obtain genetic panel when available—where original disease is unknown and particularly where there has been prior rapid allograft failure
> - Be mindful of missed paraproteinemia, Alport syndrome with anti-GBM in prior allograft, oxalosis variants with partial enzyme deficiency, Fabry disease

Co-Morbidities that Affect Post-Transplant Care

- Urinary tract abnormalities: if these are not recognized pre-transplant, they may cause: urinary obstruction (posterior urethral valve); recurrent urinary tract infection (vesico-ureteric reflux); abnormal allograft function (neurogenic/poorly functioning bladder)
- Pre-Transplant medical/social issues can interfere with adherence to medical advice and medication e.g. cognitive impairment, psychiatric illness, substance misuse
- Duration of chronic kidney disease (CKD)/end stage kidney disease (ESKD): This may increase cardiovascular risk
- Co morbidities that require special attention post-transplantion, e.g. Hypertension, diabetes mellitus, coronary artery disease, congestive heart failure including diastolic dysfunction, peripheral arterial disease, obstructive sleep apnoea, prior neoplastic disease, chronic infection, previous/prior immune suppression, opportunistic infections e.g. HHV8, HIV, hepatitis B, hepatitis C, BK virus, cytomegalovirus (CMV), Mycobacterium tuberculosis (MTB), Mycobacterium Avium Intracellulare (MAI) [1].

> **Practice Point 2**
> - Be mindful of urinary tract abnormalities in younger candidates and obtain cysto-urethrography
> - Bladder outlet obstruction in anuric dialysis patients may be asymptomatic
> - Ensure immunosuppression-free interval prior to retransplant in candidates with neoplasia related to immunosuppression and prior BK virus, CMV, MAI and HHV 8 infections and ensure clearance of Parvovirus B19 viraemia in collapsing glomerulopathy related to it
> - Invasive screening for coronary artery disease may be prudent in candidates who have uncontrolled or prolonged diabetes mellitus, other vascular diseases and/or a long dialysis vintage

Table 22.1 summarises important members of the post-transplantation multi-disciplinary team:

Table 22.1 Establishing communication among collaborative multi-disciplinary post-transplant care team

- A multidisciplinary team including a primary nephrologist, dialysis center, pre-transplant care team, transplant nephrologist and transplant surgeon, pre- and post-transplant coordinators, primary care provider
- Cardiologists and other specialists may be required for proper management in the peri- and early post-transplant period

Table 22.2 Crossmatch methods

- Pre-transplant complement-dependent cytotoxicity (CDC) crossmatch: detects alloantibody that binds and is cytotoxic to donor lymphocytes, in the presence of complement
- Flow cytometric crossmatch: detects antibody that binds to donor lymphocytes, but does not assess cytotoxicity
- Solid phase assay for donor specific antibodies: Detects the presence of antibody without additional information on lymphocyte binding or cytotoxicity
- Virtual crossmatch: Information on details of donor HLA and most current recipient antibody repertoire, without any sensitizing events in the interim allows for a 'virtual' crossmatching remotely without needing either donor or recipient tissue or blood samples.

Assessment of the Immunological Risk of Transplantation

Sensitizing events in the recipient such as blood or platelet transfusion, infections requiring hospitalization, pregnancy and prior transplants should be noted, and may lead to panel reactive antibodies, donor specific antibodies. This makes a pre-transplant virtual and/or physical cross match important, and may highlight a need for desensitization therapy. Table 22.2 summarises the different methods for Cross matching before transplantation [1].

Donor Factors that May Influence Post-Transplant Management

It is important to take into account donor related factors, that may affect outcome in the recipient, remembering that *'All kidneys are not equal'*: Consider that the best possible serum creatinine for a prospective DCD donor may be 150 μmol/L in both a tall, muscular 45-year-old male, and similarly in a short, hypertensive 65-year-old female.

Donor Related Factors that Can Influence Post-Transplant Management Include

- Live donor: HLA mismatches, age, need for desensitization, lymphocyte depleting induction
- Deceased donor: deceased cardiac death (DCD), High KDPI donor, donor age, donor CKD risk factors, cold ischemia time (CIT) and anatomical factors such as accessory renal vessel(s) and ureter(s).

Peri-Operative Events Which Affect Post-Operative Care

Cold ischemia time, delayed graft function, anatomic issues such as small accessory renal artery from the donor that could not be anastomosed, leading to loss of renal tissue, hypotension, complications such as ureteral obstruction, leak, vascular thrombosis or stenosis.

Surgical Complications that May Affect Post-Transplant Management

Transplant surgery involves anastomosis of the donor arteries and veins with those of the recipient, and the donor ureter with the recipient urinary bladder. As with any anastomosis, leaks and partial or complete blockage are the main complications. Manifestations will vary, depending on the degree and duration of leaks and the severity of stenosis. Prior condition of the recipient and donor blood vessels, recipient bladder and donor ureter, and preservation of its precarious blood supply are important factors that affect the surgical outcome. Injuries occurring to the donor prior to or during organ procurement can greatly impact the usability of the organ and complexity of the surgery. Enthusiastic cleaning of the donor ureter off its surrounding fat tissue by the procuring surgeon is often blamed by recipient surgeon for future ischemic damage to the ureter which becomes a major issue to deal with, often causing urine leak and necessitating surgical interventions. Urine leak can lead to allograft dysfunction, and sometimes resolves with placing a nephrostomy and drain from the collection, longer term bladder catheter and ureteral stent with gradual removal of the hardware over time allowing the ureter to heal. If ureteric leak is severe due to ischemic damage of long segment of donor ureter, this may necessitate re-anastomosis of the kidney to the bladder through sometimes utilizing recipients' own native ureter: a structure that surgeons often complain to be a harden to find and harder to mobilize.

An accessory renal artery to the lower pole of the donor kidney, if too small and hard to salvage during transplant surgery may be the harbinger of a compromised donor ureter.

Discharge and Education

Patient education is absolutely key to post-transplant success. Such education starts during the transplantation work-up phase, but the time in hospital after the kidney transplantation should be utilized as best as possible when patient are alert and pain-free. The following issues can be addressed prior to discharge:

1. Special attention to polypharmacy and susceptibility to medication errors
2. Transplant care being active, and complex compared to passive and relatively simple self-care during dialysis
3. The need to establish consistent and accessible contact for post-operative care and communications
4. The potential need for a care-giver with adequate skills that are complementary to the transplant recipients' own abilities
5. The need to identify barriers to optimal care, such as a language barrier, cognitive ability, comorbid psychiatric issues, transportation issues and substance mis-use (Table 22.3)
6. The need to identify and work with social determinants of health to achieve optimal outcome
7. Specific issues that need to be followed-up post-discharge, such as the need for ureteric stent removal, imaging abnormalities requiring follow-up, e.g. peri-nephric collections—all should be included in communication in the transition between inpatient and outpatient care
8. Clear and simple education and reference materials, listing post-transplant medications and the warning signs of potentially serious events that would require urgent medical attention
9. Transition of care to outpatient care teams, with a clear discharge summary and post-operative follow-up care needs

Table 22.3 Addressing Barriers to optimized care

Clinicians should be aware of:
- Cognitive impairment
- Caregiver issues
- Non-adherence with medications, medical advice and follow up visits
- Language barrier
- Psychiatric issues
- Issues with mobility and transportation
- Medical coverage and financial issues including poverty, food security and homelessness

Practice Point 3

- Establishing consistently smooth communication amongst all providers and caregivers
- The transplant recipient is integral to their optimal post-transplant care
- Ensuring a high level of adherence with medications and follow-up care is necessary for optimal outcomes in sensitized recipients, and previously known non-adherent recipients who have lost prior allografts prematurely
- Young age, prior substance mis-use, psychiatric illnesses and prior non-adherence are risk factors for non-adherence

Post-Discharge Care

The following issues should be considered during outpatient clinic visits: Whilst the COVID-pandemic has heralded a much greater demand for the flexibility and inexpensive nature of telephone consultation clinics. No doubt that the need for face-to-face consultations to help to build a good rapport and trust between patient and clinician is also acknowledged.

- Post-operative outpatient clinic schedule: Very frequent to start with 2-3 times a week and then less frequent but at regular intervals.
- Any need for post-operative home visits in-person or via Telehealth to check medication adherence, wound check, vital signs check
- Education of home care giver and collaboration with home care giver for optimized care and monitoring

- Home glucose, weight, urine put, temperature, blood pressure checks and flow sheets
- 'Pill box' filling and monitoring of adherence
- Lab test request; education regarding accurate trough level check of immunosuppressive agent
- In person home visit or Telehealth check regarding any warning signs needing to proper office visit or laboratory check/imaging study
- Coordination of care with other involved providers such as endocrinologist, cardiologist, psychiatrist, primary care giver and primary nephrologist.

Care Plan at a Post-Transplant Clinic Visit

A comprehensive post-transplant clinic visit may address all of the following over a period of time:

Acute symptoms: Fever, Pain, Urinary symptoms—dysuria, hematuria, decrease in urine output, nocturia, frequency; GI symptoms—diarrhea, constipation, nausea, vomiting, symptoms suggestive of prostatitis in males; Wound-related pain, discharge, bleeding, oedema, shortness of breath, symptoms suggestive of worsening co morbidities

Quality of life symptoms: Sleep disturbance; Activity limitation, incontinence, sexual dysfunction, driving limitations, vision changes, skin changes

Factors affecting Longevity of the recipient: Coronary artery disease, chronic infections, opportunistic infections, potentially life threatening infection

Factors affecting Longevity of the allograft: Medication adherence, achieved best allograft function, recurrent disease in the allograft, delayed allograft function, rejection episodes, closer immune monitoring of sensitized recipients; Opportunistic infections affecting allograft—BK virus, Aden, CMV, Parvo virus.

Obtaining Standardized Clinical and Laboratory Data at Each Encounter

The following clinical and laboratory data should be collected and analysed during each visit for optimal care.

Weight, urine output, blood pressure, glucose levels, medication side effects, surgical wound characteristics suggestive of healing vs. poor healing and infection

Blood counts, blood chemistry including Calcium, Phosphate, magnesium; urinalysis, urine protein/creatinine ratio; Trough levels of immunosuppressive agents—Tacrolimus, Sirolimus, Everolimus or Cyclosporin. Monitoring for opportunistic infection—BK virus PCR in blood; CMV PCR in blood following cessation of antiviral prophylaxis.

Practice Point 4

- An abnormal urinalysis with presence of blood is common immediately post-transplant, but special attention to a persistently high urine protein:creatinine ratio needs to be paid in order to recognise recurrent focal segmental glomerulosclerosis (FSGS) at the earliest possible stage

Imaging follow-up of allograft imaging post-op or previous imaging abnormalities such as lung nodules/thyroid nodules, pancreas cysts, naive kidney cysts, adrenal nodules.

Post Clinic Visit Lab Review and Follow-Up

Changes in response to immunosuppression trough levels that are sub- or supra-therapeutic; electrolyte abnormalities and changes in allograft function.

Often warranted are—Changes in immunosuppression dose, repletion of magnesium, phosphorus, potassium, managing hyperkalemia, managing hypercalcemia from hyperparathyroidism, changes in cell counts warranting changes in dosages of anti-proliferative agents when low and evaluation for possible infection when elevated. Table 22.4 summarises a typical post-transplantation clinic follow-up schedule.

Table 22.4 Post-transplantation clinic follow-up schedule

The schedule can be variable and may need to individualized; an example schedule is as follows, and may be adjusted to suit needs: • Twice weekly for the first 2 weeks post-transplant • Once weekly for weeks 1–2 • From 1st to 3rd month every 2 weeks • From the following 3 months, monthly till the end of the first year • Then every 2 months until end of second year, • Then every 3 months following 2 until 5 years • Then every 6 months lifelong

A typical model for post-transplantation clinic follow-up is illustrated in Table 22.4:

Practice Point 5

- End all post-transplant visits by summarizing any medication changes made during the visit and clarifying any doubts and establishing a time line for follow up visit based on individual circumstances
- Questions about smoking and alcohol use need to be carefully repeated at follow up visits

Common Clinical and Laboratory Abnormalities and Triage

The causes of frequently encountered clinical and laboratory abnormalities are as follows:

Clinical

- Rapid weight gain: Fluid retention: dependent oedema, elevated blood pressure, orthopnea and exertional dyspnoea. Increased risk of post-transplant new onset diabetes mellitus if non fluid weight gain
- Oedema: Fluid retention, Deep vein thrombosis, Congestive heart failure, Side effect of medications—nifedipine, amlodipine, sirolimus
- Weight loss: New onset diabetes mellitus; Poor appetite or severe diarrhea with malabsorption, Mycophenolate toxicity
- Elevated blood pressure: Need to restart antihypertensive, Tacrolimus toxicity, Acute rejection, Transplant renal artery stenosis, Fluid retention
- Low blood pressure and Orthostasis: Dehydration and hypovolemia, antihypertensive side effect, adrenal insufficiency
- Hyperglycemia: New onset or poorly controlled diabetes mellitus
- Hypoglycemia: Iatrogenic, adrenal insufficiency
- Diarrhea: Mycophenolate toxicity, Viral infection—Rota virus, Sapovirus, Clostridium difficile toxin
- Constipation: Opioid side effect; Hypothyroidism
- Abdominal Pain: Urine leak, post-operative wound infection, calculus cholecystitis, pancreatitis, cyst rupture, nephrolithiasis
- Fever: Infectious—Urinary infection, opportunistic infections, pneumonia, post-operative wound infection and abscess, Deep vein thrombosis, acute rejection, Post-transplant lymphoproliferative disorder
- Shortness of breath: pulmonary embolism, congestive heart failure, fluid retention, uncontrolled hypertension
- Increased urine output: hyperglycemia, hypercalcemia
- Urinary frequency: small bladder, prostatism, ureteric stent related
- Hematuria: Retained clots in bladder, native kidney related-cyst rupture, Urinary tract infection, ureteral stent related, BK virus infection, urinary bladder calculus
- Decreased urine output: Dehydration, Hypovolemia, low blood pressure, acute rejection
- Urinary retention: Prostatism, neurogenic bladder, bladder calculus
- Dysuria: Urinary tract infection, hematuria, ureteral stent related, Interstitial cystitis
- Stent extrusion

Practice Point 6

- Based on the time interval following transplant, prioritize enquiry during the post-transplant visit for potential major likely issues affecting allograft and patient outcome

- Special attention to quality-of-life issues as well as medication side effects and personal biases will ensure improved adherence
- New onset diabetes is easily missed in transplant recipients
- Dysuria without urinary infection is often reported in presence of haematuria.

Complete Blood Count

- Leukopenia: Viral infections—CMV, Mycophenolate toxicity, Thymoglobulin
- Leukocytosis: Bacterial infections, corticosteroid related, lymphoproliferative disorder
- Anaemia: Related to chronic kidney disease, Mycophenolate toxicity, Parvo B19 infection, T cell proliferative disorder, hemolysis, related to dapsone use, Thrombotic microangiopathy
- Erythrocytosis: Post transplant erythrocytosis, renal cell carcinoma
- Thrombocytopenia: Mycophenolate toxicity, Thymoglobulin related, Thrombotic microangiopathy

Practice Point 7

- Carefully review for trends in abnormalities and schedule shorter interval follow-up to avoid life threatening situations such as severe neutropenia or thrombocytopenia
- Special attention to decreasing haemoglobin in recipients with significant coronary artery disease
- Ensure native kidney imaging to look for renal cell carcinoma (RCC) and transplant renal artery doppler to rule out stenosis prior to initiating ACEI/ARB therapy in erythrocytosis post-transplant

Blood Chemistry

- Hyponatremia: Water intoxication, Urine leak, Hypothyroidism, Thiazide therapy
- Hypernatremia: Dehydration, osmotic diuresis from hyperglycemia, polyuria from hypercalcemia
- Hyperkalemia: Tacrolimus and cyclosporin toxicity, urinary retention, NSAID use, haemolysis, rhabdomyolysis, dehydration / hypovolemia
- Hypokalemia: Polyuria related to hyperglycemia, hypercalcemia, diuretic use
- Acidosis: Calcineurin inhibitor related Type 4 renal tubular acidosis, urinary retention, renal insufficiency
- Alkalosis: Diuretic use, hypovolemia
- Abnormal liver function tests: Elevated transaminases, bilirubin, GGT:
  - Drug induced-mycophenolate, azathioprine, calcineurin inhibitor related
  - Infection-related: CMV infection, viral hepatitis, cholecystitis, underlying liver disease
- Non-therapeutic tacrolimus/cyclosporin trough levels: Adherence issues, diarrhoea and constipation, co-intake of medications leading to interruptions, erratic absorption related to prior bowel surgery, food interactions
- Elevated creatinine: acute rejection, urine leak, urinary retention, hypovolemia, vascular issues, transplant renal artery stenosis or iliac artery stenosis, elevated calcineurin inhibitor level, Infections such as pyelonephritis, viral infections—BK virus, CMV, Adeno virus, Parvo virus
- Nephrolithiasis , bladder outlet obstruction—mechanical or functional , drug toxicity—calcineurin inhibitor, NSAIDs, contrast-related; thrombotic microangiopathy (TMA), post transplant lymphoproliferative disorder (PTLD)

Practice Point 8

- Special attention to trend in creatinine since I has low sensitivity at high GFR levels. Be mindful of rejection when Tacrolimus level is sub therapeutic with a rise in creatinine
- Careful with Tacrolimus (or Cyclosporin) and Sirolimus combination therapy since Tacrolimus toxicity can occur even with otherwise therapeutic levels
- Repletion of low magnesium (<1.5 MEq/L) or phosphorus (<2.5 MEq/L) may be due to elevated Tacrolimus level but likely need to be repleted
- An elevated Ca (>12 MeQ/L) with elevated iPTH level will necessitate increased hydration and possible treatment with Cinacalcet
- A low WBC count (<2.5) or low platelet count may necessitate adjustment or or discontinuation of mycophenolate therapy. Neutropenia if severe (<500) and persistent may warrant growth factor therapy involving GMCF.

Microbiology

- Bacteriuria, candiduria, Viral PCR for Epstein Barr virus, CMV, BK virus, West Nile virus
- Serologies: Crypto antigen, Galacto mannan, Beta D Glucan

Practice Point 9

- Check CMV PCR following discontinuation of Valganciclovir prophylaxis since this is a risky time period for CMV resurgence with clinical disease
- CMV IgG if negative is less reliable in recipient candidates since it has less sensitivity in end stage kidney disease patients

Imaging Abnormalities

Ultrasound with Doppler

- Imaging indicated for evaluation of elevated creatinine, hematuria, changes in urine output, hypertension, recurrent urinary infections, follow up of prior abnormal findings.
- Fluid collection: lymphocele, urinoma, hematoma
- Elevated velocity: Transplant renal artery stenosis, Iliac stenosis, transient post-operative
- Tardus Parvus wave form abnormality: transplant renal artery stenosis
- Elevated Resistive indices: Intrarenal pathology, acute rejection, Acute tubular necrosis
- Decreased resistive indices: Transplant renal artery stenosis, hypovolemia
- Reversal of flow in transplant renal artery: Transplant vein obstruction
- Hydronephrosis: Full calyces from distended bladder with ureteral reflux; bladder outlet obstruction, transplant ureteral obstruction from stricture, stone or edema
- Native kidney lesions: Complex cyst, neoplasm, source of recurrent urinary infection

CT scan: In further evaluation of fluid collections

PET scan: Post transplant lymphoproliferative disorder

Pharmacology of Transplant care:

Immunosuppression

Induction agents:

Lymphocyte depleting-Thymoglobulin, Campath (alemtuzumab)

Non depleting: Basiliximab

Maintenance immunosuppression:

Calcineurin Inhibitors: Tacrolimus, Cyclosporine

mTOR inhibitors-Sirolimus, Everolimus

Co stimulatory Blockade: Belatacept

Combination regimen post transplant:

Tacrolimus (Cyclosporin) + Mycophenolate (+ Prednisone)

Tacrolimus (Cyclosporin) + Sirolimus (+ Prednisone)

Belatacept + Everolimus (+ Prednisone)

Belatacept + Mycophenolate (+ Prednisone)

Belatacept + Tacrolimus (Cyclosporin)+ Mycophenolate (+ Prednisone)

Practice Point 10

- mTOR inhibitor without Calcineurin inhibitor or Prednisone (Only Sirolimus+ MMF) has been associated with a poorer long-term outcome.
- When in combination with an mTOR inhibitor, it is advised to use lower Tacrolimus (Cyclosporin) target trough levels

Immunosuppression Target Trough levels are summarized in Table 22.5.

Practice Point 11

- 2 hour post dose cyclosporin levels (C2) are used in some countries with higher target levels but lead to overall higher cyclosporin dosing and no clear benefit to improve allograft outcome

Antimicrobial Prophylaxis:

- Cotrimoxazole-Pneumocystis, urinary infection, Listeria
- Anti-fungal: Nystatin, Fluconazole, used only in special cases
- Antiviral: Valganciclovir for CMV

Practice Point 12

- 1 year (preferably indefinite) duration of prophylactic use of co-trimoxazole
- 3 months of anti-fungal prophylaxis
- 6 months of anti-CMV prophylaxis. (Dapsone or Atovoquone can be used in those allergic to cotrimoxazole
- Short term (1 year) use of Lamivudine and indefinite Entecavir or Tenofovir treatment is recommended in recipients who receive hepatitis B core antibody positive organ, and those recipients who are Hepatitis B surface antigen positive

Antihypertensive Agents:

- Calcium channel blocker—Nifedipine, amlodipine—drugs of choice in the immediate post transplant period
- Beta blockers—Metoprolol, carvedilol, atenolol, Labetalol
- Vasodilators-Hydralazine, Minoxidil
- Centrally acting-Clonidine
- ACEI/ARB: Enalapril, lisinopril, ramipril, Losartan, Valsartan, Olmesartan. To be used later ideally after 3 months when kidney function is stable.
- Diuretics: Furosemide, Bumetanide, Hydrochlorothiazide
- Alfa blockers-Tamsulosin, Doxazosin

Agents to Treat Diabetes Mellitus:

- Insulin-short acting and long acting, continuous infusion pump
- Metformin
- DPP 4 inhibitors: Sitagliptin, Linagliptin, Saxagliptin
- GLP1 agonists: Liraglutide, Exanetide, Dulaglutide

Table 22.5 Immunosuppression Target Trough Levels

Tacrolimus:	Early 8–10 ng/mL	Toxic >15 ng/mL	Minimum therapeutic level: 3 ng/mL. (With MTOR inhibitor: 2.5 ng/mL) Long term: 4–6 ng/mL
Cyclosporin:	Early 200–300 ng/mL. Toxic >350 ng/mL	Long term: 100–200 ng/mL	Minimum Therapeutic: 100 ng/mL (With MTOR inhibitor: 50 ng/mL)

- Sulfonylurea-Glipizide, Glimepiride
- Meglitinides-Repaglinide, Nateglinide
- SGLT 2 inhibitors-Canagliflozin and Empaglifozin

Practice Point 13

- Though SGLT2 inhibitors are found to have many benefits in diabetics, their use in kidney transplant recipients is yet to be widespread for fear of urinary tract infections
- Continuous glucose monitoring with or without the use of an insulin infusion pump is becoming more widespread, with obvious advantages
- If post-operative period insulin requirement is >20 units per day at discharge, it would be preferable to maintain them on a lower insulin-containing regimen on discharge initially

Other Agents:

Antiplatelet agents-Aspirin

H2 blockers and PPI: Famotidine, omeprazole, Pantoprazole

Stool softeners and Laxatives

Antimicrobials:

Antibiotics

Anti fungal agents

Antiviral agents

Note: All attempts must be made to follow any deceased donor blood, urine and any tissue cultures to inform post-transplant antimicrobial regimen especially blood and urine cultures.

Drug–Drug major interactions with Calcineurin Inhibitors (CNIs):

Rifampicin

Erythromycin, Clarithromycin

Fluconazole, Ketoconazole, Voriconazole

Food–Drug interactions with CNI are summarized in Table 22.6.

Table 22.6 Food–Drug interactions with CNI

Clinicians should be aware of the following:
Grapefruit
Fruit punch

Practice Point 14

- Always review entire medication list at each post transplant visit and have recipients carry a list of all they take including over the counter and any traditional medications such as herbal supplements

Post-Transplant Infections

The common infections associated with time post kidney transplantation are summarized in Table 22.1 [2].

Urinary Tract Infections

Bacterial: *E. coli*, Pseudomonas, Klebsiella. ESBL *E. coli* will need often parenteral therapy

Fungal: Candida-oral, esophageal, urinary tract, systemic

Recurrent, resistant and life-threatening infection should prompt additional studies including imaging, cystoscopy, reduction in immunosuppression

Pneumonia

Bacterial: Pneumococcal, Gram negatives

MTB: In endemic areas, be vigilant for resistant MTB

MAI: Ensure resolution prior to re-transplant if pre-existent

Fungal

Pneumocystis: Prevention better than treatment. Low threshold for diagnosis tests if not on prophylaxis

Aspergillus: Can be life threatening

Mucor: High mortality; Surgical approaches are often necessary for resection of infected areas

Viral

BK Virus

BK Virus infections characterized in its mild form by BK viruria and low grade transient BK viremia and in severe form interstitial nephritis and rapid loss of allograft function has become an important factor in allograft longevity.

Treatment strategy involves reduction in immunosuppression, often discontinuation of mycophenolate, addition of Leflunomide and reduced target level of Tacrolimus to minimum therapeutic levels and when recalcitrant low dose periodic infusions of antiviral agent-Cidofovir which targets virus infested kidney cells accelerating their apoptosis through P 53 pathway. Treatment strategy has to be individualized and should involve transplant professional with experience in dealing with BK virus infection. Outcome depends on the severity of allograft dysfunction at the onset, HLA mismatches and degree of alloimmune response on reducing the immunosuppression.

Cytomegalovirus

CMV infection has highly effective prophylaxis and treatment options available. Look for drug resistance and combination regimen as may be necessary. Foscarnet is nephrotoxic. Oral Valganciclovir is used for prophylaxis and treatment of mild to moderate infections and IV Ganciclovir for sever infections requiring hospitalization.

Influenza: Seasonal vaccination ; antiviral therapy with modest benefit. Can cause multi organ failure

RSV: Often associated with leukopenia necessitating discontinuation of anti proliferative agent

Coronavirus COVID 19 Pandemic saw many transplant recipients succumb to the infection with others having lung, renal and neurological sequelae

West Nile Virus: High suspicion and knowledge of endemicity can help diagnose this early and quick with potential ability to save the recipient.

Systemic Infections

MTB: In endemic areas, high suspicion. Untreated latent TB needs treatment pre transplant. Prolonged treatment and drug resistance are to be kept in mind.

Candida: Severe life-threatening infection necessitating withdrawal of Immunosuppression and systemic anti-fungal therapy can occur.

Nocardia: Can be localized or systemic ilife threatening infection often including nervous system and presenting with seizures

CMV: GI tract, lung allograft are often involved. Be vigilant immediately following cessation of prophylactic valganciclovir

Cryptococcus: Skin, lung and characteristically nervous system can be involved often necessitating prolonged treatment with anti-fungal agents.

EBV: Early post-transplant B-cell neoplastic proliferation can be associated with EBV viremia and presence in the neoplastic cells

HHV 8: Associated with Kaposi's sarcoma and resolution is necessary prior to re-transplantation

Localized Infections

Fungal: Oral candidiasis , dermatophytic fungi

Nocardia: Can be localized cutaneous, bursa

Mycobacterium marinum: Often associated with fishing related minor skin injuries

Practice Point 15

- Infections can masquerade with minimal symptoms until severe, fast progression to life threatening condition, with more difficulty in diagnosis and need prolonged treatment for response in immunosuppressed host
- High degree of suspicion, microbiology sampling of tissues and body fluids and expert infectious disease input can help

faster diagnosis and prompt and appropriate therapy

- Even with prompt diagnosis mortality is as high as 50% with infections such as Mucor
- Drastic reduction or discontinuation of immunosuppression to allow host immune system to recover is an integral treatment strategy when infection is recurrent, opportunistic and or life threatening
- Also important is the resumption of immunosuppression when the infection is controlled to prevent allograft loss
- Certain drug interactions such as with Rifampin and Tacrolimus can precipitate rejection by reducing Tacrolimus level

Evaluation of Fever in Transplant Recipient

The assessment of a febrile patient post-kidney transplant should involve:

- Physical examination
- Lab data including microbiology
- Imaging studies
- In hospital care and empirical therapy. The common causes of infection are shown in Fig. 22.1.

Practice Point 16

- Low threshold for evaluation including full physical examination and work up. Infections can produce less symptoms due to immunosuppressed star
- Consider opportunistic infections and non-infectious causes including lymphoproliferative disorder and rejection
- Plain chest radiography is less sensitive than CT for evaluating for pneumonia

Evaluation of Elevated Creatinine:

- Physical examination: signs of dehydration, fluid overload
- Laboratory studies including urine studies, BKV PCR in blood.
- Imaging studies including ultrasound with doppler and post void bladder scan
- Immunological risk evaluation: donor specific antibodies, cell free DNA, post-transplant cross match
- Allograft biopsy

Practice Point 17

- Keep in mind thrombotic microangiopathy, undiagnosed native kidney disease such as paraproteinemia

Indications for Kidney Allograft Biopsy:

- For evaluation of elevated creatinine, proteinuria
- As part of protocol in a research study
- Light microscopy, Immunofluorescence study including C4d, staining for BKV, Electron microscopy
- Standardized reporting format for features of acute rejection, antibody mediated rejection (AMR) based on Banff Schema (Fig. 22.2).
- Protocols for anti-rejection therapy for acute cellular rejection (ACR), humoral antibody-mediated rejection (AMR) which may be predominant findings on a kidney transplant biopsy
- Prompt therapy for thrombotic microangiopathy (TMA), including Apheresis and anti-complement therapies with prophylactic vaccinations.

Anti Rejection Therapies:

- Steroid pulse 250–1000 mg/dose 3–5 days
- Thymoglobulin 6–10 mg/kg in divided doses

Early Post-Transplant 0-30 Days Post-Transplant	Peak Immunosuppression 31-365 Days Post-Transplant	Late-Onset >365 Days Post-Transplant
Nosocomial Infections • MDRO: MRSA, VRE, ESLB/CRE • *C. difficile* colitis • Surgical site infections • Urinary tract infection • Catheter-related bloodstream infections • Pneumonia **Donor-Derived Infections** • Atypical post-transplant course o **Examples: LCMV, WNV, T.***cruzi*, HCV, Bacteraemia, endemic mycoses **Recipient-Derived Infections** • Incubating or colonizing o Influenza, Pseudomonas, Aspergillus	**With Prophylaxis** • Polyomaviruses • HCV • *Cryptococcus neoformans* • *M. Tuberculosis* • Strongyloides • Leishmania • PTLD **After Prophylaxis Stops** • Pneumocystis • Herpesviruses (CMV, HSV, VZV) • HBV • Listeria, Nocardia, Toxoplasmosis • Community-Acquired Infections • Urinary tract infection • Pneumonia • *C. difficile* colitis	**Opportunistic Infections** • When these occur, must consider why they are happening late • CMV • JC/PML • PTLD/EBV • Nocardia **Community-Acquired Infections** • West Nile Virus • Community-acquired Pneumonia • Urinary tract infections • Influenza • Aspergillus, atypical moulds • Hepatitis (HBV, HCV)

Fig. 22.1 Common infections associated with time since kidney transplantation [2]. Abbreviations: *C. difficile Clostideroides difficile*, *CMV* Cytomegalovirus, *EBV* Epstein-Barr virus, *ESLB/CRE* Extended spectrum beta-lactamase/carbapenem resistant enterobacteria, *HBV* Hepatitis B virus, *HCV* Hepatitis C virus, *HSV* Herpes simplex virus, *JC/PML* JC virus/progressive multifocal leukoencephalopathy, *LCMV* Lymphocytic choriomeningitis virus, *MDRO* Multi-drug resistant organism, *MRSA* Methicillin-resistant staphylococcus aureus, *M. tuberculosis Mycobacterium tuberulosis*, *PTLD* Post-transplant lymphoproliferative disease, *T. cruzi Trypanosoma cruzi*, *VRE* Vancomycin-resistant enterococcus, *VZV* Varicella zoster virus, *WNV* West Nile virus

- Apheresis (6–10 sessions over 2–3 weeks)for antibody mediated rejection (AMR)
- Rituximab (for antibody mediated rejection (AMR))
- Bortezomib (for antibody mediated rejection (AMR))
- IVIg (for antibody mediated rejection (AMR))

Re-initiation of prophylactic antimicrobial regimen including for PCP, fungal prophylaxis and CMV prophylaxis

Follow up care post rejection with shorter interval outpatient follow-up and monitoring for immunosuppression-related side-effects, e.g. infection, neoplasia

Practice Point 18

- Ensure safe allograft biopsy procedure with real time guidance, pre-biopsy studies and post-biopsy monitoring, adequate sampling and prompt reporting with clinician input for clinical context for biopsy
- Severe irreversible changes of interstitial fibrosis and tubular atrophy (IFTA) should inform and prevent over enthusiastic attempts at immunosuppression

Banff lesion score	Abbre-viation	0	1	2	3
Interstitial inflammation Tubulitis	*I* *t*	<10% None	10-25% 1-4/tubular cross section or 10 tubular epithelial cells	26-50% 5-10	>50 >10 or foci of tubular basement membrane destruction with i≥2 and t2 elsewhere
Intimal arteritis≤≥	*v*	None	<25% luminal area lost	≥25% luminal area lost	Transmural and/or fibrinoid change and medial smooth musscle necrosis
Glomerulitis Peritubular capillaritis	*g* *ptc*	None <3 leukocytes/ PTC	<25% ≥1 leukocyte in ≥ 10% of PTCs with max. of 3-4/PTC	<25%-75% ≥1 leukocyte in ≥ 10% of PTCs with max. of 5-10/PTC	>75% ≥1 leukocyte in ≥ 10% of PTCs with max. of >10/PTC
C4d Interstitial fibrosis Tubular atrophy Vascular fibrous Intimal thickening GBM double contours	*C4d* *ci* *ct* *cv* *cg*	None ≤% None None None	<10% 6-25% <25% <25%	10-50% 26-50% 26-50% 26-50% 26-50%	>50% >50% >50% >50% >50%
Mesangial matrix expansion Arteriolar hyalinosis Hyaline arteriolar thickening Total inflammation Inflammation in the area of IFTA	*mm* *ah* *aah* *ti* *i-IFTA*	None None None <10% <10%	1a: only by EM 1b: < 25% by LM ≤ 25% Mild to moderate in >1 ≥1 without circumferential 10-25% 10-25%	26-50% Moderate to severe in >1 ≥1 without circumferential 26-50% 26-50%	>50% Severe in many circumferential >50% >50%

Fig. 22.2 Synopsis of the thresholds for all Banff Lesion Scores [3]. Abbreviations: *max* Maximum, *PTC* Peritubular capillary

Thrombotic Microangiopathy

Catastrophic microvascular pathology involving injury to endothelial cells and involving fibrin in capillaries occurs from a variety of causes in post-transplant period ranging from antibody mediated injury, Calcineurin inhibitor toxicity and pre-existing genetic susceptibility involving complement. When prior knowledge of such predisposition can help in the situation in early identification of such a phenomenon, the results can still be catastrophic unless prompt actions including intensive apheresis, withdrawal and replacement of calcineurin inhibitor and institution of anti-complement therapy. Such a phenomenon can also occur with certain interventions in delayed post-transplant period such as treatment with anti-vascular endothelial growth factor (VEGF) agents.

Rapid Recurrence or Occurrence of Major Allograft Pathology

Two diseases that can quickly reoccur after transplant especially with prior recurrence are recurrent focal segmental glomerulosclerosis (FSGS) and anti-glomerular basement antibody (anti-GBM) disease in an Alport syndrome recipient. Prior knowledge of recurrence may help in early diagnosis of these, but treatment of both instances remain less than satisfactory at best. In rare cases, there has been an excellent response to an initial course of Apheresis.

Special Considerations in Post Transplant follow Up

Recipients of High-Risk Donor Organs

Recipients of high-risk donor derived organs for transmission of Hepatitis B, Hepatitis C, HIV due to well known risk factors in the donors are to be followed for these infections in the post-transplant period for unto 6 months post-transplant minimum and preferably unto 1 year. Certain seasonal/periodic testing of deceased donors are practiced, based on endemicity and seasonal or geographic variation of diseases such as Zika, Chagas disease and West Nile virus infections.

Recipients of HCV Positive Donor Organs

Recipients of known Hepatitis C infected donor organs (HCV PCR or antibody positive) are to be followed and tested by blood PCR to confirm HCV transmission and are to be treated until there is a sustained viral response using broad spectrum or genotype-specific anti-HCV regimen and are to be followed to ensure sustained viral response.

Recipients with Known Major Psychiatric Illnesses

Anxiety, depression, suicide attempts, Bipolar affective disorder, Schizophrenia are common enough to be prevalent among transplant candidates. A well thought out post-operative care plan needs to be incorporated for optimal transplant outcome in these recipients who do very well with such plans in place. Electroconvulsive therapy is particularly advantageous in conditions deemed beneficial due to its rapidity of onset of action, lack of drug interactions and ability to have a high degree of adherence. Depot preparations of antipsychotic medications are useful in those instances where pharmacotherapy is the only alternative.

Recipients with Known History of Neoplasia

Apart from ensuring being cancer free at the time of transplant with an appropriate cancer-free interval, long term monitoring plan for recurrence identification and prompt intervention is required in this group of recipients who will otherwise benefit from transplantation.

Preventive Measures

Cardiovascular Risk Reduction

Smoking cessation, daily physical activity, maintaining optimized weight, optimized control of blood pressure, cholesterol, triglycerides, blood glucose.

In those with known coronary artery disease or history of coronary re vascularization, antiplatelet therapy, beta blocker, statin and lifestyle modifications as noted above are to be ensured as appropriate [4].

Dermatology Surveillance

Skin cancer prevention by reducing sunlight exposure and dermatology follow-up and prompt treatment of any identified lesions with sometimes appropriate reduction in immune suppression in recurrent or severe cases will ensure long-term optimized outcome in this vulnerable population. While basal cell cancers are common and innocuous, squamous cell cancers that are invasive and recurrent, as well as any melanomas are more ominous and could become life threatening.

Ophthalmology Follow Up

Glaucoma and cataracts are common effects of long-term immunosuppressive regimens, including corticosteroids and the need for prompt attention to ensure vision preservation. Proactive monitoring of intra ocular pressure by eye care team is essential to early diagnose glaucoma, which may remain undetected and cause irreversible vision loss otherwise.

Cancer Screening

Age-appropriate cancer screening should continue post-transplant including prostate, breast, colon and specifically native kidneys. Though clear guidelines are lacking, an ultrasound scan every two years looking at native kidneys seems reasonable and prudent.

Vascular Access in a Successful Transplant Recipient

Whilst the decision to remove a PD catheter and tunneled dialysis catheter are fairly simple and obvious, many vascular surgeons are reluctant to obliterate functioning arteriovenous fistulae and grafts, even after a year of excellent allograft function. This needs to be seriously considered, especially in recipients with highly developed AV fistulae with considerable additional circulatory load.

Vaccination

Recommended vaccinations include influenza vaccine (yearly, seasonal, quadrivalent, high dose) and pneumococcal vaccines (every 5 years—PPSV 23 and once—PCV 13).

Varicella and measles, mumps and rubella (MMR) vaccines are to be given pre-transplant, since they are live vaccines. Varicella Zoster (VZV) vaccine, which contains live virus can be given pre-transplant; killed VZV vaccine is yet to be fully approved in kidney transplant recipients due to its high immunogenicity from the adjuvant component. Anecdotally however, the killed VZV vaccine has been administered to many transplant recipients, with no major reported harm since it has been widely available.

Travelers

Yellow fever vaccine is not recommended for transplant recipients since it is a live virus vaccine. Apart from general precautions to prevent airborne, water, food and insect-borne infections, anti-malarial prophylaxis can be safely used by traveling transplant recipients to malaria-endemic areas.

Failing Kidney Allograft and Kidney Replacement Therapy

The life of a kidney allograft is often shorter than that of the recipient, even in the best case scenario: extreme levels of adherence and gradual, silent loss of allograft function progresses with time, necessitating re-transplant when possible. It is clear re-transplant is still the treatment of choice over various form of dialysis.

Managing immunosuppression as allograft function declines is an important consideration. Recipients become less tolerant to mycophenolate as anaemia progresses, and this is often reduced or withdrawn. There are advantages to continuing Tacrolimus and prednisolone therapy for a recipient who is a re-transplantation candidate, in that it may prevention of allo-sensitization, which is a strong barrier to re-transplantation. Therefore it can be recommended to persist with these two agents through the next transplant without interruption. This is contra-indicated if there is a need for an immune suppression-free period to allow resolution of PTLD or HHV-8 infection, with or without Kaposi's sarcoma. Persistent BK viraemia despite all other strategies may also necessitate weaning of immunosuppression, as well as a curable neoplastic disease requiring chemotherapy, when only prednisone may be continued while living with a failed allograft.

These decisions are complex, individualized, and should involve the full post-transplantation MDT (Table 22.1), including transplantation specialists who are well-versed in such scenarios.

The 'Difficult-to-care-for' Kidney Transplant Patient

Transplant care is modelled on a patient-physician partnership, where honest and forthright communication is essential for a successful outcome. A sadly common scenario is one in which a patient and/or caregiver (sometimes the parents of a paediatric or transitioning allograft recipient) retains an inherent mistrust of clinical teams—manifesting in non-adherence to clinical instructions, constantly challenging and subverting the advice given—all too often leading to suboptimal patient outcomes. Where the origin of clinician mistrust may be rooted in negative childhood or other experiences, the approach in these instances should always be one of compassion and empathy, and to avoid blame—a path which the exasperated treating transplant team might otherwise follow. Whilst the learning curve may be unfavourable in some cases, such that successful re-transplantation may be either more challenging or practically impossible, it is important to nurture as positive a learning environment as possible for the patient to be able to improve their understanding and insight into their situation, and thereby optimize their care. Central to this drive amongst the paediatric and young adult transplant patient cohort are the advent of Transitional kidney care services (see chapter 25), cohorting transitioning patients in outpatient clinics, and setting up a network of 'model patients' who may have a similar background—to act as peer mentors. Similarly, kidney patient associations offer patient support to help those at risk. Ultimately all such innovations require the voluntary engagement of the patient to ultimately be reflected in improvements with adherence, and ultimately improved patient outcomes, and managed on a case-by-case basis.

Long Term Continuum of Care of Kidney Disease Patients

Optimal care of kidney transplant recipients involves seamless communication of an established team of clinicians, care providers, inpatient and outpatient providers, including primary physician, dialysis team, social worker, nutritionist, clinical pharmacist, primary nephrologist, transplant nephrologist, transplant surgeon, interventional radiologist, transplant immunologist, Apheresis team, Oncologist, gastroenterologist, Gynecologist, Urologist, Vascular surgeon, ophthalmologist and dermatologist to name a few.

Long term post-transplant follow-up care is a labour intensive, and highly involved field, where apparent stability can give way to a life-threatening situation with a short illness. With a fragile population at the risk of heart disease, neoplasia and infections both recipient and care providers have to be on guard at all times to quickly intervene before a negative situation descends out of control. With diligent care over the long term, a gratifying outcome with almost half of all kidney transplant recipients achieving a near-normal lifespan, that is both meaningful, productive and enjoyable.

Conclusions

Post-transplant management requires monitoring of kidney function, and to investigate the possible causes of any deterioration, which may be reversible. From the initial case study, the rise in serum creatinine in the 55-year-old man could have been due to rejection, CNI toxicity, recurrent IgAN; but the low haemoglobin and low platelet count instead were suggestive of a possible thrombotic microangiopathy (TMA). His tacrolimus levels was high, but despite lowering the tarcrolimus dose, his kidney allograft function did not improve: He required haemodialysis; a kidney biopsy performed a week thereafter showed features suggestive of thrombotic microangiopathy (TMA).

Questions

1. Thrombotic microangiopathy can lead to devastating injury of kidney allograft. The following statements regarding thrombotic microangiopathy are true EXCEPT:
   A. Genetic basis affecting complement system may be found in patients with thrombotic microangiopathy

B. Recipient candidates whose native kidneys failed from thrombotic microangiopathy have increased incidence of thrombotic microangiopathy compared to others when transplanted
C. Calcineurin inhibitors can cause thrombotic microangiopathy
D. Apheresis and eculizumab are therapeutic tools that may be used to manage kidney transplant recipients with thrombotic microangiopathy
E. Thrombotic microangiopathy is a contraindication for kidney transplantation

Answer: E

2. Recipients of allografts can have rapid recurrence of disease in the new kidney if the primary disease is FSGS and this can lead to graft loss. The following statements are True EXCEPT:
A. There are reports of transplanted kidney with recurrent FSGS got successfully retransplanted quickly to reverse the process
B. Management of recurrent FSGS may involve Apheresis and Rituximab
C. If native kidneys failed quickly from onset of FSGS, the risk of recurrence may be higher
D. FSGS with genetic basis does not recur in transplant recipients
E. Early detection and prompt treatment guarantees preservation of allograft function in recurrent FSGS

Answer: D

3. Features consistent with acute antibody mediated rejection in renal allograft biopsy include the following EXCEPT:
A. Acute tubular Injury
B. Thrombotic microangiopathy
C. Glomerulitis and peritubular capillaritis
D. Diffuse C4d in peritubular capillaries on immunofluorescence
E. Calcium Oxalate crystals in interstitium

Answer: E

4. The following statements regarding Calcineurin inhibitors and MTOR inhibitors are true EXCEPT:
A. Calcineurin inhibitor toxicity is enhanced by coadministration of MTOR inhibitors
B. While used concurrently with MTOR inhibitors target trough levels of Calcineurin inhibitors are lowered to avoid toxicity
C. In transplant recipients with lymphoma, Calcineurin inhibitors may be replaced by MTOR inhibitors to take advantage of their anti cancer property
D. Preexisting proteinuria in transplant recipients makes them less suitable for conversion to MTOR inhibitor based regimen from Calcineurin inhibitor regimen
E. Immediate post transplant period is the ideal time point to start MTOR inhibitors due their wound healing properties

Answer: E

5. The following statements regarding infections following kidney transplantation are true except:
A. Recurrent, life threatening and opportunistic infections can be major concerns in kidney transplant recipients
B. Risk of opportunistic infections are highest in the first month following transplantation and becomes not a concern after 6 months following transplantation
C. Prophylaxis with Valganciclovir is an excellent way to prevent life threatening CMV disease in the first 6 months following transplantation
D. Live vaccines are contra indicated in immunosuppressed kidney transplant recipients
E. EBV infection post-transplant is a risk factor for development of Post-transplant B cell lymphoma

Answer: B

6. The following statements regarding Induction therapy in kidney transplant recipients are true except
A. Thymoglobulin and Alemtuzumab are both depleting antibodies and are powerful induction agents used in kidney allotransplantation

B. Basiliximab is used for treatment of acute rejection in kidney transplant recipients who received it as an induction agent
C. Prior exposure to Thymoglobulin can lead to generation of antibodies against it making it less effective in subsequent instances.
D. Rituximab is not effective in depleting Plasma cells but can deplete anti CD 20 positive B cell lineage cells
E. Special techniques such as CD 19 crossmatch or pronase treatment are used for B cell crossmatching in transplant candidates who recently received Rituximab treatment

Answer: B

7. A question on immunological risks – which of the following statements is true?
   A. Composite tissue allograft (e.g. face, hands) are likely to induce weaker alloimmune response when compared to small intestinal allografts
   B. Liver kidney dual transplants from the same donor is more likely to induce a stronger immune response than a kidney allograft alone
   C. Male offspring donating a kidney to the biological female parent induces a weaker immune response compared to a female offspring to the biological male parent
   D. ABO incompatible donor kidney induces a stronger alloimmune response in the long term compared to HLA incompatible donor kidney
   E. Increased NK cell activity can abolish the tolerance to fetus in pregnancy and can cause spontaneous abortion

   Answer: E

8. Polycystic kidney disease is an important cause of ESKD, requiring kidney transplantation to ensure long term survival. The following statements are true regarding polycystic kidney disease EXCEPT:
   A. Polycystic kidney disease results from abnormality in ciliary function during organogenesis
   B. Native kidney nephrectomy is never advised in transplant recipients with polycystic kidneys
   C. Renal cell cancer may develop in polycystic kidneys
   D. Nephrolithiasis and recurrent urinary tract infections may complicate polycystic kidneys
   E. Siblings and parents may be considered donor candidates for recipients if they do not have genetic marker for polycystic kidneys

   Answers: B

9. Patients with Alport syndrome and end stage kidney disease may receive successful kidney transplants. However the following statements are true regarding these recipients and recipient candidates except:
   A. Alport syndrome can affect males and females
   B. Characteristic lesions seen in Alport syndrome can recur in kidney transplant recipients in their kidney allografts
   C. Anti glomerular basement disease in the allograft is a concern in recipients with Alport syndrome
   D. Immunosuppression can mitigate the development of anti GBM disease in recipient candidates with Alport syndrome
   E. Absent COL4A5 protein is a maker for Alport syndrome and can have extrarenal manifestations in the form of deafness and abnormal refraction which will not improve from receiving successful renal transplantation

   Answer: B

10. Determining presence of and significance of allo antibodies pre and post transplant forms an important advancement in in transplant immunology over the last two decades.

    The following statements about allo antibodies are true except:
    A. Anti ABO antibodies are more significant for allograft outcome than anti HLA antibodies in ABO incompatible transplants functioning after 1 year post transplant

B. Complement dependent cytotoxicity T cell crossmatch positivity suggests anti HLA antibodies that are present, binding and cytotoxic
C. Antibodies may appear denovo post transplant in HLA mismatched kidney transplant recipients and may lead to chronic allograft injury through chronic antibody mediated rejection
D. When anti HLA antibodies appear they may be accommodated by some transplant recipients and this will mitigate allograft damage from them
E. Peritubular capillaritis and diffuse C4d staining in peritubular capillaries are supportive evidence for antibody mediated allograft injury
F. Chronic injury from alloantibodies is a major cause for shortening allograft survival in HLA mismatched kidney transplant recipients

Answer: A

Test your learning and check your understanding of this book's contents: use the "Springer Nature Flashcards" app to access questions using https://sn.pub/cz9Cok. To use the app, please follow the instructions in Chap. 1.

References

1. Abramowicz D, Cochat P, Claas FH, Heemann U, Pascual J, Dudley C, Harden P, Hourmant M, Maggiore U, Salvadori M, Spasovski G, Squifflet JP, Steiger J, Torres A, Viklicky O, Zeier M, Vanholder R, Van Biesen W, Nagler E. European Renal Best Practice Guideline on kidney donor and recipient evaluation and perioperative care. Nephrol Dial Transplant. 2015;30(11):1790–7. https://doi.org/10.1093/ndt/gfu216. Epub 2014 Jul 9.
2. Agrawal A, Ison MG, Danziger-Isakov L. Long-term infectious complications of kidney transplantation. CJASN. 2022;17(2):286–95. https://doi.org/10.2215/CJN.15971020.
3. Roufosse C, Simmonds N, Clahsen-van Groningen M, Haas M, Henriksen KJ, Horsfield C, Loupy A, Mengel M, Perkowska-Ptasińska A, Rabant M, Racusen LC, Solez K, Becker JU. A 2018 reference guide to the banff classification of renal allograft pathology. Transplantation. 2018;102(11):1795–814. https://doi.org/10.1097/TP.0000000000002366. Erratum in: Transplantation. 2018 Dec;102(12):e497.
4. Chadban SJ, Ahn C, Axelrod DA, Foster BJ, Kasiske BL, Kher V, Kumar D, Oberbauer R, Pascual J, Pilmore HL, Rodrigue JR, Segev DL, Sheerin NS, Tinckam KJ, Wong G, Balk EM, Gordon CE, Earley A, Rofeberg V, Knoll GA. Summary of the Kidney Disease: Improving Global Outcomes (KDIGO) clinical practice guideline on the evaluation and management of candidates for kidney transplantation. Transplantation. 2020;104(4):708–14. https://doi.org/10.1097/TP.0000000000003137.

Complications of Kidney Transplantation

23

Mysore Phanish, Pranaw Kumar Jha, and Abbas Ghazanfar

Clinical Scenario
A 55-year-old female with IgA nephropathy, with an eGFR of 12 mL/min/1.73 m^2 received a pre-emptive, heart-beating deceased donor kidney transplantation. Her serum creatinine decreased daily till day 4, when she received her second dose of basiliximab, and was discharged home, to be followed up in the transplant outpatient clinic twice-weekly. On day 12, her serum creatinine increased by 50 μmol/L. She was admitted from the transplant clinic for further investigations and management.

Introduction

Kidney transplantation is a highly successful therapy for patients with end-stage kidney disease (ESKD). In this chapter, we focus on complications of kidney transplantation. It is important to understand that complications described in relation to kidney transplantation should be considered and analysed with reference to complications and mortality of patients on dialysis, and those on the transplant waiting list.

Immunosuppression is required to prevent alloimmune rejection of the kidney allograft. Immunosuppression is initially 'high' (induction), and then reduced gradually to a lower, maintenance immunosuppression; details of this can be found in Chap. 22.

Maintenance therapy usually consists of a calcineurin inhibitor (CNI) (e.g. Tacrolimus or Ciclosporin), oral steroids, an antimetabolite (e.g. Mycophenolate Mofetil (MMF) or Azathioprine), or mammalian target of rapamycin inhibitor (mTORi) (e.g. Sirolimus or Everolimus); There is substantial variation in immunosuppressant regimens between patients and between centres. The immunosuppressive regime and the total burden of immunosuppression is tailored according to the immune risk, and the risks of infection, cancer and diabetes mellitus. Early steroid withdrawal in selected group of patients is desirable, in order to minimise the adverse effects associated with long-term steroid therapy.

Outcomes: Patient and Graft survival

Patient and death-censored graft survival are the most widely used measures to assess success of a transplant programme. Both early and medium-term kidney allograft outcomes are excellent in

M. Phanish (✉)
Epsom and St Helier University Hospitals NHS trust, London, UK
e-mail: m.phanish@nhs.net

P. K. Jha
Department of Nephrology, Medanta Institute of Kidney & Urology, Medanta—The Medicity, Gurugram, Haryana, India

A. Ghazanfar
St George's University Hospitals NHS Foundation Trust, London, UK
e-mail: abbas.ghazanfar@stgeorges.nhs.uk

D. Banerjee et al. (eds.), *Management of Kidney Diseases*,
https://doi.org/10.1007/978-3-031-09131-5_23

most parts of the world, with steady improvement in long term outcomes, but it is widely recognised that more work needs to be done to improve long-term outcomes. For deceased donor kidney transplants, the UK national transplant registry (2019/2020) reports 94% (95% CI: 94%–95%) 1-year graft survival and 86% (95% CI: 85%–87%) 5-year graft survival; 97% (95% CI: 96%–97%) 1-year patient survival and 88% 5-year patient survival (95% CI: 87%–88%). Corresponding figures for living donor kidney transplant are 98% (95% CI: 98%–99%) 1-year graft survival and 93% (95% CI: 92%–93%) 5-year graft survival; 99% (95% CI: 98%–99%) 1-year patient survival, and 95% (95% CI: 94%–96%) 5-year patient survival. Key determinants of graft survival are donor and recipient factors. Higher risk donors are older (>60 years), have more medical co-morbidities (e.g. hypertension) and suffered a medical cause of death. High risk recipient factors are co-morbidities such as diabetes mellitus and vascular disease, poor functional capacity, second and subsequent transplants. Although age and obesity are often mentioned as high-risk recipient factors, good outcomes have been achieved in older recipients (60–75 years) and patients with high BMI (up to 38). Immunological risk, the degree of HLA matching and sensitisation status of the recipient, including presence or absence of pre-formed donor specific antibodies (DSA), development of de-novo DSAs following transplant have a key influence on rejection rates (acute and chronic) and transplant outcomes.

Surgical Complications of Kidney Transplantation

Figure 23.1 and Table 23.1 describe surgical complications following kidney transplantation. Most of the serious complications such as haemorrhage,

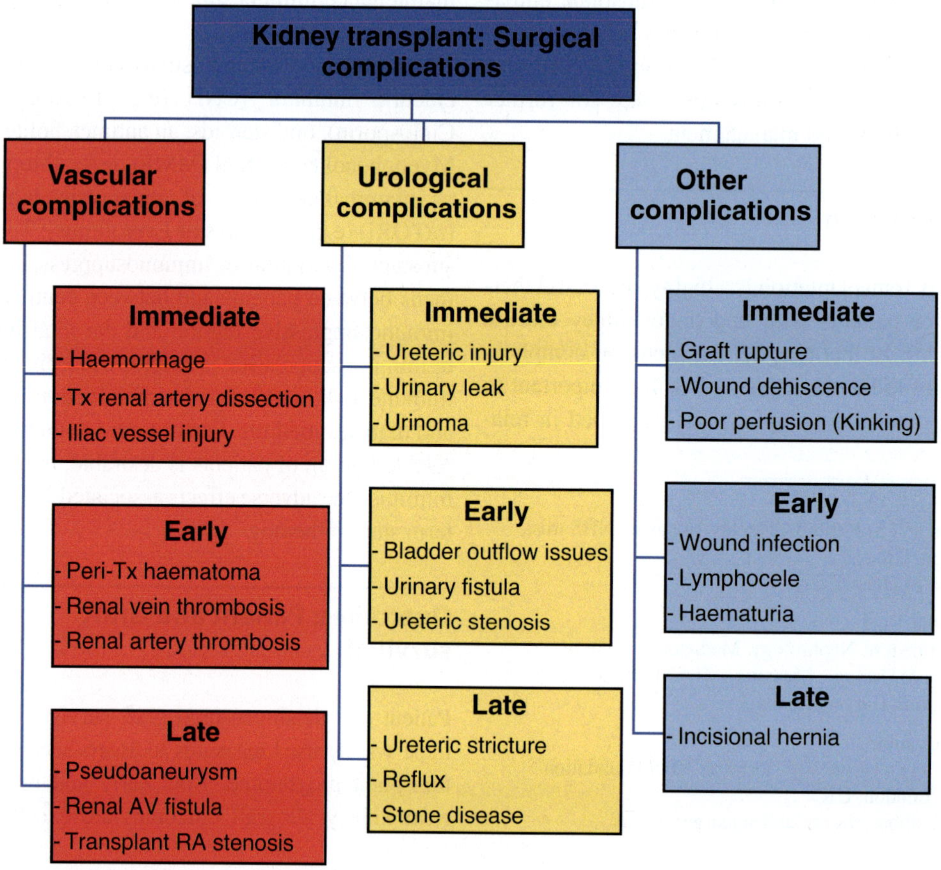

Fig. 23.1 Surgical Complications

Table 23.1 Surgical Complications

Presentations and causes		Examination & Investigations	Management
Vascular Complications			
Immediate Haemorrhage (minutes to hours)	**Presentations:** – Shock – Sudden swelling at site of kidney transplant – Frank blood in drain **Causes:** – Anastomotic rupture – Anastomotic leak – Vein rupture ***Clinical diagnosis***	**Look:** – Signs of shock – Oozing from wound – High drain output **Feel:** – Pulse – BP – Abdomen ***Remember:*** *Clamp drain to cause tamponade effect*	**Immediate action:** – Clamp the drain – ABCD – Urgent blood for transfusion – Call for help – Transfer to operation theatre **Surgical exploration** – Repair by suturing – Explant and reimplant – Pack and re-explore – Nephrectomy
	Technical tips: – *Have kidney back bench perfusion equipment ready for possible exploration and cold perfusion* – *First partially open the muscles of wound and if there is sudden pooling of fresh blood pack the wound and go higher to take control of common iliac artery. May need transabdominal approach in rare cases*		
Early Haemorrhage (hours to days)	**Presentations:** – Pain and tenderness – Swelling around transplant site – External bruising – Dropping urine output – Increase drain blood – Dropping Hb **Causes:** – Anastomotic leak – Biopsy site bleed – Bleeding from surgical bed and kidney hilum	**Look:** – Subcutaneous swelling around wound – Bruising around abdomen mainly flanks and thigh – Penile and scrotal bruising and haematoma **Feel:** – Transplant site – Abdomen with scrotum **Listen:** – Bruit over transplant kidney – Bowel sounds **Investigations:** – Transplant US – Plan abdominal CT – CT Angiogram – Catheter angiogram ***To look for:*** – *Graft perfusion* – *Peri Transplant haematoma* – *Compression on vessels*	**General management:** – Arrange blood – Dialysis if required – Stabilize the patient **Specific management:** *(depends on cause)* – ***Anastomotic leak*** – *Exploration and surgical repair/suturing* – ***Biopsy site bleed*** – *Interventional Radiology for percutaneous transluminal coiling* – *Exploration and surgical repair by direct suturing or using "plug technique".* ***Peri-Transplant bleed*** – *No compression on vessels/ small to medium size haematoma: Usually no intervention* – *Compression on vessels/ Medium to large haematoma: Surgical exploration for evacuation of haematoma*
	Technical tips: – Plug technique: When biopsy site is more than 2 mm in size suturing the kidney directly can cause sutures to cut through the tissue and makes bleeding worse and the damaged area bigger. Therefore, plug technique is more useful as it does not cause tension in sutures. In this technique first take some interrupted prolene sutures throughout the length of biopsy hole. Take a piece of fat from subcutaneous or intraabdominal fat and make a plug to seal the biopsy hole. Then tie all interrupted sutures without tension		

(continued)

Table 23.1 (continued)

Presentations and causes		Examination & Investigations	Management
Late Haemorrhage (days to weeks)	**Presentations:** – Sudden onset pain – Haematuria – Shock **Causes:** – Biopsy site bleed – Mycotic Pseudoaneurysm – Secondary infection ***Remember:*** *Patients with fungal positive culture in organ preservation fluid require routine follow-up with US/CT scans to exclude development of mycotic pseudoaneurysm*	**Look:** – Subcutaneous swelling around wound – Bruising around abdomen mainly flanks and thigh – Penile and scrotal bruising and haematoma **Feel:** – Transplant site – Abdomen with scrotum **Listen:** – Bruit over transplant kidney – Bowel sounds **Investigation:** – Transplant US – CT scan angiogram – Conventional angiogram – MRI for pseudoaneurysm ***To look for:*** – *Graft perfusion* – *Peri-transplant haematoma* – *Compression on vessels* – *For pseudoaneurysm looking for site, size and flow with proximal and distal vascular flow*	**Mycotic pseudoaneurysms** – Majority of mycotic pseudoaneurysms are picked on routine scans. – Antifungal treatment – Interventional Radiology procedure like stenting and/or coiling – Surgical exploration – Repair – Excision and interposition graft – Excision, interposition graft and auto-transplant – Femoral-femoral crossover graft – Nephrectomy – Nephrectomy with repair of arterial defect with prosthetic patch – Pseudoaneurysm can present as acute rupture. The management is same as management of shock and acute haemorrhage – Management of biopsy site bleed is as described above
	Technical tips: – For Mycotic Pseudoaneurysm cases consult with vascular surgical team and have them on board. – Keep back bench cold perfusion ready in case of exploration – Take control of proximal and distal vessels as high as possible before mobilising the kidney and/or examining the pseudoaneurysm		
Transplant Renal Arterial Dissection	**Presentations:** – Intraoperative poor perfusion of kidney – Rarely post operatively presenting as signs and symptoms of transplant renal artery thrombosis (see below) **Causes:** – Missed retrieval injury to kidney artery at the time of back bench preparation – Missed iatrogenic injury at time of transplant surgery	**Look:** – Poor and/or patchy perfusion of transplanted kidney **Feel:** – Pulsation in Transplant artery **Listen:** – Intra-operative doppler **Investigation:** – Transplant US – Contrast CT scan	**General management:** – Arrange blood – Dialysis if required **Specific management** – Urgent surgical exploration – Graft nephrectomy

Table 23.1 (continued)

Presentations and causes		Examination & Investigations	Management
Transplant Renal Artery Thrombosis	**Presentations:** – Within hours to days (usually within 3–4 days) post transplantation. – Acute reduction in urine output/anuria, rising creatinine, may or may not have graft tenderness, Hyperkalemia and raised LDH. **Causes/Risk factors:** – Iatrogenic arterial injury – Problems with anastomosis – Hypercoagulability/ Pro-thrombotic state – Hypotension – Malposition of kidney – multiple donor arteries	**Look:** – Usually, no external signs **Feel:** – Tenderness over graft **Investigation:** – Transplant US – Contrast CT scan – Isotope renogram ***Remember:*** *Time is very crucial in management. Any delays in surgical exploration is associated with reduced chances of organ salvage*	**General management:** – Arrange blood – Dialysis if required – IV Heparin **Specific management** – Urgent surgical exploration – Commonly graft nephrectomy – Rare, graft rescue by explanting, back bench perfusion, reimplantation
Transplant Renal Vein Thrombosis	**Presentations:** – Reduction in urine output and rising creatinine usually within 7 days post transplantation. – Pain, swollen graft and tenderness – Dropping urine output/anuria if occlusive thrombus. Non-occlusive thrombus may present more insidiously. – Painful swollen ipsilateral leg – Hyperkalemia. **Causes/ Risk factors:** – Haematoma, lymphocele, Urinoma causing compression – Iatrogenic venous injury – Problems with anastomosis – Hypercoagulability – Malposition of kidney, renal vein kink – Ipsilateral ileo-femoral DVT	**Look:** – Swollen transplant site – Swollen ipsilateral leg **Feel:** – Tenderness over graft – Tender thigh or calf **Investigation:** – Transplant US – Contrast CT Urogram with arterial and venous phases	**General management:** – Arrange blood – Dialysis if required – IV Heparin **Specific management** – Radiological drainage of compressing fluid collection – Urgent surgical exploration – Commonly graft nephrectomy – Rare, graft rescue by explanting, back bench perfusion, reimplantation
	Technical tips: [Transplant RA or RV thrombosis] – Keep back bench cold perfusion ready in case of exploration. Use heparin in perfusion fluid. Generally, 10,000 U in 1L of Soltran solution. Perfuse kidney under pressure (100–120 mmHg)		

(continued)

Table 23.1 (continued)

Presentations and causes		Examination & Investigations	Management
Transplant Renal Artery Stenosis	**Presentations:** – Within months to years – Worsening or new onset hypertension, fluid retention – Graft dysfunction in the absence of rejection, drug toxicity, ureteric obstruction and infection **Causes:** – Suture technique – Atherosclerotic arterial disease in donor or recipient – Arterial trauma during organ procurement or transplant – Prolonged cold ischemia – Arterial kinking – Chronic antibody mediated rejection – Cytomegalovirus infection	**Look and Feel:** – Generally, no signs. May have signs of fluid retention, difficult to control blood pressure. **Listen:** – Bruit over transplant site **Investigations:** – Transplant artery doppler USS (Velocity of >200–250 cm/s in Tr A usually indicates significant stenosis) – Contrast CT angiogram – Magnetic resonance angiography – Catheter angiogram ***To look for:*** – *Site of stenosis* – *Single or multiple* – *Extrinsic Compression on vessels*	**General management:** – Blood pressure control. **Specific management** – Percutaneous transluminal balloon angioplasty (PTA) – Percutaneous transluminal balloon angioplasty (PTA) with stenting – Surgical intervention – High risk procedure – Bypass grafting – Stricturoplasty – Reimplantation ***Remember:*** *PTA with or without stenting is treatment of choice*
Urological Complications			
Urethral Injury	**Presentations:** – Difficult male catheterisation at the time of surgery. **Causes:** – Unknown enlarged prostate not presented before due to oligo-anuria. – Unknown pre-existing urethral stricture.	**Investigation:** – If known before, retrograde urethro-cystogram. – At time of surgery can do flexible cystoscopy.	**Management:** – Attempt catheterisation, if not possible use cystoscopy and guidewire technique. If not possible, consider supra-pubic catheterisation. – Urology referral ***Remember:*** *Do not attempt forced catheterisation*

Table 23.1 (continued)

Presentations and causes		Examination & Investigations	Management
Urinary Leak / Urinary fistula / Urinoma	**Presentations:** – Urinary leak: High drain output during early post-operative period. – Urinary fistula: Presenting early as above or after taking the ureteric stent out in which case presents with raising creatinine and US finding of fluid collection. **Causes:** – Commonly anastomotic leak. – Iatrogenic bladder injury. – Iatrogenic transplant kidney renal pelvic or ureteric injury	**Look and Feel:** – Wound examination **Investigations:** – Drain fluid for creatinine levels [will be much higher (mmol/L) compared to serum creatinine (μmol/L). – Transplant kidney and pelvic US – Contrast CT urogram – Retrograde cystogram to demonstrate contrast leak, not usually required – Technetium-99m MAG3 nuclear medicine test. ***Remember:*** *Drain fluid creatinine level is key test to differentiate between urinary leak and lymphocele*	**General management:** – Wound care, stoma bag. Large defects can have portable vac dressing. **Specific management** – Insert urinary catheter if not already in. Usually for small to medium size leaks with drain output upto <500 mL/24 h settles down with few weeks of bladder catheterisation. – Nephrostomy will be helpful but difficult due to lack of hydronephrosis. – If there is large urinoma with pressure effects, it will need per-cutaneous drain. Avoid inserting drain for small collections as there is significant infection risk. – Antegrade or retrograde (uncommon) ureteric stenting for ureteric or pelvi-ureteric injuries. – Surgical exploration, ureteric repair and neo uretero-vesical anastomosis which may require a Boari bladder flap or utilisation of native ureter for new anastomosis
	Technical tips: – Small urinary leaks can be treated with bladder catheterisation. Leave the ureteric stent in-situ until the leak is resolved. – During surgery retrograde controlled filling of urinary bladder with saline coloured with methylene blue dye usually helps to identify the area of leak.		
Bladder outflow issues	**Presentations:** – Urinary retention. **Causes:** – Enlarged prostate not presented before due to oligo-anuria – Pre-existing urethral stricture. – Reduced urinary bladder capacity due to long periods of oligo-anuria whilst on dialysis- Usually leads to marked frequency and urgency of urination.	**Look and Feel:** – Tender supra pubic area due to distended bladder. – Dull percussion note. – PR examination for prostate. **Investigation:** – Urinary bladder scan to assess urinary volume. – Transplant and bladder US. – Trans-rectal US for prostate. – Check PSA	**General management:** – Urinary catheterisation. – Trial without catheter. **Specific management** – Consider alpha blockers. – Urology referral.

(continued)

Table 23.1 (continued)

Presentations and causes		Examination & Investigations	Management
Ureteric stenosis/ stricture	**Presentations:** – Acute presentation: After removal of ureteric stent, sudden drop in urine output and raised creatinine. – Chronic presentation: Gradual slow increase in serum creatinine with or without noticeable change in urine output. **Causes/Risk factors:** – Stenosis at the level of Ureteroneocystostomy. – Pelvi-ureteric junction stenosis. – Ureteric stenosis or stricture, mainly distal ureter (usually ischaemic due to ligation/ sacrifice of lower pole donor artery, rarely in association with BK Virus infection) – Ureteric kinking	**Look and Feel:** – Generally, no signs. – Graft tenderness. **Investigations:** – Transplant US – Nephrostomy with nephrostogram is gold standard investigation. – Isotope renogram – CT urogram ***To look for:*** – *Site of stenosis/ stricture* – *Length of stenosis/ stricture* – *Single or multiple*	**General management:** – Ensure safe K^+ **Specific management** – Nephrostomy to bypass obstruction and decompress pelvicalyceal system – Antegrade ureteric stent for 6–8 weeks followed by surgery – Recent transplants or allografts with good function will require ureteric reimplantation, which, depending on length of the stricture, may require a Boari bladder flap or utilisation of native ureter for new anastomosis – Allografts with poor function or short graft life expectancy can be managed by dilatation and antegrade stenting ***Remember:*** *Ureteric reconstruction surgery is often very challenging therefore there should be reasonable graft life expectancy to attempt this procedure. Generally, allograft GFR >20 mL/min with slow yearly decline rate*
	Technical tips: – When planning for surgery, where possible, pre-operative insertion of an anterograde ureteric stent is helpful for identifying ureter during surgery		

Table 23.1 (continued)

Presentations and causes		Examination & Investigations	Management
Lymphocele	**Presentations:** – High drain output. – External swelling at transplant site. – Swollen ipsilateral leg (Due to venous compression±DVT) – Urinary symptoms frequency and urgency (Due to bladder compression) – Allograft dysfunction – Incidental finding **Causes:** – Lymph leak from transplant bed dissection. – Lymph leak from renal hilum/donor kidney lymphatics. – mTOR inhibitors (Sirolimus/ Everolimus) increase the risk of Lymphocele	**Look and Feel:** – Generally, no external signs. – External swelling or ipsilateral lower limb swelling. **Investigation:** – Drain fluid for creatinine. – Transplant US to assess size of collection. – CT scan. ***Remember:*** *Mild to moderate size collections not causing compression on vessels can be managed conservatively.*	**General management:** – Wound care is key. If controlled area can put a stoma bag. Large defects can have portable vac dressing. – Drain care. **Specific management** – If picked up after taking the drain out: US or CT guided drain insertion depending upon size, site and any compression effects on surrounding structures particularly renal transplant vessels and iliac vessels. – Low output <250 mL/24 h: Can be managed with radiological drainage +/– sclerotherapy. – Moderate output between 250–500 mL/24 h: Drainage with sclerotherapy +/– surgery. - High output >500 mL/24 h usually requires surgical fenestration/marsupialization either laparoscopic or open. Laparoscopic creation of 'window' in to peritoneal cavity
	Technical tips: – Sclerotherapy: 5% povidone-iodine percutaneous sclerotherapy is commonly used. Through drain under strict antiseptic measure gently aspirate the lymphocele fluid as much as possible. Slowly inject 5% povidone-iodine solution into lymphocele cavity (commonly between 50and 100 mL). Clamp the drain and observe the patient. If clinically well keep clamp between 15 and 30 min and then leave it for free drainage. Repeat the process 5–6 times over a period of week to 10 days		

(continued)

Table 23.1 (continued)

Presentations and causes		Examination & Investigations	Management
Stone in renal transplant	**Presentations:** – Acute obstruction with graft dysfunction. – Transplant pyelonephritis or recurrent UTI. – Urinary symptoms frequency and urgency. – Allograft dysfunction – Incidental finding **Risk factors/Causes:** – Previous history of recurrent stones in the recipient with persistent metabolic abnormalities (Hyperparathyroidism, hyperoxaluria, hypercalciuria, low urinary citrate) – Ureteral obstruction or chronic urinary stasis – Foreign body (especially nonabsorbable suture material) – Pre-existing stone or tubular defects in donor kidney	**Look and Feel:** – Generally, no external signs except tenderness over graft. **Investigation:** – Plane Xray of transplant site. – Transplant kidney US to look for hydronephrosis. – CT scan KUB with contrast. – Stone profile studies ***Remember:*** *Transplant hydronephrosis is an emergency that requires nephrostomy to decompress the system and preserve allograft function*	**General management:** – Analgesia. – Nephrostomy where required. – Small non obstructing stone can be managed conservatively. – Maintain fluid intake of around 3 L/day and salt restrict. Do not restrict dietary calcium. **Specific management** – Extracorporeal shock-wave lithotripsy (ESWL) – Percutaneous nephrolithotripsy (PCNL) – Ureteroscopy and stone removal – Open surgery
Wound infection	– Uncommon, encourage weight loss and a BMI of <30 pre-transplant to reduce the risk – Diabetes, obesity and previous kidney transplant, high level of immunosuppression are risk factors – mTOR inhibitors (Sirolimus and Everolimus) are associated with poor wound healing	– Look for signs of wound infection, routine blood tests including CRP – Wound swab for culture and sensitivity – Blood culture – US scan to look for any peri-transplant collections	**Management:** – Wound care – Antibiotics – Optimise glycaemic control – Radiological drainage of infected collections as clinically indicated
Incisional Hernia	**Risk factors** Obesity, diabetes mellitus, wound infection		**Management:** – Usually surgical repair as clinically indicated

transplant kidney artery and vein thrombosis are very rare. It must be noted that allograft dysfunction following kidney transplant can be due to surgical complications such as a ureteric leak, or poorly perfused kidney, or due to medical complications, such as acute rejection or tacrolimus toxicity, with minimal clinical signs apart from a rising serum creatinine. Therefore, simultaneous consideration of surgical and medical causes of complications, with systematic clinical, laboratory and radiological assessments are essential to make the correct diagnosis, and initiate appropriate treatment.

Kidney transplantation is becoming a common procedure for the management of patients with end stage kidney disease [ESKD]. Over recent years, the incidence of surgical complications has dropped significantly from as high as 20% between 1960 and 1980 [1, 2], to a current incidence of around 5% [3, 4]. The surgical complications can generally be divided into three major categories: vascular, urological and other complications. Each of these can be further subclassified into immediate, early and late, according to the timing of their occurrence (Fig. 23.1).

Urological Complications

Urologic complications are the commonest surgical complication after kidney transplantation, causing significant morbidity and mortality.

In the early era of kidney transplantation, the incidence of urological complications was as high as 10–25% [5]; this has reduced significantly—to 5–7% in recent years [4]. Urinary leak/fistulae are the most common surgical complications, followed by ureteric strictures and reflux. The majority of urinary leaks present with a high drain output. Early leaks are commonly due to technical challenges; a small capacity, very thick or thin-walled urinary bladder, with a short length transplant ureter is a common scenario. Small leaks are usually from a neo-ureterocystostomy, and can be managed with prolonged urethral catheterisation, however results of early exploration and surgical repair are also good. Large leaks are commonly due to ureteric necrosis, and requires skillful surgery. Ureteric stenosis or strictures can present early due to ischaemic injury, or late due to chronic scarring, or BK virus infection. Kidneys with poor allograft function are often managed by antegrade dilatation and stenting or long-term nephrostomy, whereas good functioning allograft kidneys require surgical reconstruction. Depending on the length of the remaining healthy donor ureter, the surgical options include resection and neo-ureterocystostomy, psoas hitch surgery, Boari flap, or uretero-ureteric drainage.

High drain output post kidney transplant surgery

This a common complication, illustrated in Practice Points 1 and Fig. 23.2:

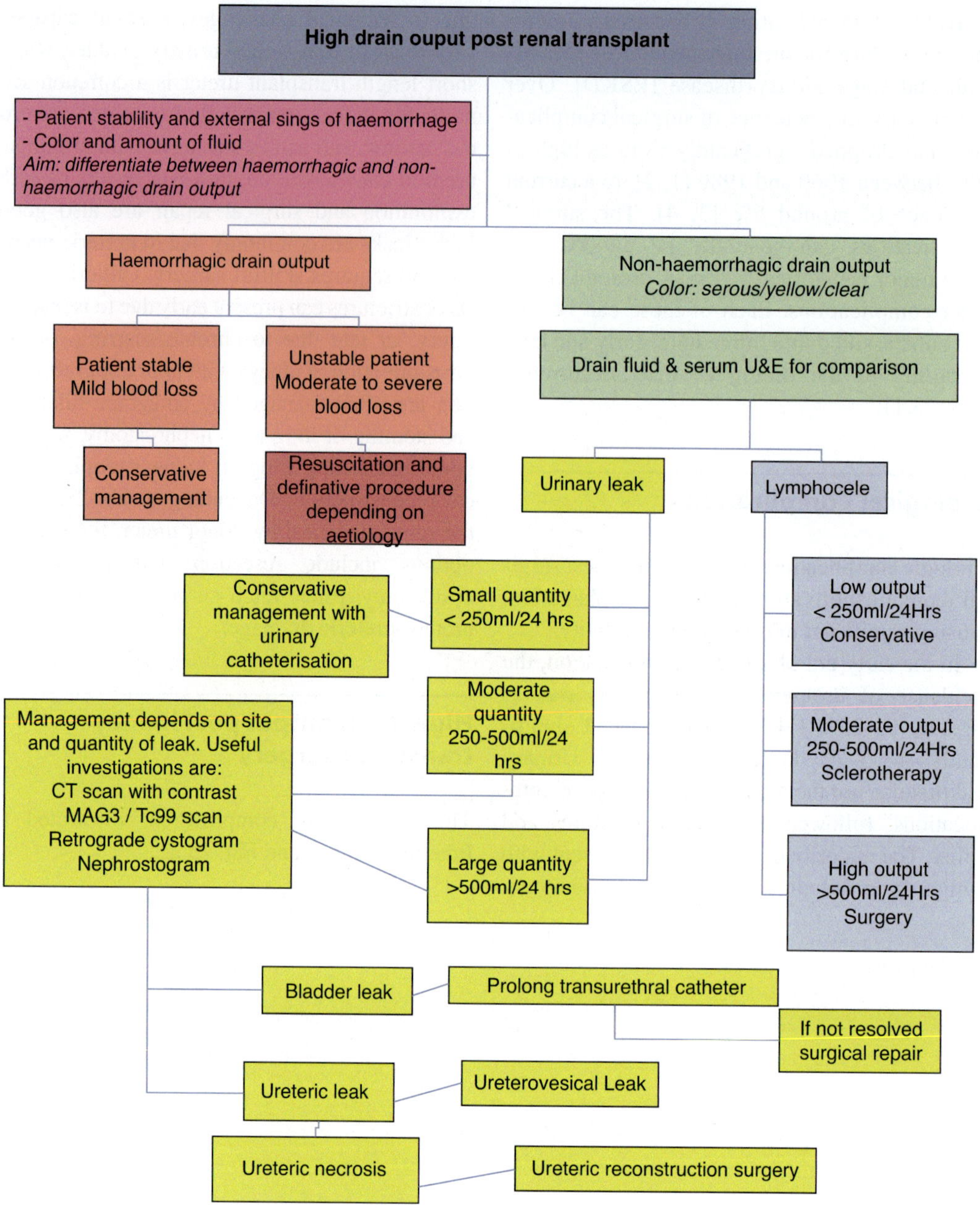

Fig. 23.2 Proposed management algorithm for high drain output post kidney transplant

Practice Point 1

High drain output post kidney transplant surgery

Clinical Scenario:

A 43-year-old female patient with a ***BMI of 38 kg/m²*** on ***peritoneal dialysis***, having a history of ESKD secondary to ***ADPKD*** received her first live donor kidney transplant from a 58-year-old genetically unrelated ABO-compatible donor. The donor kidney had a ***small lower polar***

artery, in addition to a main renal artery, which was separately anastomosed. She had uneventful transplant surgery, with immediate graft function. From immediately post transplantation, she had a ***high drain output***, which failed to settle over the ensuing days

Challenges:

This is a common presentation after kidney transplantation: iatrogenic ***missed peritoneal membrane injury*** or ***injury to a native kidney cyst*** can confuse the common differential diagnosis of urinary leak or lymphocoele. A smaller lower polar artery, if thrombosed, can increase the risk of ***distal ureteric necrosis, resulting in a urinary leak***. A ***high BMI is a risk factor for lymphocoele.***

Examination

Haemodynamically stable patients with no additional symptoms except heaviness around the transplant site. There were no external clinical signs, apart from mild wound tenderness due to recent surgery. There was straw coloured fluid in the drain.

Investigations

Good allograft function with a stable Hb. Drain fluid showed creatinine of 156 μmol/L, compared to a serum level of 147 μmol/L, which excluded a urinary leak. An ultrasound of her transplant kidney showed a large peri-transplant collection, which was drained:

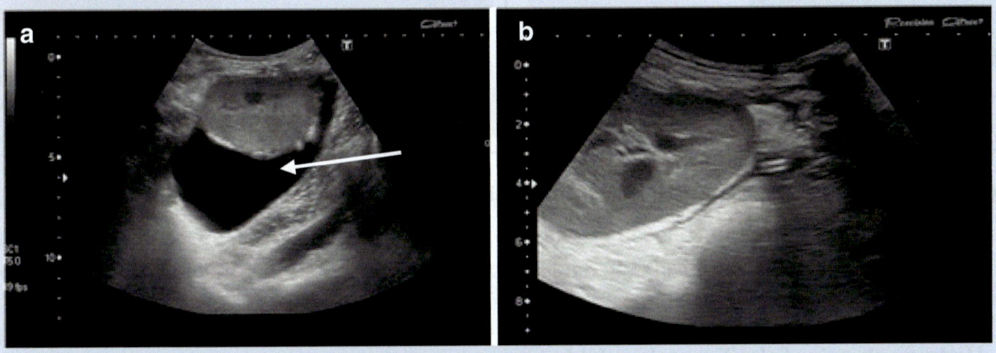

Image shows a kidney transplant ultrasound scan, demonstrating a large peri-transplant collection (a, white arrow), which resolves post drainage (b):

Management

The case was initially managed with instillation of 5% povidone-iodine solution through the drain, which did not lead to a reduction in drain output, hence surgical laparoscopic fenestration was successfully undertaken at 28 days post transplantation

Hydronephrosis of the Transplant Kidney

This complication is uncommon, and is illustrated in Practice Points 2 and Fig. 23.3

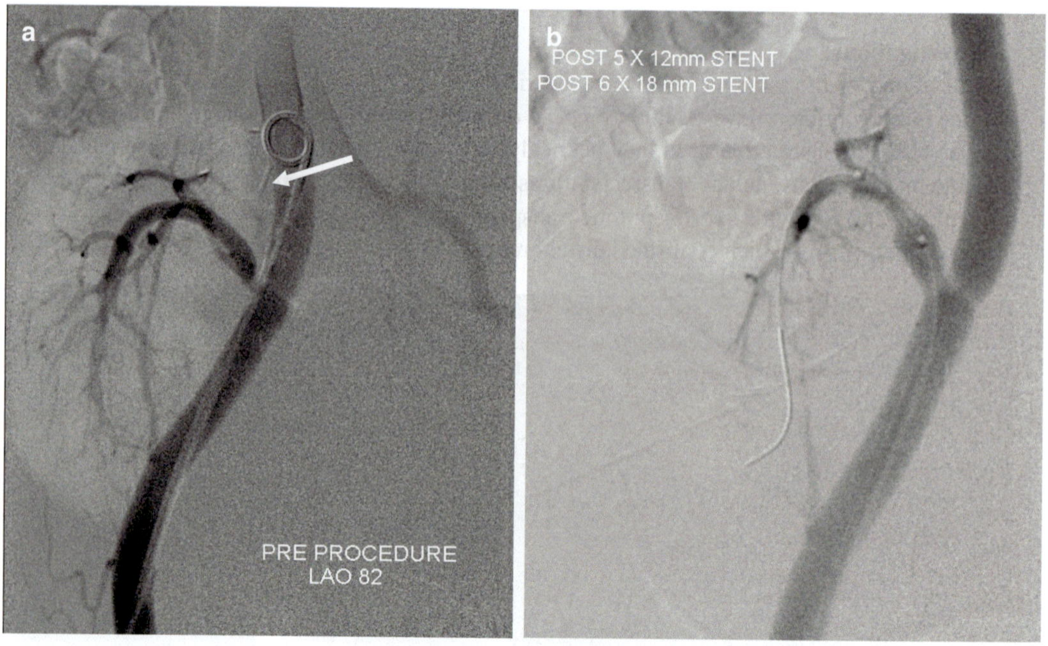

Fig. 23.4 Stenting of a transplant renal artery post-transplant. (**a**) Transplant renal artery stenosis demonstrated (white arrow) and post stenotic vessel dilatation pre-procedure on selective arteriography. (**b**) Post transplant renal artery stenting procedure—good flow and run-off distal to the stricture is demonstrated

Practice Point 3

Oliguria post kidney transplant

Clinical Scenario:

A 59-year-old female patient with ESKD secondary to FSGS, with a previous history of unprovoked DVT, received a cadaveric kidney transplant following donation after brain death (DBD) from a 49-year-old male donor, with a history of acute kidney injury (AKI) Stage 2 at the time of donation. The surgery was uneventful, but the patient suffered delayed graft function. On the 7th post-operative day, she had a percutaneous transplant biopsy. The procedure was uneventful, but on the same night, she presented with sudden severe pain over her transplanted kidney, and anuria.

Challenges:

The real challenge in this case is to differentiate between a vascular event, or simple acute tubular necrosis due to donor AKI. Risk factors for thrombosis are a history of unprovoked DVT, and potential post biopsy bleeding, compressing on the kidney transplant hilum, causing renal vein thrombosis.

Investigations: Transplant coloured doppler US remains the first investigation to look for organ perfusion, vascular flow and haematoma. In equivocal CT angiogram, or MAG3 nuclear scans can be helpful. In this case, her US showed flow in the renal transplant artery, with reversal of diastolic flow. There was no flow detectable in the renal vein.

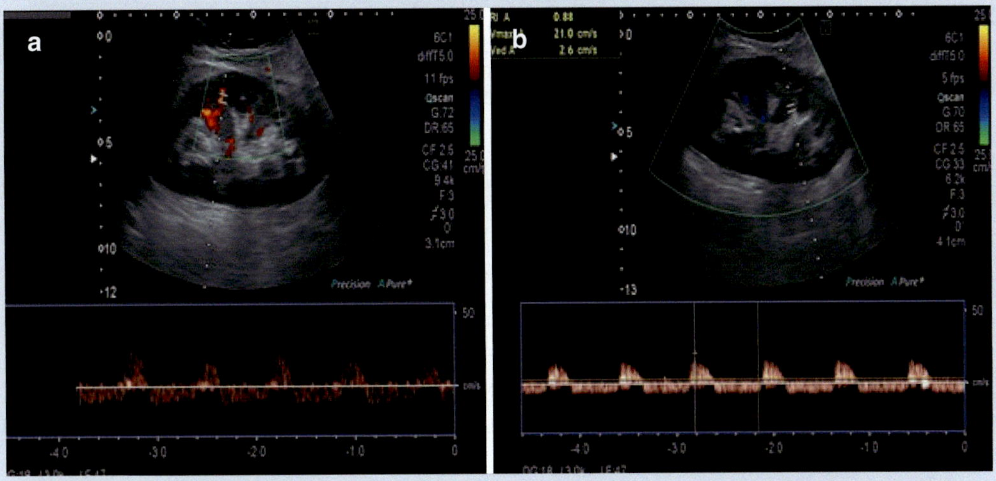

Images shows a colour doppler scan of a transplanted kidney. US showed flow in the renal transplant artery, with reversal of diastolic flow (a). There was no flow detectable in the renal vein (b).

Management:

Once a diagnosis or suspicion of transplant renal vein or renal artery thrombosis is made, it requires immediate exploration. Any chance of graft salvage depends on how quickly organs can be re-perfused. In the majority of cases, graft nephrectomy is the only option. Small to medium sized haematomas, not compressing on kidney vasculature, can be managed with a conservative approach. In the above case the patient had transplant renal vein thrombosis, which was not salvageable, and culminated in graft nephrectomy

Oliguria post kidney transplant

Oliguria or anuria with AKI post-transplant is common, but rarely due to surgical causes. This is described with a management plan with Practice Points 3 and Fig. 23.5:

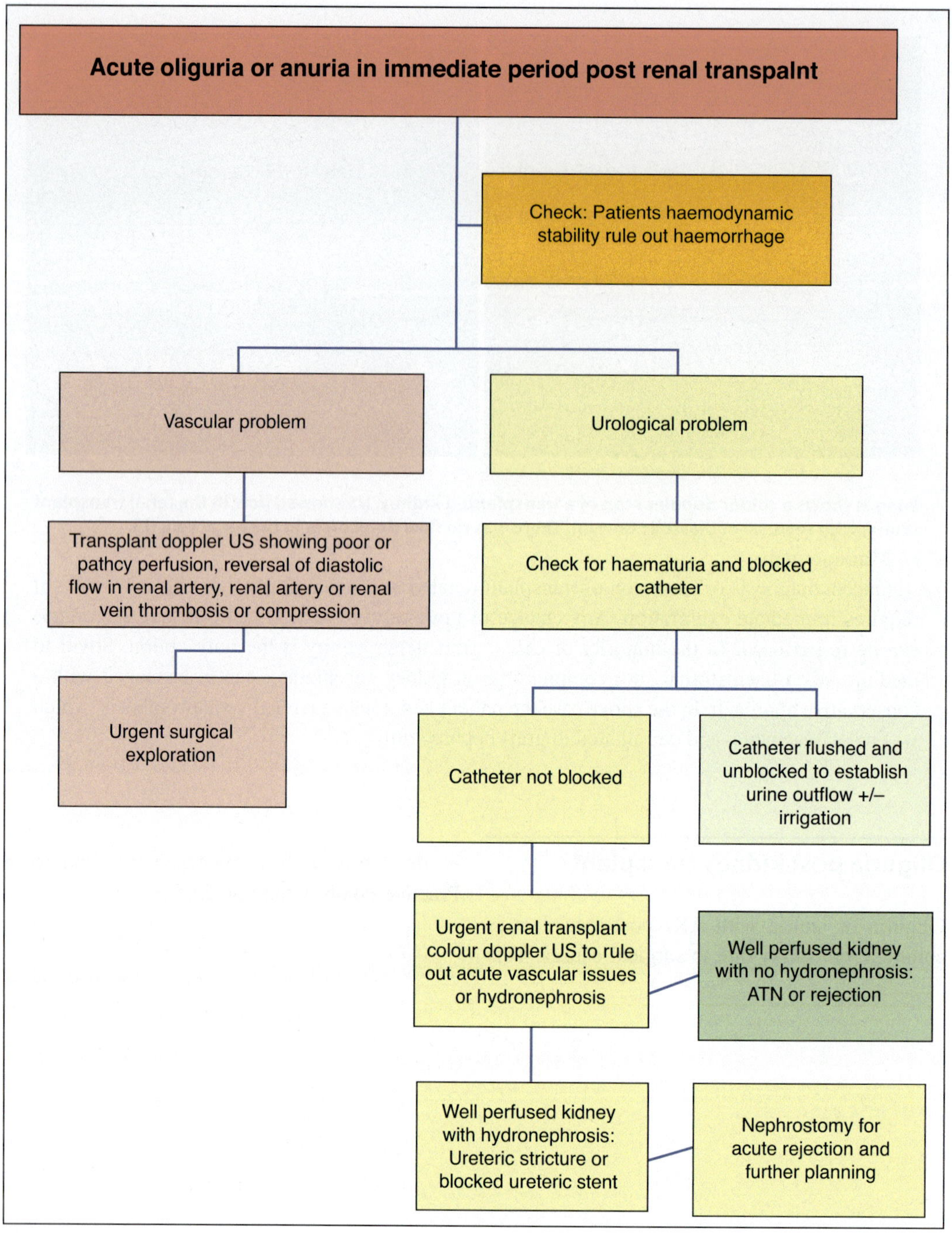

Fig. 23.5 Management of oliguria and anuria post kidney transplant

Medical Complications of Kidney Transplantation

Infections

- Infections are more common in transplant recipients due to both immunosuppression and commonly associated co-morbidities, such as diabetes mellitus. One should consider the overall immunosuppressive burden of the patient (including immunosuppression the patient might have received for their native kidney disease, as well as immunosuppression given on induction and maintenance treatment following kidney transplantation), while assessing infection risk.
- The infections can be typical or atypical bacterial infections (including mycobacterial infections), viral and fungal infections acquired either in healthcare or community settings, or reactivation of endogenous infections such as cytomegalovirus (CMV), varicella zoster virus (VZV) or latent Tuberculosis. Typical early infections are perioperative bacterial infections: wound infections, urinary tract infections (often in association with bladder catheter or ureteric stent) and pneumonia. Opportunistic fungal infections (Pneumocystis Jirovecii, Aspergillus, Cryptococcus) and viral infections such as CMV usually occur between 1 and 6 months post transplantation.
- Early removal of the bladder catheter and ureteric stent removal between 2 and 4 weeks post-transplant is recommended to reduce the risk of urinary tract infections.
- In a post-transplant patient with abnormal liver function tests, consider CMV infection, Hepatitis B, C, A and E infections.
- Presentation can be atypical in an immunocompromised host. Every attempt should be made to obtain an organism from appropriate specimen for early diagnosis and treatment. This may include bronchoscopy and bronchoalveolar aspirate, radiological drainage of collections, viral PCRs (polymerase chain reaction) from blood samples in addition to routine blood, urine and sputum cultures.
- Antimicrobial prophylaxis with Sulfamethoxazole-Trimethoprim (480 mg once a day) is primarily used for prevention of Pneumocystis pneumonia but it also provides some protection against urinary tract infections. CMV prophylaxis with Valganciclovir is given where the donor is seropositive and the recipient is seronegative (D+/R−). In some centres, seropositive recipients (irrespective of donor CMV status) are given Valganciclovir prophylaxis, and no prophylaxis is given where both donor and the recipient are CMV seronegative.
- Viral and fungal infections tend to be more common in patients who receive lymphocyte depleting antibody induction such as anti-thymocyte globulin (ATG), and in particular those who receive higher doses (>3–4 mg/kg).

Cytomegalovirus (CMV)

In kidney transplant recipients, symptomatic disease due to CMV is either due to reactivation of latent disease, donor-derived new infection, or infection with an exogenous strain (community acquired). CMV disease in uncommon in the first 4 weeks post-transplantation, but not unknown. Those at highest risk of developing high-grade viraemia and CMV disease are D+/R− patients, hence this is the population targeted to receive Valganciclovir prophylaxis. There are two approaches to prevent and treat CMV infection in transplant recipients: The first is regular surveillance blood PCR screening to detect CMV viraemia, and to treat pre-emptively if viraemia is detected, or give valganciclovir prophylaxis in selected recipients, and treat viraemia detected on clinical grounds. Our practice is to give Valganciclovir prophylaxis to D+/R− patients for minimum of 90 days, and do active CMV PCR surveillance in seropositive recipients (D+/R+ and D−/R+) for 3 months. The immunosuppressive burden has usually lowered by 3-months post-transplantation, enabling cessation of Valganciclovir prophylaxis and surveillance. Coupled with minimisation of immunosuppression in low/standard immunological risk transplant recipients (steroid withdrawal on D7, reduction in mycophenolate mofetil dose from 1 g BD to 500 mg BD after 30 days, long term dual immunosuppression in the majority of the patients), we have found that this approach results in low CMV infection rates (5–8%), and is cost-effective. Some centres continue prophylaxis for 200 days in D+/R– patients and also use prophylaxis for all patients except for D-/R– patients.

CMV can present in kidney transplant recipients as either asymptomatic CMV viraemia or CMV disease. CMV disease is defined as the presence of CMV virus in blood or tissues (usually detected in blood by CMV PCR), along with clinical features of organ involvement. Usual clinical manifestations are hepatitis, colitis (diarrhoea, with or without blood and mucus), and haematological (leucopenia). Other rare manifestations in severe disease include pneumonitis and meningoencephalitis, but these are uncommon in the current era of kidney transplantation, where immunosuppressive burden is usually kept at modest levels.

Diagnosis is either made by demonstrating CMV antigenaemia to detect CMV proteins (pp65) in peripheral blood leukocytes (isolated from buffy coat fraction of blood sample) or by PCR in peripheral blood sample (obtained in an EDTA tube). At our centre, the diagnosis is made by CMV PCR from whole blood. Higher viral loads are often associated with CMV disease, so it is important to have close links with virology laboratory as reporting units (DNA copies/mL or units/mL) vary widely between laboratories.

Treatment is a reduction of immunosuppression, with or without antiviral therapy. We usually manage asymptomatic CMV viraemia with immunosuppressive reduction alone (usually dose reduction or withdrawal of mycophenolate mofetil), but in some patients deemed at high risk of rejection we treat with oral valganciclovir without altering their immunosuppression. In patients with high grade viraemia associated with CMV disease, we treat with reduction in immunosuppression and oral valganciclovir. The treatment is continued until complete resolution of signs and symptoms of CMV disease and there is absence of CMV viraemia in two blood PCRs performed at least one week apart. The typical duration of therapy is 2–4 weeks. Upon completion of treatment, the options are either stop valganciclovir and do monthly CMV PCR surveillance for a further 3–4 months or continue prophylactic dose for 3–4 months. If the viremia fails to respond to Valganciclovir, viral ganciclovir resistance should be suspected, and appropriate resistance gene mutation studies should be done. Both the treatment and prophylactic dose of valganciclovir should be adjusted to estimated creatinine clearance or estimated GFR (eGFR). Patients with severe disease may require treatment with intravenous ganciclovir for the first 48–72 h. Options are limited for gancicloivir resistant CMV disease and these include Foscarnet (toxic drug) and other newer/experimental antiviral drugs such as Marabavir.

There are two approaches to prevent CMV disease: either routine prophylaxis (usually with oral valganciclovir) or routine monitoring for evidence of viraemia with pre-emptive treatment.

Epstein–Barr Virus (EBV) and Post-Transplant Lymphoproliferative Disorders (PTLD)

Acute infection with EBV is not usually a clinically relevant problem after adult kidney transplantation, but an important long-term complication of EBV infection is the development of post-transplant lymphoproliferative disease (PTLD), with an incidence of 0.5–1%. Although it is usually described that most cases of EBV-driven PTLD occur within one year post transplant, cases can occur at any time following transplantation. The more intense the immunosuppression used (in particular, lymphocyte depleting antibody induction), the greater the risk of PTLD, and the earlier it tends to occur. There is an increased risk of PTLD amongst EBV-negative recipients of EBV-positive donor organs. The majority of PTLD develops as a result of EBV-driven uncontrolled B-cell proliferation, on a background of suppressed cytotoxic T cells due to immunosuppression.

A small proportion of post-transplant lymphomas (around 10%) are from EBV-negative B-cells, and these behave clinically like non-Hodgkin's lymphoma (NHL). The presentation may be typical of NHL, with symptoms or systemic signs such as fever, unexplained weight loss, anaemia, fatigue, lymphadenopathy, gastrointestinal symptoms (including obstruction), hepatosplenomegaly, central nervous system symptoms or pulmonary symptoms (often with nodules on chest X ray). An atypical presentation in a transplant patient could be unexplained graft dysfunction due to lymphoma infiltrating the transplant kidney, in the absence of generalised lymphadenopathy or hepatosplenomegaly. This can be mis-interpreted as cellular rejection, and special immunocytochemical stains would be needed to differentiate between the two. Usually, the interstitial infiltrate is extensive and diffuse in PTLD. Blood PCR usually reveals high grade EBV viraemia. Treatment consists of withdrawal or marked reduction of immunosuppression accepting the risk of rejection and graft loss. Rituximab alone, or in combination with other standard NHL chemotherapy regimen is often used to treat PTLD. A close liaison with haemato-oncology is essential while managing these patients.

BK Virus (BKV)

BK virus belongs to the family of polyomavirus group and causes tubulointerstitial nephritis and rarely ureteric strictures in kidney transplant recipients.

BK virus infects urothelial (transitional epithelium) and tubular epithelial cells, with no clinical features of systemic involvement outside the urinary tract. The virus either comes with the donor kidney, which harbours latent infection, with re-activation following transplantation due to immunosuppression, or from re-activation of latent virus in the recipient genitourinary system. The risk factors for BK virus infection include the degree of immunosuppression, trauma to the urinary tract and male gender. With a low immunosuppressive burden (early steroid withdrawal and reduced mycophenolate mofetil exposure), we observe low BKV rates of around 2–5%.

BK viruria post-transplant is common, and doesn't always mean a viral infection of the transplant kidney (BK virus nephropathy, BKVN). BKVN is usually associated with high grade viremia (positive BKV PCR in blood of >10,000–20,000 DNA copies/mL), but we have seen cases of BKVN with low grade viremia, and occasionally, absence of a positive viral stain on kidney transplant biopsy specimens in the presence of high grade viraemia, which can be due to the patchy nature of the pathology and sampling error. The diagnosis in such cases can often be made with repeat biopsy from a different site. The diagnostic yield is higher if the cortico-medullary junction or medulla is included in the biopsy, since BKV has a predilection for the kidney medulla.

The clinical presentation of BKVN is a rising creatinine, with no other clinical features or rarely, a ureteric stricture causing hydronephrosis of the transplant kidney. The transplant kidney biopsy remains the definitive test to diagnose BKVN and immunohistochemical staining for BKV (SV40 large T antigen, SV40T stain) should be the standard practice. The histological features include tubulointerstitial inflammation (can be very similar to rejection) and positive SV40T stain. An early improvement in serum creatinine with methylprednisolone does not exclude BKVN, as suppression of inflammation associated with viral infection can improve kidney function transiently. Concomitant acute rejection can occur, but treatment should be directed towards BKVN once diagnosis is proven with reduction in immunosuppression with further changes dictated by clinical course and where necessary, further transplant kidney biopsy.

Various BKV screening protocols have been advocated as viraemia often predates clinical graft dysfunction by several weeks or even months. One should bear in mind that low grade viraemias (usually <2000 copies/mL) detected on surveillance PCRs may not be clinically relevant and reduction in immunosuppression without a biopsy diagnosis of BKVN could lead to rejection. Therefore, a biopsy is recommended to confirm the diagnosis of BKVN before altering immunosuppression.

Urine PCR for BKV is not recommended for the diagnosis or monitoring of BKVN. The other test often mentioned in the literature is 'decoy' cells in the urine. These are tubule cells infected with BKV, and shed in the urine, identified by their morphology of 'large irregular nuclei' due to viral inclusions but this test is not widely used in clinical practice.

The main treatment of BKV is a reduction of immunosuppression. We usually stop mycophenolate mofetil, maintain the patient on tacrolimus monotherapy while monitoring BKV viral load in blood with 2–4 weekly PCRs and add small dose of prednisolone (5 mg once a day) once reductions in viral load is achieved. There is no specific antiviral treatment for this condition and no randomised trials. The drugs that have been tried are a 2-week course of ciprofloxacin and more recently leflunomide. The leflunomide has in vitro antiviral properties and is immunomodulatory, is well tolerated and we have observed stabilisation of graft function in patients with BKVN upon treatment with this drug along with reduction of immunosuppression. Other approaches that have been tried are- switching calcineurin inhibitor (CNI) to mTOR inhibitor (Sirolimus/Everolimus) and intravenous immunoglobulin.

Pneumocystis Jiroveccii (Carinii)

Pneumocystis pneumonia (PCP/PCJ) is a potentially life-threatening pulmonary infection that occurs in immunocompromised individuals.

Transplant patients are at highest risk in their first 3 months post-transplant due to higher levels of immunosuppression, but the infection can occur at later stages in patients maintained on higher levels of immunosuppression, and those receiving treatment for rejection episodes. In the transplant patient, PCJ typically presents as hypoxic type1 respiratory failure, associated with fever and dry cough, with diffuse and bilateral pulmonary interstitial infiltrates on chest X ray and CT scan. The index of suspicion should be high and often treatment is commenced before obtaining microbiological proof, but every attempt should be made to demonstrate the organism from sputum (difficult in practice, usually need to be induced with saline inhalation) and bronchoscopic aspirate. Diagnostic yield is enhanced by performing PCR from respiratory tract secretions, in addition to conventional staining and microscopy.

PCJ in immunosuppressed recipients can be life threatening and therefore, prompt commencement of treatment upon high clinical suspicion is required. The treatment consists of high therapeutic dose trimethoprim/sulfamethoxazole orally in mild to moderate disease or intravenously in patients with severe disease. In those in whom trimethoprim/sulfamethoxazole is contraindicated, alternative drugs include clindamycin/primaquine, trimethoprim/dapsone, atovaquone and pentamidine.

It is routine clinical practice worldwide to give prophylactic co-trimoxazole at a standard dose of 480 mg once a day for 3–6 months to all kidney transplant patients. With this regime, there have been marked reductions in the incidence of PCJ infections in kidney transplant patients.

Mycobacterium Tuberculosis (MTB)

Mycobacterium Tuberculosis (MTB) is an important opportunistic infection in kidney transplant recipients, with significant variation in prevalence in different parts of the world, based on community prevalence of the disease. Managing tuberculosis in transplant recipients is challenging in view of the non-specific clinical presentation, interaction of anti-MTB medicines with immunosuppressive medications, and higher incidence of anti-MTB medicine-related adverse effects. The risk factors include a previous history of incompletely treated MTB, underlying chronic lung disease, fungal co-infections, diabetes mellitus, poor nutritional status and high immunosuppressive burden in particular, one that includes lymphocyte depleting antibody induction. MTB in a kidney transplant patient could be: (a) endogenous reactivation of latent tuberculosis infection (LMTB) in the post-transplant period (b) donor-derived tubercular infection (rare) (c) de-novo infection due to exposure to MTB bacilli in the post-transplant period. The presentation can be a typical respiratory presentation of cough, fever, haemoptysis and weight loss, or an atypical presentation with intermittent fevers, weight loss and predominantly extrapulmonary disease.

Pre-transplant Screening for Latent Mycobacterium Tuberculosis (LMTB)

Latent mycobacterium tuberculosis (LMTB) infection has been defined by the world health organization (WHO) as "a state of persistent immune response to stimulation by Mycobacterium Tuberculosis antigen, with no evidence of clinically manifest active MTB disease". The concern in patients with undetected LMTB who get transplanted, is that immunosuppression could lead to re-activation of the disease. Various guidelines recommend screening for the prospective kidney transplant recipients, who are deemed to be a higher MTB risk for LMTB pre-transplant, and treating it. The options are:

1. Screen everyone in high prevalence areas of the world and treat if positive.
2. Screen selected high risk population in low prevalence areas of the world (<20 per 100,000 population) and treat if positive (for e.g. close contact with TB cases, recently arrived from high endemic regions, spend a significant amount of time in high prevalence parts of the world).
3. Do not screen anyone in high prevalence parts of the world, as exposure would continue to occur following completion of treatment, and using one or two agents to treat latent TB in these regions would promote resistance, which already is a significant issue in these areas of the world. This option is often favoured in these regions where clinicians opt to treat clinically active MTB pre-transplant where possible and watch for any signs of active MTB post-transplant and treat as appropriate.
4. Treat with Isoniazid alone (300 mg once a day), along with pyridoxine for 6 months, starting at the time of transplant in high- risk patient population in low prevalence areas of the world, without prior screening for latent TB.

At our centre in the UK, we currently adopt option 4. It must be emphasised that option chosen should be based on local prevalence and incidence of the disease and one should follow local expertise and guidelines.

The two commonly used tests for screening for LMTB, include tuberculin skin test (TST) and interferon gamma release assay (IGRA). In the IGRA test, cytokine interferon (IFN)-gamma is measured as the readout of effector-T cell stimulation upon exposure to mycobacterium tuberculosis antigen in vitro. In immunocompromised patients, it has the advantage of differentiating anergy from a true negative test. It is also more specific than TST when used in BCG vaccinated individuals.

Active tuberculosis must be ruled out in all the patients undergoing transplant, evaluation as well as in the post-transplant setting. A detailed history and clinical examination concentrating on symptoms such as chronic cough, weight loss, unexplained fever, night sweats should be followed by a thorough lab workup, including microscopy for acid fast bacilli (AFB), tubercular culture in appropriate samples (sputum, urine, pleural fluid etc.), needle aspirate or biopsy histology, Gene Xpert for MTB assay and imaging such as x-ray chest, ultrasound and CT scan. More invasive procedures like bronchioalveolar lavage, pleural and lung biopsy may be required.

Treatment of latent and active Mycobacterium Tuberculosis (MTB)

Whenever feasible LTB treatment should be completed pre-transplant while the patient is on waitlist and the treatment of choice is Isoniazid and Rifampicin for 3 months.

As far as the active tuberculosis is concerned, the ideal scenario would be to completely treat it prior to kidney transplantation, as per the WHO or the local guidelines. However, this may not be feasible always especially in high prevalence areas where the dialysis infrastructure is poor and continuing dialysis could be associated with frequent complications and higher morbidity and mortality. Successful outcomes have been achieved when transplantation was done after completing the initial intensive phase (2 months) pre-transplant and then continuing the maintenance phase in the post-transplant period. Standard regime includes 4-drug combination of Isoniazid, Rifampicin, Pyrazinamide and Ethambutol for 2 months of initiation phase followed by 4-month continuation phase with Isoniazid and Rifampicin. Patients with extra pulmonary tuberculosis require longer duration of treatment. Treatment of active MTB in the post-transplant setting is challenging in view of the interaction of anti-tubercular and immunosuppressive medications, in particular Rifampicin, which is a potent enzyme inducer and it is very difficult to achieve adequate tacrolimus levels with concomitant Rifampicin treatment. Therefore, to treat active MTB post-transplant, often non-Rifampicin-based regimen would be required which may make the treatment less effective.

Fungal Infections in Kidney Transplant Recipients

Fungal infections are a serious infectious complication of kidney transplant recipients in certain parts of the world where environmental factors contribute significantly in addition to host factors. Some of the fungal infections such as histoplasmosis, blastomycosis, coccidioidomycosis, para-coccidioidomycosis are endemic in some geographical areas of the world, and some are opportunistic fungal infections more widespread all over the world, affecting immunocompromised hosts (candidiasis, aspergillosis, cryptococcosis, mucormycosis). In most series, candidiasis is the most common invasive fungal infection followed by aspergillosis, cryptococcosis, endemic fungi and zygomycosis. Candida and aspergillus are the common causes in the first three to six months when the immunosuppression tends to be at a higher level awhile cryptococcal and endemic fungal infections tend to occur at later stages. Various risk factors for getting fungal infections in post-transplant period include the net state of immunosuppression, use of anti-thymocyte globulin (ATG) for induction, diabetes mellitus, prolonged and indiscriminate use of antibiotics, central venous catheter, intravenous cannulae left in for long durations and prolonged urinary catheterisation.

The clinical picture varies, depending upon the sites affected and can include gastrointestinal tract, lung, urinary tract, respiratory tract, blood stream and central nervous system involvement. The commonest form of candidiasis in a kidney transplant recipient is that of mucosal involvement leading to oral thrush, oesophageal candidiasis and candidal vaginitis. Severe forms can present as candidemia with hematogenous spread to various organs. *Candida albicans* is the most common cause of invasive candidiasis, followed by non-albicans such as *glabrata* and *krusei*. Pulmonary aspergillosis is the most common presentation of invasive aspergillosis in kidney transplant recipients. Aspergillus *fumigatus* and *flavus* are the commonest causes, followed by rare types like *terreus*. The patient with pulmonary aspergillosis presents with cough, dyspnoea, low-grade fever and haemoptysis. Due to its angio-invasive nature, it can lead to organ infarction and dissemination to other organ systems. Aspergillosis of urinary tract and vascular anastomotic site can happen rarely due to infected graft-associated transmission. *Cryptococcosis* is another common fungal infection in kidney transplant recipients. Most common organism is *Cryptococcus neoformans,* but cases with C. *gattii* have been increasingly reported now. Presentation is usually 6 months after transplantation. The most common site of presentation is central nervous system (CNS). Cryptococcal meningitis presents with unexplained headache, fever and altered consciousness level. Unexplained skin involvement can be another form of presentation.

Mucormycosis is an angio-invasive fungal infection. Rhino-paranasal sinus-cerebral mucormycosis is the most common presentation. Other forms including pulmonary, cutaneous, gastrointestinal tract (GIT), graft kidney and disseminated disease. Due to the angio-invasive nature the dissemination of fungus is rapid with high fatality rate reaching up to 75% despite appropriate and timely surgical and medical treatment.

Endemic mycosis has varied presentation. Histoplasmosis presents as fever, weight loss, pancytopenia, and lymphadenopathy due to lympho-reticular system involvement. Disseminated infection with CNS involvement may be seen. Blastomycosis can involve pulmonary system causing acute respiratory distress syndrome (ARDS) and can also involve musculoskeletal system. Coccidioidomycosis may have similar presentations.

Diagnosis and Management of Fungal Infections

A high index of suspicion is important in diagnosing fungal infections, as the symptoms might be non-specific. Main principles of management are reducing immunosuppression, removing/replacing intravenous cannulae and urinary catheter. A combination of appropriate fungal stains and culture on suitable body fluids, molecular diagnostic methods and imaging would be needed to make a diagnosis. Always work closely with microbiology department to facilitate appropriate investigations. A blood 1,3 beta-D-glucan is useful as a screening test for invasive fungal infections, but it is non-specific. Cryptococcal meningitis is diagnosed by CSF examination by India ink stain and gram stain. Cryptococcal antigen detection in CSF has excellent sensitivity and specificity and it is one of the best tests for a rapid diagnosis. PCR to detect fungal nucleic acid improves the diagnostic yield.

Treatment depends upon the nature of the fungus and severity of the illness. Oral Candidiasis may just require nystatin suspension whereas Esophageal candidiasis would need Fluconazole which interacts with Tacrolimus increasing the levels due to the inhibition of CYP3A4 cytochrome isoenzyme. Tacrolimus level needs to be monitored closely in these patients and a dose reduction is often needed. In severe, invasive fungal infections and fungaemia, drugs such as caspofungin (An Echinocandin) or Anidulafungin and liposomal amphotericin B would be needed along with drastic reductions or complete withdrawal of immunosuppression. Cryptococcal meningitis is treated with liposomal amphotericin B plus flucytosine followed by prolonged periods of oral fluconazole. Invasive mucormycosis will need treatment with IV liposomal amphotericin B with posaconazole as stepdown treatment if there is response.

The prognosis of kidney transplant patients with invasive fungal infections remains poor and therefore, measures to prevent or minimise the risk of these infections are of paramount importance.

COVID-19 Infection and Kidney Transplant Recipients

COVID-19, a respiratory disease caused by the coronavirus SARS-CoV-2 was declared a global pandemic in March 2020. The disease has affected millions of people globally with a case fatality ratio of 25–30% in hospitalised kidney transplant patients infected with the virus. The current strategies to combat the virus include societal measures to minimise the risk of aerosol transmission, hand hygiene, wearing masks in closed spaces and vaccination. The management options available at the time of this writing in March 2021 are supportive measures, respiratory support, reduction in immunosuppression (reduction or withdrawal of mycophenolate mofetil depending on disease severity, continuation of tacrolimus and steroids in most of the cases, dexamethasone in suitable patients as per RECOVERY trial evidence, Remdesivir as per local guidelines, Tocilizumab in severe cases as per local and national guidelines along with participation in clinical trials testing new therapies. AKI is common in kidney transplant patients with COVID-19 but most of the patients do recover their graft function. The reduction in immunosuppression may result in rejection of the kidney but this is not common in our experience.

Other Common Infections and Vaccinations Post-Transplant

In addition to common bacterial chest infections and urinary tract infections, Infections with Herpes family of viruses can occur post-transplant causing genital herpes infections and shingles. Treatment is with Aciclovir or Valaciclovir. It is important to screen waitlisted patients for Varicella-Zoster (VZV) antibodies and immunise with VZV vaccine in those who are antibody negative. As this is a live vaccine, it must be given to patients before transplantation. It is recommended that all kidney transplant patients receive annual influenza vaccine and pneumococcal vaccine once every 5 years. It is also recommended that transplant patients receive SARS-CoV-2 vaccine to protect against Covid-19. Live vaccines should be avoided in kidney transplant recipients, and they should only have inactivated (killed) vaccines.

Post-Transplant Diabetes

New-onset diabetes after transplantation (NODAT) or Post Transplant Diabetes Mellitus (PTDM) occurs in 5–20% patients following kidney transplantation, depending on pre-transplant patient characteristics, post-transplant weight gain and the immunosuppressive regime. The immunosuppressive drugs Tacrolimus and corticosteroids both increase the risk of diabetes post transplantation. Early steroid withdrawal results in low incidence of PTDM, and this should be considered in suitable recipients with appropriate immunological risk stratification. The presence of PTDM is associated with an increased risk of graft loss, cardiovascular disease and mortality. Although tacrolimus is associated with higher risk of diabetes compared to cyclosporine A, given the better tolerability and lower risk of rejection with tacrolimus, routine switch from Tacrolimus to Cyclosporine A to improve glycaemic status is not recommended.

Management of diabetes in the longer-term post-transplantation (whether new onset or not) follows similar strategies to those of the general population that include diet and lifestyle advice to enable weight loss and drugs. Late steroid withdrawal or an attempt to run low tacrolimus levels to achieve better glycemic control are not recommended as these measures often result in acute or chronic rejection with reductions in graft survival or further increase in steroid exposure due to treatment of rejection episodes. To treat diabetes post transplantation, all the usual oral agents can be used (Metformin remains a drug of choice), following the usual modifications to account for kidney transplant function. Insulin can be used as needed. The SGLT2 inhibitors are likely to be of significant renal and cardiovascular benefit for overweight kidney transplant recipients, similar to their beneficial effects observed in non-transplant population but these drugs haven't been systematically tested in kidney transplant patients. Concerns are potential increased risk of infections, in particular genitourinary infections in women, risk of dehydration leading to volume depletion and AKI when used in association with ACEI/ARBs. It is unlikely that the latter would be a significant clinical issue.

Acute and Chronic Rejection

Acute or chronic alloimmune injury results in rejection of the allograft. This may be acute, chronic, acute on chronic, cellular (T-cell driven), antibody-mediated or in many cases, mixed T-cell and antibody-mediated rejections. Hyperacute rejection, where severe vascular rejection occurs driven by preformed donor specific anti-HLA antibodies is almost an unknown entity in the modern era of kidney transplantation where recipients are screened carefully for donor specific anti-HLA antibodies with Luminex technology along with crossmatch techniques that incorporate flowcytometry and CDC methods.

- Acute rejection typically occurs within 3–4 months post-transplantation but it can occur anytime. Steroid resistant rejections and recurrent episodes of rejections confer poor prognosis. Usually, there are no clinical features associated with transplant rejection except for severe cases where there could be graft tenderness.
- Suspect rejection in following situations: An increase in serum creatinine of ≥20–25% from baseline *OR* a serum creatinine that is stable but higher than expected following transplantation *OR* a creatinine that stops decreasing further following initial decline post- transplant OR delayed graft function with dialysis dependence post- transplant.

Rejection can only be definitely diagnosed by graft biopsy and histopathology. The Banff grading system is updated and modified regularly to include histological patterns, mechanisms of rejection, acute Vs chronic rejection, activity and chronicity index within a given histological sample. The commonly known 'acute cellular rejection' is a T-cell mediated process characterised by interstitial lymphocytic infiltrates and infiltration of tubular epithelium by lymphocytes (tubulitis) severity of which is graded depending upon the percentage of cortex covered by cellular infiltrates and number of lymphocytes per cross section of tubule (Type IA and 1B rejection in 1997 Banff grading; Category 4, TCMR 1A and 1B in 2017 Banff grading). If blood vessels are involved by lymphocytic infiltration it would be classed as more severe 'vascular' rejection graded based on the extent of intimal involvement or transmural involvement (Type IIA, B and III in 1997 Banff grading; Category 4, TCMR IIA, IIB and III in 2017 Banff Grading). These categories are T cell mediated rejection that often respond to IV methylprednisolone but cases with vascular involvement (in particular, grade IIB and III) often require Anti-thymocyte globulin (ATG).

The second main category of rejection is acute/active antibody mediated rejection (AMR, category 2 in 2017 Banff grading system) which requires demonstration of microvascular inflammation in peritubular capillaries (PTC) or glomerulus (neutrophilic infiltrates in endothelium and vessel wall), C4D staining in peritubular capillaries, thrombotic microangiopathy and presence of donor specific anti HLA antibodies. C4D negative AMR is now well-recognised.

It must be emphasised that cellular (T-cell driven), and Antibody mediated rejections (AMRs) often occur together.

Additional categories belong to 'chronic rejection' and both chronic antibody mediated rejection (transplant glomerulopathy, multilayering of peritubular capillary basement membrane seen on electron microscopy, C4D staining in PTCs, arterial intimal fibrosis) and chronic T cell mediated rejection (Chronic TCMR, characterised by varying degrees of tubular atrophy/interstitial fibrosis (IFTA) along with interstitial inflammation, chronic allograft vasculopathy- arterial intimal fibrosis with mononuclear inflammatory cells) are now recognised and these are important causes of chronic allograft dysfunction and eventually, graft failure. Chronic rejection, in particular chronic AMR/transplant glomerulopathy is usually associated with significant proteinuria and progressively increasing proteinuria of >1 g/day is an indication to perform a kidney biopsy to diagnose chronic AMR or recurrent glomerular disease.

Late rejection episodes (occurring more than 6 months after transplantation) are often due to inadequate immunosuppression either due to poor adherence and non-compliance with immunosuppressive medications or due to inappropriate reductions in tacrolimus dose aiming for low levels to minimise CNI toxicity or inappropriate late steroid withdrawals. The tacrolimus levels should be maintained between 5 and 7 ng/mL (with exception of PTLD and other malignancies where lower levels may be desirable) long term to minimise the risk of de-novo DSA formation, reduce the risk of late acute and chronic rejections. Table 23.2 summarises the differences between acute T-cell mediated (cellular) rejection (ACR/Acute TCMR) and acute antibody-mediated rejection (AMR).

Maintenance of adequate immunosuppression, particularly maintaining tacrolimus levels in range most of the time reduce the risk of chronic TCMR as well as chronic AMR. While keeping patients on triple immunosuppression (Tacrolimus, mycophenolate mofetil and pred-

Table 23.2 Differences between acute T cell mediated (cellular) rejection (ACR/Acute TCMR) and acute antibody-mediated rejection (AMR) and management options

	ACR (Acute TCMR)	Acute AMR
• **Interstitial lymphocytic infiltration, Tubulitis**	Present	Absent (Can occur when there is concomitant TCMR)
• **Vascular mononuclear inflammation, fibrinoid necrosis**	Present	Absent
• **Donor-specific antibody in serum**	Absent	Present
• **Neutrophilic infiltrates in glomerular and peritubular capillaries with or without microvascular thrombosis (TMA), histological and electronmicroscopic evidence of endothelial injury**	Absent	Present
• **C4d staining in peritubular capillaries (PTC)**	Absent	Present
	Absent	Present
• **Primary therapy**	Pulse methylprednisolone, rabbit anti-thymocyte globulin (ATG) (for vascular T-cell rejection, grade IIB and above), increase in baseline immunosuppression, consider assessing mycophenolic acid exposure and adjust the dose.	Plasmapheresis (PEx) (Usually 5 sessions), intravenous immunoglobulin, pulse steroids. ATG if concomitant severe T cell mediated cellular/vascular rejection. Optimise Tacrolimus levels. Consider assessing mycophenolic acid exposure and adjust the dose. Eculizumab is an option in severe cases of AMR. Rituximab has been used with limited evidence and the efficacy remains unclear. IvIg and ATG should be given post-PEx.

nisolone) long term seems like best option to reduce the risk of chronic rejection, there is no evidence that this is the case compared to long term dual immunosuppression (Tacrolimus, mycophenolate mofetil OR tacrolimus, prednisolone; which is our usual practice for majority of our standard risk transplant recipients) and long-term triple immunosuppression is likely to be associated with higher rate of infections and malignancies.

The optimal immunosuppression long-term remains unclear and it should be individualised as much as possible taking in to account the immunological (rejection) risk, infection risk, cancer risk and patient preferences to achieve best long-term outcomes.

Some of the new developments in this field include: non-invasive diagnosis of rejection with urinary cell transcriptomics, urinary biomarker (free and exosomal proteins, miRNA) panels diagnostic of rejection, circulating cell free donor DNA to detect allograft damage and rejection in early stages, routine molecular analysis of biopsy specimen, Safe CNI free regimen with co-stimulatory blockade, protocols designed to develop transplant tolerance and evidence base for utilisation of DSAs as biomarkers to optimise long term outcomes. In addition to these, there is a need for good quality clinical research to identify optimal long term immunosuppressive regimes, treatment protocols that are effective and safe for acute AMR and chronic rejection (cAMR and cTCMR), treatments that work for recurrent glomerular diseases, in particular, recurrent IgAN.

Calcineurin Inhibitor Nephrotoxicity

Whilst the CNIs ciclosporin and tacrolimus revolutionized the world of solid organ transplantation by prolonging graft survival, they are potentially nephrotoxic agents. CNIs can lead to both acute kidney injury (AKI), which is due to dose dependent reversible vasoconstriction of glomerular afferent arterioles leading to drop in GFR and chronic toxicity (vasculopathy and tubulointerstitial fibrosis) which is largely irreversible. However, as described in previous section on rejection, very similar histopathological changes of vascular sclerosis and tubulointerstitial fibrosis do occur secondary to chronic TCMR and chronic AMR and it can be quite difficult to distinguish between these entities. Electron microscopic features of PTC multilayering, interstitial inflammation and C4D positivity are suggestive of chronic rejection whereas striped interstitial fibrosis without inflammatory infiltrates is suggestive of chronic CNI toxicity.

Acute CNI nephrotoxicity is common is early post- transplant period and rise in creatinine due to high tacrolimus levels usually settles down within 48h-72h of dose reduction and achieving therapeutic target levels. If the creatinine levels remain high with tacrolimus dose reduction, a biopsy should be performed.

Thrombotic microangiopathy can be a manifestation of CNIs toxicity which can occur at any dose or plasma level. Treatment often is withdrawal of CNI and replacing CNI with mTOR inhibitor such as sirolimus/everolimus or maintaining on mycophenolate mofetil/prednisolone combination. Belatacept is another option in these patients to keep them CNI free. CNIs can lead to hyperkalaemia with a mild acidosis due to type IV renal tubular acidosis. Other electrolyte disturbance due to CNI toxicity include hypomagnesemia and hypophosphataemia although the latter is more often likely due to parathormone induced phosphate loss in patients with underlying secondary or tertiary hyperparathyroidism before transplantation.

Chronic allograft dysfunction attributed to CNI induced graft fibrosis can be managed by switching to mTOR inhibitors. Unfortunately, these drugs may not be well tolerated which often leads to switching back to tacrolimus but in those who tolerate these drugs, GFR tends to stabilise and improve. Usual guideline for switching is: eGFR >35 mL/min and proteinuria <1 g/day (lesser the better). Hyperlipedemia, worsening proteinuria and thrombocytopenia are potential side effects of mTOR inhibitors. These drugs should be stopped 2 weeks before any elective surgery and patient switched back to tacrolimus as wound healing can be markedly impaired if operations are done while on mTOR inhibitors.

Delayed Graft Function (DGF)

DGF refers to poor transplant kidney function in the immediate post-transplantation period and can be caused by donor events before or during retrieval that leads to ischaemic kidney injury, older donor age (and other extended criteria donor), DCD (donation after cardiac death) kidneys, warm ischaemia or trauma to blood vessels at the time of organ retrieval, prolonged cold ischaemia or perioperative hypotension. The most common definition of DGF is the need for dialysis within one week of transplantation. The management is to run tacrolimus levels slightly low, transplant kidney biopsy to exclude rejection after making sure perfusion of the kidney is fine with patent renal vein and support the patient with dialysis and optimal fluid balance while waiting for the kidney to open up.

Chronic Allograft Failure

Over a period of years, the transplant kidney function declines leading to progressive CKD and eventually graft failure requiring kidney replacement therapy. There is often combination of factors that lead to chronic inflammation and fibrosis in the transplant kidney leading to graft failure. These include, chronic allograft nephropathy (A term used to describe immunological and non-immunological causes of graft damage), chronic rejection (cAMR and cTCMR), hypertension and vascular disease with or without diabetes mellitus, recurrent glomerular disease, recurrent episodes of acute rejection, recurrent episodes of urinary tract infections with or without obstructive uropathy in transplant kidney, calcineurin inhibitor (CNI) toxicity and BKV nephropathy. It is important to focus on and optimise management of cardiovascular risk factors including appropriate management of hyperlipidaemia, hypertension and diabetes along with smoking cessation and weight management. The optimal management of these non-immunological risk factors play a vital role in long-term patient and graft survival. Chronic rejection and CNI toxicity have been discussed in previous section.

Recurrent glomerular disease is an important cause of graft dysfunction and failure. Primary focal segmental glomerulosclerosis (FSGS), mesangiocapillary, MCGN (membranoproliferative, MPGN) and IgA nephropathy are the primary glomerulonephritidis most likely to recur in transplant kidney. Other glomerular disorders such as membranous glomerulonephritis can recur in the transplant kidney but this is not a common clinical problem. ANCA positive vasculitis and anti-glomerular basement membrane (GBM) disease very rarely recur in the transplant kidney. De-novo anti-GBM disease has been reported in patients with Alport's syndrome receiving a kidney from a donor with no Alport like collagen abnormalities. De-novo glomerulonephritis has been reported but these are rare. Thrombotic microangiopathy (renal limited, systemic or both) can affect the transplant kidney in acute, subacute and chronic forms. Usually this is due to CNI toxicity (non-dose dependent), acute or chronic active AMR or combination of the two. Atypical haemolytic uraemic syndrome (aHUS) can recur in early post-transplant period resulting in systemic thrombotic microangiopathy, systemic complement abnormalities, glomerular microthrombi and graft dysfunction which can lead to rapid graft loss. The management consists of plasmapheresis and consideration of Eculizumab. Recurrent MCGN is often difficult to distinguish from chronic antibody mediated rejection (cAMR) as glomerular histological pattern can be similar in these conditions. Positive C4D staining in peritubular capillaries, peritubular capillary basement membrane multilayering on electron microscopy and positive donor-specific HLA antibodies in serum favour the diagnosis of cAMR, whereas absence of these features and systemic complement abnormalities favour the diagnosis of recurrent MCGN. Primary FSGS can recur in early post-transplant period with severe nephrotic range proteinuria and graft dysfunction or recur with a more indolent course. Management of aggressive recurrent FSGS includes plasmapheresis (usually 5 sessions) followed by Rituximab. These therapeutic measures may need repeating at regular intervals depending upon clinical response and tolerability. Recurrent IgA nephropathy is common after kidney transplantation with most of the transplant kidneys demonstrating mesangial IgA deposits 3–5 years post-transplant usually resulting in chronic allograft dysfunction but more aggressive recurrences with necrotising and crescentic glomerulonephritis is also known. Unfortunately, there is no specific treatment for this common recurrent disease in transplant kidney.

Cancer

Cancer rates are higher in transplant recipients compared to general population. This is particularly true for skin cancers and cancers driven by viral proliferation such as PTLD (EBV), Kaposi's sarcoma (human herpes virus 8, HHV8) and cervical cancer (human papilloma virus). There is a modest increased risk of other cancers such as lung and gastrointestinal cancers while there seem to be no increased risk of other common cancers such as breast and prostate malignancies.

The higher levels of immunosuppressive burden over a period of time increases the risk of cancers. The mTOR inhibitors have been associated with lower rates of cancer but higher incidence of side effects and poor tolerance have prevented their widespread use. However, in selected cases of cancers, for eg, recurrent squamous cell skin cancers, a switch to sirolimus or everolimus should be considered. The management of cancers consists of running immunosuppression as low as possible along with specific treatment for a given malignancy.

Practice Point 4

- Kidney Transplantation is the best form of long -term kidney replacement therapy in suitable recipients
- Both living and deceased donor transplants offer excellent short to medium term results with room for improvement in long term outcomes. Compared to patients remaining on dialysis, kidney transplant patients have lower mortality and better quality of life
- Recipient work-up for kidney transplantation includes surgical, immunological and non-immunological assessments to optimise outcomes and minimise complications
- Surgical complications are rare and include arterial/venous thrombosis, bleeding, ureteric leak, wound infections and lymphocele
- Medical complications include acute and chronic rejection, higher rate of typical and atypical infections and malignancies secondary to immunosuppression and post-transplant diabetes mellitus

Questions

1. A 45-year-old man with Type 2 Diabetes Mellitus, hypertension and CKD Stage G5 on maintenance haemodialysis, received a living donor kidney transplant, with his wife as a donor. The induction consisted of thymoglobulin (ATG), with maintenance immunosuppression of Tacrolimus, MMF and prednisone. Seven months post-transplant, he developed a headache and fever. On examination, there was neck stiffness. A CT brain scan showed a granulomatous lesion. Lumbar puncture revealed 70 cells/high power field, with 90% lymphocytes, glucose 50 mg/dL (blood glucose value was 100 mg/dL), protein 65 mg/dL, and increased ADA (Adenosine deaminase) (25 IU/L)

   All of the following are true except:

   A. Background history of Diabetes Mellitus and use of ATG and Tacrolimus are risk factors for development of tuberculosis in him
   B. The source of infection could be donor derived, endogenous reactivation of disease or a de-novo infection
   C. Treatment should include initiation phase of 2 months of HRZE followed by 10 months of continuation phase of HR
   D. Rifampicin based regime should be avoided in view of its interaction with tacrolimus
   E. Rifampicin based regime would be necessary, in spite of its interaction with tacrolimus

   Answer – D This patient has CNS tuberculosis. In cases of CNS tuberculosis, a prolonged maintenance phase of at least 10 months will be required, and the rifampicin should be included in the treatment regime, since a rifampicin sparing regime would not be sufficient in severe cases like this. The dose of tacrolimus will need adjustment (a higher dose will be needed), in view of the interaction with rifampicin

2. A 64-year-old man presents to the Transplant service five months after his migration from Bangladesh to London, UK. He has a history of CKD Stage 5 and hypertension. He was placed on the waiting list for a kidney transplant

   All of the following are true except:

   A. He should be screened for latent tuberculosis as he is coming from a high endemic region or given Isoniazid prophylaxis post- transplant
   B. A tuberculin skin test will be more sensitive and specific compared to interferon gamma release assay to detect latent tuberculosis in him
   C. In case of a positive test for latent tuberculosis, he should be treated for the same while he is on the waitlist
   D. The treatment course may be interrupted and continued post-transplant in case the patient receives a deceased donor kidney while on the waitlist

Answer – B An interferon gamma release assay will be more sensitive and specific in this patient than the tuberculin skin test. It will also help in differentiating anergy from a true negative test

In the UK, and in other developed parts of the world, the usual practice is to complete the treatment for TB before transplantation, especially when a Rifampicin-based regime is used to treat latent tuberculosis. In parts of the world where transplantation is highly desirable compared to keeping the patient on dialysis, option D may be used—and is therefore not the correct answer

3. A 55-year-old man, with known Type 2 Diabetes Mellitus, hypertension and ESKD. He underwent a deceased donor kidney transplant one year ago. Basiliximab was used as an induction agent, and he was on maintenance triple immunosuppression of Tacrolimus, MMF and prednisone. His blood glucose control has been poor lately. He presented with headache of 10 days' duration. On examination, he had tenderness over his bilateral maxillary sinuses. An ENT examination showed a blackish material, which on histopathological examination revealed broad non-septate hyphae, suggestive of mucormycosis

   All of the following statements are true except:

   A. IV liposomal amphotericin B should be started immediately, and MMF should be stopped
   B. Immunosuppressive medications and poorly controlled Diabetes Mellitus are important risk factors for mucormycosis
   C. Surgery has no role in the management and medical management with IV liposomal amphotericin B, followed by posaconazole gives a good cure rate
   D. Mucormycosis is an angio-invasive disease, with high rates of mortality

Answer – C Extensive debridement to remove the infected material is an important step in containing the infection. Amphotericin B and posaconazole are used to treat the infection and reduction of immunosuppression is an important component of overall management. Prognosis is poor

4. Ms. YK, a 46-year-old female presented with a history of headache and low-grade fever for one week. She had known hypertension, hypothyroidism and ESKD. She underwent an unrelated living donor kidney transplant eleven months previously; her husband was the kidney donor. Her induction regimen was thymoglobulin (ATG); her maintenance immunosuppression consisted of Tacrolimus, MMF and prednisone. On examination, she had neck stiffness. Her CT brain scan was normal. A lumbar puncture was performed, and her CSF analysis showed 42 cells, 70% lymphocytes, glucose of 50 mg/dL and protein of 98 mg/dL. CSF staining for India ink was positive, as was her cryptococcal antigen stain

   All of the following are true except:

   A. Cryptococcal infections are commoner in kidney transplant recipients and may clinically mimic tuberculosis
   B. Presentation is usually six months post-transplantation
   C. The most commonly affected organ is the lung
   D. IV liposomal amphotericin B and flucytosine are used in treatment in the induction phase, followed by fluconazole in the consolidation and maintenance phases

Answer – C The most common site of involvement in cryptococcal infection is central nervous system

5. A 55-year-old female with a functioning deceased donor kidney was seen in the kidney transplant follow-up clinic. Her serum creatinine levels increased from 90 μmol/L to 170 μmol/L between days 30 and 40 post transplantation. Her blood tacrolimus levels were high between 18 and 20 ng/mL between days 30 and 40. He had a kidney biopsy

   What are the features suggestive of tacrolimus toxicity on kidney biopsy?

   A. Glomerular mesangial expansion
   B. Lymphocytic infiltrates in the interstitium
   C. Lymphocytic infiltration into blood vessel

D. Vacuolation of tubular cells
E. Oedema in the interstitium
Answer – D

6. A 65-year-old female developed a tender swelling over the right iliac fossa lateral to the scar for her deceased donor kidney transplantation five days prior. Her serum creatinine improved from 465 μmol/L to 260 μmol/L. The collection on ultrasound which caused the swelling was drained with ultrasound guidance. The drain fluid was yellow had a creatinine of 270 μmol/L

What is the most likely cause of the swelling?
A. Haemorrhage
B. Infection
C. Lymphocele
D. Lipoma
E. Urine leak
Answer – C

7. A 45-year-old female with a functioning second deceased donor kidney transplant was seen in the kidney transplant follow-up clinic. Her serum creatinine levels had increased from 100 μmol/L to 150 μmol/L between days 20 and 25 post transplantation. Her blood tacrolimus levels were as expected, between 8 and 10 ng/mL. She had a kidney transplant biopsy. Both she and her donor were negative for CMV before transplantation

What is the most likely cause of her acute kidney injury?
A. Acute rejection
B. Acute tubular necrosis
C. Tacrolimus toxicity
D. CMV infection
E. BK virus infection
Answer – A

8. A 45-year-old female with a functioning second deceased donor kidney transplant, was seen in the kidney transplant follow-up clinic. Her serum creatinine levels increased from 100 μmol/L to 150 μmol/L between days 20 and 25 post transplantation. Her blood tacrolimus levels were as expected between 8 and 10 ng/mL. She had a kidney transplant biopsy. Both she and her donor were negative for CMV before transplantation

What is the most likely finding on the kidney biopsy?
A. Glomerular mesangial expansion
B. Lymphocytic infiltrates in the interstitium
C. Striped fibrosis of the interstitium
D. Vacuolation of tubular cells
E. Oedema in the interstitium
Answer B

9. A 43-year-old female patient with BMI of 38 kg/m^2 on peritoneal dialysis with a history of end stage kidney disease secondary to adult polycystic kidney disease received her first live donor kidney transplant from a 58-year-old genetically unrelated, ABO compatible donor. The donor kidney had a small lower polar artery, in addition to a main renal artery, which was anastomosed separately. She had an otherwise uneventful transplant surgery, with immediate allograft function on the table. She continued to have a high drain output from immediately post-operatively, which has failed to settle

What is the most important next investigation?
A. Transplant kidney ultrasound
B. Measure drain fluid creatinine
C. Drain fluid microscopy, culture and sensitivities
D. Repeat haemoglobin
E. Immediate serum urea and electrolytes measurement

Answer – B The above case is a common presentation after renal transplant. Iatrogenic missed peritoneal membrane injury or injury to a native renal cyst can confuse the common differential diagnosis of urinary leak or lymphocele. Smaller lower polar artery, if thrombosed increased the risk of distal ureteric necrosis resulting in urinary leak. High BMI is a risk factor for lymphocele. The key initial investigation here is creatinine level in drain fluid to establish diagnosis of urinary leak or lymphocele

10. A 63-years old male patient with history of end stage kidney disease secondary to diabetic nephropathy received a kidney from a 69-years old deceased donor after circulatory arrest (DCD donor). After initial period of

delayed graft function, he had good kidney allograft function. He had double J ureteric stent removal at 6 weeks, following which his creatinine started to go up with dropping urine output

What is the most likely cause?

A. Ureteric stricture
B. Acute Cellular Rejection (ACR)
C. Antibody Mediated Rejection (AMR)
D. Transplant urinary infection
E. Fluid depletion

Answer – A This is most likely to be a case of a lower ureteric stricture due to ischaemia, that has manifest after ureteric stent removal

Test your learning and check your understanding of this book's contents: use the "Springer Nature Flashcards" app to access questions using https://sn.pub/cz9Cok. To use the app, please follow the instructions in Chap. 1.

References

1. Mundy AR, Podesta ML, Bewick M, Rudge CJ, Ellis FG. The urological complications of 1000 renal transplants. Br J Urol. 1981;53(5):397–402. https://doi.org/10.1111/j.1464-410x.1981.tb03216.x.
2. Leapman SB, Vidne BA, Butt KM, Kountz SL. Elective and emergency surgery in renal transplant patients. Ann Surg. 1976;183(3):266–70. https://doi.org/10.1097/00000658-197603000-00009.
3. Ayvazoglu Soy EH, Akdur A, Kirnap M, Boyvat F, Moray G, Haberal M. Vascular complications after renal transplant: a single-center experience. Exp Clin Transplant. 2017;15(Suppl 1):79–83. https://doi.org/10.6002/ect.mesot2016.O65.
4. Eufrásio P, Parada B, Moreira P, Nunes P, Bollini S, Figueiredo A, Mota A. Surgical complications in 2000 renal transplants. Transplant Proc. 2011;43(1):142–4. https://doi.org/10.1016/j.transproceed.2010.12.009.
5. Kocak T, Nane I, Ander H, Ziylan O, Oktar T, Ozsoy C. Urological and surgical complications in 362 consecutive living related donor kidney trans- plantations. Urol Int. 2004;72:252–6.

24 An Approach to Obstetric Nephrology

Anita Banerjee, Serene Thain, and Brenda Sequeira Dmello

Clinical Scenario 1

A 32 year old woman with Type I diabetic for the past 16 years presents to the preconception clinic. She is planning her 4th pregnancy. Her serum creatinine is 122 μmol/L and her urine protein:creatinine ratio (uPCR) is 142 mg/mmol. Her HbA1c is 88mmol/mol. She is on basal bolus insulin: Novorapid and Levemir.

- ***What pre-pregnancy counselling would you offer her?***
- ***What would be the treatment target for her blood pressure in pregnancy?***
- ***How would you recognize the development of superimposed pre-eclampsia?***

Introduction

Physiological adaptations of the kidney in pregnancy are marked by significant volume expansion and vasodilation. Renal plasma flow increases up to 80% and the glomerular filtration rate increases by 50% compared with non-pregnant levels. The resulting decrease in serum creatinine levels lead to an average creatinine in pregnancy of 53 mmol/L [1, 2]. Serum creatinine levels should therefore not be interpreted in the same way as in non-pregnant women. Similarly, because of these haemodynamic changes, estimated glomerular filtration rate (eGFR) measurements, widely used in non-pregnant adults have not hitherto been validated in pregnant women.

Aside from acute kidney injury in pregnancy, women can also enter pregnancy with pre-existing chronic kidney disease (CKD). The presence of CKD increases the risk of adverse obstetric, maternal and perinatal outcomes such as preterm birth, foetal growth restriction, hypertensive disorders of pregnancy such as gestational hypertension or pre-eclampsia, and stillbirth. Pregnancy can potentially worsen pre-existing CKD, and lead to further deterioration in kidney function, that may or not recover fully back to baseline in the postpartum period.

This chapter will aim to discuss the management of CKD in pregnancy, including transplant recipients, as well as the diagnostic work-up and differentials for acute kidney injury (AKI) in pregnancy.

A. Banerjee (✉)
Women's Services, Guy's and St Thomas' Hospitals NHS Foundation Trust, London, UK
e-mail: anita.banerjee@gstt.nhs.uk

S. Thain
Department of Maternal & Fetal Medicine, KK Women's and Children's Hospital, Singapore, Singapore
e-mail: serene.thain.p.t@singhealth.com.sg

B. S. Dmello
Medical College, Aga Khan University, Dar es Salaam, United Republic of Tanzania

D. Banerjee et al. (eds.), *Management of Kidney Diseases*,
https://doi.org/10.1007/978-3-031-09131-5_24

Chronic Kidney Disease

CKD affects 0.1 to 3% of all pregnancies. The prevalence of CKD is rising, likely contributed by the changing obstetric landscape worldwide with increasing number of advanced maternal age pregnancies, increasing incidence of diabetes mellitus and obesity. Individualised pre-pregnancy counselling and optimisation for every single woman of childbearing age with CKD is an important aspect not to be forgotten.

Traditionally, many nephrologists have advised women with CKD to avoid pregnancy. However, this paternalistic approach can and should no longer hold true. All women of childbearing age should be involved in shared decision-making with health professionals regarding future planning for pregnancies. The risks of pregnancy and progression of maternal CKD need to be considered. Pre-existing hypertension, proteinuria and kidney impairment are associated with an increased risk for adverse pregnancy outcomes in women with CKD. Other factors contributing to outcomes include that of disease aetiology, severity of the disease, rate of decline outside of pregnancy and previous obstetric history. An additional factor associated with adverse pregnancy outcomes independent of kidney disease is that of superimposed pre-eclampsia (PET). The responsibility of the healthcare professional is to facilitate an autonomous and informed decision-making process.

With regard to the optimal timing for conception, the aim would be to strive for quiescence and stability of kidney disease before trying to conceive. Entering a pregnancy with kidney disease that has been *quiescent for six months* prior to conception has been shown to improve outcomes. For women with mild CKD, the risk of significant loss of kidney function at the end of pregnancy is possible, though not likely. For those with more advanced CKD however, the potential for loss of kidney function must not underestimated, and women should be counselled appropriately, and implications discussed before embarking on pregnancy.

The common causes of CKD in women of childbearing age are described in Table 24.1,

Table 24.1 Risks of various causes of chronic kidney disease on pregnancy and pregnancy-specific aims and targets

Type of kidney disease	Pregnancy-specific aims and targets	CKD-specific obstetric risks
Adult polycystic kidney disease (APKD)	• Intensify targets for blood pressure control	• Pre-existing hypertension is a risk factor for adverse pregnancy outcomes, others include • Infection (pyelonephritis) • Kidney calculi • Kidney cyst complications (rupture, haemorrhage)
IgA nephropathy (IgAN)	• Intensify targets for blood pressure control	• Pre-existing hypertension is a risk factor for adverse pregnancy outcomes • Presence of >1 g of protein a day is associated with an increased risk of loss of residual function, independent of pregnancy
Diabetic nephropathy (DN)	• Intensify targets for blood pressure control and glucose pre-pregnancy and throughout pregnancy • Individualise when to stop renin-angiotensin-aldosterone system (RAAS) blockade pre-pregnancy or at time of positive pregnancy test with appropriate switch in medications if required	• Pre-existing hypertension is a risk factor for adverse pregnancy outcomes • Risk of acceleration of kidney disease • Diabetes mellitus is a risk factor for adverse pregnancy outcomes such as birth defects, pre-eclampsia, growth restriction, foetal macrosomia, stillbirth (risk correlated with glycemic control) • Proteinuria increases the risk for venous thromboembolism
Lupus nephritis (LN)	• Anti Ro and La antibodies (if present) can cross the placenta and confer a 2% risk of congenital heart block (CHB) and 5% risk of neonatal cutaneous lupus	• Pregnancy can trigger a relapse • Increased risk for adverse pregnancy outcomes • Proteinuria (if present) increases the risk for venous thromboembolism

along with targets to be achieved and specifics pertaining to each condition.

Preparation for Pregnancy

Pre-pregnancy counselling is essential, and each consultation with a woman with CKD is an excellent opportunity to optimise and prepare for a future pregnancy. Lifestyle modifications include smoking cessation, weight management and regular exercise. The importance of achieving disease stability and conversion of potentially teratogenic medications to pregnancy favourable medications should be discussed at the preconception visit in conjunction with the relevant specialists, with clinical decisions individualised based on the factors such as the underlying kidney condition, degree of kidney impairment or proteinuria and the likelihood of continued quiescent disease with change in medications.

Important preconception supplements include at least 400 μg of folic acid, or high dose 5 mg folic acid for women with diabetes, as well as vitamin D supplementation. Folic acid should ideally be initiated 3 months prior to conception. Anaemia is a common complication in CKD patients and this should be addressed and optimised prior to pregnancy. The importance of optimisation of blood pressure control prior to conception should also be reiterated.

For genetic kidney conditions such as adult polycystic kidney disease (APKD) or Alport syndrome, women should be counselled on the risk of inheritance for their offspring. Timely genetic work-up if not previously performed and genetic counselling is key. Consideration for preimplantation genetic testing (PGT) for some genetic conditions may be possible, although access to PGT may be limited depending on location, and the indications for PGT and policies policing it also vary widely in different parts of the world.

Table 24.2 summarises the common drugs used in pregnancy for women with CKD.

Clinical Scenario 1

A 32 year old woman with Type I diabetic for the past 16 years presents to the preconception clinic. She is planning her 4th pregnancy. Her creatinine is 122 μmol/L and her urine protein:creatinine ratio (uPCR) is 142 mg/mmol. Her HbA1c is 88mmol/mol. She is on basal bolus insulin: Novorapid and Levemir.

Table 24.2 Safety profile of medications for kidney disease during pregnancy and breastfeeding

Medication	Pregnancy	Breastfeeding
Azathioprine	Safe	Compatible
Steroids	Safe but increased risks of gestational diabetes, hypertensive disorders of pregnancy, infection, preterm delivery	Compatible
MMF	Teratogenic. Avoid in pregnancy and stop at least 6 weeks before a planned pregnancy.	Avoid
Calcineurin inhibitors (CNI) e.g. tacrolimus, cyclosporin	Safe but increased risks of gestational diabetes and hypertensive disorders of pregnancy	Compatible
Cyclophosphamide	Teratogenic, Avoid in pregnancy. Can be considered for use in the 2nd and 3rd trimester if required as no adverse effects have been observed in observational studies.	Limited data
Rituximab	Stop 6 months prior to conception. Although limited evidence has not shown it to be teratogenic, 2nd and 3rd trimester exposure is associated with neonatal B cell depletion.	Limited data
Biologics e.g. eculizumab	Safe	Compatible
Hydroxychloroquine	Safe	Compatible

- ***What pre-pregnancy counselling would you offer her?***
  - *Advise her regarding the increased risk of deterioration of her kidney disease with any future pregnancies and the implications of this*
  - *Counsel her on the importance of achieving optimal blood glucose and blood pressure control prior to conception*
  - *Advise her to continue effective contraception until her glycaemic control has improved as the risk of congenital anomaly increases with increasing HbA1c level.*
  - *Advise her to remain on Ramipril 2.5 mg until she has a positive pregnancy test*
  - *Commence 5 mg folic acid three months prior to conception to reduce the risk of congenital anomaly*

Antenatal Care

An early review by the multidisciplinary team (MDT) comprising nephrologists, maternal foetal medicine specialists, obstetric physicians and midwives is important for timely individualisation of care and surveillance.

Women with CKD are at higher risk of developing pre-eclampsia (PET). There is strong evidence that low dose aspirin 75–150 mg taken from 12 to 36 weeks of pregnancy reduces the risk of PET. A recent randomised clinical trial found a 62% reduction in preterm PET in women taking aspirin 150 mg nocte from 11–14 weeks to 36 weeks of gestation as compared with placebo [3]. In addition, women with significant baseline proteinuria of >100–150 mg/mmol should be risk stratified for venous thromboembolism, with consideration to initiating low molecular weight heparin (LMWH) prophylaxis during pregnancy and up to 6 weeks postpartum.

With regard to foetal surveillance for pregnancies complicated by CKD, women with CKD exposed to teratogenic drugs in the first trimester should be referred to a specialist foetal medicine unit, with appropriate detailed anomaly scan done to assess for foetal defects. Pregnancies complicated by CKD should also have serial growth scans in the third trimester for monitoring of foetal well-being.

With regard to maternal surveillance for pregnancies complicated by CKD, monthly kidney function tests and urine protein:creatinine ratio (uPCR) measurement is recommended. Increasing the frequency of monitoring in the third trimester can be considered, especially if there is a suspicion of superimposed PET or progression of kidney disease, so that decisions regarding timing of delivery can be made whilst balancing maternal and foetal health. It is also important to continue treatment of maternal anaemia and optimising the haemoglobin throughout pregnancy, and especially around the time of delivery for maternal and foetal benefits.

Management of Hypertension in the Preconception, Antenatal and Postnatal Period

The recommended first-line choice of antihypertensives drugs in pregnancy include labetalol and nifedipine. Methyldopa, which had traditionally been used widely in pregnancy in the past, is less commonly used now because of its association with antenatal and postnatal depression. Angiotensin-converting enzyme inhibitors (ACE-I) and angiotensin II receptor blockers (ARBs) used in renin-angiotension-aldosterone system (RAAS) blockade are contraindicated in pregnancy, except in the rare event of a scleroderma renal crisis (Table 24.3). For women with diabetic nephropathy, the timing of discontinuation of RAAS blockade, e.g. either during the preconception period or at time of a positive urine pregnancy test, should be individualised based on the severity of proteinuria or kidney function impairment. In making these decisions, it is important also to understand that women with CKD may experience reduced fecundity and may require a longer time to conceive.

Table 24.3 Common anti-hypertensive medications used during pregnancy and breastfeeding

Class of drug	Risk of Teratogenicity	Breast Feeding	Anti-hypertensive medication used in hypertensive emergencies
Calcium channel blockers e.g. nifedipine MR, amlodipine	None	Limited data No adverse effects reported with amlodipine	Nifedipine MR oral *(Risk of headaches)*
Β-blockers e.g. bisoprolol α/β blockers e.g. labetalol	None	Limited data-widely used Compatible	Labetalol infusion *(Risk of nausea and dizziness)*
Central α-adrenergic e.g. Methyldopa	None	Compatible	
α-adrenergic blockers e.g. doxazosin, prazosin	None	Not recommended for routine use in pregnancy unless no alternatives available	
Peripheral arterial vasodilator e.g. hydralazine	None	Compatible	Hydralazine infusion *(Risk of maternal tachycardia & hypotension)*
ACE-inhibitors e.g. enalapril, captopril	Yes Lowest incidence of birth defects with exposure in the 1st trimester Risk of foetal anomalies in the 2nd and 3rd trimester e.g. foetal kidney damage	Compatible	

With regard to blood pressure targets used in pregnancy, the Control of Hypertension in Pregnancy Study (CHIPS) trial published in 2015 demonstrated that targeting a tighter diastolic blood pressure of <85 mmHg had benefits of a reduced likelihood of developing accelerated maternal hypertension, without increasing the risks of adverse foetal outcomes as compared to less tight (100 mmHg) control [4]. Although the CHIPS trial did not include women with proteinuria, there is increasing expert consensus that hypertension in pregnant women with CKD should be treated to a target blood pressure of <130/80 mmHg [5].

Clinical Scenario 1

A 32 year old woman with Type I diabetic for the past 16 years presents to the preconception clinic. She is planning her 4th pregnancy. Her creatinine is 122 µmol/L and her urine protein:creatinine ratio (uPCR) is 142 mg/mmol. Her HbA1c is 88mmol/mol. She is on basal bolus insulin: Novorapid and Levemir.

- ***What would be the treatment target for her blood pressure in pregnancy?***
  – *There is increasing expert consensus that hypertension in pregnant women with CKD should be treated, with a target average blood pressure of <130/80 mmHg* [5]. *In addition, the results of the CHIPS trial found that targeting a tighter diastolic blood pressure of <85 mmHg was associated with a reduced likelihood of developing accelerated maternal hypertension and its risks, without increasing the risks of adverse foetal outcomes as compared to less tight (100 mmHg) control* [4]. *The results of the CHIPS trial may not be entirely reproducible in women with CKD as this study did not include women with proteinuria.*

Diagnosing Pre-Eclampsia in the Context of Pre-Existing Kidney Disease

The traditional definition of pre-eclampsia is that of new onset of hypertension and proteinuria after the 20th gestational week. It can therefore be very challenging to make a diagnosis of pre-eclampsia in women with pre-existing hypertension, kidney impairment, proteinuria—a combination that is frequently seen in women with CKD. An important point to note is that newer definitions of pre-eclampsia, such as that from the International Society of the Study of Hypertension in Pregnancy (ISSHP) recognise that even in the absence of proteinuria, if there is new onset hypertension associated with either systemic effects in the form of biochemical derangements (e.g. deranged liver function tests, raised serum creatinine levels) or evidence of placental insufficiency (e.g. foetal growth restriction), a diagnosis of pre-eclampsia can be made. This is further illustrated in the later part of the chapter, discussing pre-eclampsia. Other biochemical markers and foetal growth should therefore come into the picture when establishing a diagnosis of pre-eclampsia in women with CKD.

A clinical practice guideline on pregnancy and kidney disease published by The UK Kidney Association has made recommendations to help with the above clinical conundrum [6]. This guideline recommends that a diagnosis of superimposed pre-eclampsia be considered:

- In a woman with non-proteinuric CKD, if she develops new hypertension (systolic BP >140 mmHg and/or diastolic BP >90 mmHg) and proteinuria (uPCR >30 mg/mmol or uACR >8 mg/mmol) or maternal organ dysfunction after 20 weeks' gestation.
- In a woman with proteinuric CKD if she develops new hypertension (systolic BP >140 mmHg and/or diastolic BP >90 mmHg) or maternal organ dysfunction after 20 weeks' gestation.
- In a woman with chronic hypertension and proteinuria, if she develops maternal organ dysfunction after 20 weeks' gestation.

As for women with chronic hypertension and proteinuria, the guideline recommends that the development of sustained severe hypertension (systolic BP >160 mmHg and/or diastolic BP >110 mmHg or doubling of antihypertensive agents) and/or a substantial rise in proteinuria (doubling of uPCR or uACR compared to early pregnancy) should prompt clinical assessment for superimposed pre-eclampsia.

The guidelines also make mention of the role of angiogenic markers, namely placental growth factor (PlGF) and soluble fms-like tyrosine kinase-1 (sFlt-1), as adjuncts to diagnose superimposed pre-eclampsia. This is further elaborated in the section on pre-eclampsia later in this chapter.

Clinical Scenario 1

A 32 year old woman with Type I diabetic for the past 16 years presents to the preconception clinic. She is planning her 4th pregnancy. Her creatinine is 122 μmol/L and her urine protein:creatinine ratio (uPCR) is 142 mg/mmol. Her HbA1c is 88mmol/mol. She is on basal bolus insulin: Novorapid and Levemir.

- ***How would you recognize the development of superimposed pre-eclampsia?***
  - *Regular blood pressure monitoring with attention to the development of any new onset hypertension (systolic blood pressure >130 mmHg and/or diastolic BP >80 mmHg), monitoring for maternal organ dysfunction in the form of biochemical parameters and symptoms, and surveillance of foetal growth are crucial steps to making a diagnosis of superimposed pre-eclampsia. In this particular case, where the mother has significant pre-existing proteinuria, a diagnosis of superimposed pre-eclampsia should be considered if she develops new onset hypertension or any evidence of maternal organ dysfunction or uteroplacental dysfunction after 20 weeks' gestation. The diagnosis of superimposed pre-eclampsia should also be considered if there is a substantial rise in proteinuria e.g. doubling of uPCR com-*

pared to early pregnancy values. Adjuncts such as the use of placental growth factor (PlGF) can also be useful in ruling out superimposed pre-eclampsia in the correct clinical context.

Dialysis and Pregnancy

The indications for kidney replacement therapy (KRT) in pregnancy are similar to those in the non-pregnant population and include metabolic acidosis, hyperkalemia, and fluid overload refractory to medical treatment. However, in addition to that in the context of pregnancy would be raised urea levels (> 17mmol/L) despite medical management as significant urea levels can lead to foetal diuresis and polyhydramnios and foeto-toxicity.

Pregnancy rates in women on peritoneal dialysis (PD) are lower than on those on haemodialysis.

Studies have shown increased dialysis frequency e.g. daily haemodialysis are associated with lower rates of preterm delivery and low birthweight babies. There is a paucity of data for the precise duration of dialysis needed to optimize outcomes. Women who initiate dialysis during pregnancy have improved outcomes compared with those who conceive on dialysis. In general, the current expert consensus is that dialysis should be initiated when maternal urea reaches levels of 17–20 mmol/L [6].

Erythropoietin stimulating agents (ESAs) are safe for use in pregnancy, and can be an important adjunct in maintaining optimal haemoglobin levels, which is important for mother and foetus.

Kidney Transplantation and Pregnancy

More women are now successfully achieving conception after kidney transplantation, particularly over the past two decades, due to advances in treatments and surgery, as well as better access to transplant centres. The management of pregnancy in kidney transplant recipients remains challenging, although the risks with pregnancy are greater in women with very advanced CKD compared with women with a kidney transplant. In helping to decide on suitability for conception, a detailed review of allograft function, stability of serum creatinine post-transplant and immunosuppressant medications is required. Stability for at least one year prior to conception after a transplant is advised. The risk of deterioration in kidney function should be discussed in the preconception period, and women on teratogenic medications such as mycophenolate mofetil (MMF) should be switched to alternative medications that are more compatible with pregnancy. The recommended maintenance immunosuppression drugs for pregnant women are calcineurin inhibitors (CNIs) (e.g. tacrolimus, cyclosporine), azathioprine, and prednisolone. Risk factors associated with an increased risk of adverse pregnancy outcomes include pre-existing hypertension, a serum creatinine level of more than 124 μmol/L, history of more than 2 kidney transplants, as well as proteinuria.

Women with a kidney transplant should book for their antenatal care at the earliest possible opportunity, once pregnancy is confirmed. Close attention to kidney function and monitoring of immunosuppressant trough levels of tacrolimus or cyclosporine throughout pregnancy is important: women may require higher doses of cyclosporine and tacrolimus during pregnancy. Post-delivery, the levels of tacrolimus and cyclosporine should continue to be monitored, as dose reductions will likely be required if the dose had been increased in pregnancy. Regular review of blood pressure and proteinuria is advised so that deterioration in kidney function or superimposed PET can be identified.

In addition, women on steroids or calcineurin inhibitors have a higher risk of developing gestational diabetes mellitus (GDM). It is important to screen for GDM with an oral glucose tolerance test and optimise the blood sugar profile if GDM is diagnosed.

Contraception in Women with CKD

All healthcare professionals should have a clear understanding of options for contraception in women with CKD. Decision-making on appropriate contraception needs to be individualised based on risks, acceptability to the patient and likelihood of compliance. In general, oestrogen-containing contraceptive methods (e.g. combined oral contraceptive pills, contraceptive patch) should be avoided because of its association with increased blood pressure, as well as increased risks for thrombotic or vascular events. Progestogen-only contraception [e.g. progestogen-only pill, intramuscular Depo-Provera® contraceptive injection, intrauterine system (Mirena®), implant (Nexplanon®)] are favoured for women with CKD as they are safe and effective. Barrier methods are acceptable options as well, although its effectiveness and reliability with typical use is much lower compared to other forms of contraception. Sterilisation (female and male) is effective but irreversible, and can be considered if the couple has completed their family or is certain that future conception is not desired.

Acute Kidney Injury (AKI) in Pregnancy

Clinical Scenario 2

A 29 year old primiparous woman presents at 24 weeks' gestation feeling unwell with a blood pressure of 180/95 mmHg. Her serum creatinine level is 222 μmol/L, and her platelet count is 22×10^9/L.

- ***What are your differential diagnoses?***
- ***What focused investigations would you consider performing?***
- ***How would you manage her?***

The current international consensus definitions for acute kidney injury (AKI) in the general population have not been validated for pregnancy. It has been suggested that a new creatinine level of > 77umol/L should be the diagnostic threshold for kidney injury in pregnancy [7]. AKI is associated with increased morbidity and mortality for both the mother and foetus regardless of the underlying cause which can be either pregnancy specific (e.g. pre-eclampsia, acute fatty liver of pregnancy) or non-pregnancy specific (e.g. sepsis, hypovolemia). The causes of AKI in pregnancy can be divided into three groups as listed in Table 24.4: pre-renal, renal and post-renal or obstructive causes. These aetiologies may be overlapping and therefore AKI in pregnancy is a heterogeneous syndrome, defined as occurring during pregnancy, labour and the postpartum period

There are usually multiple co-existing factors for the development of AKI in pregnancy, with pregnancy-specific complications such as PET, postpartum haemorrhage and sepsis. High vigilance is required.

Clinical Scenario 2
A 29 year old primiparous woman presents at 24 weeks' gestation feeling unwell with a blood pressure of 180/95 mmHg. Her serum creatinine level is 222 μmol/L, and her platelet count is 22×10^9/L.

Table 24.4 Causes of acute kidney injury in pregnancy and the postpartum period

Pre-renal	• Sepsis e.g. pyelonephritis, chorioamnionitis, septic abortion • Dehydration e.g. hyperemesis gravidarum • Hypovolemia e.g. antepartum or postpartum haemorrhage
Renal	• Drug-related causes e.g. non-steroidal anti-inflammatory drug (NSAID)-induced AKI • Pre-eclampsia • Haemolysis, elevated liver enzymes, low platelets (HELLP) syndrome • Acute Fatty Liver of Pregnancy (AFLP) • Atypical Haemolytic Uraemic Syndrome (aHUS) • Thrombotic Thrombocytopenic Purpura (TTP) • New onset glomerulonephritis
Post-renal	• Obstruction • Ureteric injury (intra-operatively during caesarean delivery) • Neuropathic bladder with retention

- ***What are your differential diagnoses?***
  - Pre-eclampsia
  - Haemolysis, elevated liver enzymes, low platelets (HELLP) syndrome
  - Atypical Haemolytic Uraemic Syndrome (aHUS)
  - Thrombotic Thrombocytopenic Purpura (TTP)
  - New onset glomerulonephritis

Investigations for AKI in pregnancy should be performed in a timely and focused manner. Table 24.5 discusses the common investigations performed as part of the diagnostic workup for AKI in pregnancy.

Clinical Scenario 2

A 29 year old primiparous woman presents at 24 weeks' gestation feeling unwell with a blood

Table 24.5 Investigations for AKI in pregnancy

Type of test	Specific test	Rationale for test	Pregnancy specific changes
Blood	Full blood count (FBC)	• To look for anaemia that may be a result of chronic kidney disease or acute causes such as blood loss or haemolysis	• Expansion in plasma volume leads to a fall in haemoglobin levels. (Hb of 100–110 g/L considered normal for pregnancy) • Platelet count tends to fall progressively during normal pregnancy, hence significant thrombocytopenia is considered if the platelet count is less than 100×10^9/L
	Urea, creatinine, electrolytes	• To assess the degree of severity of the kidney function and determine the need for dialysis • To assess for electrolyte abnormalities associated with AKI and correct as necessary	• Serum creatinine levels decrease in pregnancy. If this is not observed, it could potentially be a red flag as there is an absence of normal renal physiological adaptation
	Liver function test (LFT)	• Presence of transaminitis may point towards HELLP syndrome or acute fatty liver of pregnancy (AFLP)	• Pregnancy ranges for transaminases ALT and AST are largely similar to non-pregnant individuals
	Lactate dehydrogenase (LDH)	• To assess for the presence of haemolysis	• Reference ranges does not change in pregnancy
	Peripheral blood film	• To assess for signs of microangiopathic haemolytic anaemia (MAHA)	• No pregnancy related changes in pregnancy
	Clotting studies	• Can be deranged in severe pre-eclampsia, HELLP syndrome, acute fatty liver of pregnancy (AFLP) and disseminated intravascular coagulation (DIC)	• Levels of factors VIII, IX and X are increased • Fibrinogen levels are increased • Antithrombin, protein S & protein C levels decrease
	ADAMTS-13* activity	• Significantly low levels of ADAMTS-13 activity (<10%) can be diagnostic for thrombotic thrombocytopenic purpura (TTP)	• This is slightly reduced in pregnancy
Urine	Protein measurement (urine protein:creatinine ratio (uPCR))	• To assess for the presence of proteinuria which can be associated with pre-eclampsia especially if new onset • If detected, quantifying the proteinuria may be useful in guiding decisions regarding thromboprophylaxis	• uPCR ≥50 mg/mmol can be suggestive of PET if there had been no proteinuria prior to conception

(continued)

Table 24.5 (continued)

Type of test	Specific test	Rationale for test	Pregnancy specific changes
	Urine microscopy and culture	• To look for urinary tract sepsis	• Urinary stasis in the dilated collecting system • predisposes pregnant women with asymptomatic bacteriuria and can lead to pyelonephritis. • All asymptomatic bacteriuria should be treated
	Urine phase contrast microscopy	• The presence of abnormal urinary sediment such as red blood cell casts may indicate an underlying kidney pathology	• Reference ranges does not change in pregnancy
Imaging	Ultrasound kidneys MRI CT KUB	• Exclude obstruction as a cause for AKI • Bilateral small kidneys may be indicative of underlying CKD • MRI (non-contrast) and CT imaging modalities are safe in pregnancy and during lactation. CT contrast may exacerbate existing AKI, hence the benefits versus risks of performing the test should be individualised	• Increased renal blood flow leads to an increase in renal size of 1–1.5 cm • Commonly, right-sided pelvicalyceal prominence due to the anatomical circumstances of the right ureter crossing the iliac and ovarian vessels at an angle before entering the pelvis
Histology	Kidney biopsy	• Rarely required for diagnostic workup of AKI in pregnancy • Reserved for severe pregnancy-related AKI or nephrotic syndrome warranting a definitive diagnosis with established therapy or when prolongation of pregnancy is a priority e.g. in the 1st or 2nd trimester • Risks of kidney biopsy in the form of bleeding risk are higher in pregnancy (7%) compared to outside of pregnancy (1%) [8].	

pressure of 180/95 mmHg. Her serum creatinine level is 222 μmol/L, and her platelet count is 22×10^9/L.

• ***What focused investigations would you consider performing?***

Urgent

– Full blood count, renal profile, liver profile, clotting profile
– Urine protein:creatinine ratio (uPCR)
– Peripheral blood film
– ADAMTS-13* activity

Specific Conditions and Their Management

Pre-eclampsia

Pre-eclampsia is a multisystem disorder that complicates 3–8% of pregnancies and constitutes a major source of morbidity and mortality worldwide. In Latin America and the West Indies, hypertensive disorders contribute to almost 26% of maternal deaths. In Africa and Asia they contribute to 9% of all maternal deaths. Traditionally, pre-eclampsia is defined as new-onset hypertension developing after 20 weeks of gestation in the presence of proteinuria. Newer definitions in recent years have recognised that even in the absence of proteinuria, new-onset hypertension associated with other maternal organ dysfunction or uteroplacental dysfunction would similarly qualify as a diagnosis of pre-eclampsia. The revised International Society for the Study of Hypertension in Pregnancy (ISSHP) definition of pre-eclampsia is reflected in Table 24.6 [9].

Placental growth factor (PLGF) based testing can be used as a diagnostic adjunct and a confirmatory test in women with suspected PET. The PELICAN Study demonstrated that the negative predictive value of PlGF using a cut-off value of more than 100 picograms/mL in women presenting with suspected pre-eclampsia between 20 weeks and 34 weeks plus 6 days of gestation was 98% [10].

Pre-eclampsia leads to AKI in around 1.5–2% of cases [11]. The presence or absence of AKI in pre-eclampsia can be used as a marker of severity which may affect obstetric decisions such as timing of delivery.

The principles of management of pre-eclampsia are:

(a) Control of blood pressure
(b) Prevention of convulsions (eclampsia)
(c) Fluid management
(d) Timely delivery

Table 24.6 The revised ISSHP Definition of Pre-eclampsia [9]

Hypertension developing after 20 weeks' gestation and the coexistence of one or more of the following new onset conditions:
1. Proteinuria
2. Other maternal organ dysfunction
(a) Kidney insufficiency (creatinine > 90 μmol/L)
(b) Liver involvement (elevated transaminases and/or severe right upper quadrant or epigastric pain)
(c) Neurological complications (e.g. eclampsia, altered mental state, blindness, stroke or more commonly hyperreflexia when accompanied by clonus, severe headaches when accompanied by hyperreflexia, persistent visual scotoma
(d) Haematological complications (thrombocytopenia, disseminated intravascular coagulopathy (DIC), haemolysis)
3. Uteroplacental dysfunction
(a) Foetal growth restriction

(a) Control of blood pressure

A blood pressure reading of 160/110 mmHg is an obstetric emergency. The goal of treatment is to aim for a systolic blood pressure of <140 mmHg to reduce the risk of intracerebral haemorrhage. Commonly used anti-hypertensive agents for the control of blood pressure at this time include oral nifedipine MR and intravenous labetalol and hydralazine. Common side-effects with intravenous labetalol include nausea and dizziness. With hydralazine, common side effects include maternal tachycardia and hypotension which can be reduced by adequate hydration prior to administration.

(b) Prevention of convulsions (eclampsia)

Magnesium sulphate is recommended for the prevention of eclampsia in women with severe pre-eclampsia and is the drug of choice for neuroprotection for the foetus before 32 weeks of gestation. This is administered as a loading dose of 4 g IV over 5–15 mins followed by a maintenance dose of 1 g/h by continuous infusion for 24 h or until 24 h after delivery or last convulsion, whichever is later. In cases with underlying kidney impairment, administering the same bolus dose of magnesium sulphate and then halving the maintenance dose to 0.5 g/h with regular surveillance of serum magnesium levels would be the recommended approach. Further dose adjustments may be required to avoid maternal toxicity, and in cases of anuria, may require cessation entirely.

(c) Fluid management

Endothelial damage as a result of pre-eclampsia can also lead to pathologic capillary leak that can present in the mother as oedema, rapid weight gain, haemoconcentration and pulmonary oedema. Oliguria may be observed in pre-eclampsia because of intrinsic kidney disease (including acute tubular necrosis), and may not respond to plasma volume expansion. Excessive intravenous hydration in women with pre-eclampsia can potentially lead to complications such as pulmonary oedema. It is recommended for women with pre-eclampsia to avoid aggressive fluid resuscitation, with fluid restriction of 85–100 mL/h recommended in the peripartum period. Regular review and judicious assessment and management of fluid status is paramount.

(d) Timely Delivery

Delivery leads to eventual resolution of the disease progression for pre-eclampsia. Decisions regarding timing of delivery in pre-eclampsia requires consideration of the potential neonatal risks of prematurity versus maternal risks for severe morbidity or mortality in continuing the pregnancy. Shared decision-making using a multidisciplinary approach is required.

Women with pre-eclampsia should be followed up closely in the postpartum period, and assessment for resolution of proteinuria and normalization of blood pressure should be performed. Complete resolution of the effects of pre-eclampsia can take up to 12 weeks post-delivery. In cases of persistent proteinuria, consideration for referral to a Nephrologist for further diagnostic workup should be made. It is important to know that even in individuals who have completely recovered from pre-eclampsia, they go on to have a higher risk for hypertensive and cardiovascular disorders, not just in future pregnancies, but also in later life outside of pregnancy. In addition, pre-eclampsia, particularly early pre-term pre-eclampsia, has been found to be strongly associated with several chronic kidney disorders later in life [12]. Women with pregnancies complicated by pre-eclampsia should be counselled on the risk of recurrence of hypertensive disorders of pregnancy in future pregnancies, and advised about lifelong regular blood pressure surveillance.

HELLP Syndrome

HELLP syndrome is a complication of pregnancy characterised by haemolysis, elevated liver enzymes and low platelets, and is typically associated with severe pre-eclampsia. It occurs in 0.5–0.9% of all pregnancies and 10–20% of severe pre-eclampsia, and may not always present as full blown HELLP syndrome with all features, but can present as an incomplete HELLP syndrome with only some of the features. The majority of patients with HELLP syndrome will present with hypertension and proteinuria, but the condition may also occur without these symptoms and manifest only later on.

The incidence of kidney impairment is higher in HELLP syndrome than in pre-eclampsia, with AKI complicating 3–15% of cases. The risk of AKI increases if complications associated with HELLP occur, such as abruption, disseminated intravascular coagulation (DIC), haemorrhage, intrauterine death or sepsis, and AKI in the context of HELLP syndrome worsens prognosis.

Laboratory abnormalities of HELLP syndrome typically worsen after delivery and peak at 24-48 hours postpartum. Haematological and biochemical abnormalities should be expected to gradually return to pre-pregnancy values thereafter. If these laboratory abnormalities do not recover after delivery, and if AKI and thrombocytopenia dominate the clinical picture, then consideration for alternative diagnoses of thrombotic microangiopathies such as thrombotic thrombocytopenic purpura (TTP) and atypical haemolytic uremic syndrome (aHUS) should be considered.

The management of HELLP syndrome is largely supportive, and mirrors that of pre-eclampsia. Delivery is the definitive management for this condition. In general, if the pregnancy is less than 34 weeks' gestation, provided that maternal and foetal condition remains stable, delivery can be performed after completion of steroids for foetal pulmonary maturation. For pregnancies beyond 34 weeks of gestation, women with HELLP syndrome should generally be delivered soon after maternal stabilisation.

Thrombotic Microangiopathies (TMAs)

Thrombotic thrombocytopenic purpura (TTP) and atypical haemolytic uremic syndrome (aHUS) are thrombotic microangiopathies that may both masquerade as and co-exist with pre-eclampsia in pregnancy. Although these three conditions have similar clinical features, they are in actual fact very distinct entities. with distinct etiologies, pathogenesis and treatment, which lends point to the importance of being able to distinguish between them. Although TTP and aHUS are not commonly seen conditions, each with an incidence of only 1 in 25,000 pregnancies, both can potentially lead to significant maternal and foetal morbidity, and even mortality. It is therefore important to have a high index of suspicion for these conditions in the correct clinical context, so that early recognition and treatment can be achieved.

Thrombotic Thrombocytopaenic Purpura (TTP)

TTP is typically characterised by the pentad of fever, microangiopathic anaemia, thrombocytopenia, kidney failure and neurologic findings. However, not all individuals with TTP will have the full pentad—only 40% may present with all 5 clinical manifestations. The median age of presentation with acute TTP is in the 3rd to 4th decade of life, typically affecting women. TTP in pregnancy can be acquired (90%) or may manifest as an initial, delayed presentation of congenital TTP disease (10%). Severe ADAMTS-13 deficiency is defined as less than 10% of normal activity, with this having an approximately 90% sensitivity and specificity for the diagnosis of TTP. Pregnancy can trigger the onset of TTP, as von Willebrand factor increases with gestation, whilst ADAMTS-13 activity reduces in the 2nd and 3rd trimester of pregnancy. The mainstay of treatment for TTP is plasma exchange, which may allow for prolongation of pregnancy if time required for foetal maturation is desired. Recognition of the diagnosis, together with active monitoring and management during pregnancy results in positive pregnancy outcomes [13].

The risk of recurrence of TTP in future pregnancies is 92% for women with congenital TTP, 47% for women with acquired idiopathic TTP, and 45% for acquired pregnancy-associated TTP [14]. Women with a previous history of TTP should undergo appropriate pre-pregnancy counselling by a multidisciplinary team. They should be monitored closely for development of TTP in their next pregnancies. With regard to the management of women who had previous pregnancies complicated by TTP, regular 2-weekly plasma exchange, starting from the 1st trimester of pregnancy, with a view to increasing the frequency from the late 2nd trimester to 3rd trimester as guided by FBC and LDH levels, can be a suitable approach.

Atypical Haemolytic Uraemic Syndrome (aHUS)

Atypical HUS is a type of TMA characterized by intravascular haemolysis, thrombocytopenia, and acute kidney failure, with the underlying pathophysiology being that of uncontrolled complement activation. Although the majority (80%) of women with aHUS are diagnosed in the postpartum period, with potential triggers being infection or postpartum haemorrhage, it can present in any gestation of pregnancy as well, even as early as the 1st trimester. The treatment of aHUS is largely supportive, comprising of red cell transfusion, blood pressure control, and dialysis (if required). Specific treatment for aHUS includes the use of eculizumab, a humanized IgG monoclonal therapy that is a potent inhibitor of C5 cleavage, and aids in overall complement inhibition. Safety data for use of eculizumab in pregnancy is extrapolated from its use in treatment of paroxysmal nocturnal haemoglobinuria (PNH) in pregnancy, where foetal mortality and miscarriage rates have been demonstrated to being comparable or better than untreated pregnant women with PNH [15].

Postpartum Haemorrhage (PPH)

Postpartum PPH can be divided into primary and secondary PPH, with the former referring to PPH

Table 24.7 Definition of Postpartum Haemorrhage (PPH)

Primary PPH	Bleeding per vagina > 500mL within 24 h of delivery
Secondary PPH	Bleeding per vagina >500 mL more than 24 hours but less than 6 weeks after delivery
Minor PPH	Loss of 500–1000 mL of blood from the genital tract after the birth of a baby
Major PPH	Loss of >1000 mL of blood from the genital tract after the birth of a baby
Massive PPH	Postpartum blood loss >2000 mL or lesser amounts resulting in changes in haemodynamic parameters which lead to moderate or severe hypovolemic shock

occurring within the first 24 h of delivery, and the latter referring to PPH at any time point after the first 24 h up to 6 weeks after delivery. Table 24.7 lists the various definition and severity classification of PPH. It is important to remember that individuals with pre-existing anaemia (e.g. those with anaemia secondary to CKD) have a lower tolerance to blood loss in general.

The common causes of postpartum haemorrhage can be divided into the 4Ts:

- **T**one—uterine atony is the most common cause of PPH
- **T**rauma—tears in vagina, cervix, vulva
- **T**issue—retained placental tissue
- **T**hrombin—DIC/HELLP/coagulation disorders

Healthcare providers have a tendency to underestimate blood loss and efforts at visual quantification does help standardize the amount of blood loss, especially in low resource settings [16]. It is also important to recognise how differences in maternal weight with its corresponding estimated total blood volume can contribute to varying severity and impact on the individual. Table 24.8 demonstrates this.

Management of PPH requires early diagnosis, a team approach to simultaneously minimise or arrest the bleeding and maintain circulating blood volume through replacing blood products if blood loss more than 1000 mL and ongoing or any patient triggers that indicate impending hypovolemic shock. The aim of management is to prevent progression of mild PPH to major or massive haemorrhage, that carries a worse prognosis and increased risk of AKI or permanent kidney damage.

Table 24.8 Table of maternal weight when estimating blood loss and its consequences

Maternal weight	Estimated total blood volume	15% blood loss (mL)	30% blood loss (mL)	40% blood loss (mL)
50 kg	5000	750	1500	2000
60 kg	6000	900	1800	2400
70 kg	7000	1050	2100	2800
80 kg	8000	1200	2400	3200

In low resource settings, approaches to minimise blood loss and mitigate the effects of massive haemorrhage include bimanual uterine compression, aortic compression, and applying clamps to arrest bleeding from cervical and vaginal tears before referral or whilst waiting to be transferred to the operating theatre. These should be done concurrently along with measures to maintain circulation.

Clinical Scenario 2

A 29 year old primiparous woman presents at 24 weeks' gestation feeling unwell with a blood pressure of 180/95 mmHg. Her serum creatinine level is 222 μmol/L, and her platelet count is 22×10^9/L.

- ***How would you manage her?***
  - *Admit to a high dependency unit*
  - *Intravenous access*
  - *Treat blood pressure appropriately*
  - *Assess for microangiopathic thrombotic causes such as HELLP syndrome, atypical haemolytic uremic syndrome (aHUS) or thrombotic thrombocytopenia purpura (TTP) by performing appropriate investigations*
  - *Treat based on likely diagnosis. If HELLP syndrome is diagnosed, delivery after stabilisation is recommended. If TTP is confirmed, treatment with plasma exchange should be initiated.*

Conclusions

Case 1 highlights the importance of pre-pregnancy counselling and surveillance of chronic kidney disease during pregnancy. Case 2 highlights the importance of timely investigations and recognition of AKI in pregnancy. The worldwide burden of CKD and AKI in pregnancy and the inequalities in access to point of care testing and novel treatment options make a compelling demand to develop more global collaboration and understanding of kidney disease in pregnancy.

Questions

1. In the management of a patient with Chronic Kidney Disease in pregnancy, the following are true except:
   A. Maintaining the Diastolic Blood Pressure less than 85 mmHg improves
   B. A serum creatinine of 100 μmol/L is considered abnormal in pregnancy
   C. Pregnancy is inadvisable in a woman with CKD
   D. Pre-pregnancy counselling, multivitamins, management by a multidisciplinary team, replacement of teratogenic drugs for pregnancy safe drugs improves outcomes
   E. Aspirin 75–150 mg from 12 weeks reduces the risk of superimposed pre-eclampsia

Answer: B

2. The obstetric risks of chronic kidney disease in pregnancy include the following except:
   A. Miscarriage
   B. Placental abruption
   C. Postpartum haemorrhage
   D. Sepsis

Answer: B

3. The maternal risks of chronic kidney disease in pregnancy include the following EXCEPT:
   A. Depression
   B. Gestational diabetes mellitus
   C. Mortality
   D. Pre-eclampsia
   E. Progression of chronic kidney disease-
   Answer: A
4. The perinatal risk for chronic kidney disease in pregnancy include the following, except:
   A. Fetal growth restriction
   B. Hypercalcaemia
   C. Lower birth weight
   D. Perinatal mortality
   E. Stillbirth

Answer: B

5. Investigations at booking for a patient with diabetic nephropathy in pregnancy include the following:
   A. Brain natriuretic peptide (BNP)
   B. Bone profile
   C. Erythrocyte sedimentation rate (ESR)
   D. Renal profile
   E. Renin-aldosterone ratio

Answer: D

6. Surveillance for ongoing antenatal review of pregnancy include the following EXCEPT:
   A. Blood pressure
   B. Oxygen saturation
   C. Schober test
   D. Signs and symptoms of heart failure
   E. Urine dipstick for proteinuria**Answer: C**
7. Concerning dialysis in a pregnant woman, the following are true:
   A. Indications include maternal urea concentration is 10–15 mmol/L
   B. Pregnant women with acute kidney injury due to massive haemorrhagic shock do not require dialysis
   C. AKI complicating HELLP syndrome may benefit from early dialysis
   D. Increased frequency of dialysis is required for patients on dialysis who get pregnant
   E. Peritoneal dialysis is preferred over haemodialysis

Answer: D

8. Individual risk factors for pre-eclampsia include the following EXCEPT:
   A. Cervical cerclage
   B. Hypertension
   C. In vitro fertilization

D. Obesity
E. Multiple pregnancy

Answer: A

9. Complications of pre-eclampsia includes the following EXCEPT:
   A. Intrauterine foetal death
   B. Multi-organ failure
   C. Acute Kidney Injury
   D. HELLP Syndrome
   E. Gestational diabetes mellitus

Answer: E Gestational diabetes mellitus

10. Postnatal follow-up after pre-eclampsia include the following EXCEPT:
    A. Blood pressure
    B. Contraception
    C. Kidney function
    D. Six minute test
    E. Urine dipstick for proteinuria

Answer: D

Test your learning and check your understanding of this book's contents: use the "Springer Nature Flashcards" app to access questions using https://sn.pub/cz9Cok. To use the app, please follow the instructions in Chap. 1.

References

1. Dunlop W. Serial changes in renal haemodynamics during normal human pregnancy. Br J Obstet Gynaecol. 1981;88(1):1–9.
2. August P. Preeclampsia: a "nephrocentric" view. Adv Chronic Kidney Dis. 2013;20:280–6.
3. Rolnik DL, et al. Aspirin versus placebo in pregnancies at high risk for preterm preeclamspia. N Engl J Med. 2017;377:613–22.
4. Magee LA, et al. CHIPS Study Group (2016). The CHIPS Randomized Controlled Trial (Control of Hypertension in Pregnancy Study): Is Severe Hypertension Just an Elevated Blood Pressure? Hypertension. 2016 Nov;68(5):1153–9.
5. Wiles KS, Nelson-Piercy C, Bramham K. Reproductive health and pregnancy in women with chronic kidney disease. Nat Rev Nephrol. 2018;14(3):165–84.
6. Wiles K, Chappell L, Clark K, et al. Clinical practice guideline on pregnancy and renal disease. BMC Nephrol. 2019;20:401.
7. Wiles K, et al. Serum creatinine in pregnancy: a systematic review. Kidney Int Rep. 2019;4:408–19.
8. Piccoli G, Daidola G, Attini R, Parisi S, Fassio F, Naretto C, Deagostini M, Castelluccia N, Ferraresi M, Roccatello D, Todros T. Kidney biopsy in pregnancy: Evidence for counselling? A systematic narrative review. BJOG. 2013;120 https://doi.org/10.1111/1471-0528.12111.
9. Brown MA, Magee LA, Kenny LC, et al. International Society for the Study of Hypertension in Pregnancy (ISSHP). The hypertensive disorders of pregnancy: ISSHP classification, diagnosis & management recommendations for international practice. Pregnancy Hypertens. 2018;13:291–310.
10. Chappell LC, Duckworth S, Seed PT, et al. Diagnostic accuracy of placental growth factor in women with suspected preeclampsia: a prospective multicentre study. Circulation. 2013;128:2121–31.
11. Gammill HS, Jeyabalan A. Acute renal failure in pregnancy. Crit Care Med. 2005;33(Suppl 10):S372–84.
12. Kristensen JH, Basit S, Wohlfahrt J, Damholt MB, Boyd HA. Pre-eclampsia and risk of later kidney disease: nationwide cohort study. BMJ. 2019;365:l1516.
13. Scully M, Thomas M, Underwood M, Watson H, Langley K, Camilleri RS, Clark A, Creagh D, Rayment R, Mcdonald V, Roy A, Evans G, McGuckin S, Ni Ainle F, Maclean R, Lester W, Nash M, Scott R, Brien O. collaborators of the UK TTP Registry. Thrombotic thrombocytopenic purpura and pregnancy: presentation, management, and subsequent pregnancy outcomes. Blood. 2014;124(2):211–9.
14. Fyfe-Brown A, Clarke G, Nerenberg K, Chandra S, Jain V. Management of pregnancy-associated thrombotic thrombocytopenia purpura. AJP reports. 2013;3(1):45–50.
15. Kelly RJ, et al. Eculizumab in Pregnant Patients with Paroxysmal Nocturnal Hemoglobinuria. N Engl J Med. 2015;373:1032–9.
16. Bose P, Regan F, Paterson-Brown S. Improving the accuracy of estimated blood loss at obstetric haemorrhage using clinical reconstructions. BJOG. 2006;113:919–24.

Transitional Care of Adolescents and Young Adult Patients with Kidney Disease

25

Joyce Popoola and Christopher Esezobor

Clinical Scenarios

(a) *An 18-year-old female was seen in the adult kidney transplant clinic. She had first developed kidney disease due to haemolytic uraemic syndrome five years prior to this, in Portugal. She had then spent 2 years on haemodialysis, before going on to receive a deceased donor kidney transplant. At that time, she had excellent subsequent allograft function, reflected by a baseline serum creatinine of 90 μmol/L (1.02 mg/dL). At the age of 16 years, she had relocated with her parents to the UK, maintaining her transplant function with her new paediatric transplant clinic team. Now 18, she had recently started university in a new city, away from her parents, and returned during the holidays to the adult transplant clinic for her follow-up appointment. Her serum creatinine was found to be 203 μmol/L (2.3 mg/dL).*

She reported challenges combining her university studies and keeping up with her friends: caring for her kidney transplant on top of this was overwhelming for her, and she just didn't feel that there was any support for people in her position: by the end of the academic year, her kidney allograft had failed, and she was re-established on haemodialysis.

A stormy period restarting haemodialysis ensued, as she suffered with recurrent infections, and challenges in keeping to her dialysis time slots. Recurrent hospital admissions led her to defer her university studies. Multiple donor-specific antibodies proved a challenge to re-transplantation, but this was eventually achieved two years later, when her mother was able to donate a kidney via the kidney sharing scheme, and she received the same.

She was able to return to university studies at the age of 22; this time living at home, and studying at a more local university.

Reflections:

What support could have been offered to this patient, and how could this have been tailored along her timeline?

How can periods of transition and their potential impact in a young person's journey be identified?

(b) *A 17-year-old male was preparing to transfer his care to an adult kidney unit. He had been born with prune belly syndrome: with dysplastic kidneys, complicated by vesicoureteral reflux, he had undergone extensive reconstructive surgery at the age of*

J. Popoola (✉)
Department of Nephrology and Transplantation, St George's University Hospitals NHS Foundation Trust, London, UK

St George's University of London, London, UK
e-mail: joyce.popoola@stgeorges.nhs.uk

C. Esezobor
Department of Paediatrics, Faculty of Clinical Sciences, College of Medicine, University of Lagos, Idi-Araba, Lagos, Nigeria

D. Banerjee et al. (eds.), *Management of Kidney Diseases*,
https://doi.org/10.1007/978-3-031-09131-5_25

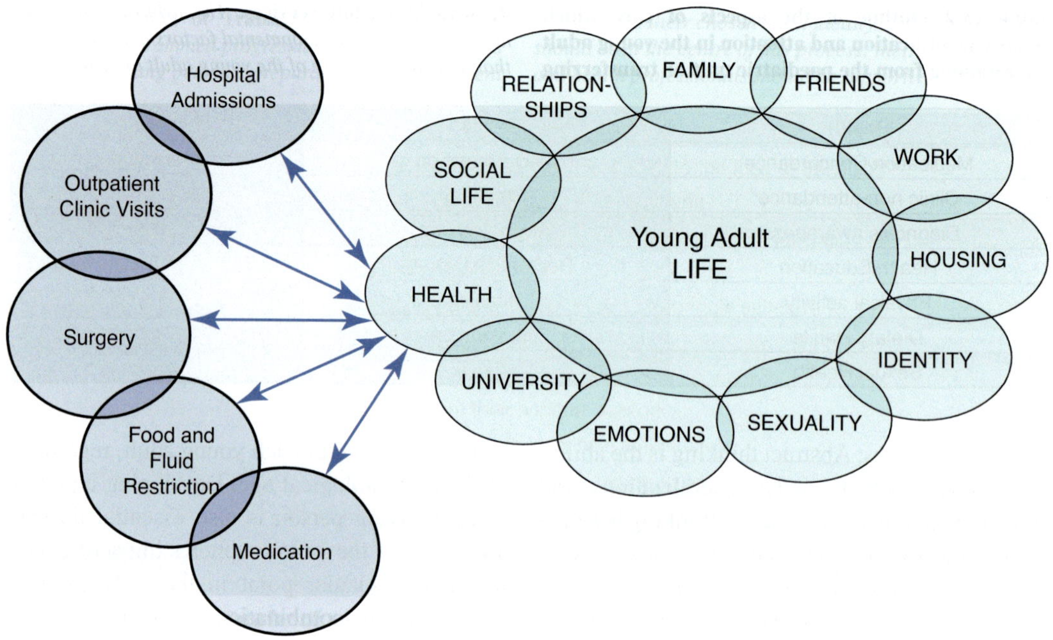

Fig. 25.1 The Impact of Kidney Disease on a Young Adult Life. *Bubble diagram illustrating factors influencing the life of a typical adolescent moving into young adulthood (turquoise), and the additional factors that can impact the life of a young adult with kidney disease (blue)*

with a mixture of supportive and medical management [13]. Their kidney function may alternatively be on a trajectory heading toward end stage kidney disease, and the need for kidney replacement therapy (KRT). The young person may already be on kidney replacement therapy: the majority (73%) in this group will have a functioning kidney transplant, although up to 35% of young adults lose a successfully functioning kidney transplant within 36 months of moving to adult services—this is a significantly increased rate of allograft loss compared with children and older adults [14].

Young people are particularly aware of their body image, hence peritoneal dialysis and haemodialysis catheters, arteriovenous fistulae, and the impact of fluid retention and medications such as steroids and calcineurin inhibitors, which are all such clear and common clinical signs in kidney medicine—can also compound a young kidney patient's frustrations [15].

Adolescents and young adults are thus twice as likely to demonstrate concordance issues when compared with the wider adult population [16]. Non-adherence with kidney transplant medications amongst young adults, for instance, is four times greater than in the general adult. Failure to engage properly with adult services has been shown to be associated with increased morbidity [17, 18].

How Can We Improve Outcomes for Young People in the Kidney Unit?

Tailored psychological and social support is required, alongside direct medical care of their kidney disease, and any other co-morbidities, and support for them when they are acutely unwell. Interestingly, young kidney patient and healthcare workers' perspectives as to the impact of kidney disease do differ markedly: A survey of over a 100 young adults with kidney disease carried out at St George's Hospital reported keeping active & exercising, limits on food & drink, and going out with friends as their top three major challenges. By contrast, their caring healthcare workers felt that Limits on food and drink, attending dialysis

Table 25.3 Perceptions of Challenges to Daily Living for Young Adult Patients with Kidney Disease. *Breakdown of the top three challenges to daily living reported by young adult patients with kidney disease, compared with perceived limitations reported by caring staff, and age-matched medical students. Aspects of medical care and issues directly related to their clinical condition were relatively low on their priority list even though they were perceived by health care workers as a priority for the young adults*

Rank	Young Adult Patients with Kidney Disease	Caring Staff	Age-matched Medical Students
1	Keeping active & exercising	Limits on food and drink	Attending dialysis
2	Limits on food and drink	Attending dialysis	Limits on food and drink
3	Going out with friends	Attending hospital appointments	Attending hospital appointments; spending time with friends

and hospital appointments were their three biggest challenges (Table 25.3). Whilst both lists display an awareness of the patients' loss of autonomy, it highlights the importance of identifying and helping to address patient reported factors, rather than merely staff perceptions.

In order to achieve full engagement with their direct medical care, young adults require mental, emotional and social support, to enable them manage their physical and medical needs [19]. The way in which young adults present to adult service, and their subsequent management can make a profound impact on their short, medium and long-term outcomes. Planning and support therefore needs to take into account whether the young person has presented directly to adult services as an acute admission or via clinic, or as a planned transfer from paediatric services. Embracing a methodical approach, such as embracing a toolkit to guide their care can help provide a structure, and uniformity of approach (Table 25.4).

Young persons are likely to need additional support in order to minimise hospital admissions, since not understanding their perspective can lead to prolonged inpatient stays, particularly if they are perceived as not co-operating, and the quality of communication is poor, or even absent. Discharge planning for a young adult requires early reflection, as it is not uncommon for them to have complex discharge needs, particularly as they may have concomitant long term disabilities, and other social and/or mental health concerns. Emphasis needs to be given to preventing readmission, and shortening hospital stays, since young people with kidney disease are likely to spend a considerable proportion of their life in and around healthcare settings.

The young person may require additional support around procedures such as surgery, dialysis catheter insertions and investigations. Establishing a link surgeon, and anaesthetists with experience in dealing with young people and children can be invaluable, in particular to deal with the slight nuances required to consent, where the next of kin, or an alternative independent witness may be required where a patient lacks competence to consent. Of course, there are other situations in which an adolescent under 16 years of age may be deemed competent to consent through *Gillick or Fraser competence.*

Nursing staff and other members of the multidisciplinary team need to be educated, and be provided with the tools around the nuances of caring for and supporting young persons in kidney units. An invaluable addition to the workforce is a Young Adult Worker, and identification of a Transition and Young Adult Consultant lead. It is beneficial if the latter has experience in paediatrics to facilitate as seamless a transition as possible.

Young adult workers (YAW) can offer an invaluable resource: when available, they should be involved in every aspect of the young persons' pathway—for instance in their inpatient stay and discharge planning (Appendix 1). They serve as the advocate and a liaison across the various specialties particularly to help overcome the young

Table 25.4 **A Toolkit for Transitional Care.** *The elements required to ensure a smooth and effective transition from paediatric to adult services*

Toolkit	Tool Components
Care Plan	• Detail of young person's care needs, who will support them in the adult service • Young person should be involved in service, design, delivery and evaluation • Focus should be what is possible for the young adult
Personal Folder	• One page profile (or portable, accessible electronic summary) • Information about health condition & medications • History of unplanned admissions • Preferences about parent/carer involvement • Emergency care plans • Strengths, achievements, hopes for the future and goals
Young Adult Worker	• Works with young adult in adult service to help them use the service • Explore alternative ways to help the Young Person meet their care needs early on
General or Family Practitioner	• All young adults must be registered with a medical practitioner in the community • Especially important to review if young adult has moved • Central point for prescription medications
Identified Community Support network	• Family, carers, social workers, members of educational institutions etc

person's challenges around articulating their needs, with a view to ultimately enabling self-empowerment of the young adult. The YAW provides 1:1 support tailored to the individual young person they are able to relate in a maturity appropriate way to the young person and provide continuity of care. They also assist in co-ordinating appointments, investigations, support in the community, as well as create social opportunities through buddies and peer support networks. They signpost the young person to educational and career opportunities: interview/application/grant opportunities as young people with kidney disease often miss schooling and examinations, leading to poor performance, which can prevent them from reaching their educational goals, and thus limit their career potential. Social Support Services maybe required—this is often practical to assist the young person with daily living, sorting out benefits, housing and social support. It is important to bear in mind that young adults may themselves have young dependent children, or have independent carers where this is required, or require additional reasonable adjustments to take account of their individual disabilities.

Adherence and concordance to treatment schedules often requires innovation—for instance charts, medication cards, electronic reminders, dosette boxes or blister packs, one-on-one training sessions with a pharmacist to talk about each of their medications, the involvement of a 'buddy' (peer support), and other members of their support network [11].

Establishing integrated paediatric and young adult clinics are an important aspect of young adult services. Such dedicated clinics promote more engaged young adults and provide the opportunity for the young adults to be seen in the same clinic. They work best where they incorporate named members of the multidisciplinary team as this enables continuity and more focused care of young people in a youth friendly supported environment [20]. The Young adult clinic provides a unique opportunity to break down feelings of isolation and promote support networks, as the attendees are more likely to meet contemporaries when they are seen as a cohort.

Harnessing peer support can also have a positive impact on adherence to treatments such as dialysis for instance cohorting young adults on the same shift. The provision of peer support with other young adults for instance on dialysis leads to improved adherence to scheduled treatment and improved wellbeing [21]. There is a need to be mindful that peer pressure can cause emotional upheaval, which can be from other young adults a partner and a desire to form intimate relationships, family (parents, siblings), lectures or teachers or friends. Provision of emotional support is best achieved by discussing issues with the young adults as they arise before they evolve. The young adult with disabilities such as deafness, blindness, mobility issues, or learning difficulties may require additional support—as may those whose parental culture or language may present a challenge to their receiving optimal healthcare.

Impact of Young Adult Care and Transition on Caregivers

As resources are channelled into the care of young people, it is important that the central role of family, caregivers, and supporters is also highlighted: whilst healthcare providers may experience snapshots of a young adult's clinical presentation, caregivers are closely involved in the day-to-day support of the individual: in certain circumstances, this can be unrelenting and stressful, particularly in situations where the young adult patient has cognitive, behavioural, mental health and/or significant physical disabilities.

Young persons with kidney disease may have siblings: competition between siblings for attention, parental feelings of guilt, overlaid with other negative emotions, can lead to a challenging home environment. The many difficulties of bringing up a child with a chronic illness may not infrequently lead to the breakdown of the family unit—such that young adult patients may live in a single-parent home. Financial strain is also common—consequent upon both the added expense of supporting young adult patients, and because carers may be have to give up gainful employment, or work flexibly around the young person's needs. There are also situations where care is provided either wholly or in combination with a care institution: whilst this may be associated with greater costs for a family, and create a more confusing and unstable home environment for the young adult patient, careful work to mitigate for these aspects may provide an optimal long-term care environment for patients.

Feelings of inadequacy can arise in caregivers, as they not only negotiate the milestones of normal transition from childhood to adulthood, alongside other competing life events, but are also faced with the challenges of caring for a child with chronic illness: overseeing the daily administration of medications, supporting patients through procedures and treatments, attending other hospital appointments, and acting as patient advocate—all whilst maintaining an outwardly positive outlook. Concurrently, they may experience conflicts around letting go, enabling and allowing the young person to transition into adult life, and developing the skills required for independent self-care.

Where clinical staff may witness individual challenging episodes from a young adult patient, caregivers may by contrast experience constant, sometimes bewildering outbursts or challenging behaviours—the cause of which may not be clear: caregivers frequently know best how to manage these situations, and in a similar way, should be recognised as key players in working out how to achieve the best outcome for the young person—whilst adopting a passive, or more active role over the course of the young person's care.

Caregivers may themselves require support, and they should be signposted as to how to obtain it accordingly: this may include receiving direct support from a psychologist, and/or a social worker—for their own personal care, beyond that of the young adult patient. There may also be the need to help enable caregivers to apply for grants and other sources of financial support, to help the young adult patients and their families cope. Similarly to their charges, caregivers may also benefit from peer support or 'buddying', to help them work out solutions to every-day challenges.

The importance of facilitating a healthy dynamic—not only for the young adult patient, but also their caregivers—cannot be overemphasised.

Global Perspectives of Young Adult Care and Transition

The provision of healthcare varies enormously across the world: this has led to enormous gaps in healthcare provision for large sectors of society—which are particularly marked in developing nations, and are reflected in healthcare outcomes when comparing developed and developing nations.

Financial allocation for healthcare are complex and multi-layered: very young <16 years (paediatrics) and older >65 years (geriatrics) patients frequently have dedicated services to support them; the majority of general care is geared towards the middle aged (40–65), who constitute the highest number using healthcare resources. The majority of funds are deployed to treat older patients in developed nations, where there is a higher age expectancy, culminating in better survival, with increased numbers of co-morbidities amongst this demographic.

The idea of medical care specifically catering for young adults is a relatively undescribed area, with little targeted funding or legislation, even in some of the more developed nations. In the continents of Asia and Africa, care for young adults constitutes even more of an enigma: there is significant variation in practice: the definition of an adult for timing of transition is as young as 12 years in some developing nations, 16 years in parts of North America [22], and 18 years in most parts of Europe. To overcome the shortfall of targeted care for this patient group, it is important that there is enhanced cross-working between paediatric and adult nephrology specialists—to ensure that the best care is provided to this vulnerable group. The aim should be that despite the presence of a chronic medical condition, the young person should, in addition to being provided with age-appropriate medical care, be enabled to reach their maximal potential socially, mentally and emotionally, whilst minimising morbidity and mortality.

Practice Points

- Liaise closely with your paediatric nephrology colleagues to ensure that adolescent and young adult kidney patients are engaged in the transition process early
- Get to know who the different members of the transition team in your kidney unit are
- Identify all additional members of your patient's support network
- Agree sensible, achievable therapeutic goals with your adolescent/young adult kidney patient
- Some adolescent/young adult kidney patients, presenting directly to adult kidney services, may also benefit from dedicated and coordinated support from a young adult team

Conclusions

It is useful to reflect on the four very different clinical scenarios from the beginning of the chapter—each very complex in nature. Both cases A and B were well-known to their respective paediatric nephrology teams, but patient A's transition was complicated by her move to a new country, and subsequently starting higher education in a new university environment, away from home. This led to a loss of continuity in support, and co-incident failure of her kidney allograft—with a heavy cost in terms of a deferment in her university education of four years, and a clinical pathway complicated by infection on resumption of dialysis. Patient B's carefully planned approach to transition, and adapted educational support throughout his childhood, allowed for a smoother pathway to a second transplant, and resumption of his university education. Patient C's devastating story reflects the bold intentions of a young man attempting independently to find a constructive pathway out of a mutually physically and emotionally erosive life at home. Complicated by end stage kidney disease, and the absence of an available support network—and without the engagement of dedicated young adult or mental health services, his life on kidney replacement therapy rapidly spiralled downward, culminating in him taking his own life. Patient D's case highlights the vast difference in health care access, and differing definitions as to who is a competent adult, and thus who is responsible for his care. The 13-year-old being treated as an adult, with no healthcare insurance, has huge—potentially life-limiting implications on his morbidity and mortality: this is the story of many, particularly in the developing world.

The issues around transitional care for adolescent and young adult kidney patients have only relatively recently been highlighted, particularly by inferior clinical outcomes and engagement when compared with adult care. Improving awareness of the common issues, and identifying collective solutions can go a long way to addressing these—in the UK, the Department of Health (DOH), the National Institute for Health and Care Excellence (NICE) and the Care Quality Commission (CQC) all support a model that provides a tailored, patient-centred service, led by a multi-disciplinary team. We might optimally call for this model to include adult and paediatric nephrologists, trained nurse specialists, and all other members of the multidisciplinary kidney care team, coordinated by a dedicated young adult worker, liaising closely with each other, the patient and their individual care network, with the shared goal of providing holistic, mutually satisfying care, incorporating physical, mental and social health—both throughout transition, and into the patient's adult life beyond this.

Appendix 1: The Transitional Care Referral Form

A sample referral form for the transfer of care of a young adult from paediatric to adult kidney services

REFERRAL FORM FOR YOUNG ADULT KIDNEY PATIENTS TO TRANSITIONAL CARE

Demographics Name: Date of birth: Ethnicity: Religion (Spiritual beliefs):
Medical Problems Renal Diagnosis Other relevant co-morbidities
Renal Status Transplant Peritoneal dialysis Haemodialysis
Relevant Social Issues (and key worker where relevant)
Relevant Psychological Issues (and key worker where relevant)
Disabilities or learning difficulties (and key worker where relevant)

Questions

1. According to the World Health Organisation, adolescents make up which age group?
   A. 10–15 years
   B. 10–19 years
   C. 11–21 years
   D. 16–29 years
   E. 15–21 years

Answer B: Whilst there are arguments that adolescence should encompass the mid 20's, the World Health Organisation (WHO) defines adolescence as 10–19 years. Those age between 15 and 24 are regarded as 'Youth' and 'Young People' covers those between 10 and 24 years.
   A. False
   B. True
   C. False
   D. False
   E. False

2. An 18 year old female with end stage kidney disease secondary to IgA nephropathy is referred to the adult transplant follow up clinic 1 year following her deceased donor transplant. Her baseline serum creatinine is 90 µmol/L (1.02 mg/dL), and her urinalysis remains negative for protein and blood. Which of the following is true?
   A. The risk of recurrence of IgA nephropathy in her transplant kidney is 3%
   B. The risk of her losing her kidney allograft in the next three years is up to around 35%
   C. Her risk of graft failure would be significantly reduced if she had been transplanted at a younger age
   D. She should be followed up on an annual basis in the kidney transplant clinic
   E. The likelihood of her kidney allograft remaining functional at 5 years is 98%

Answer B: The risk of her losing her kidney allograft in the next three years is up to 35%
   A. False. The risk of recurrence of IgA nephropathy in the graft is 6–20%, although may be as high as 58% depending on the rate of biopsy and the length of follow-up. The risk of graft loss due to recurrent IgAN is 1.6–16%
   B. True. The risk of young adult kidney transplant recipients losing their kidney allograft within three years of transitioning to adult services is up to around 35%
   C. False. Her risk of graft failure is not altered by age at transplantation
   D. False. UK Kidney association clinical practice guidelines suggest 3–6 monthly follow up after 12 months—this may need to be adapted to the individual patient setting.
   E. The likelihood of her kidney allograft remaining functional at 5 years is 75% post deceased donor transplantation, although it may be lower than 65% (see B).

3. An eighteen-year-old, Caucasian male with CKD Stage 3 due to IgA Nephropathy has moved from the North of England to London as he is keen to make his own way in life following the divorce of his parents. Which of the following need to be taken into consideration following his transfer to a new renal unit?
   A. Paid employment
   B. Social isolation
   C. Independent living
   D. Educational opportunities
   E. All of the above

Answer E: Despite this young man having plans of living independently he may not have means or the awareness and may have in fact been dependent on one or both of his parents for support in managing his medical condition. At his initial consultation it would be essential to take a holistic approach to his care exploring whether he is prepared for independent living in the community in addition to his ability to take responsibility for his medical condition.

4. What age should the transition process ideally start for the young person moving from paediatric services to adult services considering WHO guidelines from the choices below
   A. 14 years
   B. 15 years
   C. 16 years
   D. 17 years
   E. 18 years

Answer A: Transition should be a seamless process not only for the young person concerned but also for the caregivers and healthcare professionals. This can only be achieved if the transition process starts early in the pathway of the young adult with chronic illness in order that they becoming familiar and don't feel isolated in their journey through healthcare systems. In order to achieve the preparation and transition process needs to start as early as possible sometimes this can be as early as 12 years.

5. The following need to be taken in to consideration in relation to the registered carer if they are the parent of a transitioned eighteen-year old autistic adult with renal disease who is wheelchair bound with multiple disabilities with the exception of.

A. Has the ability to care for the young person
B. Is willing to care for the young person beyond 18 years
C. Tertiary Education of the carer
D. Works or plans to do so
E. Training in communication skills

Answer C: Carers need to be adequately equipped even if they are the parents of a child. It should not be assumed that they have the ability or will be the carers of the child after the age of 18 years particularly in situations where the child has complex needs. There are some environments where there is not the infrastructure to meet such a young person's needs and this may require focus in the future as more infants with complex needs are starting to survive in to adult hood. Provision of tertiary care such as university education to the carer is not a direct support to the young person's care.

6. A fifteen-year old secondary school student presents to the Accident and Emergency department while on a day trip in Wales with severe abdominal pain, she has acute kidney injury and an obstructing renal calculus. Who of the following cannot give consent for surgery.
   A. The parents
   B. The legal guardian
   C. The student
   D. None of the above
   E. All of the above

Answer D: All of the listed can give consent for the procedure including the young person in the event they are considered mature enough to understand the process and potential risks and benefit. This is through *Gillick Competence* a term used in medical law to determine if a child less than sixteen can consent independently to their medical care. In circumstance where this is not possible due to for instance disability or immaturity and neither parents or legal guardians are available consent be provided by medical professionals in an emergency by making the young person a ward of the court.

7. A twenty-one-year old with a live donor transplant from her Father 5 years ago attends the local university and turns up for an emergency review in your clinic complaining of abdominal pain over the transplant feeling tired and haematuria. The creatinine has gone from her baseline of 1.1 mg/dL to 2.3 mg/dL (97 μmol/L to 204 μmol/L). You have never seen her before although this is her second semester at the university. High on your differential diagnosis must include
   A. Urinary tract infection
   B. Acute rejection
   C. Direct Trauma
   D. Recurrent disease
   E. Chronic Allograft Nephropathy

Answer B: Rejection must be high on the list of differentials and quickly diagnosed or excluded due to the potential consequences of undiagnosed rejection and the fact that if detected early it is reversible. Often a further history around adherence can assist with making the diagnosis. Transplant loss in young people in transition phases for instance hospitals and education is common particularly when appropriate checks and balances are not implemented to assist prevention.

8. Which of the following is the most common concern among adolescent and young adults with renal conditions?
   A. Taking medications
   B. Social networks
   C. Educational opportunities
   D. Dietary restrictions
   E. The nature of their renal disease

Answer B: Interestingly healthcare providers have very different perspectives to what is most important for young adults and their general wellbeing. While maintaining social networks with friends is the predominant concern of young adults, healthcare professionals seem tend to assume that the health condition of the young adults is their predominant concern.

9. One of your young adults—a 23-year-old Indo-Asian female—recently got married, following her diagnosis of lupus one month earlier. She has been started on mycophenolate mofetil (MMF) and steroids, and is starting to show good response. She is keen to

start a family straight away, as she is being subjected to pressure from both her parents and her in laws. How would you manage her case?

A. Do nothing
B. Stop the immunosuppressive therapy
C. Change her immunosuppression therapy immediately
D. Refer for preconception counselling
E. None of the above

Answer D: It is common to receive queries from young adults hoping to get pregnant on potential teratogenic agents, in this case mycophenolate mofetil. This patient is starting to respond to therapy and we would normally aim for the lupus to stabilise prior to pregnancy. Preconception counselling can prove invaluable particularly if it involves the partner, as it is an opportunity to make as safe a planned pregnancy as possible, with improved concordance consequent upon an improved understanding, and ultimately providing an optimal outcome for the young person, and their chances of a successful pregnancy with minimal complications.

10. A Young Adult Worker can take on the following roles except

A. Advocacy for young people
B. Prescribing for young people
C. Enpowerment of young people
D. Creation of peer support opportunities for young people
E. Support co-ordination of clinics for young people

Answer B: It would be unusual for a young adult worker to take on the role of prescribing medications for young people unless they had specific training from another role which they carried a license for. A young adult worker has a supportive role assisting the transition of the young adult and their subsequent care with in the adult facility with the aim that the young person is not inhibited from reaching their maximal potential in all spheres of life despite their medical condition.

11. The following strategies can be used to promote medication adherence among young adults

A. Reduction of bill burden
B. Highlighting potential side effects prior to prescribing
C. Use of a dossette box or blister pack
D. Enlisting a buddy or peer supporter
E. All of the above

Answer E: Adherence is an age old problem and one of the commonest causes of poor response to treatment. All of the above strategies can be adopted other strategies include setting alarms, using electronic pill counters for monitoring. Ideally the aim of the transition years is to reduce the dependence on the carer so avoiding strategies that depend on the guardian to maintain adherence should be avoided.

12. One of your young adults—a nineteen-year-old male, had been hoping to receive a pre-emptive renal transplant from his mother. Unfortunately, his mother was found to have a low GFR 59 and cystic changes to one of her kidneys. The mother is insistent that she donate to help her son regardless, as she would do anything for her child. The following would be the least appropriate approach:

A. Explore potential interim dialysis options
B. Activate on the deceased transplant waiting list
C. Arrange referral of mother to donor surgeon
D. Explore other potential donors
E. Arrange counselling for patient and mother

Answer C: Where the care of young people is concerned, it is not uncommon for parents or carers to want to take the place of their child in relation to the young person's illness. In this situation the mother would not be the best donor for her son: for a young person, the ideal donor offers as healthy a donor organ as possible: additionally, it would lead her toward a more significant renal impairment, which could culminate in ESKD. Counselling, and in some cases psychological input can have a vital role to help deal with feelings of guilt and disappointment.

Test your learning and check your understanding of this book's contents: use the "Springer Nature Flashcards" app to access questions using https://sn.pub/cz9Cok. To use the app, please follow the instructions in Chap. 1.

References

1. Albon L, Vaughan L. Adolescents and young adults on the acute medical unit: how might we do it better? Clin Med. 2015;14:618–22.
2. Hargreaves DS, Viner RM. Children's and young people's experience of the National Health Service in England: a review of National Surveys 2001-11. Arch Dis Child. 2012;97:661–6.
3. Transition getting it right for Young People National Framework Department of Health; 2006.
4. Transition from children's to adults' services for young people using health or social care services NICE Guidelines (NG43) Published 24 February 2016.
5. You're Welcome: Quality criteria for young people friendly health services; DoH 2005 & April 2011.
6. Nagra A, McGinnity PM, Davis N, Salmon AP. Implementing transition: ready steady go. Arch Dis Child Educ Pract Ed. 2015;100(6):313–20.
7. Sawyer SM, Drew S, Yeo MS, Britto MT. Adolescents with a chronic condition: challenges living, challenges treating. Lancet. 2007;369(9571):1481–9.
8. https://www.gov.uk/government/publications/early-adolescence-applying-all-our-health/early-adolescence-applying-all-our-health. Updated December 16th 2020.
9. Steinberg L. Cognitive and affective development in adolescence. Trends Cognitive Sci. 2005;9(2):69–74.
10. Freitas AL, Gollwitzer P, Trope Y. The influence of abstract and concrete mindsets on anticipating and guiding others' self-regulatory efforts. J Exp Soc Psychol. 2004;40(6):739–52.
11. Popoola J, Greene H, Kyegombe M, MacPhee IA. Patient involvement in selection of immunosuppressive regimen following transplantation. Patient Preference and Adherence. 2014;8:1705–12.
12. Watson AR. Non-compliance and transfer from paediatric to adult transplant unit. Paediatr Nephrol. 2000;14:469–72.
13. Lost in transition: moving young people between child and adult health services; RCN 2008.
14. Foster BJ. Heightened graft failure risk during emerging adulthood and transition to adult care. Pediatr Nephrol. 2015;30:567–76.
15. Hamilton AJ, Casula A, Ben-Shlomo Y, et al. The clinical epidemiology of young adults starting renal replacement therapy in the UK: presentation, management and survival using 15 years of UK Renal Registry data. Nephrol Dial Transplant. 2017;32:1434–5.
16. From the Pond to the Sea: Children's transition to adult health services Care Quality Commission—June 2014.
17. Department of Health GoU. Quality criteria for young people friendly health services. http://www.gov.uk/government/publications/quality-criteria-for-young-people-friendly-ealth-services. 2011.
18. Blum RWM, Garell D, Hodgman C, Jorissen T, Okinow N, Orr D, et al. Transition from child-centered to adult health-care systems for adolescents with chronic conditions. J Adolesc Health. 1993;14:570–6.
19. Hamilton AJ, Caskey FJ, Casula A, Ben-Shlomo Y, Inward CD. Psychosocial health and lifestyle behaviours in young adults receiving renal replacement therapy compared to the general population: findings from the SPEAK study. Am J Kidney Dis. 2019;73(2):194–205.
20. Harden PN, Walsh G, Bandler N, Bradley S, Lonsdale D, Taylor J, et al. Bridging the gap: an integrated paediatric to adult clinical service for young adults with kidney failure. British Medical Journal. 2012;344
21. Turner ML, Matthews J, Cronin H, Sinclair F, Popoola J. Modification of Young Adult Outcomes on Haemodialysis...Changing "Our" Practice. Pediatr Nephrol. 2017;32:1648. https://doi.org/10.1007/s00467-017-3753-x.
22. Fernandez HE, Foster BJ. Long-term care of the pediatric kidney transplant recipient. CJASN ePress. 2021;(17) https://doi.org/10.2215/CJN.16891020.

26 Conservative Care for Patients with Chronic Kidney Disease

Helen Alston and Katie Vinen

Clinical Scenario

An 85 year old man is seen in the advanced kidney care clinic. He has an eGFR of 14 mL/min/1.73 m^2 which is falling by 2 mL/min/1.73 m^2 per year and a serum albumin of 30 g/L. He can walk 200 m slowly, but needs a stick to help with balance. He meets friends weekly to play bowls and is a keen gardener, although now needs help with this. He enjoys a good quality of life though his wife has disabling dementia. He has two children and five grandchildren, two of whom live abroad. His daughter has noticed some early memory difficulties. He has recently transferred to the Advanced Kidney Care Clinic so that he "can prepare for dialysis when the time comes".

Introduction

What is Conservative Care?

When first developed, dialysis was offered only to young non-diabetic patients. As it became clear that it could benefit many other patients, in countries where resources allow, it was extended to older complex patients, including those over 70. Whilst many benefit, for others the burdens of dialysis out-weigh the benefits. An alternative, non-dialysis care pathway has therefore been developed, called Conservative Care (CC).

Comprehensive Conservative kidney care can be defined as planned, holistic, patient centered care for those with stage 5 chronic kidney disease, that does not involve kidney replacement therapy (KRT). It includes interventions to delay progression of the disease and minimise complications, but focuses predominantly on: management of symptoms; psychological, social, cultural, and spiritual support; and advance care planning [1, 2].

This chapter aims to describe:

- key elements of the conservative care pathway for patients with CKD
- approaches to assessment, and when this pathway may be appropriate
- tools to aid optimal delivery of this pathway.

We acknowledge the relative paucity of data in this area, and therefore highlight a practical approach to delivering CC. We note key areas of knowledge which are currently being actively researched, supported by patients who see CC as a top research priority.

H. Alston · K. Vinen (✉)
Kings College Hospital NHS Foundation Trust, London, UK
e-mail: helen.alston@nhs.net; katie.vinen@nhs.net

D. Banerjee et al. (eds.), *Management of Kidney Diseases*,
https://doi.org/10.1007/978-3-031-09131-5_26

Why do we Require a Conservative Care Pathway?

In high income countries (all treatment options for CKD 5 available): Choice driven conservative care:

In high income countries, the development of CC is a response to changing demographics of the end-stage kidney disease (ESKD) population. Many patients are older or highly co-morbid, and may benefit from or choose to have care which avoids the burdens and medicalisation associated with KRT. Care may involve a combination of nephrological, care of elderly and palliative input.

Improved treatments have also supported another population of patients (some relatively young) who begin dialysis in good health, but over years of treatment become frailer. Their care may change to focus on symptom control, reduced tablet burden and sometimes reduced dialysis frequency. Care focuses on maintaining quality of life and planning for end-of-life. These interventions overlap CC but are delivered in parallel with KRT—this is often called supportive care but is outside the scope of this chapter.

In middle and lower income countries (treatment choices may be restricted): Choice restricted conservative care:

In lower income countries, CC may be offered as a choice-restricted option when resources do not allow provision of KRT for all patients. Here the population receiving CC may be younger, with fewer co-morbidities. Where resources are limited, only certain aspects of CC may be available.

Variations in Conservative Care Provision

In 2019, an ISN global survey on care for ESKD found that CC was offered in 124 (81%) of 154 countries [3]. In 66 countries (43%), this option was choice-restricted, whilst in 77 (50%) countries, CC availability was driven by patients' choice or medical guidance, and not limited by resources.

CC was offered in all countries in north, east, and south Asia, and most countries in eastern and central Europe (95%, 18/19), Oceania and South East Asia (93%, 14/15), western Europe (90%, 18/20), the Middle East (82%, 9/11), and Africa (80%, 33/41). However, CC was offered by fewer than half of countries in Latin America (44%, 8/18), and just over half of countries in newly independent states, Russia (57%, 4/7) and North America (67%, 6/9).

Although some provision of CC was provided at similar levels (75-85%) in countries of all income levels, the provision of medically advised CC did rise with income level. Income also appeared to affect the elements of CC that were offered; only 37% of 154 countries offering CC adopted a multidisciplinary team approach and only 26% used shared decision-making tools (e.g. practice guidelines for providers and patient decision aids). Whilst systematic symptom management of advanced kidney failure was provided in 52% of countries, only 29% were able to provide psychological, cultural, and spiritual support within CC.

What Are the Key Elements of the Conservative Care Pathway?

Whilst the key elements of comprehensive CC are defined, their relative importance varies over time and, even in affluent health systems, there remains variation in elements of the pathway offered.

Where choice-driven CC is provided, early priorities include honest prognostic information, excellent communication, and understanding the patient's own beliefs and wishes. Preservation of function (physical, cognitive and renal), excellent symptom control, reduction in treatment burdens (including maximising hospital-free days), and an effective network of professional support can then be offered. Ensuring a "good death" and providing support for family before and after death are important later aspects of CC.

In countries only able to offer choice-restricted CC, the focus of resources will be less on supporting decision-making, and more on later aspects such as symptom control. Key elements are summarised in Table 26.1.

Table 26.1 Key elements of the Conservative Care pathway

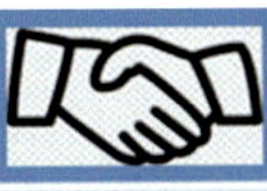	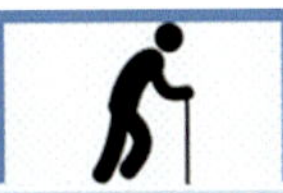	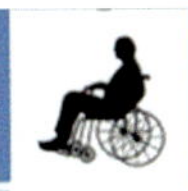	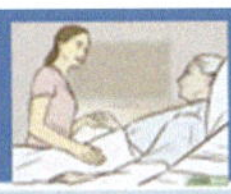	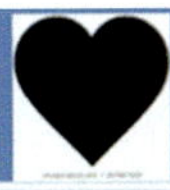
Decision making	Stability	Increasing symptoms	End of life care	Care after loss
Assessment	Patient and family education	Patient and family education	Patient and family education	Family support
Education				
Choice	Preservation of kidney function	Preservation of kidney function	Optimisation of quality of life	Memorial events
Shared decision making	Optimisation of physical and cognitive function	Optimisation of physical and cognitive function		
	Symptom control	Symptom control	Symptom control	
		Creation of community care network	Increasing use of network of community care	
	Introduction of advance care planning	Creation of advance care plan	Enactment of advance care plan	
		Crisis plan	Crisis plan	

Training and Empowering the Clinical Team

Many patients and clinicians feel uncomfortable discussing later life care. Whilst the prognosis associated with ESKD) is often worse than that of some cancers, many patients believe that kidney failure is curable with transplantation, and indefinitely treatable with dialysis. Few patients understand the true burden of dialysis, and some falsely believe that dialysis will help dementia or cure poor mobility. Studies suggest that patients want to have their prognosis discussed but this is rarely done. Overly-optimistic estimates of prognosis on dialysis can accidentally lead to overemphasis on disease-directed care.

Staff sometimes have a poor understanding of limited prognostic information, little time or knowledge to use systematised assessment tools, and poor training in communication skills. Any CC programme is based on well-informed staff who are skilled and confident to deliver difficult and complex information sensitively. Links to staff training resources are included in the key tools table at the end of the chapter [4].

Assessment, Education, Choice and Shared Decision Making

Helping patients make meaningful choices requires cognitive, functional and physical assessment to reveal multi-morbidity or functional decline previously unrecognised in short nephrology appointments. Initial assessment is time-consuming but vital to true shared decision-making (SDM).

Education necessitates practical information about what treatment pathways entail and realistic prognostic guidance for patients and families about survival and quality of life associated with each choice. Some patients may actively choose to forgo dialysis whilst for others the decision may be consensus-driven, due to frailty or cognitive impairment.

Table 26.2 shows possible assessment tools which may help the clinician to guide realistic choices. Where resources allow, these tools should not be used to deny a patient their treatment choice but to inform the SDM process.

Initial treatment discussions may focus on age and trajectory of GFR decline, to establish likelihood of

Table 26.2 Clinician Tools which help guide older frailer ESKD patients through treatment choices

Indicator	Tools	Relevance	Evidence	Limitation
Age	Chronological age	Easy to measure and understand May improve discussions realism	Observational data suggest those > 70 with significant co-morbidity and those simply > 80 may gain little survival advantage on RRT	Only ever predicts average survival in people of same age - may not reflect the individual No RCT data yet available (NIHR PREPARE study awaited)
Trajectory of decline of kidney function	Trajectory of GFR Proteinuria	Shorter life associated with rapid decline in kidney function may alter treatment choice.	Kidney Failure Risk Equation (KFRE)—internationally-validated tool to calculate 2 and 5yr risk of ESRF https://kidneyfailurerisk.com/	Does not allow for acute events precipitating sudden decline in renal function.
Estimated survival tools after RRT start (derived from large renal databases).	US Renal Data system French REIN registry New England HD clinics (sometimes called Cohen tool) https://qxmd.com/calculate/calculator_135/6-month-mortality-on-hd#	Use a mixture of demographic, functional, biochemical and clinician instinct in predictor scores to assess possible survival at 3 and 6 months after dialysis initiation	Large national and regional renal databases from Europe and USA.	Only exist for some populations Need constant updating

Physical frailty	Clinical frailty Score (CFS) https://www.scfn.org.uk/clinical-frailty-scale Charlson score	Quick and easy for MDT to use Co-morbidity based scale more suitable for remote assessment Higher Charlson scores are associated with increased 2 years mortality in renal patients	Higher CFS (≥5) scores predict a greater likelihood of hospitalization and death Nursing home patients have only 13% chance of being alive and at same level of function 1 year after RRT start	Not developed for use in patients <65 years More complex to calculate
Cognitive deficit	MoCA 4AT	Significant deficit may affect ability to contribute to treatment choice Progressive deficit my impede ability to receive treatment (unable to sit still) or to travel to unfamiliar dialysis unit	Approximately 30-70% of haemodialysis patients have some degree of cognitive impairment. Incidence of cognitive impairment has been associated with both severity of chronic kidney disease and with rate of CKD decline and albuminuria. Visuospatial and executive functions disproportionately affected in ESRF. NHANES III found slower learning speeds and impaired visual concentration even in younger CKD patients (aged 20-59), compared with standardised populations. Implications for pre-dialysis counselling, patient education and treatment compliance. https://www.mocatest.org/ https://www.the4at.com/	Requires literacy/vision to complete tests. Potential language barrier for some languages (though some MoCA translations exist).
Surprise question	Would I be surprised if this patient died in the next 6–12 months.	Uses synthesis of all knowledge about patient.	Nephrologists had a positive predictive power of 67%, with higher levels of accuracy when there was agreement between several clinicians	Best used by experienced clinician who knows patient well.

ESKD in the near future for older patients (some of whom have low but very slowly declining function).

For those with a clear GFR decline, most patients initially focus on length of survival. However, with limited data, discussions are often dominated by the possibility (rather than probability) of life prolongation (sometimes driven by the family not the patient).

Limited observational data has shown that for those over 70 with a WHO performance status of ≥3, those over 75 with ≥2 co-morbidities, or those over 80 regardless of co-morbidity, there may be little to no survival benefit in starting dialysis. Higher clinical frailty scores predict an increased risk of hospitalisation and death in a renal population, whilst starting dialysis from a nursing home is associated with only a 13% chance of one-year survival with a maintained level of functional status (with 87% of patients dying or declining).

Formal prediction tools may help patients to understand their comparative six-month survival chance were they to start dialysis. Co-morbidity should also be considered, as data suggest that for those patients who enter CC, only about 50% die of uremia (with others dying from non-kidney related causes). Patients often perceive that death on the CC pathway will occur shortly after they would have started dialysis. In fact, uremic death rarely occurs until later, with a median survival of 6 months even after GFR has fallen to 6–7 mL/min/1.73 m^2.

Formal cognitive assessment aids clinical judgement of a patient's ability to understand complex choices and management of practical aspects such as possible disorientation in an unfamiliar dialysis unit.

Factors that may help patients to consider treatment options are shown in Fig. 26.1. In addition to overall survival, patients need support to

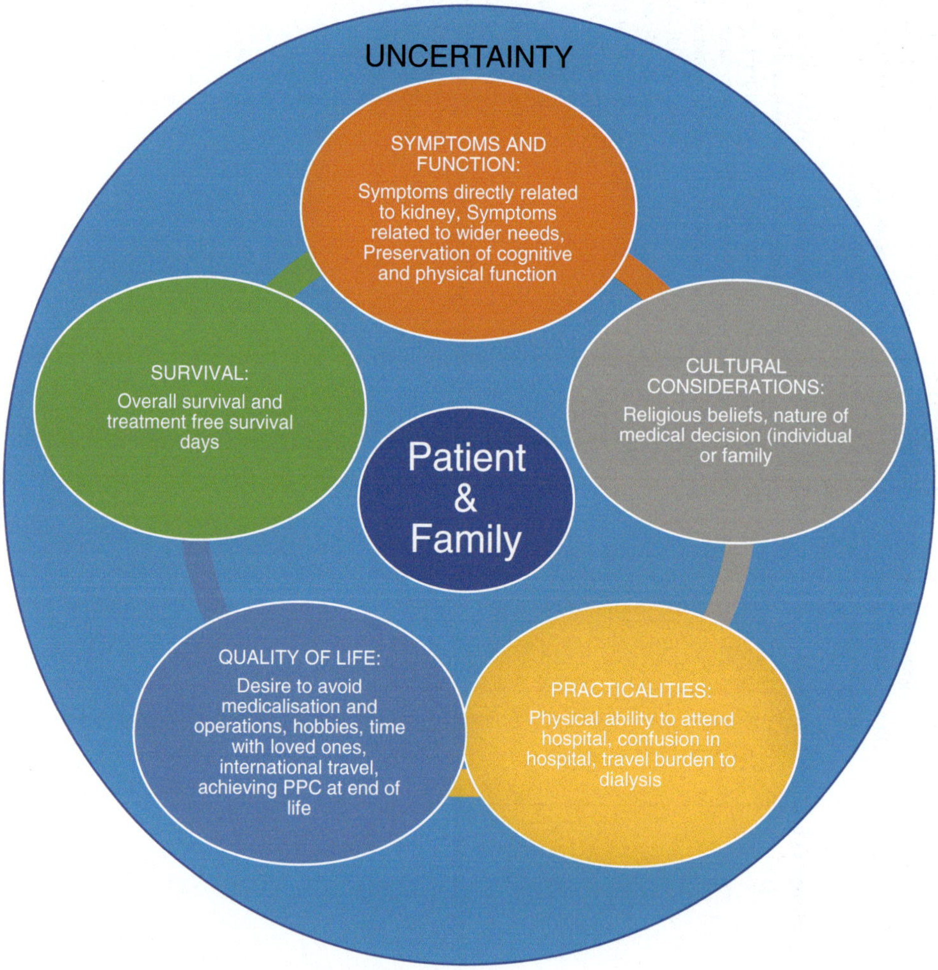

Fig. 26.1 Factors affecting patients' treatment decisions

consider hospital-free days, symptom burden, freedom to travel, and the likelihood of achieving a preferred place of death (which has been shown to be more likely in those choosing CC).

Limited studies have assessed quality of life on CC. One important longitudinal study compared QOL in late CKD 4 and CKD 5 patients who had chosen a CC pathway, with those who had chosen dialysis. Whilst the patients choosing CC were older, frailer and more co-morbid than those on dialysis, they maintained QOL, whereas for those choosing dialysis, life satisfaction scores deteriorated after starting dialysis. All patients, especially those with cognitive impairment, may find it hard to understand the intrinsic uncertainty surrounding treatments for the frail and elderly in ESKD. Any decision support tool must allow for this.

Data to support these difficult discussions are largely based on small observational studies. The British NIHR-supported PREPARE study is the first ever randomized control trial to look at outcomes in older frailer patients, comparing those who prepare to receive KRT with those who receive CC. Due to report in 2024, it will be a significant step forward in information available.

Measures to Prevent Progression of CKD

Measures such as cessation of smoking, optimal diabetic and blood pressure control and avoidance of nephrotoxins are documented elsewhere in this book. Factors that may receive attention in younger patients (because they have long term sequelae) may be less relevant for those in later life (e.g. high phosphate levels), or may need to balance competing priorities e.g. high potassium (arrhythmia risk) versus quality of life (enjoyment from eating). Risk factors may benefit from more pragmatic targets, e.g. the balance of tight blood pressure or diabetic control against the risk of falls due to postural symptoms or hypoglycaemia. There are no internationally agreed treatment targets for CC patients, but pragmatically the authors use the suggested values shown in Table 26.3.

Table 26.3 CKD treatment targets modified for CC Population

Measure	Target	Comments
Blood pressure	≤160/90 mmHg	European Society of Hypertension 2018 Guidelines >80 years Many hypertension studies focus on long term benefit rarely relevant in CC
Diabetic control	HbA1c >7.5%	Hypoglycaemia is greater risk in CC
Cholesterol	No target	No evidence of relevance in frail elderly.
Acidosis	Serum bicarbonate >22 mmol/L	Evidence that acidosis may contribute to fatigue, muscle wasting and malnutrition
Anemia	9.5–11.5 g/L	If the patient is asymptomatic, lower levels of haemoglobin may be acceptable
High potassium	<6.5 mmol/L	More relaxed targets may allow improved nutrition/QOL
Calcium and phosphate management	Immediate symptom benefit to keeping calcium within normal range (eg avoidance of fitting). No specific target suggested for phosphate—balance of QOL and better nutrition with relevant symptoms	May help myalgia, pseudogout and restless legs Seeking to normalize values to reduce vascular calcification less relevant for shorter prognosis
Fluid and sodium restriction	Sodium and total fluid intake may be limited where volume overload and breathlessness are significant symptoms	Where fluid overload not significant, less restriction may improve nutrition.

Excellent Symptom Control

Although patients in CC show considerable symptom burden (with on average 6–17 symptoms per patient), studies show that symptoms are often under-reported. Systematic use of assessment tools such as the POS-s renal are recommended.

Some symptoms clearly relate to deteriorating renal function (such as itching or nausea) and may come in clusters (such as pain relating to poor sleep and depression relating to QOL), so improvements in one may affect an entire cluster [5].

Depression is common amongst kidney patients, occurring in 20–30% of patients. Formal assessment using tools such as the Hospital Anxiety and Depression Scale (HADS) can help to reveal hidden depression which if left untreated is associated with higher morbidity and mortality, higher functional dependence, and worse quality of life. Symptoms, together with possible therapies, are listed in Tables 26.4 and 26.5. As no international guideline exists, we have included pragmatic guidance as used by the authors.

Studies have shown that with the input of a supportive care clinic, 57% of patients on CC can maintain similar or improved symptom scores and 58% have similar or improved QOL. Other non-renal symptoms such as mobility or memory

Table 26.4 Common symptoms in CKD stage 5, and suggested therapeutic approach

Symptom	% of CC patients with symptom	Possible contributing factor for correction	Non-pharmacological approach	Pharmacological approach
Fatigue, weakness, and sleep disturbance	Fatigue 70% sleep disturbance: 39%	Vit D deficiency Metabolic acidosis Hypo or hyperthyroidism Anxiety and depression. Medication toxicity e.g. Benzodiazepine, anti-depressants, opioids	Exercise Energy conservation strategies Optimise sleep hygiene	Sleep disturbance Gabapentin 50–300 mg at night* Amitriptyline 5 mg at night gradually increasing to a maximum of 25 mg Zopiclone 3.75–5 mg at night
Nociceptive pain	62%	Investigate and treat underlying cause of pain	Physiotherapy Nerve blocks Trigger point injections	As per modified WHO analgesic ladder Step 1 Paracetamol to maximum dose of 1 g 4 times per day Step 2 Tramadol to maximum 50 mg twice daily (watch for toxicity of accumulation) Step 3 Transdermal buprenorphine starting at 5 ucg per hour release
Neuropathic pain	62%	Investigate and treat underlying cause of pain	Physiotherapy Nerve blocks Trigger point injections	Gabapentin 50–300 mg per 24 h* Amitriptyline 10–25 mg per day Tramadol 25–50 mg (max 100 mg per 24 h) Buprenorphine transdermal patch increasing gradually from 5 mcg per hour
Uraemic pruritis	55%	Anemia and iron deficiency Allergies, infestation, contact dermatitis Dry skin Heat	Emollients with high water content Camphor 0.25%/menthol 0.25% emollient Avoid skin warming such as hot baths and electric blankets Short nails Night-time gloves	Gabapentin 50–300 mg daily 1–2 h before sleep*. Tricyclic anti-depressants e.g. amitriptyline 10–25 mg before bed Anti-histamines—although little evidence well tolerated and easy to judge if effective e.g. cetirizine

Table 26.4 (continued)

Symptom	% of CC patients with symptom	Possible contributing factor for correction	Non-pharmacological approach	Pharmacological approach
Anorexia	49%	Over -restrictive renal diet advice Chronic nausea Poor gastric emptying due to drug toxicity eg opiods Depression/social isolation/fatigue	Loosen diet See below Drug review See below	No convincing pharmacological interventions
Breathlessness	39%	Anxiety Correct Anaemia Correct Acidosis Treat Pulmonary oedema Treat Infection	Sit up Humid environment Salt and fluid advice	Frusemide 40–500 mg per 24 h. Erythropoietin Sodium bicarbonate (balance correction of acidosis against sodium load)
Anxiety and depression	Anxiety 34% Depression 28%	Sleep disturbance Untreated pain	Psychological support	Sertraline 50 mg od Amitriptyline 10–25 mg at night Citalopram 10 mg at night
Restless-leg syndrome	28%	Anemia and iron deficiency	r/o alcohol, caffeine, stimulants	Gabapentin 50–300 mg daily 1–2 h before sleep* Pramipexole and rotigotine dermal patch (require very slow titration) Clonazepam 500 mcg nocte if RLS associated with sleep disturbance
Nausea and vomiting	27%	Metabolic disturbance GI disturbance eg delayed gastric emptying Review medications (opioids and anti-depressants)	Treat constipation Small frequent meals	Ondansetron 4–8 mg per 8 h PRN Metoclopramide 10 mg up to three times per day before meals. Haloperidol 0.5 mg every 8 h (can be increased to max 5 mg per 24 h in severe refractory cases)

*Increase dose gradually, with long interval to minimize toxicity due to accumulation

Table 26.5 End of life symptom management in CKD stage 5

Mild pain, or fevers	Paracetamol/acetaminophen, 650–1000 mg QDS (max 4 g/24 h)
Pain Pain is not a common feature of ESKD, but may be caused by other comorbidities. The starting doses shown are for opioid-naïve patients—if a patient is already taking opioid painkillers, the dose should be converted to take account of this (see BNF, or local palliative care conversion tables)	Opioids: fentanyl and oxycodone generally better tolerated, with fewer side effects, than morphine and codeine Starting doses: Oxycodone po/sc 2.5–5 mg 2–4 hourly, titrate up as required or Fentanyl sc 25 mcg 2–4 hourly prn, titrated as required
Nausea	Cyclizine 50 mg tds (max 150 mg/24 h) or Ondansetron 4–8 mg 2–3 times daily or Metaclopramide 10 mg tds or Haloperidol 0.5–1 mg bd or (intractable nausea) Levomepromazine 6mg nocte orally, or 2.5–5 mg by subcutaneous injection

(continued)

Table 26.5 (continued)

Mild pain, or fevers	Paracetamol/acetaminophen, 650–1000 mg QDS (max 4 g/24 h)
Shortness of breath	Furosemide—very high doses (250–500 mg per day) may be required in end stage renal disease Fluid restriction <750 mLs/day (and salt restriction to manage thirst) Opioids, such as fentanyl or oxycodone
Secretions	Glycopyrronium 400–600 mcg (max 2.4 mg in 24 h) or Hyoscine hydrobromide 400 mcg qds
Agitation	Midazolam 0.5–1.0 mg every 4–6 h or Haloperidol 0.5–1.0 mg bd
Itch, dry skin This is a common symptom, often at higher eGFRs (<15 mL/min). Often blamed on high serum phosphate levels, there is no evidence that use of phosphate binders reduces uraemic itch, and tight dietary restrictions may not be appropriate at end of life. Lifestyle modification to avoid triggers, and use of emollients/topical creams is often sufficient to manage symptoms.	Emollients and other measures such as soap substitutes and avoiding triggers such as hot baths, or dry air (use a humidifier) Antihistamines Menthol 0.25%/camphor 0.25% in emollient cream Capsaicin 0.025% cream Gabapentin 100 mg nocte, or pregabalin 25 mg nocte Consider referral to dermatology for UVB phototherapy

difficulties, however, may relate to the wider health needs of the aging, frail patient; these are addressed in a later section.

Drug Chart Review

Many CC patients have acquired long burdensome drug lists. Some have little prognostic value for later life, others have significant side effects (e.g. anti-cholinergic drugs). Some are no longer indicated but have remained on charts, whilst others previously carried a clear indication but have been ineffective.

Regular reviews using tools such as STOPP-START can minimise both tablet burden and side effects.

Wider Needs Assessments

When kidney disease is advanced and drug management more specialised, a kidney clinic is often the principal source of support for CC patients. However, many suffer with geriatric syndromes, so ideally teams should build networks of care including access to comprehensive geriatric assessment (CGA) [6].

The CGA assessment process has been shown to improve outcomes in older clinically frail patients when assessed during hospital admissions, as measured by an improved chance of living in their own home one year after hospitalisation. It identifies medical, social and functional needs and uses an MDT approach to create a coordinated care plan. Key domains of assessment may include depression/anxiety, falls risk, cognition, polypharmacy, continence, skin integrity, nutrition, ADLs and social issues, with relevant referrals and signposting to services such as memory and falls clinic, or occupational and physiotherapy service. Such wider needs enquiries may also help patients and families to understand that correcting renal function alone is unlikely to improve quality of life, and time may be better spent on other interventions including advance care planning (ACP).

Creating a Network of Care

Nephrology services can offer excellent symptom management and psychological support for patients and their families, but true 24 h holistic end of life care requires involvement of the wider multidisciplinary community team, including inter-agency working (Fig. 26.2).

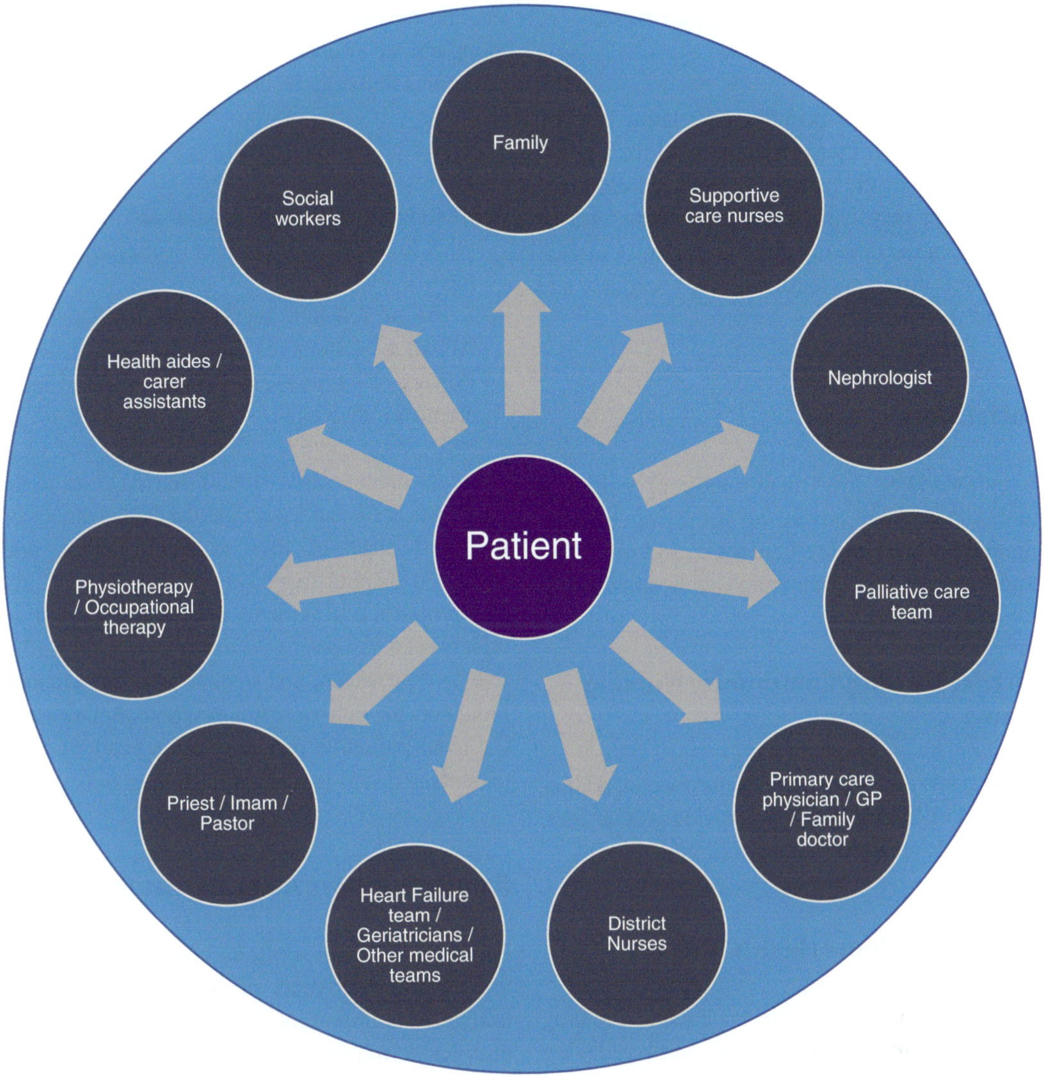

Fig. 26.2 Elements of a Network of Care

An existing network of care will ease the transition from secondary care to community end of life care, and reduce the chances of poor communication. Local health service arrangements will dictate precisely which other agencies need to be involved, but consider creating links with the following teams:

Palliative Care Teams

The palliative care team may provide community symptom management, help with creating Advance Care Planning documents (ACP), and support for families.

Primary Care/General Practitioners/ Family Medicine

Involvement of the primary care team is vital, both for community prescribing, and for a holistic overview of the patient's other medical problems. They may carry out home visits, and be involved in the drawing up of community DNAR (Do Not Attempt Resuscitation) orders and ACPs.

Social Work

Social workers, from nephrology or palliative care, can provide advice on accessing benefits entitlements, arranging homecare, and obtaining equipment such as commodes and hospital beds.

District Nursing/Community Nursing Teams

These teams may administer Erythropoetin, administer end of life medications, provide wound care, and provide pressure area monitoring.

Social Care/Home Health Aides

These provide personal care to patients, allowing them to stay in their own homes, while relieving some of the burden on family members. Good home care is essential to prevent unnecessary hospital admissions.

Advance Care Planning

Creating an Advance Care Plan allows patients to express their wishes about the end of life.

In many countries, ACPs are not legally binding, but are a useful way to structure a patient's thoughts and discussions about priorities, and how they envisage the end of their life. It is important that families, particularly surrogate decision-makers and next-of-kin, are involved in these discussions and are aware of the contents of an ACP.

Topics that may be covered include:

- preferred place of death,
- spiritual beliefs
- treatments that they would and would not wish to undergo (including resuscitation),
- next-of-kin
- a list of relevant legal documents such as Advance Directives, or medical Lasting Powers of Attorney, so that the medical team are aware they exist.

A recent meta-analysis found that creation of an ACP was associated with greater achievement of preferred place of care at death (PPC), and increased hospital-free days in the last year of life. The proportion of patients completing an ACP is widely seen as a surrogate marker for good palliative care provision, and is used as a performance indicator (the only performance outcome measure for renal palliative care services agreed by both patients and staff in a recent Delphi exercise).

Family Support After Bereavement

Patients and families often know the nephrology team well, after years of renal care. Seamless transition is important so that patients and their families do not feel "abandoned" by the move to community end of life care.

As well as formal grief counselling and support, which may be available via the primary care and/or community palliative care teams, some centres send a condolence card, or organise an annual departmental Service of Remembrance for patients who have died in the last twelve months (often appreciated by nephrology staff).

This is also important from the perspective of other patients within the department. If they feel that deceased patients are "brushed away" and forgotten, they may worry that the same will happen to them when they die.

Conclusions

For the 85 year old gentleman referred for consideration of kidney replacement therapy, his survival advantage with dialysis is very limited [e.g using Cohen's tool, his chance of surviving the first six months on dialysis is just 50%]. A better option for his further management may be for personalised conservative care to delay progression of his CKD, symptom control and advanced care planning.

Despite huge advances in renal care, evidence suggests that not all kidney patients genuinely benefit from kidney replacement therapy. The alternative conservative care pathway offers a high-quality holistic pathway for those in whom there will be no benefit, or for those who choose not to undergo the complexities of kidney replacement therapy in their frailer years.

Focusing on symptom control and addressing their wider needs (often related to co-morbidity), as well as building an excellent network of care and planning for the last days of life are all vital elements. It is always the duty of a professional to enable a patient to live well, but it is equally important to ensure patients approaching end of life are also able to die well (Table 26.6).

Questions

1. An 81 year old comes to AKCC with her grandson. She has an eGFR of 12 mL/min/1.73 m^2 and is of Indian heritage. She manages well, living with a supportive family and has no professional carers. She has not noticed any memory difficulties but no longer does her own banking. Which aspects of assessment may help you guide her through her treatment choices ?
   A. Clinical frailty score alone
   B. MoCA alone
   C. Assessment of patient's current priorities
   D. Consideration of rate of GFR decline
   E. All of the above

E. Despite the patient managing well without professional carers, a high level of family support may mask mobility or other practical difficulties which might impact on her ability to travel to a dialysis facility. Patient are not always aware of or willing to disclose memory difficulties; the fact that she no longer does her banking may hint at some loss of cognitive function which may impact on her ability to understand complex treatment choices. Her own priorities are vital as recognition that regular trips to see a beloved sister in India several times a year are a top priority may make a relatively constraining treatment such as dialysis less attractive. Her rate of GFR decline will directly impact her estimated survival if she chooses conservative kidney management so is a vital part of early assessment.

2. She chooses conservative care. You meet her later when she has developed more symptoms particularly neuropathic pain, poor sleep and low mood. How do you approach this problem.
   A. Tell her this is not related to her kidneys, and she should see her GP
   B. Explain it is a normal part of ageing, and she shouldn't expect to feel as healthy as she did when she was a girl.
   C. Carry out a comprehensive assessment of her symptoms, and institute a management plan which may involve both pharmacological and non-pharmacological interventions.
   D. Start gabapentin 300 mg nocte for her neuropathic pain, diazepam 10 mg nocte for her poor sleep, and mirtazapine 15 mg nocte for her low mood.
   E. Start a buprenorphine patch for her pain

C. The causes of her pain, poor sleep and low mood may be multifactorial, and may also be inter-related. For example, if she is anxious about her renal prognosis, this may be causing her low mood and poor sleep, and this may increase the intrusiveness of her pain. Careful and thorough history-taking is important to unpick the many aspects of her symptoms.

Renal patients experience high levels of medication side-effects, due to both polypharmacy, and accumulation of renally-

Table 26.6 Tools available to support conservative care (CC) programmes

Tool /programme	Focus	Link
Staff training		
Vital talk	Teaching resource for staff communication training	https://www.vitaltalk.org/
CKM Care	Resources of conservative kidney management programme developed by Alberta Health Service, Canada.	HYPERLINK "http://www.ckmcare.com " www.ckmcare.com
Kidney Supportive Care: Core Curriculum 2020	CPD covering all aspect of Conservative Care	See Gelfand et al. [4]
ACP toolkit	NHS/British Geriatric Society resources to help staff start the ACP process	https://ihub.scot/project-toolkits/anticipatory-care-planning-toolkit/anticipatory-care-planning-toolkit/guidance-for-health-and-social-care-professionals/ https://www.bgs.org.uk/sites/default/files/content/attachment/2018-04-18/Advance%20Care%20Planning%20Guideline.pdf https://www.goldstandardsframework.org.uk/advance-care-planning
Patient assessment tools		
Clinical Frailty Score	Simple visual scale that can be used by all members of MDT to assess level of frailty	https://www.nice.org.uk/guidance/ng159/resources/clinical-frailty-scale-pdf-8712262765
Charlson Comorbidity Index	Scoring system for comorbidity, higher scores associated with worse mortality	https://www.mdcalc.com/charlson-comorbidity-index-cci
Edmonton Frail Scale	Detailed assessment of frailty—includes physical and cognitive assessment	https://www.cgakit.com/fr-1-edmonton-frail-scale
WHO performance status	Scored from 0 (asymptomatic) to 5 (dead)	https://www.nice.org.uk/guidance/ta121/chapter/appendix-c-who-performance-status-classification
Karnofsky Performance Scale (KPS)	Scored from 100 (well) to 0 (dead)	https://www.mdcalc.com/karnofsky-performance-status-scale
BGS Clinical Frailty toolkit	Toolkit containing practical resources for assessing frailer patients	https://www.england.nhs.uk/rightcare/wp-content/uploads/sites/40/2019/07/frailty-toolkit-june-2019-v1.pdf
Decision support tools		
Alberta Health Services	Tool to help patients decide whether CC or RRT is right for them	www.ckmcare.com
YoDDA (Yorkshire Dialysis Decision Aid)	Accurate and balanced information about RRT/non-RRT options	http://www.yodda.leeds.ac.uk/Survey/Information
Symptom assessment tools		
POS-S Renal	Palliative care symptom assessment tool adapted to include common symptoms of CKD	https://www.ncbi.nlm.nih.gov/portal/utils/pageresolver.fcgi?recordid=5ff1be23bdb3052f32e0c7cf
Treatment guidance tools		
STOPP START tool	Toolkit to help clinicians reduce polypharmacy	https://www.cgakit.com/m-2-stopp-start

excreted metabolites. Many prefer to "put up with" symptoms in order to reduce pill burden. Non-pharmacological treatments such as sleep hygiene, gentle exercise and counselling for low mood and lethargy, distraction techniques and medicated emollients for pruritis and neuropathic pain, and simply addressing her health-related concerns directly in a gentle and reassuring way, may reduce many of her symptoms to a more manageable intensity.

GPs often shy away from prescribing in CKD stage 5, and it is the responsibility of the nephrology team to provide guidance on medications which are and are not safe to use in these patients, with appropriate dose reductions where necessary.

It is true that "she should not expect to feel as healthy as she did when she was a girl", but it is also unhelpful and does nothing to address her very treatable symptoms. Neither does it foster a good doctor-patient relationship.

Gabapentin certainly has an important place in the management of neuropathic pain, but 300 mg nocte is too high a starting dose and is likely to lead to over-sedation, which will also increase her falls risk. Prescribing gabapentin in combination with diazepam and mirtazapine, in a naïve patient with CKD stage 5, would be extremely dangerous.

Buprenorphine is not indicated for first-line management of neuropathic pain.

3. Her symptoms improve but 12 months later with an eGFR of 7 mL/min/1.73 m^2, her family ask for her to be seen urgently as she has "changed her mind and wishes to have dialysis". How do you approach this request?
   A. Arrange an urgent dialysis start
   B. Suggest a trial of dialysis
   C. Decline the request as she has previously made a choice for to follow a conservative management pathway
   D. Meet the patient with her family, confirm that she does wish to change her treatment pathway and organise line insertion to start dialysis.
   E. Meet the patient with her family, and find out what has prompted this change of decision before making any hard-to-reverse changes to her management plan.

E. It is important to establish why she has changed her mind—have her symptoms worsened, or do her family believe that she will live longer if she chooses to have dialysis? She has attended with her grandson in the past, but he may not be the family's main decision-maker. Ensure her whole family have a clear understanding of what dialysis can and cannot achieve, and understand that her life expectancy is limited either with or without dialysis.

Manage any new symptoms, and reassure her that she will not be in any pain or discomfort (fluid overload is particularly difficult for patients to tolerate, and is a frequent trigger for decisions to change modality, but can often be managed well without dialysis).

Alternatively, she may have chosen CC in the past, to avoid dialysis "unless I really need it"—many patients, particularly those who are older, are extremely keen to avoid upheaval and change in their lives, and may choose to delay dialysis discussions for the time being by choosing conservative management. Others, with executive function impairment, may have been unable to make a decision about modality until a crisis point has been reached. Families will often report "she didn't really understand what she was agreeing to". A trial of dialysis may seem a good option but can often extend for several months. Such longer trials can lead to loss of native function so that if she subsequently decides to stop, she may have a shorter life expectancy than if she had not commenced dialysis.

4. Three months later, she and her family are happy with Conservative Care, but she and her family still want her to be resuscitated. How do you approach this?
   A. Accept that it is her right to request CPR, even if it would be futile.
   B. Seek advice from the hospital legal team about lack of concordance of views in CPR status
   C. Agree to CPR for her and her family's peace of mind.

D. Explain that CPR is a medical decision, and complete a DNAR order for her.
E. Talk to her about her understanding of CPR, and her ideas about end of life in general.

E. Many people, particularly older patients, worry that agreeing not to be resuscitated means that they will not receive any medical care at all. Reassure her that this is not the case. Explain what is involved in resuscitation, and what CPR can and cannot do. Explore her plans for end of life (preferred place of death, degree of medicalisation, etc), and whether CPR would align with those goals. Help her to complete an ACP document which sets out her wishes. Whilst it is important to be up to date with the legal position in your own health care system, these situations generally reflect communication difficulties, which should be addressed first.

5. She confirms that she does not want to be resuscitated, and wishes to die at home with her family. Six months later, you are called by her daughter. She has been in bed for the past two weeks, and has been sleeping for most of the day. Tonight, she has woken and is very restless and agitated. Her daughter is distressed, and asks for help. What do you suggest?
   A. Bring her in to the Emergency Department for an assessment.
   B. Tell her daughter it sounds like she needs to start dialysis
   C. She has chosen supportive care, so is no longer a renal patient—they should call her GP in the morning
   D. This sounds like terminal agitation, and they need urgent palliative care input to manage her symptoms
   E. Explain that you will write a referral to the local hospice team.

D. The history of increasing sleepiness and lethargy suggest that this lady is approaching end of life. She has now developed symptoms (agitation and restlessness), which are not controlled by her current medications, and which are causing her and her family some distress.

Ideally, the community palliative care team (or local equivalent) would already be involved in her care. If not (perhaps because this deterioration was unanticipated), an urgent referral should be done.

An emergency home visit needs to be made, this evening, by either the renal team, palliative care team, or family doctor (the most appropriate person will depend on the structure of local services), and a full assessment of her symptoms and care needs should be made. It is not reasonable to leave her in distress until the following day.

It is also not reasonable ask a family to bring a dying woman to the ED, as there is a high chance of her either dying during the journey, or in a distressing environment such as the busy ED treatment area, instead of at home as she wished.

For symptoms such as terminal agitation, a combination of either midazolam or haloperidol, plus fentanyl, may be added to a syringe driver to manage her symptoms overnight. A full assessment of her care needs (physical, emotional, spiritual, and family support needs) can be made once the immediate crisis has passed.

Test your learning and check your understanding of this book's contents: use the "Springer Nature Flashcards" app to access questions using https://sn.pub/cz9Cok. To use the app, please follow the instructions in Chap. 1.

References

1. Davison SN, Levin A, Moss AH, et al. Executive summary of the KDIGO Controversies Conference on Supportive Care in Chronic Kidney Disease: developing a roadmap to improving quality care. Kidney Int. 2015;88(3):447–59.
2. Brown EA, Brown E, Chambers EJ, Eggeling C. End of life care in nephrology: from advanced disease to bereavement. OUP Oxford; 2007.
3. Hole B, Hemmelgarn B, Brown E, et al. Supportive care for end-stage kidney disease: an integral part of kidney services across a range of income settings around the world. Kidney Int Suppl. 2020;10(1):e86–94.
4. Gelfand SL, Scherer JS, Koncicki HM. Kidney supportive care: core curriculum 2020. Am J Kidney Dis. 2020;75(5):793–806.
5. Raghavan D, Holley JL. Conservative care of the elderly CKD patient: a practical guide. Adv Chronic Kidney Dis. 2016;23(1):51–6.
6. Nixon AC, Brown J, Brotherton A, et al. Implementation of a frailty screening programme and Geriatric Assessment Service in a nephrology centre: a quality improvement project. J Nephrol. 2020;

27 Electrolytes & Acid Base Disorders

Gates B. Colbert, Ajay Kher, Kareem Genena, and Edgar V. Lerma

Clinical Scenario

A 48-year-old man with a past medical history of Heart Failure with Reduced Ejection Fraction (HFrEF) 25% and Chronic Kidney Disease Stage III (CKD) is referred to the emergency room from CKD Clinic. He has been struggling with volume overload and his diuretic Torsemide has been increased from 20 mg per day to 100 mg per day. He reports weight loss of about 10 kg and improvement in his edema. The patient has been urinating large volumes for several weeks and reports increased fatigue. His vital signs were within normal ranges, but outpatient labs returned abnormal with Na 121 mEq/L, K 2.9 mEq/L, Cl 95 mEq/L, HCO_3 38 mEq/L, BUN 44 mEq/L, and Cr 1.5 mg/dL.

Introduction

Volume management is a difficult clinical problem for patients with HFrEF and CKD. Patients frequently retain sodium and water, due to decreased kidney perfusion and increase renin-angiotensin activation from both disease states. Electrolyte balance can be difficult with both Hyper- and Hypo- electrolyte conditions due to diet, medications, and treatments of HFrEF and CKD. This chapter will address the electrolyte imbalances above, as well as the opposing high or low electrolyte clinical scenarios.

Hyponatremia

Hyponatremia is defined as a serum sodium concentration, Na <135 mEq/L, and is encountered in up to 30% of hospitalized patients (Table 27.1) [1, 2]. A few key concepts should be reviewed to facilitate the management of this disorder (Table 27.2).

1. Serum Na is determined by the sum of total body exchangeable sodium and potassium divided by total body water [3]. In fact, most disorders of Na are secondary to changes in total body water rather than changes in total body sodium.
2. Serum Na is the major determinant of serum osmolality and is tightly regulated by an inter-

G. B. Colbert
Texas A&M College of Medicine at Dallas, Dallas, TX, USA
e-mail: Gates.Colbert@BSWHealth.org

A. Kher
Vishwasth Clinic, Noida, Uttar Pradesh, India
e-mail: ajay@vishwasth.com

K. Genena
Baylor University Medical Center, Dallas, TX, USA

E. V. Lerma (✉)
Section of Nephrology, University of Illinois at Chicago College of Medicine/Advocate Christ Medical Center, Oak Lawn, IL, USA

D. Banerjee et al. (eds.), *Management of Kidney Diseases*,
https://doi.org/10.1007/978-3-031-09131-5_27

use of desmopressin with 3% saline is advocated for by some and has been shown to reduce the incidence of overcorrection.

Hypernatremia

Etiology

Hypernatremia is defined as a serum Na > 145 mEq/L, and could be secondary to water deficit (most common), solute excess, or water shift into cells (Tables 27.3 and 27.4). Hypernatremia results in hypertonicity and normally stimulates the thirst mechanism with ADH release and subsequent production of a concentrated urine. Restricted or insufficient water intake is necessary for hyponatremia to develop. Even individuals with complete diabetes insipidus (DI) maintain near-normal [Na] if access to water is not restricted. Rarely, a hypothalamic disorder impairing thirst is the culprit in hypernatremia. The predominant symptom of hyponatremia is thirst. Altered mental status has been associated in severe cases.

Diagnosis

Two primary diagnostic questions can help solve a case of hypernatremia:

1. Is there a loss of water?
2. Why is the patient not drinking appropriately?

Non-kidney water loss is evident from the patient's history. Kidney water loss is manifested as polyuria and is divided into 2 main categories: diabetes insipidus and osmotic diuresis. The kidney's ability to concentrate urine in cases of non-

Table 27.3 Causes of Hypernatraemia

A. Water Deficit	*Non-Kidney water loss*	Vomiting
		Diarrhea
		Sweat
		Insensible losses
	Kidney water loss	Central diabetes insipidus
		Nephrogenic diabetes insipidus
		Osmotic diuresis
	Adipsia	
B. Solute Excess		Ingestion of salt
		Infusion of hypertonic solution
		Mineralocorticoid excess
C. Shift of Water into Cells		Seizures
		Excessive exercise

Table 27.4 Causes of Kidney water loss

Central Diabetes Insipidus	Mutations in vasopressin
	Pituitary tumors and infiltrative disease
	CNS infections
	Neurosurgery and trauma
	Anoxic encephalopathy
	Idiopathic
Nephrogenic Diabetes Insipidus	Mutations in V2 receptor or aquaporin 2
	Drugs (e.g., lithium, amphotericin B, demeclocycline)
	Kidney interstitial disease
	Obstructive uropathy
	Hypokalemia
	Hypercalcemia
Osmotic Diuresis	Glucose
	Urea
	Mannitol

kidney water loss is usually preserved and the urine osmolality is typically >600–800 mosm/kg. The urine osmolality in central and complete nephrogenic DI is usually <300 mosm/kg but could be higher in partial nephrogenic DI. Response of the urine osmolarity and volume to exogenous desmopressin differentiates central from nephrogenic DI. In cases of osmotic diuresis, the daily osmole excretion (urine osmolality x urine volume) typically exceeds 1000 mosm/day. In states of solute excess, the extracellular space is usually expanded and urine Na is typically >100 mmol/L (Fig. 27.1).

Limited access to water is often due to altered mental status or physical debility. A hypothalamic lesion impairing the thirst mechanism should be suspected in alert patients with free access to water.

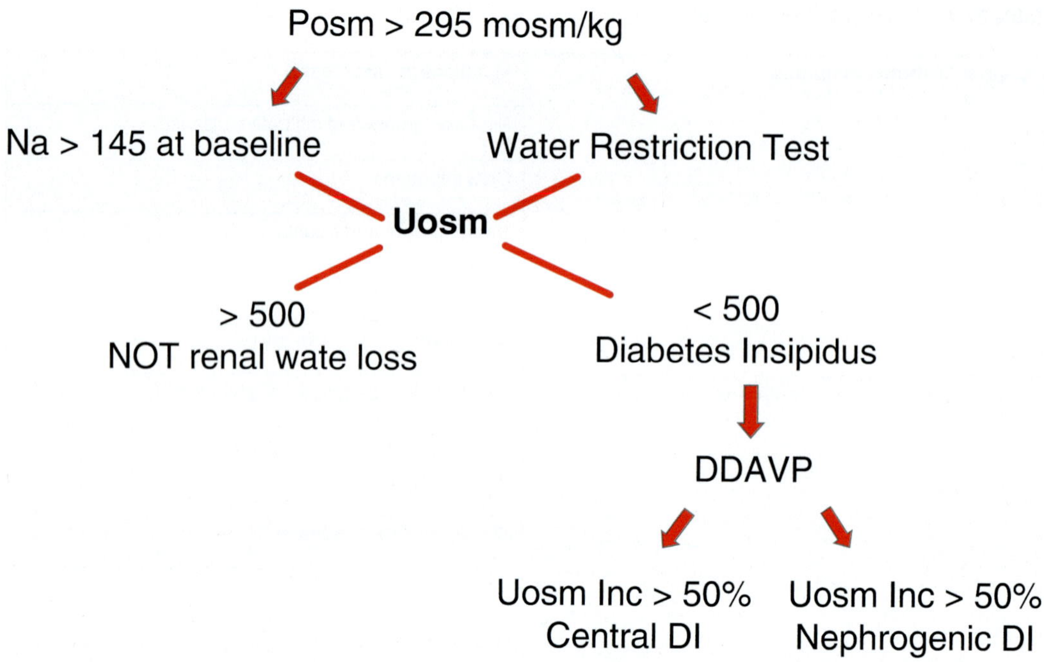

Fig. 27.1 Algorithm for determining central vs nephrogenic diabetes insipidus

Treatment of Hypernatraemia

The water deficit can be estimated from the equation: {(serum [Na] − 140)/140} × total body water. The rate of correction should be limited to 12 mEq/L per day. One liter of dextrose 5% water provides 1 L of free water, while 1 L of 0.45% saline provides 500 mL of free water. Concomitant volume depletion should be treated with isotonic fluids before the water deficit is replaced with hypotonic fluids.

Non-kidney water loss: The source of water loss should be addressed if possible.

Osmotic diuresis: Hyperglycemia should be treated. High protein feeding should be modified.

Central DI: Treated with desmopressin acetate. Usual maintenance dose is 10–20 mcg intranasally once or twice daily.

Nephrogenic DI: Electrolytes abnormalities should be corrected, and offending medications should be discontinued if possible. A low-salt and low-protein diet reduces the obligate kidney water loss since the urine osmolality is fixed at a low value. Thiazide diuretics impair the distal tubule's diluting capacity. Amiloride can be used in lithium-induced DI.

Adipsia: Forced water intake with monitoring of weight, urine output and point of care [Na] when available.

Solute excess: Loop diuretics together with free water.

Hypokalemia

The majority of potassium is intracellular and initial buffering (intracellular shifts) of potassium absorbed from diet is critical to ensure that extracellular potassium does not have large shifts post meals (Fig. 27.2). Any alterations in these mechanisms can lead to hypokalemia or hyperkalemia (Table 27.5).

Kidney elimination of potassium is critical for maintaining potassium homeostasis. Kidney

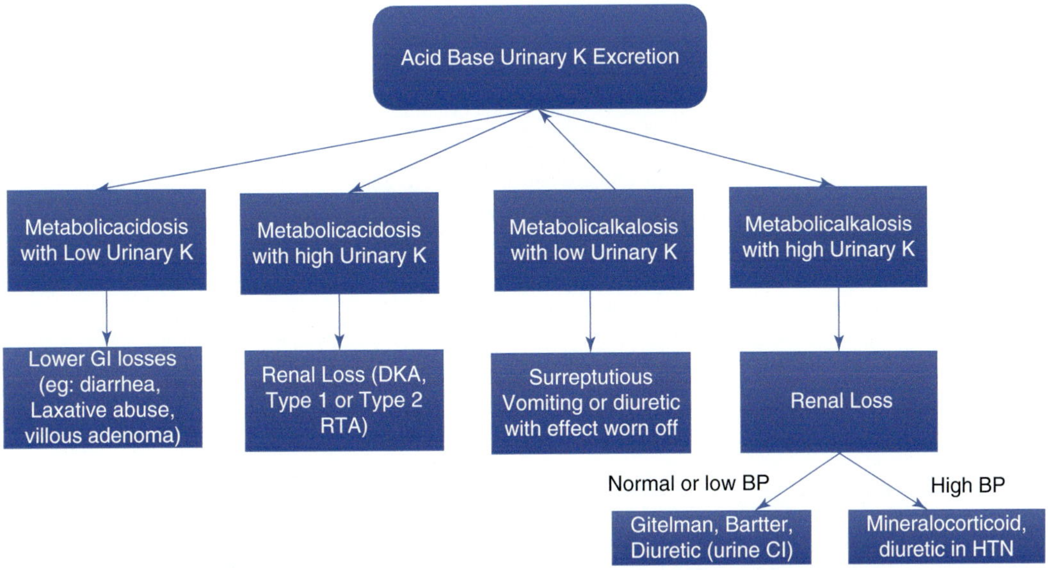

Fig. 27.2 Diagnostic algorithm for hypokalemia

elimination is determined by the following factors: adequate distal tubular delivery, serum potassium, and the presence of aldosterone. Due to the huge adaptability of the kidney excretion of potassium (20 meq–400 meq), diet alone is seldom a cause for hypokalemia or hyperkalemia, though it can be a contributing factor. Changes in distal delivery, Aldosterone, or kidney function can lead to hypokalemia or hyperkalemia.

Signs and symptoms of hypokalemia are listed in Table 27.6. The three most common causes of hypokalemia are vomiting, diarrhea, and diuretics and these are usually self evident on history and examination (Table 27.5). However, if etiology is not clear a systematic evaluation requires a combination of acid- base status (metabolic acidosis/metabolic alkalosis) with kidney potassium excretion (low or high potassium excretion) to provide the answer (Fig. 27.2).

Table 27.5 Causes of Hypokalemia

Low potassium dietary intake	(not usually sole cause)	
Transcellular shift of potassium	Increased pH (metabolic alkalosis)	
	Increased insulin	
	Increased Beta adrenergic activity (stress or medications)	
	Periodic paralysis	
	Cell Turnover (treatment of megaloblastic anemia/ GM-CSF)	
	Pseudohypokalemia	(eg: AML, post blood collection)
	Others	Barium intoxication Chloroquine intoxication
Renal Loss of potassium	Loop and thiazide diuretics	
	Gitelman and Bartter Syndrome	
Increased mineralocorticoid activity	Primary Mineralocorticoid excess	Primary Hyperaldosteronism (adenoma, hyperplasia, carcinoma) Cushings disease Exogenous Mineralocorticoid (fludrocortisone) Hyperreninism (Renal artery stenosis, Renin producing tumor) Glucocorticoid remediable hyperaldosteronism Hypersecretion of Deoxycorticosterone or other mineralocorticoid Licorice or other mineralocorticoids
	Liddle's Syndrome	
	Amphotericin B Hypomagnesemia	
Increased distal delivery/flow	Polyuria	
	Salt wasting nephropathies	
Non kidney causes	Vomiting (urinary K loss contributes)	
	Diarrhoea	
	Dialysis	

Table 27.6 Signs and symptoms of hypokalemia

Muscle weakness	Starts with lower extremity and can progress to trunk and upper extremity
	Respiratory failure– respiratory muscle weakness
	Intestinal Ileus (Pseudo-obstruction)
	Rhabdomyolysis
Cardiac Arrhythmias	ECG changes: Delayed Ventricular repolarization, Depression of ST segment, decrease in amplitude of T waves and increase in amplitude of U waves (esp V4-V6)
	Premature atrial or ventricular beats, sinus bradycardia, atrioventricular blocks, Ventricular tachycardia or ventricular fibrillation.

Treatment of Hypokalaemia

The goals of treatment in hypokalemia are to prevent or treat life threatening complications (arrhythmias, paralysis and rhabdomyolysis), replace potassium loss (if actual deficit and not due to transcellular shifts) and diagnose and treat underlying cause. It is important to recognise whether the hypokalemia is due to transient potassium loss (kidney or gastrointestinal) for which potassium replenishment and resolution of underlying cause is appropriate or whether this a steady state (Bartter, Gitelman, hyperaldosteronism, stable diuretic doses with need for continued use) where supplementation is unlikely to correct the hypokalemia and hence potassium sparing diuretics (amiloride/triamterene) or mineralocorticoid antagonists (spironolactone/ eplerenone) are more appropriate. Another important aspect is the amount of potassium deficit (if not due to transcellular shift) required to cause a serum potassium of 3 meq/L is 200–400 meq and 2 meq/L is 400–800 meq (Table 27.7).

Table 27.7 Treatment of hypokalemia

Principle	Degree or cause	Treatment
1. Prevent or treat life threatening complications	**Severe Hypokalemia**	Intravenous Potassium Chloride (20-40 meq/L of saline solution or dextrose). Usually at rate not more than 10 meq/hour (central vein). Avoid dextrose if possible as this will increase endogenous insulin and lead to transcellular shift of potassium and worsen hypokalemia. Additional oral potassium should be provided as larger quantities can be provided through this route. Likely deficit fora K of 3 meq/L is 200-400 meq and for a K of 2 meq/L is 400-800 meq. Frequent monitoring is needed as ongoing losses are not accounted in deficit estimate.
	Mild - moderate Hypokalemia (3-3.5 meq/L)	Usually, oral potassium chloride of 60-80 meq/day. However, larger amounts may be needed if potassium loss is expected to continue.
2. Diagnose and correct underlying cause	**Low dietary intake**	Augment diet
	Transcellular shift	Correct shift, supplement potassium only if severe symptoms (eg: paralysis) as likely overshoot later.
	Kidney Elimination	
	Diuretics	Stop if possible, if ongoing need then add potassium sparing diuretics (amiloride/triamterene/spironolactone/eplerenone)
	Mineralocorticoid	Remove mineralocorticoid if possible (eg: adenoma, licorice) or add Mineralocorticoid antagonist or potassium sparing diuretic (amiloride/triamterene) Supplementing with oral or IV potassium is unlikely to significantly alter potassium as these patients are at "steady state"

Hyperkalemia

Hyperkalemia results from increased potassium out of the intracellular space and into the plasma space (Table 27.8). The vast majority of total body potassium is intracellular. When potassium remains outside of the cell, hyperkalemia results without prompt ability of the body to eliminate the excess potassium.

Potassium buffering: It is important to recognize the vital role played by buffering in daily potassium management of the body (Figs. 27.3, 27.4, 27.5).

The signs and symptoms of hyperkalemia are listed in Table 27.9.

Treatment of hyperkalemia is focused on 3 steps: (Tables 27.10, 27.11)

1. If membrane instability (ECG changes as in Figure B) then stabilize the membrane (IV calcium gluconate/calcium chloride)
2. Shift potassium intracellularly, if membrane instability and need time to implement/derive benefit from step 3.
3. Remove potassium from body

Table 27.8 Causes of Hyperkalaemia

High potassium dietary intake		(not usually sole cause)
Transcellular shift of potassium		Decreased pH (Metabolic acidosis)
		Insulin deficiency
		Beta- adrenergic blockade
		Periodic paralysis
		Cell lysis/Tissue catabolism Severe exercise
		Pseudohyperkalemia (during collection – repeated clenching with tourniquet, hemolysis or post collection – cell lysis)
		Others: Succinylcholine Digitalis overdose
Decreased renal excretion of potassium		Impaired kidney excretion (acute or chronic)
Decreased mineralocorticoid activity	**Decreased RAAS:**	Hyporeninemic hypoaldosteronism NSAIDS ACE-inhibitors/ARBs Calcineurin inhibitors
	Decreased Adrenal synthesis :	Low cortisol (primary adrenal insufficiency, congenital adrenal hyperplasia) Normal cortisol (heparin, isolated hypoaldosteronism, post adrenal adenoma removal)
	Aldosterone resistance:	Potassium sparing diuretics Pseudohypoaldosteronism
		Selective potassium secretion defects
		Type 4 Renal Tubular Acidosis
Decreased distal delivery		Volume depletion (true or effective)

NSAID: non-steroidal anti-inflammatory drugs, ACE: angiotensin converting enzyme, ARB: angiotensin receptor blocker

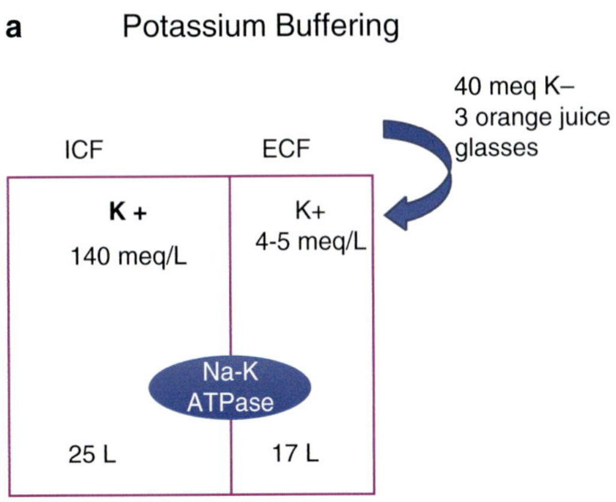

Fig. 27.3 Potassium Buffering 1. Figure represents the potassium distribution of the body and the person is about to drink 3 glasses of orange juice (net K load 40 meq)

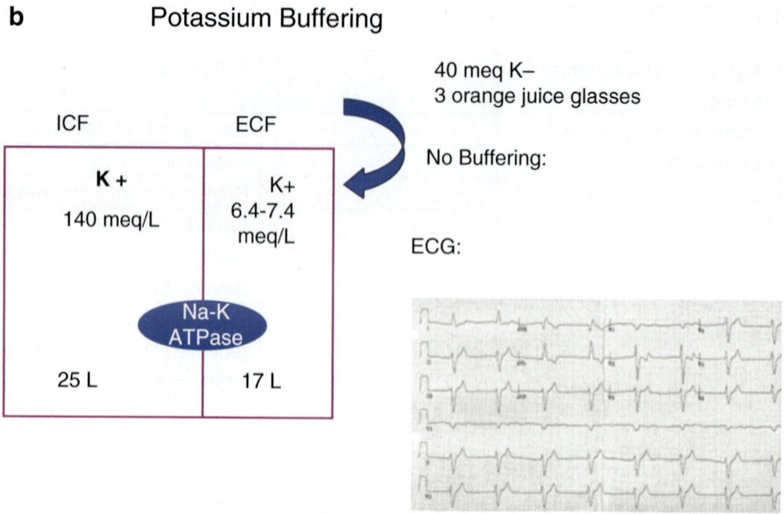

Fig. 27.4 Potassium buffering II. *Diagram illustrates what would happen if there was no buffering of the potassium to the intracellular compartment, significant increase in potassium and lead to bradycardia as shown in the ECG*

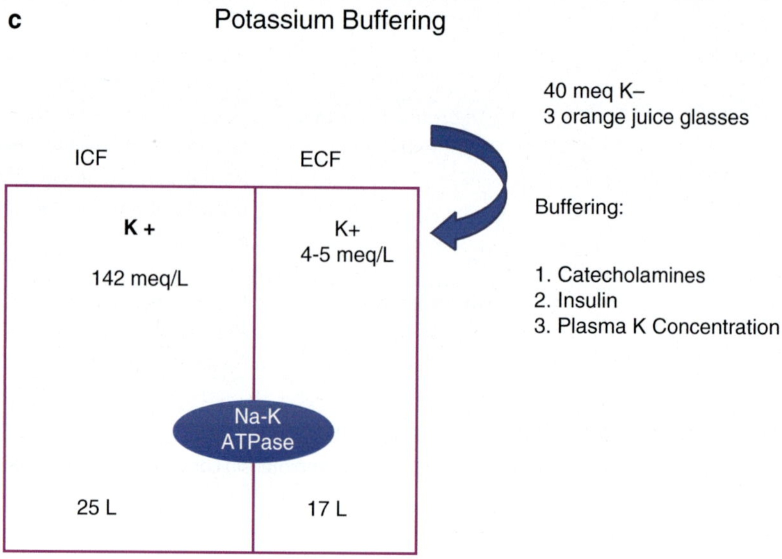

Fig. 27.5 Potassium Buffering III. *Diagram illustrates that buffering due to the serum potassium level, Insulin and catecholamines, leads to a limited increase in serum potassium*

Table 27.9 Signs and symptoms of hyperkalemia

Muscle Weakness	Begins with lower extremity and ascends to trunk and upper extremity
	Paralysis
Cardiac Arrhythmia	ECG Changes (Figure 3)
	Sine-wave or cardiac standstill
	Ventricular fibrillation
Asymptomatic	

Table 27.10 Treatment of hyperkalemia

Step 1. Stabilize the membrane. (If no ECG changes and hyperkalemia is not severe, can skip step 1)	IV calcium gluconate or Calcium Chloride Usual dose 10ml of 10% calcium gluconate	Give if there are ECG changes as demonstrated in Figure B. Continue to monitor ECG and continue to repeat calcium every 5 minutes till ecg changes reversed. Calcium chloride has 3 times the calcium of calcium gluconate but requires a central line for administration
Step 2. Shift Potassium into the cell (to buy time till step 3 can work) **If hyperkalemia is not severe and there is enough time for step 3 to work, then can skip step 2**	Glucose and insulin IV Usual Dose: 10 units of regular insulin with 30-50gm of glucose	Impact starts in minutes, peaks at 1 hours and lasts 4-6 hours with a lowering of 0.5-1.5meq/L (if hyperglycemia is present, can give insulin alone)
	Sodium Bicarbonate IV Usual dose: 50meq given over 5 mins	Impact starts in 1 hour and lasts 4-6 hours, with lowering of 0.5meq/L Impact is low in patients with kidney failure and those who don't have metabolic acidosis
	Beta 2 adrenergic agonists (inhaled) Usual dose: anti-hyperkalemic dose is 10-20mg of albuterol over 10 mins	Impact starts in 60-90 minutes and lasts 4-6 hours with a lowering of 0.5-1.5 meq/L Tachycardia and angina can be precipitated and so avoid in active coronary disease
Step 3. Removal from the body	Diuretics	Loop or thiazide diuretics or their combination, if there is enough kidney function If not volume overloaded then may combine with IVF (normal saline or bicarbonate) to increase distal delivery
	Cation exchange resins	Sodium polystyrene, Patiromer, Sodium zirconium cyclosilicate Take time to act and need active gut motility, risk of intestinal necrosis, hence avoid in conditions listed in Table 7
	Dialysis Treatment	May be needed for those with limited or no renal function

Table 27.11 Exchange resins for hyperkalemia

Potassium Binding Agent	Usual Dosing	Exchanges	Concerns
Sodium Polystyrene Sulfonate	15g given 1-4 times a day	Exchanges potassium for sodium. Also binds magnesium and calcium	Intestinal necrosis. Electrolyte abnormalities (hypokalemia). Fluid overload if sensitive to sodium. GI symptoms
Patiromer	8.4g daily and increase dose in 8.4g increments	Exchanges potassium for calcium. Also binds magnesium	Hypomagnesemia, hypokalemia. GI symptoms
Sodium Zirconium Cyclosilicate	10g thrice a day for first 48 hours, maintenance doses from 5g alternate day to 15g daily (adjust in 5g increments)	Exchanges potassium for hydrogen and sodium.	Edema Hypokalemia

Metabolic Alkalosis

Getting back to our patient with metabolic alkalosis and a serum HCO_3 38. Metabolic alkalosis is defined as a rise in serum bicarbonate concentration above 30 mEq/L, and usually accompanied by an increase in the serum pH. This state is usually prevalent when two conditions occur: a process leading to the increase in bicarbonate concentration, and a situation that prevents excess bicarbonate excretion through the kidneys [5]. Normal kidney function allows for complete excretion of excess bicarbonate that the body does not require to maintain pH around the normal 7.40 range. Several processes increase serum bicarbonate concentration and can be seen in Table 27.12. Some common situations are hydrogen loss from gastric secretions, excess urinary acid loss from diuretics in the kidney, a shift of hydrogen ions into the cell, and exogenous sodium bicarbonate or equivalent ingestion.

Measurement of urine chloride levels can be helpful to determine the etiology of metabolic alkalosis (Table 27.13).

Treatment of metabolic alkalosis should be targeted at two main causes, the source of bicarbonate generation and reversal of diminished kidney excretion. Treating the underlying cause or condition is paramount if it is reversible. Limiting conditions of vomiting, excess gastric secretion removal, halting loop or thiazide diuretics can make a quick impact. Gastric loss of acid can be treated with medications that reduce gastric acid (HCl) secretion such as H2 blockers or proton pump inhibitors that may improve serum alkalosis. Exogenous sources and ingestions of alkali should be stopped. Bicarbonate salts such as sodium bicarbonate or potassium bicarbonate should be held, as well as any anions that are metabolized to bicarbonate such as citrate or lactate.

Kidney excretion of excess bicarbonate should be optimized to return serum bicarbonate to normal levels. Restoring EABV will promote bicarbonaturia, as well as correcting chloride depletion, hypochloremia, and hypokalemia. Improvement in raising EABV is most effectively achieved with chloride containing solutions such as isotonic saline 0.9% which not only restores volume but provides adequate chloride

Table 27.12 Common causes of metabolic alkalosis

Gastrointestinal acid loss	Kidney acid loss	Hypokalemia	Alkali administration with reduced kidney function	Contraction alkalosis
Vomiting	Primary mineralocorticoid excess conditions	Villous adenoma	Calcium-alkali syndrome	
Gastric suction	Licorice ingestion	Malnutrition	Bicarbonate infusion	
Congenital chloride diarrhea	Liddle syndrome	Laxative abuse	Bicarbonate salt ingestions	
	Apparent mineralocorticoid excess state			
	Loop or thiazide diuretics			
	Bartter or Gitelman syndrome			
	Post chronic hypercarbia state			

Table 27.13 Causes of metabolic alkalosis utilizing a urine chloride level

Low urine Chloride (<20 mEq/L)	Normal Urine Chloride (>20 mEq/L)
Vomiting or nasogastric suction	Primary hyperaldosteronism
Diuretic-induced alkalosis	Liddle's syndrome
Laxative abuse	Excess licorice ingestion (glycyrrhizic acid)
Cystic fibrosis with sweat loss	Apparent mineralocorticoid excess syndrome
Congenital chloride diarrhea	Bartter syndrome
	Gitelman syndrome
	Hypokalemia

to the serum [6]. Improvement in heart failure, nephrotic syndrome, and cirrhosis exacerbations can improve effective blood volume out of the so called "third space". Improving the EABV will restore the kidney's ability to reduce reabsorption of sodium and chloride and allow bicarbonate losses in the urine. The increased filtrate delivery to the distal tubule will allow acid secretion through the type B intercalated cells as well. Once this is achieved, bicarbonaturia can be measured with a urinary pH above 7 (Table 27.14).

Patients with impaired kidney function have great difficulty with bicarbonaturia generation. In some patients with markedly elevated serum bicarbonate levels, dialysis may be needed to remove the excess bicarbonate. Low bicarbonate baths are usually used but have a high floor usually much higher than a normal HCO_3 of 24 mEq/L. Continuous renal replacement therapy (CRRT) may be used as more tailored dialysate baths are available that could contain lower amounts of sodium bicarbonate, and some preparations are made with sodium lactate. Severe and rare cases of metabolic alkalosis of bicarbonate levels greater than 50 mEq/l and/or pH greater than 7.55 may need acid infusion [7]. Intravenous HCl or precursors such as ammonium chloride can be infused as a 0.1 N(100 mEq/L) solution of HCl in normal saline.

Table 27.14 Management of metabolic alkalosis

Source of HCO3 excess	Treatments	MOA	Limitations
Vomiting	Anti-emetic medications	Limits gastric HCl loss and HCO3 generation	Does not restore volume lost
Gastric suction	Stop suction	Limits gastric HCl loss and HCo3 generation	Does not restore volume lost
	H2 blocker or proton pump inhibitors	Limits gastric HCl loss and HCO3 generation	Must tolerate oral therapy
Exogenous sources	Stop bicarbonate salts (bicarbonate, citrate, lactate)	Halts exogenous HCO3 excess	May have stomach upset if known ulceration or GI disease
True volume depletion	Restore volume with intravenous and oral fluid - Recommend isotonic saline 0.9%	Halts HCO3 reclamation in proximal tubule, promotes bicarbonaturia	Need to avoid volume overload
Inadequate EABV	Correct disease exacerbations such as heart failure, nephrotic syndrome, cirrhosis	Pulls volume into vascular space and improves oncotic pressure	Disease severity is variable and may not be correctable
	Potassium chloride	Offsets Cl losses	May cause hyperkalemia or metabolic acidosis
	Acetazolamide	Carbonic anhydrase inhibitor in proximal tubule of nephron	Sulfa based medication, hypokalemia, cannot be used in cirrhosis, chronic lung disease or late stage CKD
Post hypercapnic metabolic state	Acetazolamide	Carbonic anhydrase inhibitor in proximal tubule of nephron	Sulfa based medication, hypokalemia, cannot be used in cirrhosis, chronic lung disease or late stage CKD
Life threatening metabolic alkalosis	Dialysis therapy	Removes excess bicarbonate	Need for dialysis catheter, machine, and staffing resources, High cost
	Intravenous HCl or ammonium chloride	Offsets HCO3 by giving exogenous acid	Necrosis of tissues, toxicity, metabolic acidosis

Metabolic Acidosis

Metabolic acidosis is a frequent problem with patients experiencing both acute kidney injury (AKI) and chronic kidney disease (CKD). While regional and cultural diets are highly variable, those consuming a typical Western Hemisphere diet consume 15,000 mmol of carbon dioxide and 50–100 mEq of nonvolatile acid are produced each day. To maintain appropriate serum acid-base balance, the lungs and kidneys work together to excrete both these elements. The kidney must excrete acid as a combination of hydrogen ions with titratable acids, particularly phosphate and ammonia. Ammonia (NH_3) conversion to ammonium NH_4^+ is an adaptive response from metabolism of glutamine and the process can be increased as needed during episodes of acid loading [8].

Metabolic acidosis is defined as a process that increases the concentration of hydrogen ions in the body, thus lowering the bicarbonate concentration. Acidemia is defined as a lower arterial serum pH <7.35, which can result from pathologic processes of metabolic acidosis, respiratory acidosis, or both. Metabolic acidosis can be measured with a low serum bicarbonate usually <23 mEq/L [9]. Interestingly not every patient with a metabolic acidosis will have a lower arterial pH. Both the pH and hydrogen ion concentration depend upon the coexistence of other acid-base disorders. Therefore, the pH in each individual patient will vary depending on the level of metabolic acidosis and other clinical factors.

While the pathophysiology of each is beyond the scope of this chapter, treatment depends on determining which category is leading to the acidotic state. Causes of metabolic acidosis, separated as those causing an anion gap and those without a gap, are listed in Table 27.15. A common mnemonic used to list the causes of an anion gap metabolic acidosis is GOLDMARK [10].

Treatment recommendations vary depending on the disease state or condition leading to the acidosis. Underlying conditions of diabetic ketoacidosis, lactic acidosis, acute kidney injury, or diarrheal illness should be corrected as they may be the primary causes of the acidosis. Ingestions such as aspirin, methanol and ethylene glycol should be stopped once recognized. Acute metabolic acidosis and chronic metabolic acidosis are generally treated as separate entities. Acute metabolic acidosis should be treated with bicarbonate therapy with severe acidemia indicated by a pH <7.1. It is also suggested to treat with bicarbonate if pH <7.2 in patients who have severe AKI, as there may be survival and kidney function improvement. Clinical impact of treating severe acute metabolic acidosis remains contro-

Table 27.15 Causes of metabolic acidosis both anion gap and normal gap

Mechanism of acidosis	Increased Anion Gap	Normal Anion Gap
Increased acid production	Lactic acidosis	
	Ketoacidosis	
	Diabetes Mellitus	
	Starvation	
	Alcohol	
	D-Lactic acidosis	Potential co-existence due to urinary D-lactate as Na and K salts
Ingestions	Ethylene glycol	
	Aspirin	
	Methanol	
	Toluene	Toluene
	Diethylene glycol	
	Propylene glycol	
	Pyroglutamic acid (5-oxoproline)	
Loss of bicarbonate		Diarrhea or GI losses
		Type II RTA (proximal)
		Post Treatment of ketoacidosis
		Carbonic anhydrase inhibitors
		Ureteral diversion
Decreased renal acid excretion	Chronic kidney disease	Nephron damage (but preserved eGFR)
		Type I RTA (distal)
		Type IV RTA (hypoaldosteronism)

versial due to conflicting data. Most studies of sick patients with acute MA have been from animal or tissue experiments, while human studies of cardiovascular benefits have not been replicated. Still many clinicians agree that starting bicarbonate therapy when measured serum HCO_3 is <5 meq/L with pH below 7.1 is prudent.

Bicarbonate therapy is administered in the form of oral sodium bicarbonate tablets, baking soda powder, or intravenous sodium bicarbonate diluted in a hypotonic solution. $NaHCO_3$ is the most commonly used alkalinizing agent, as compared with giving lactate, citrate, potassium bicarbonate, or ketoacid anions (Table 27.16). Intravenous sodium bicarbonate is usually delivered as 8.4 percent (50 mEq/50 mL) 50 mL vials or ampules. It is expected that if normal body water weight is present, one 50 mEq/L vial will raise the HCO_3 concentration between 1.3 and 1.5 mEq/L in a patient weighing 70 kg. If more than 1 vial is to be administered, hypotonic water solution should be used to avoid hypernatremia as the bicarbonate will deliver a large quantity of sodium.

Treating chronic metabolic acidosis is less controversial as there are known consequences in patients with CKD including decreased muscle mass, bone health, and worsening eGFR. For long term maintenance treatment, potassium salts with bicarbonate can be effective for patients with hypokalemia.

Metabolic acidosis exists as both an acute and chronic problem. Patients usually can accommodate acid loading, but when kidney function is impaired, or gastrointestinal bicarbonate losses are high, the serum pH and HCO_3 balance can quickly become out of homeostasis. Treatment of existing underlying conditions combined with the appropriate therapy of alkaline solution can improve serum HCO_3, raise pH to normal levels, and improve long term clinical status of patients.

Conclusions

Returning to the patient at the beginning of the chapter—the 48-year-old man with a past medical history of Heart Failure with Reduced Ejection Fraction (HFrEF) 25%, and Chronic Kidney Disease Stage G3, who has been struggling with volume overload, and had recently been prescribed an increased dose of his loop diuretic. Whilst his 10 kg weight loss is reflected in the improvement in his edema, he has noted large volumes of urination, and concomitant increased fatigue. The case, and his blood test results highlight the importance of understanding that the likely cause of his hyponatremia is a result of an inability to excrete free water, and may be exacerbated by his diuretics. This is frequently seen amongst CKD patients with heart failure. His hypokalemia and metabolic alkalosis are also frequent complications of loop diuretic use.

Broadly, understanding electrolyte and acid base disorders requires a thorough assessment of

Table 27.16 Oral alkali preparations for treating metabolic acidosis

Product	Concentration	Base Concentration
Potassium Citrate (Polycitra)	500 mg per 5 mL	2 mEq per 1 mL
Sodium Bicarbonate	325 or 650 mg tablets	4 mEq per 325 mg tablet
Citric Acid (Shohl's Solution)	140 g per 1000 mL	1 mEq per 1 mL
Sodium Citrate (Bicitra)	500 mg/334 mg per 5 mL	1 mEq per 1 mL
Baking Soda (sodium bicarbonate)	1 tsp, 5000 mg powder	60 mEq per tsp
Enteric coated Sodium Bicarbonate (Bicarbi)	650 or 1300 mg tablets	8 mEq per 650 mg tablet

the likely cause, which in turn will direct the best approach to treatment.

Questions

1. A 21-year-old woman is brought to the Emergency Department (ED) after she suffered a tonic-clonic seizure outside of a party. She has no significant medical history and takes no medications. Friends who also attended the party reported that "recreational" drugs were at the party. On arrival to the ED, her vital signs were notable for a temperature of 38.6 °C, pulse of 89 beats/min, and blood pressure of 141/76 mmHg. Her examination was notable for some confusion and lethargy. Otherwise, her physical examination was within normal limits.

   Laboratory studies revealed: Serum sodium: 121 mEq/L Serum potassium: 4.3 mEq/L Serum bicarbonate: 21 mEq/L Serum chloride: 92 mEq/L Urine osmolality: 466 mOsm/kg

   Which of the following is the MOST likely etiology of this patient's presenting symptoms and laboratory findings?

   A. Primary polydipsia
   B. Synthetic marijuana
   C. "Bath Salt" intoxication
   D. Cocaine intoxication
   E. "Ecstasy" intoxication

   Answer: E. "Ecstasy" intoxication

   A. Primary polydipsia—Incorrect. A patient with primary polydipsia should have a very dilute urine in the acute setting of water intoxication with urine osmolality less than 100 mOsn/kg
   B. Synthetic marijuana—Incorrect. This is not associated with hyponatremia with elevated urine osmolality
   C. "Bath Salt" intoxication—Incorrect. This is not associated with hyponatremia with elevated urine osmolality
   D. Cocaine intoxication Incorrect. This is not associated with hyponatremia with elevated urine osmolality
   E. "Ecstasy" intoxication—Correct. Ecstasy causes a SAIDH picture with ADH release leading to inappropriately concentrated urine osmolality. Additionally, frequently at parties young people are encouraged to drink fluids such as alcohol, water, and flavored drinks leading to further hypotonic ingestion.

2. A 32-year-old man is referred for evaluation of hypertension. He believes that his hypertension was first diagnosed at age 15 but he was never told what the etiology may be. Of note, his father died at age 43 with a stroke, and he has a brother age 25 with hypertension. On physical examination, he is normal appearing with a blood pressure of 182/90 mmHg, and his fundoscopic examination reveals mild arteriolar narrowing. There are no abdominal bruits. Laboratory studies revealed: Serum sodium: 145 mEq/L Serum potassium: 3.0 mEq/L Serum chloride: 108 mEq/L Serum bicarbonate: 30 mEq/L Serum creatinine: 1.1 mg/dL Urine potassium: 90 mEq/24 h Plasma aldosterone: 7 ng/dL Plasma renin activity: 0.6

   Which of the following would be the MOST likely cause of his hypertension and associated laboratory findings?

   A. Gordon's syndrome
   B. Liddle's syndrome
   C. Bartter's syndrome
   D. Gitelman's syndrome
   E. Primary hyperaldosteronism

   Answer: B Liddle's Syndrome

   A. Gordon's syndrome—Incorrect. This syndrome is associated with hyperkalemia, hypertension and metabolic acidosis
   B. Liddle's syndrome—Correct. This syndrome is associated with normal or suppressed plasma aldosterone and renin as there is inappropriate uptake of urine sodium at the distal tubule. Patients frequently have hypertension, hypokalemia, and normal or suppressed plasma and renin levels
   C. Bartter's syndrome—Incorrect. This syndrome is associated with hypokalemia,

hypotension, and increased serum renin and aldosterone levels

D. Gitelman's syndrome—Incorrect. This syndrome is associated with hypokalemia, hypotension, increased serum renin and aldosterone levels, and hypercalcemia

E. Primary hyperaldosteronism—Incorrect. This syndrome is associated with a high aldosterone level and suppressed renin leading to an elevated aldosterone renin ratio (ARR).

3. A 60-year-old man undergoes neurosurgery for a craniopharyngioma. Postoperatively, his urine output is noted to be high for 2 days, and he is given two doses of intravenous desmopressin. Replacement doses of hydrocortisone are prescribed, and he is discharged from the hospital. Two days later, he is readmitted with lethargy and a serum sodium of 118 mEq/L.

   Which of the following is the MOST likely cause of the hyponatremia?

   A. Mineralocorticoid deficiency
   B. A persistent effect of desmopressin
   C. Adrenocorticotropic hormone (ACTH) deficiency
   D. Degenerating hypothalamic neurons

Answer: D. Degenerating hypothalamic neurons

A. Mineralocorticoid deficiency—Incorrect. No evidence related to deficiency with clinic picture

B. A persistent effect of desmopressin—Incorrect. Desmopressin last for less than 12 hours whether endogenous or exogenous.

C. Adrenocorticotropic hormone (ACTH) deficiency—Incorrect. ACTH deficiency would not cause hyponatremia this quickly in a patient who can tolerate a diet and consume appropriate fluids.

D. Degenerating hypothalamic neurons—Correct. Desmopressin hormone is stored in the posterior pituitary. During surgery causing injury, the pituitary necroses and slowly releases the desmopressin stored likely causing the hyponatremia.

4. A 67-year-old man with bipolar disorder managed for 25 years with lithium carbonate is admitted for acute appendicitis. Postoperatively, his urine output is replaced milliliter for milliliter with 0.9% saline. The next day, he is lethargic, and his serum sodium concentration is found to be 162 mEq/L.

   Which of the following about his condition is TRUE?

   A. Lithium is not associated with hypernatremia
   B. A patient on lithium only has electrolyte changes in early stages
   C. The patient will likely have a very concentrated urine
   D. The patient should have hypotonic fluid given now such as 0.45% saline
   E. 0.9% normal saline is an appropriate fluid to give a patient with hypernatremia

Answer D: The patient should have hypotonic fluid given now such as 0.45% saline

A. Lithium is not associated with hypernatremia- Incorrect. Lithium frequently is associated with hypernatremia as it causes a nephrogenic diabetes insipidus

B. A patient on lithium only has electrolyte changes in early stages—Incorrect. Lithium is most associated with electrolyte changes in the chronic setting of exposure

The patient will likely have a very concentrated urine—Incorrect. The patient is likely to have a dilute urine as lithium leads to an insufficient concentrating defect and nephrogenic diabetes insipidus

C. The patient should have hypotonic fluid given now such as 0.45% saline—Correct. The patient cannot concentrate urine correctly and is needing a hypotonic fluid replacement to return serum sodium back to normal range

D. 0.9% normal saline is an appropriate fluid to give a patient with hypernatremia—Incorrect. 0.9% sodium has a Na of 154 mEq/L and therefore does not have the best capacity to bring serum sodium into normal range. A hypotonic fluid is more appropriate and effect per mL of volume.

5. A 32-year-old pregnant woman is being treated for pre-eclampsia and is noted to have a serum calcium of 7.5 mg/dL and a serum phosphate of 5.3 mg/dL, with a normal serum albumin. She has a BUN of 21 and a creatinine of 1.9 mg/dL.

   Which of the following is the likely cause of the hypocalcemia?
   A. Chronic kidney disease
   B. Hyperphosphatemia
   C. Hypermagnesemia
   D. Hyperkalemia
   E. Hypernatremia

Answer: C Hypermagnesemia

   A. Chronic kidney disease—Incorrect. This is not the best answer as Cr is not sufficiently high to be associated with a late stage CKD which is associated with hypocalcemia
   B. Hyperphosphatemia—Incorrect. The phosphate level in this patient is within the upper limits of normal.
   C. Hypermagnesemia—Correct. Patients with preeclampsia are frequently placed on a magnesium infusion as prevent of moving into eclampsia. This patient likely has an undiagnosed elevated serum magnesium leading to hypocalcemia.
   D. Hyperkalemia—Incorrect. Hyperkalemia does not directly cause hypocalcemia and would not correlate with the clinical scenario
   E. Hypernatremia—Incorrect. Hypernatremia does not directly cause hypocalcemia and would not correlate with the clinical scenario

6. A 38 year man with heart failure with reduced ejection fraction, CKD stage IV presents to clinic for follow up. He has lower extremity edema on exam and mild rales at the bases of his lungs on auscultation. You advise the patient based on guidelines to maintain a 2400 mg/day sodium restriction. He is on Lisinopril 50 mg, Furosemide 20 mg twice a day, carvedilol at 12.5 mg twice a day. Labs show Na 136 mEq/L, K 5.7 mEq/L, HCO_3 21 mEq/L and Cr 2.8 mg/dL.

   Which oral potassium binder or treatment does not expose the patient to further sodium loading?
   A. Patiromer
   B. Sodium zirconium cyclosilicate
   C. Polystyrene sulfonate (Kayexalate)
   D. Normal saline IV push with furosemide treatment
   E. Sodium bicarbonate

Answer: Patiromer

   A. Patiromer—Correct. The only oral potassium binder not bound to sodium. Patiromer is bound with calcium.
   B. Sodium zirconium cyclosilicate—Incorrect. This potassium binder is bound with sodium.
   C. Polystyrene sulfonate—Incorrect. This potassium binder is bound with sodium.
   D. Normal saline IV push with furosemide treatment- Incorrect—Normal saline has 9 g of sodium per 1 L bag.
   E. Sodium bicarbonate—Incorrect. Sodium bicarbonate is bound with sodium

7. A 24 year old woman presents to the emergency room with altered mental status. Her initial labs are drawn and she is found to have an anion gap of 22. Which medical condition or ingestion is not associated with a high anion gap acidosis?
   A. Ethylene glycol
   B. Diabetic ketoacidosis
   C. Isopropyl alcohol
   D. Metformin overdose
   E. Acetaminophen overdose

Answer: Isopropyl alcohol

   A. Ethylene glycol—Incorrect. This ingestion causes a high AG and is frequently ingested accidentally or during a suicide attempt.
   B. Diabetic ketoacidosis—Incorrect. Ketoacidosis leads to a high anion gap and is part of the GOLDMARK acronym for AG diagnoses.
   C. Isopropyl alcohol—Correct. Isopropyl alcohol is not associated with a high anion gap but causes an elevated osmolar gap.
   D. Metformin overdose—Incorrect. Metformin overdose leads to lactic acidosis type

B. Lactic acidosis causes a high anion gap.
E. Acetaminophen overdose—Incorrect. Acetaminophen is associated with a high anion gap due to propylene glycol.

8. A 32 year old man presents to CKD clinic for follow up. He has CKD Stage V and suffering with chronic metabolic acidosis. His serum HCO_3 is 17 mEq/L on recent lab. He is started on Sodium bicarbonate therapy twice a day and on follow up 3 months later his serum bicarbonate level has improved to 22 mEq/L. Which therapeutic advantages with his improving acidotic state will the patient experience?
   A. Lower Mortality
   B. Improved bone strength
   C. Slower eGFR loss
   D. Hyperkalemia prevention
   E. All of the above

Answer: E. All of the Above
   A. Lower mortality—Incorrect. Lower mortality is associated with improving acidosis but is not the only correct answer.
   B. Improved bone strength. Incorrect. Improved bone strength is associated with improving acidosis but is not the only correct answer.
   C. Slower eGFR loss—Incorrect. This answer is associated with improving acidosis but is not the only correct answer.
   D. Hyperkalemia prevention—Incorrect. Hyperkalemia prevention is associated with improving acidosis but is not the only correct answer.
   E. All of the above—Correct. All answer choices are correct.

9. Which anti-hypertensive treatment is associated with hyponatremia in some patients?
   A. Amlodipine
   B. Spironolactone
   C. Hydrochlorothiazide
   D. Losartan
   E. Carvedilol

Answer: C. Hydrochlorothiazide
   A. Amlodipine—Incorrect. Calcium channel blockers are not commonly associated with hyponatremia.
   B. Spironolactone—Incorrect. Spironolactone is not commonly associated with hyponatremia.
   C. Hydrochlorothiazide—Correct. Thiazide and thiazide like diuretics are associated with hyponatremia. Usually this is reversible once the medication is stopped.
   D. Losartan—Incorrect. Angiotensin receptor blockers are not commonly associated with hyponatremia.
   E. Carvedilol—Incorrect. Beta blockers are not commonly associated with hyponatremia.

10. A 29 year old woman presents to the emergency room with altered mental status. Her Na is 109 mEq/L, K 2.9 mEq/L and Cr 0.7 mg/dL. You determine that you would like to give her a 3% saline bolus to improve her serum sodium level and improve mental status. During the initial phase of hyponatremia treatment, what is the recommended rate of rise in the first 24 h to prevent osmotic demyleniation syndrome (ODS)?
   A. 2–4 mEq/L rise in serum Na
   B. 4–6 mEq/L rise in serum Na
   C. 8–10 mEq/L rise in serum Na
   D. 10–12 mEq/L rise in serum Na
   E. No limitation is recommended

Answer: B. 4-6 mEq/L rise in serum Na
   A. 2–4 mEq/L rise in serum Na—Incorrect. A rise of 6 mEq/L is usually considered safe to prevent ODS symptoms while still allowing mental status symptoms to improve. This is too low.
   B. 4–6 mEq/L rise in serum Na—Correct. A rise of 6 mEq/L is usually considered safe to prevent ODS symptoms while still allowing mental status symptoms to improve.
   C. 8–10 mEq/L rise in serum Na—Incorrect. A rise of this magnitude in the first 24 h of treatment has been shown to be associated with ODS symptoms.

D. 10–12 mEq/L rise in serum Na—Incorrect. A rise of this magnitude in the first 24 h of treatment has been shown to be associated with ODS symptoms.
E. No limitation is recommended—Incorrect. Uncontrolled rise of sodium in hyponatremia is directly related to ODS symptoms.

Test your learning and check your understanding of this book's contents: use the "Springer Nature Flashcards" app to access questions using https://sn.pub/cz9Cok. To use the app, please follow the instructions in Chap. 1.

References

1. Verbalis JG, Goldsmith SR, Greenberg A, Korzelius C, Schrier RW, Sterns RH, Thompson CJ. Diagnosis, evaluation, and treatment of hyponatremia: expert panel recommendations. Am J Med. 2013;126(10 Suppl 1):S1–42. https://doi.org/10.1016/j.amjmed.2013.07.006.
2. Spasovski G, Vanholder R, Allolio B, Annane D, Ball S, Bichet D, Decaux G, Fenske W, Hoorn EJ, Ichai C, Joannidis M, Soupart A, Zietse R, Haller M, van der Veer S, Van Biesen W, Nagler E, Hyponatraemia Guideline Development Group. Clinical practice guideline on diagnosis and treatment of hyponatraemia. Eur J Endocrinol. 2014;170(3):G1–47. https://doi.org/10.1530/EJE-13-1020. Erratum in: Eur J Endocrinol. 2014 Jul;171(1):X1.
3. Edelman IS, Leibman J, O'Meara MP, Birkenfeld LW. Interrelations between serum sodium concentration, serum osmolarity and total exchangeable sodium, total exchangeable potassium and total body water. J Clin Invest. 1958;37(9):1236–56. https://doi.org/10.1172/JCI103712.
4. Kraut JA, Madias NE. Re-evaluation of the normal range of serum total CO2 concentration. Clin J Am Soc Nephrol. 2018;13(2):343–7.
5. Furst H, Hallows KR, Post J, Chen S, Kotzker W, Goldfarb S, Ziyadeh FN, Neilson EG. The urine/plasma electrolyte ratio: a predictive guide to water restriction. Am J Med Sci. 2000;319(4):240–4. https://doi.org/10.1097/00000441-200004000-00007.
6. Schwartz WB, Ypersele V, de Strihou KJP. Role of anions in metabolic alkalosis and potassium deficiency. N Engl J Med. 1968;279(12):630–9.
7. Mehta AN, Emmett JB, Emmett M. GOLD MARK: an anion gap mnemonic for the 21st century. Lancet. 2008;372(9642):892.
8. Luke RG, Galla JH. It is chloride depletion alkalosis, not contraction alkalosis. J Am Soc Nephrol. 2012;23(2):204–7.
9. Frick PG, Senning A. The treatment of severe metabolic alkalosis with intravenous N /10 or N /5 hydrochloric acid. Germ Med Monthly. 1964;9:242.
10. Garibotto G, Sofia A, Robaudo C, Saffioti S, Sala MR, Verzola D, Vettore M, Russo R, Procopio V, Deferrari G, Tessari P. Kidney protein dynamics and ammoniagenesis in humans with chronic metabolic acidosis. J Am Soc Nephrol. 2004;15(6):1606–15.

28 The Role of Renal Registries

Mogamat Razeen Davids, Fergus J. Caskey, and John B. Eastwood

Clinical Scenario

A 54-year-old male haemodialysis patient, with end stage kidney disease secondary to diabetes mellitus, has recently learned that data from all kidney patients in the unit are being sent to a national database. At his next clinic appointment, he asks what is happening to his data.

What will you say?

Introduction

The combined burdens of non-communicable diseases, infectious diseases, exposure to environmental toxins and acute kidney injury (AKI) related to trauma and childbirth are driving a global epidemic of kidney disease. It is estimated that there are over 850 million people worldwide who have kidney disease, and approximately 3.9 million of these individuals have kidney failure (end stage kidney disease/ESKD), which is being treated with kidney replacement therapy (KRT) [1].

National kidney disease registries provide valuable information, that can inform the planning of services for kidney care and enhance the arguments for better resource allocation. They also allow audit of the delivery and quality of care, and the monitoring of the impact of interventions. Most registries focus on patients with kidney failure who are treated with KRT, especially dialysis, and there are few countries with registries for chronic kidney disease (CKD) or AKI.

In this chapter, we give a brief overview of renal registries in different parts of the world, describe the elements involved in establishing a renal registry, consider the research questions which could be addressed by renal registries and describe examples of the impact of registry data on clinical practice and access to kidney care.

Renal Registries Around the World

Most developed countries have national renal registries, that provide critical information to support the planning, delivery and evaluation of dialysis and transplantation services. The European Renal Association (ERA) Registry is the world's oldest renal registry and was started in 1964 [2, 3]. The ERA Registry publishes an annual report and several scientific papers each

M. R. Davids (✉)
Division of Nephrology, Stellenbosch University and Tygerberg Hospital, Cape Town, South Africa
e-mail: mrd@sun.ac.za

F. J. Caskey
Population Health Sciences, University of Bristol, Bristol, UK
e-mail: fergus.caskey@bristol.ac.uk

J. B. Eastwood
Department of Renal Medicine, Institute of Medical and Biomedical Education, St. George's, University of London, London, UK
e-mail: jbeastwo@sgul.ac.uk

D. Banerjee et al. (eds.), *Management of Kidney Diseases*,
https://doi.org/10.1007/978-3-031-09131-5_28

year. It also offers courses in epidemiology and training in data analysis.

Many other registries have followed, including the Australia and New Zealand Dialysis and Transplant Registry (ANZDATA, established in 1977), the Canadian Organ Replacement Register (CORR, 1981), the Japanese registry (1983) [4], the United States Renal Data System (USRDS, 1988), the Scottish Renal Registry (1991), the Malaysian Renal Registry (1992) and the UK Renal Registry (1995).

The international comparisons chapter of the US Renal Data System annual report is an excellent resource, which collates information on the treatment of kidney failure worldwide [5]. The highest annual incidences of treated kidney failure in 2018 were reported from Jalisco, Mexico (594 per million population (pmp)), Taiwan (523 pmp), Hungary (508 pmp) and the US (395 pmp). The lowest rates were reported from South Africa (16 pmp), Ukraine (40 pmp) and Bangladesh (61 pmp). The highest prevalence rates in 2018 were from Taiwan (3587 pmp), Japan (2653 pmp), the US (2354 pmp) and Singapore (2255 pmp). The lowest rates were reported from Bangladesh (119 pmp), South Africa (186 pmp) and Ukraine (227 pmp).

The lack of renal registries in many low- and middle-income countries means that there are few reliable statistics on kidney failure and KRT. For example, in Africa, registry data have been published mainly by North African countries, starting with Egypt and Tunisia in 1975, followed by South Africa in 1977, and thereafter by Libya, Algeria and Morocco. Most of these registries failed due to resource constraints, and in recent years only the re-established South African Renal Registry [6, 7] has published regular reports, starting with its analysis of 2012 data. In 2015, the African Association of Nephrology (AFRAN) established the African Renal Registry [8] and to date, six countries have joined this initiative and are using its online data capture platform.

The International Society of Nephrology (ISN) has a project under its advocacy theme called SHARing Expertise to support the set-up of Renal Registries (SharE-RR) [9]. SharE-RR supports countries without registries and promotes shared learning among countries with established surveillance systems. One of its first activities was to conduct a survey of kidney health surveillance systems. Of the 85 responding organisations (Fig. 28.1), 99% collected adult haemodialysis data, 92% collected peritoneal dialysis data and 74% collected transplant data. Paediatric haemodialysis, peritoneal dialysis and transplant data were collected by 75%, 66% and 60%, respectively. Data on CKD were collected by 22% and data on AKI by 9%, respectively [9].

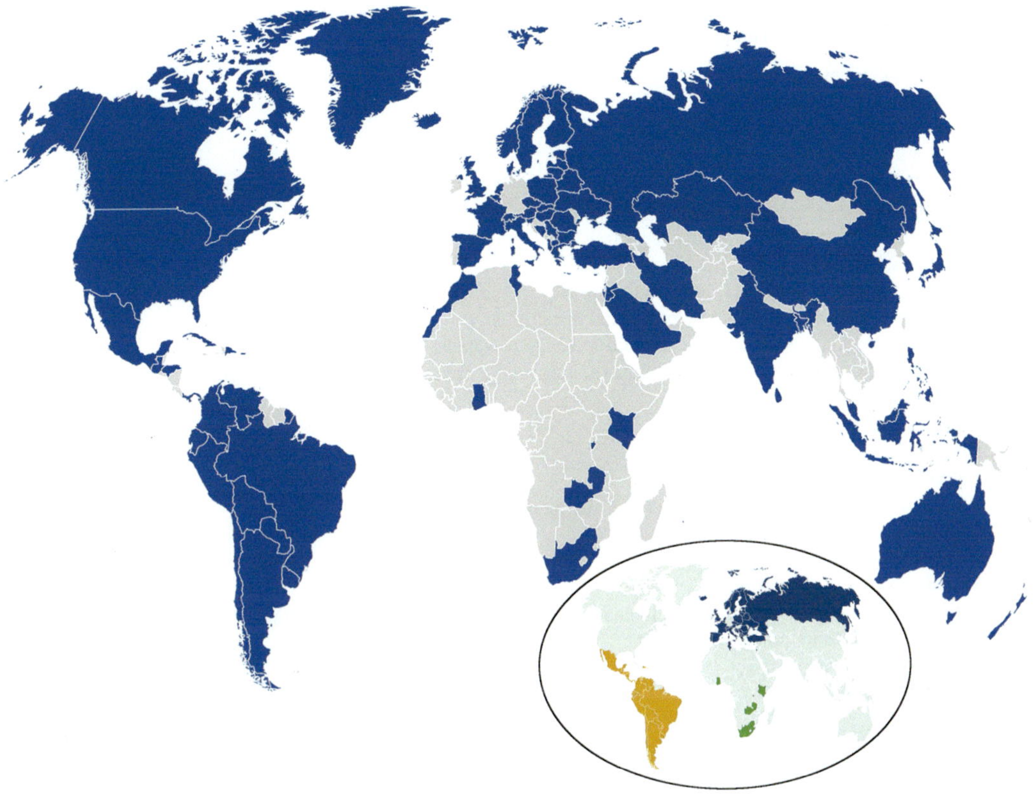

Fig. 28.1 Countries reporting renal registries in the SHARing Expertise to support the set-up of Renal Registries (SharE-RR) survey. Dark blue indicates countries with registries. The inset shows coverage of the regional registries in South America (Sociedad Latinoamericana de Nefrología e Hipertensión, SLANH; yellow), Europe (European Renal Association, ERA; blue) and Africa (African Association of Nephrology, AFRAN; green). From Hole et al. [9].

Which Questions Can Be Answered by Renal Registries?

Renal registries collect a well-defined set of health and demographic data with the aim of generating information on the main causes and the incidence of kidney failure, and information on the prevalence, treatment and outcomes of patients on KRT. Table 28.1 summarises the questions that might be readily answered using data collected by renal registries.

In most countries, especially low- and middle-income countries (LMICs), the incidence of KRT will not be the same as the incidence of kidney failure, because of the variable access to dialysis and transplantation services. The prevalence of KRT is determined by the burden of the disease, access to treatment and survival on KRT. The extremely wide variation in reported prevalence is mainly a reflection of differing access to dialysis and transplantation [11]. This is particularly relevant in LMICs, where transplantation services are limited, and where dialysis may have to paid for out of pocket by patients and their families [11]. Most patients in such a situation are unable to afford dialysis treatments beyond the first few months [12].

Table 28.1 Some questions that can be addressed by renal registries. Focused on patients with kidney failure (stage 5 CKD/ESKD). Adapted from Davids et al. [10]

Epidemiology of kidney failure – incidence of CKD stage 5 – incidence of patients accessing KRT – aetiology – prevalence of KRT – KRT modalities
Patient characteristics and disparities in access to KRT – age, sex, ethnicity – comorbid diseases—diabetes, infections with HIV, hepatitis B or hepatitis C – geography—urban/rural, regional/provincial disparities – socio-economic status, medical insurance, access to private vs. public sector services – access to medications such as erythropoietin, intravenous iron, immunosuppressive agents
Primary outcomes – patient survival – modality/technique survival Other outcomes – causes of death or reasons for cessation of treatment – hospitalisations – dialysis adequacy – vascular access in HD patients – laboratory data such as those related to anaemia management, bone-mineral disease, etc. – rejection episodes in transplant patients Patient-reported outcomes – quality of life – employment – travelling and distances to treatment centres
Outcomes in sub-populations of interest – children – the elderly – people with HIV – people treated with supportive/palliative care, without KRT

Abbreviations: HD, haemodialysis; HIV, human immunodeficiency virus; KRT, kidney replacement therapy; PD, peritoneal dialysis

Establishing Renal Registries

Information for nephrologists or nephrology societies wanting to establish a renal registry is available via the SharE-RR pages on the ISN website (https://www.theisn.org/initiatives/data-collection/#SharE-RR). Some of the important elements to consider when starting a new registry are briefly mentioned below [8, 9].

Identifying Stakeholders and Building the Registry Team

Renal registries are often established by national nephrology societies, with the support of government. The governance and oversight plans need to be clear. Registry teams usually include nephrologists, data managers and data capturers, epidemiologists or statisticians, administrators and software developers/database managers. Some registries also employ nurses or unpaid volunteers [9]. Advisory committees may include patient representatives, and representatives from industry and funding organisations.

Clarifying the Purpose, Scope and Minimum Outputs

The purpose is usually to generate information on the prevalence, incidence and causes of kidney failure in patients on KRT and, to a variable extent, additional information on the treatment and outcomes. A small set of epidemiologic data is collected over many years. Unnecessary complexity should be avoided, as this will drive up costs and decrease compliance with data submission.

Defining and Finding Cases

All patients who receive KRT for kidney failure should be included, including those who do not survive to 90 days. It is important to report on those patients who discontinue dialysis for financial reasons and those "crash landers" who present very late and die soon after commencing KRT. The use of multiple sources of information increases completeness and may include the patient's doctor, treatment centres, laboratories, funders, and suppliers of medications or consumables.

A Minimum Dataset and the Data Dictionary

Many registries focus their annual follow-up data collection on 31 December. A typical minimum dataset would include the following:

- Country, region and centre
- Patient unique identification number and name
- Date of birth and sex
- Primary kidney disease
- Date and modality of first treatment
- Changes of doctor, centre
- Current treatment modality
- Changes of treatment modality since last census, including cessation of treatment or loss to follow-up
- Death details

Optional data might include more aspects of the treatment, indicators of treatment quality and additional outcomes such as hospitalisations and quality of life.

The data dictionary describes the elements to be collected and specifies the data type (categorical, numerical), precision (number of decimal points), range of acceptable values, etc. Definitions should conform to those used by well-established registries to facilitate comparisons and to allow the aggregation of data. For example, the coding of the primary kidney disease should use an established system such as the ERA Registry coding scheme [13].

Collecting Data and Ensuring Data Quality

This is the most resource-intensive aspect of running a registry. Well-documented processes should guide data collection and ensure data quality. Where possible, data should be collected directly from health information systems. Quality control must focus on data completeness, the prevention of duplicates, validity and accuracy, timeliness, usefulness of items and the accuracy of data interpretation and reporting [14].

Data Ownership and Access, and Dissemination of Findings

The question of who owns the data should be clarified at the start. Making anonymised information widely available is a principle common to many registries and requires data access and publication policies for responding to requests for data while safeguarding patient confidentiality. Routine outputs might include annual reports, presentations at academic meetings, publications in medical journals and the release of datasets.

Ethical Considerations

Consideration of ethical aspects and privacy and data protection legislation is extremely important for registries. Many registries have obtained waivers of individual informed consent to facilitate including all patients in the registry while taking the necessary precautions to protect patients' personal information. Examples include the UK, Scottish, French and South African registries.

Impact of Registries

Improving Access to Care

Renal registries can aid efforts to prevent, detect and treat the earlier stages of CKD by identifying the most important causes of kidney failure in each country. Where access to treatment is restricted on economic grounds, registry data can highlight disparities in the provision of KRT services within and between countries. This may encourage governments and other funders to increase their support. Registries can identify sub-groups with reduced access to treatment or poor outcomes and monitor the adoption and impact of evidence-based interventions. A few examples of the impact of renal registries are provided below.

The Tunisian dialysis registry has had a major impact on the country's development of KRT [15]. Registry data influenced decisions to increase the number of nephrologists, develop a new transplant programme, start new dialysis units and develop a kidney disease prevention programme. The rate of new patients starting KRT in Tunisia increased from 82 pmp in 1992–3 to 159 pmp in 2000–1.

The Thailand Renal Replacement Therapy Registry was instrumental in building the case for their "*PD First*" programme [16], which saw a marked increase in access to peritoneal dialysis as the initial modality of treatment. The registry provided essential quality assurance data on peritonitis rates and peritoneal dialysis technique survival [17].

The National Renal Registry of the Malaysian Society of Nephrology reports on treatment rates and modality, quality standards, patient reported outcomes and kidney biopsy data. They also serve as an excellent example of how registry data was used to argue for increased funding of KRT as their country's national wealth increased [18].

In South America, the Latin American Dialysis and Transplant Registry [19] has contributed to the development of national registries and allowed participating countries to report their treatment rates and outcomes in the context of geographically, culturally and economically similar neighbours, challenging treatment modality preferences and highlighting the importance of primary and secondary prevention in CKD [19].

In South Africa, the first report of the re-established South African Renal Registry [6] revealed a markedly uneven distribution of KRT across provinces and large differences in prevalence rates between the resource-constrained public healthcare sector and the well-resourced private sector (73 vs. 620 pmp). This generated prominent media coverage and led to the national health minister convening a summit on "*An effective approach to chronic kidney disease in South Africa*", in 2015. It is hoped that a comprehensive approach and more resources will eventually flow from this initiative. More recently, Jardine et al. [20] have used registry data to demonstrate that the 1-year survival of incident South African patients on KRT (90.4%) is comparable with that of better-resourced countries. There was no difference in survival between patients treated in the public and private sectors and the authors argue that these findings should encourage government to increase access to KRT in the public sector.

Embedding Interventional Studies in Renal Registries

Traditional clinical trials have become increasingly expensive and may have limited generalisability among the populations of patients on KRT. A more pragmatic approach is now being adopted that makes better use of routine data, such as that collected by renal registries [21]. Registries may be used to identify potentially eligible participants, provide the baseline data and provide much or all of the follow-up data, including some of the safety monitoring data. This "efficient study design" greatly reduces the burden and cost of trials. Two examples of registry trials are presented below.

In the UK, the Campath, Calcineurin inhibitor reduction, and Chronic allograft nephropathy (3C) study randomised kidney transplant recipients to tacrolimus or sirolimus maintenance therapy [22]. Researchers were able to obtain follow-up data on graft function, patient survival, cancer and cause-specific mortality for one of the randomisation arms by linking to routine databases including Hospital Episode Statistics, the Office for National Statistics, UK Transplant and the UK Renal Registry.

In Australia and New Zealand, the Better Evidence for Selecting Transplant Fluids (BEST-Fluids) trial is evaluating the effect of intravenous therapy with Plasmalyte® versus 0.9% saline on delayed graft function following deceased donor kidney transplantation. Participants will be enrolled, randomised and followed up using ANZDATA, the Australia and New Zealand Dialysis and Transplant Registry [23].

Practice Points

- Involving your patient in a national renal registry is central to improving kidney care for all patients
- Where there is no current national renal registry—particularly in LMICs, there is international support available to develop one

Conclusions

The importance of kidney health surveillance systems has been recognised in the ISN's integrated end-stage kidney disease (ESKD) strategy [24]. Most high-income countries have a renal registry, but this is not yet the case for LMICs, where the impacts of kidney failure can be catastrophic at the human and societal level. Registry data is critical to inform the planning of nephrology services and to argue for more resources for comprehensive kidney care. More recently, registries are increasingly being used in pragmatic clinical trials to reduce the costs and improve the generalisability of the research findings.

Returning to the clinic, and our 54-year-old gentleman on haemodialysis, who wishes to know what is happening to his data at the national renal registry. His question highlights an important and common ethical concern over ownership and sharing of personal data. It may be useful for him to understand how the data collated from all units across the country helps to drive and maintain improvements in dialysis care at his unit. He can be reassured that collating anonymised data from all patients receiving kidney care in the country, whilst ensuring the safety of all identifiable personal data, is central to the role of the national renal registry. He may also be interested to learn about how certain research studies have been delivered more effectively with the support of national renal registries. Finally, he may like to see an example of the data report—which is made freely available to clinicians and patients alike.

Questions

1. What is the estimated global prevalence of kidney disease?
   A. 200 million
   B. 350 million
   C. 500 million
   D. 850 million
   E. 1000 million

Answer D. The "single number" paper of Jager et al. estimated that the total number of people with acute or chronic kidney disease exceeds 850 million (Kidney Int. 2019; 96:1048–1050).

2. Which is the world's oldest renal registry?
   A. Australia and New Zealand Dialysis and Transplant Registry (ANZDATA)
   B. European Renal Association (ERA) Registry
   C. Malaysian Renal Registry
   D. US Renal Data System (USRDS)
   E. The South African Renal Registry

Answer B. The ERA Registry was the first, established in 1964.

3. Which are the most important benefits of a renal registry?
   A. Informs the planning, delivery and evaluation of nephrology services
   B. Helps to direct the care of individual patients

C. Collects comprehensive information for research projects
D. Tracks expenditure related to kidney replacement therapy
E. Compares the performance of nephrologists and treatment centres

Answer A: Providing critical information for the planning, delivery and evaluation of nephrology services is the main purpose. A registry will not typically help to direct an individual patient's care, although including an individual patient's data may help inform the care of future patients with a similar condition. Some well-established registries do report centre-based data, but this is not common and could lead to reduced participation by nephrologists and treatment centres when establishing a new registry.

4. What is the likely reason for the low prevalence of patients on kidney replacement therapy in South Africa (186 pmp in 2018)?
   A. The burden of kidney disease is low
   B. Data capture is incomplete and there is substantial under-reporting
   C. The South African registry does not include patients with a kidney transplant
   D. The South African registry does not include patients treated in private treatment centres
   E. Access to kidney replacement therapy is low because of limited resources

Answer E: Access to KRT in the poorly resourced public healthcare sector is the main reason; this sector provides care for 85% of the population and, unfortunately, there has been no real increase in access to KRT over the past two decades. The South African Renal Registry has country-wide coverage, in both public and private healthcare sectors, and includes all modalities of KRT.

5. Which are the important initial steps when setting up a renal registry?
   A. Identifying stakeholders, assembling the team and clarifying the purpose, scope and outputs
   B. Finding cases, collecting data and ensuring data quality
   C. Developing a database and an online data capture system
   D. Drafting policies for data access and publications
   E. Securing funding for the registry

   Answer: A. All the above are important, but identifying stakeholders, assembling the team and clarifying the purpose, scope and outputs are the priorities at the start.

6. Should registries strive to access multiple data sources?
   A. Only data submitted by the patient's doctor should be used
   B. Only data submitted by the patient's treatment centre should be used
   C. Only data submitted by the patient's doctor or treatment centre should be used
   D. Yes, using multiple sources would improve data completeness and quality
   E. Patients should be consulted and data collection adapted accordingly

Answer D. The strength of a registry lies in capturing accurate data on all (or almost all) patients. Accessing multiple data sources would improve data completeness and quality.

7. What should be included in the dataset collected by new registries?
   A. A minimum dataset: demographics, primary disease, treatment start/end and modality
   B. Basic data plus data on treatment aspects such as dialysis adequacy, vascular access, etc.
   C. Basic data plus data on treatment aspects, laboratory tests and hospitalisations
   D. Data as above, plus data patient reported outcomes, such as quality of life
   E. Comprehensive data to facilitate research projects

Answer A. New registries are advised to keep the dataset to the minimum to reduce the administrative burden and increase compliance with data submission, especially where this is not mandatory. Once regular data submission has been established, additional information can be requested.

8. Please indicate whether each of the following statements about renal registries are true or false.
   A. Renal registries can aid efforts to prevent, detect and treat the earlier stages of CKD by identifying the most important causes of kidney failure in each country
   B. Renal registry data allows the nephrologist to predict the exact cause of death in a patient who has been on kidney replacement therapy for four years
   C. Registry data can highlight disparities in the provision of KRT services within and between countries
   D. A patient can request to have his/her identifiable data deleted from the registry
   E. Renal registries can identify sub-groups with reduced access to treatment or poor outcomes and monitor the adoption and impact of evidence-based interventions
   A. True
   B. False - Registry data reports on groups of patients and can generate the probabilities of outcomes of interest, but these cannot be expected to always apply in individual patients
   C. True
   D. True – If possible, suggest that your patient considers the option of having only the identifiable information deleted, or replaced by a code, so that all the information is not lost. Explain the importance of including everyone's information and the measures being taken to keep it safe.
   E. True
9. Please indicate (True/False) whether each of the following are real-life examples of questions answered by a renal registry.
   A. Establishing the Tunisian dialysis registry led to an increase in the number of nephrologists, development of a new transplantation programme, new dialysis units, and a kidney disease prevention programme
   B. The Thailand Renal Replacement Therapy Registry was instrumental in building the case for the "*PD First*" programme, which saw a marked increase in access to peritoneal dialysis as the initial modality of treatment.
   C. Data from the Malaysian Renal Registry was used to successfully argue for increased funding of KRT as their country's national wealth increased
   D. The 3C study randomised kidney transplant recipients to tacrolimus or sirolimus maintenance therapy, with follow-up data on graft function, patient survival, and mortality obtained by linking to routine databases including the UK Renal Registry
   E. In South Africa, the first report of the re-established South African Renal Registry revealed a markedly uneven distribution of KRT across provinces and large differences in prevalence rates between the resource-constrained public healthcare sector and the well-resourced private sector (73 vs. 620 pmp).

   Answers: A–E are all True.
10. Which aspects of a registry facilitate comparisons of aggregate data?
    A. Careful capturing of data from the notes of the treating doctor
    B. Avoiding methods other than online data capture
    C. Obtaining ethical approval for data sharing
    D. Ensuring that duplicate entries are avoided
    E. A data dictionary which uses well-established definitions and coding systems

    Answers: E. The data dictionary describes the elements to be collected and specifies the data type (categorical, ordinal, numerical), precision (number of decimal points), range of acceptable values, etc. Definitions should conform to those used by well-established registries to facilitate comparisons and to allow the aggregation of data. For example, the coding of the primary kidney disease should use an established system such as the ERA Registry coding scheme.
11. The majority of existing renal registries report on which group of patients predominantly?

A. Patients with a genetic kidney disease
B. Patients with ESKD treated with dialysis or transplantation
C. All patients with CKD of any cause
D. Patients with AKI
E. Only those patients with an unknown aetiology of their kidney disease

Answer: B. Patients with ESKD treated with dialysis or transplantation

A. Patients with a genetic kidney disease—incorrect—all causes of kidney disease are considered, not solely those with a genetic kidney disease
B. Patients with ESKD treated with dialysis or transplantation—correct—Most registries report on patients with kidney failure who are treated with dialysis or transplantation—there are few countries with registries for CKD or AKI
C. All patients with CKD of any cause—incorrect—Most registries report on patients with kidney failure who are treated with dialysis or transplantation—there are few countries with registries for CKD or AKI
D. Patients with AKI—incorrect—Most registries report on patients with kidney failure who are treated with dialysis or transplantation—there are few countries with registries for CKD or AKI
E. Only those patients with an unknown aetiology of their kidney disease—incorrect, the registry will include patients with both known and unknown aetiologies of their kidney disease.

12. It is recognised that the reported prevalence of kidney replacement therapy varies widely between countries. Which of these factors is likely to contribute *most significantly* to this variation?
    A. Differing access to dialysis and transplantation
    B. Variations in the data collection
    C. Different patterns of disease prevalence
    D. Many registries do not collect data on transplants
    E. The exclusion of adults on peritoneal dialysis from most registries

Answer: A. Differing access to dialysis and transplantation

A. Differing access to dialysis and transplantation—correct—in LMICs in particular, access to dialysis and transplantation may be limited, thus giving an artificially low reported prevalence.
B. Variations in the data collection process—incorrect—The extremely wide variation in reported prevalence is mainly a reflection of differing access to dialysis and transplantation
C. Different patterns of disease prevalence—incorrect—while the burden of kidney disease will indeed vary globally, the access to dialysis and transplantation amongst patients with ESKD makes a more significant contribution.
D. The majority of registries do not collect data on transplants—incorrect—According to SharE-RR, 74% of registries do collect transplant data.
E. The exclusion of adults on peritoneal dialysis from most registries—incorrect—According to SharE-RR, 92% of registries collect data on peritoneal dialysis.

Test your learning and check your understanding of this book's contents: use the "Springer Nature Flashcards" app to access questions using https://sn.pub/cz9Cok. To use the app, please follow the instructions in Chap. 1.

References

1. Jager KJ, Kovesdy C, Langham R, Rosenberg M, Jha V, Zoccali C. A single number for advocacy and communication—worldwide more than 850 million individuals have kidney diseases. Kidney Int. 2019;96:1048–50.
2. Alberts C, Drukker W. Report on regular dialysis in Europe. Proc Eur Dial Transplant Assoc. 1965;2:82–7.
3. Jager KJ, Wanner C. Fifty years of ERA-EDTA Registry—a registry in transition. Kidney Int Suppl. 2015;5:12–4.
4. Teraoka S, Toma H, Nihei H, Ota K, Babazono T, Ishikawa I, et al. Current status of renal replacement therapy in Japan. Am J Kidney Dis. 1995;25:151–64.
5. 2020 USRDS Annual Data Report: Epidemiology of kidney disease in the United States. Bethesda, MD: National Institutes of Health, National Institute of Diabetes and Digestive and Kidney Diseases; 2020. https://adr.usrds.org/2020. Accessed 25 November 2020.
6. Davids MR, Marais N, Jacobs JC. South African Renal Registry Annual Report 2012. Cape Town: South African Renal Society; 2014. https://sa-renal-society.org/registry/. Accessed 25 November 2020.
7. Davids MR, Jardine T, Marais N, Jacobs JC, Sebastian S. South African Renal Registry Annual Report 2018. Afr J Nephrol. 2020;23:185–96.
8. Davids MR, Eastwood JB, Selwood NH, Arogundade FA, Ashuntantang G, Benghanem Gharbi M, et al. A renal registry for Africa: first steps. Clin Kidney J. 2016;9:162–7.
9. Hole BD, Evans KM, Pyart R, Davids MR, Bedat CG, Hanafusa N, et al. International collaborative efforts to establish kidney health surveillance systems. Kidney Int. 2020;98:812–6.
10. Davids MR, Caskey FJ, Young T, Balbir Singh GK. Strengthening renal registries and ESRD research in Africa. Semin Nephrol. 2017;37:211–23.
11. El Nahas M. The global challenge of chronic kidney disease. Kidney Int. 2005;68:2918–29.
12. Arogundade F, Sanusi A, Hassan M, Akinsola A. The pattern, clinical characteristics and outcome of ESRD in Ile-Ife, Nigeria: Is there a change in trend? Afr Health Sci. 2011;11:594–601.
13. Venkat-Raman G, Tomson CR, Gao Y, Cornet R, Stengel B, Gronhagen-Riska C, et al. New primary renal diagnosis codes for the ERA-EDTA. Nephrol Dial Transplant. 2012;27:4414–9.
14. Couchoud C, Lassalle M, Cornet R, Jager KJ. Renal replacement therapy registries—time for a structured data quality evaluation programme. Nephrol Dial Transplant. 2013;28:2215–20.
15. Counil É, Cherni N, Kharrat M, Achour A, Trimech H. Trends of incident dialysis patients in Tunisia between 1992 and 2001. Am J Kidney Dis. 2008;51:463–70.
16. Morad Z, Choong HL, Tungsanga K, Suhardjono. Funding renal replacement therapy in southeast Asia: building public-private partnerships in Singapore, Malaysia, Thailand, and Indonesia. Am J Kidney Dis 2015; 65:799-805.
17. Dhanakijcharoen P, Sirivongs D, Aruyapitipan S, Chuengsaman P, Lumpaopong A. The "PD First" policy in Thailand: three-years experiences (2008-2011). J Med Assoc Thai 2011; 94 Suppl 4:S153-S161.
18. Lim TO, Goh A, Lim YN, Morad Z. Use of renal registry data for research, health-care planning and quality improvement: what can we learn from registry data in the Asia-Pacific region? Nephrology. 2008;13:745–52.
19. Rosa-Diez G, Gonzalez-Bedat M, Pecoits-Filho R, Marinovich S, Fernandez S, Lugon J, et al. Renal replacement therapy in Latin American end-stage renal disease. Clin Kidney J. 2014;7:431–6.
20. Jardine T, Wong E, Steenkamp R, Caskey FJ, Davids MR. Survival of South African patients on renal replacement therapy. Clin Kidney J. 2020;13:782–90.
21. Caskey FJ, Jardine T, Davids MR. Embedding randomised controlled trials in renal registries. Afr J Nephrol. 2019;22:54–9.
22. The 3C Study Collaborative Group. Campath, calcineurin inhibitor reduction, and chronic allograft nephropathy (the 3C Study) - results of a randomized controlled clinical trial. Am J Transplant. 2018;18:1424–34.
23. Collins MG, Fahim MA, Pascoe EM, Dansie KB, Hawley CM, Clayton PA, et al. Study protocol for Better Evidence for Selecting Transplant Fluids (BEST-Fluids): a pragmatic, registry-based, multicenter, double-blind, randomized controlled trial evaluating the effect of intravenous fluid therapy with Plasma-Lyte 148 versus 0.9% saline on delayed graft function in deceased donor kidney transplantation. Trials. 2020;21(428).
24. Harris DC, Davies SJ, Finkelstein FO, Jha V, Donner J-A, Abraham G, et al. Increasing access to integrated ESKD care as part of universal health coverage. Kidney Int. 2019;95:S1–S33.

Index

D. Banerjee et al. (eds.), *Management of Kidney Diseases*,
https://doi.org/10.1007/978-3-031-09131-5

D

L

M

N

GPSR Compliance

The European Union's (EU) General Product Safety Regulation (GPSR) is a set of rules that requires consumer products to be safe and our obligations to ensure this.

If you have any concerns about our products, you can contact us on ProductSafety@springernature.com

In case Publisher is established outside the EU, the EU authorized representative is:

Springer Nature Customer Service Center GmbH
Europaplatz 3
69115 Heidelberg, Germany

Batch number: 10753456

Printed by Printforce, the Netherlands